CLINICAL DRUG THERAPY
Rationales for Nursing Practice

ANNE COLLINS ABRAMS
R.N., B.S.N., M.S.N.

Assistant Professor, Department of Baccalaureate Nursing, College of Allied Health and Nursing, Eastern Kentucky University, Richmond, Kentucky

CONSULTANTS

TRACEY L. GOLDSMITH, Pharm. D.

Assistant Professor, College of Pharmacy, University of Kentucky, Lexington, Kentucky

WILLIAM R. OUTMAN, Pharm. D.

Clinical Pharmacy Fellow in Infectious Disease, Hartford Hospital, Hartford, Connecticut

VINCENT J. PEAK, Pharm. D.

Pharmacy Resident, College of Pharmacy, University of Kentucky, Lexington, Kentucky

K. ANN PATTERSON, Pharm. D.

Assistant Professor, Adjunct Series, College of Pharmacy, University of Kentucky, Lexington, Kentucky

J. B. LIPPINCOTT COMPANY Philadelphia

London · Mexico City · New York · St. Louis · São Paulo · Sydney

CLINICAL DRUG THERAPY

Rationales for Nursing Practice

SECOND EDITION

Sponsoring Editor: Joyce Mkitarian
Manuscript Editor: Virginia M. Barishek
Indexer: Barbara Farabaugh
Design Director: Tracy Baldwin
Design Coordinator: Don Shenkle
Designer: Katharine Nichols
Production Manager: Kathleen Dunn
Production Coordinator: Caren Erlichman
Compositor: TAPSCO, Inc.
Printer/Binder: The Murray Printing Company

Second Edition

6 5 4 3 2

Library of Congress Cataloging-in-Publication Data

Abrams, Anne Collins.
Clinical drug therapy.

Includes bibliographies and index.
1. Chemotherapy. 2. Drugs. 3. Nursing.
I. Goldsmith, Tracey L. II. Title. [DNLM: 1. Drug—nurses' instruction. 2. Drug Therapy—nurses' instruction. QV 55 A161c]
RM262.A27 1987 615.5'8 86-15238
ISBN 0-397-54627-0

The author and publisher have exerted every effort to ensure that drug selection and dosage set forth in this text are in accord with current recommendations and practice at the time of publication. However, in view of ongoing research, changes in government regulations, and the constant flow of information relating to drug therapy and drug reactions, the reader is urged to check the package insert for each drug for any change in indications and dosage and for added warnings and precautions. This is particularly important when the recommended agent is a new or infrequently employed drug.

This second edition is dedicated to all health care providers who strive to learn and to use their knowledge to improve patient care

PREFACE

Few areas related to nursing practice expand as rapidly as the area of drug therapy. Many new drugs are marketed yearly. Some of these are different from current drugs; most are new members of expanding families of drugs. In fact, some drugs are commonly referred to as second or third generations of drug groups. In addition to new drugs, there are changes in clinical uses of both newer and older drugs as a result of research and experience. A concerted effort has been made to reflect these additions and changes in this second edition.

The organizational framework of the first edition has been retained, for the most part. The book is divided into ten sections. The first section covers the basic knowledge and skills required for safe and effective drug therapy. Specific topics include drug effects on the body, factors that influence drug effects, guidelines for studying pharmacology, methods of drug administration, and nursing responsibilities in relation to drug therapy. In subsequent sections, drugs are categorized and discussed mainly according to their therapeutic effects on particular body systems; also, separate sections take up nutritional products, drugs used in treatment and prevention of infections, and drugs used in specific situations: neoplastic disease, ophthalmic and dermatologic disorders, and uterine motility. Most sections begin with a brief chapter that reviews the physiology of a body system; others begin with introductory material related to the condition for which drug therapy is given.

Within chapters there are four major organizational categories: *a description and a list of uses of the therapeutic class of drugs, a list of individual drugs within the class, principles of therapy, and nursing actions with rationale.* Groups of drugs are first discussed in terms of their general characteristics, including their effects on the body; clinical indications for use, including descriptions of the conditions in which the drugs are used (*e.g.,* pain, congestive heart failure); and contraindications. Then individual drugs are discussed.

"Principles of Therapy" provides information on nursing assessment of the client's condition in relation to the drug group, measures to prevent or minimize the need for drugs, guidelines for the choice of drug, dosage, and route of administration, and guidelines for using drugs in specific populations (*e.g.,* geriatric clients), when appropriate.

In each chapter the nursing actions related to drug therapy are categorized in five general functions: "Administer Drugs Accurately," "Observe for Therapeutic Effects," "Observe for Adverse Effects," "Observe for Drug Interactions," and "Teach Clients."

In this edition, every chapter has been thoroughly reviewed; some chapters have been extensively revised. New tables have been added to present content in a more meaningful way, and considerations related to pediatric, pregnant, or geriatric clients have been expanded. The nursing process is delineated and emphasized to a greater extent, especially in the chapter sections entitled "Principles of Therapy."

A unique feature of *Clinical Drug Therapy* remains the inclusion of rationales for nursing actions. The rationale for many nursing actions can be deduced with enough knowledge about the drug being administered and the condition of the person receiving it. However, this is a time-consuming process, and time is usually limited for both student and professional nurses. In addition, some nursing actions do not bear a clearly defined relationship to drug actions or the recipient's condition. Such situations promote reliance on memory rather than understanding and knowledge. If reasons for nursing actions are not understood, the nurse cannot readily alter actions when circumstances change. An explicit statement of the rationale, on the other hand, enhances understanding and promotes knowledgeable monitoring of drug therapy.

The overall purpose of this book is to promote rational, safe, and effective drug therapy. The author strongly believes that the study of drugs is important to nurses primarily in relation to drug effects on people. Thus, safe and effective drug therapy requires knowledge about both the drug and the person receiving the drug. Other beliefs and assumptions include the following:

- Knowledge and understanding of drug effects on people allow the nurse to predict both therapeutic and adverse effects of drug therapy.
- Therapeutic effects can be enhanced by nursing interventions.
- Adverse effects may be prevented or minimized by nursing interventions.
- If effective, non-drug-related interventions are generally safer than drug therapy.
- All drugs may cause adverse effects.
- Nursing responsibility includes observation of client responses to drug therapy and teaching clients about drug therapy as well as accurate administration of drugs.

Anne Collins Abrams, R.N., B.S.N., M.S.N.

ACKNOWLEDGMENTS

Four clinical pharmacists reviewed content for the second edition. Tracey Goldsmith distributed revised chapters among the group, collected them, and returned them to the author for final corrections before their submission to the publisher. All members of the group completed their reviews well within deadline dates. Their contributions are gratefully acknowledged to be essential and invaluable in this book.

Several people kindly reviewed selected chapters of the first edition and made helpful suggestions for the second edition. Much appreciation is expressed to the following people:

John D. Cronin, M.D.
Lexington Clinic, Lexington, Kentucky

L. Mae McPhetridge, R.N., M.A.
Clinical Nurse Specialist, Endocrinology, Veterans Administration Medical Center, Lexington, Kentucky

Raymond B. Otero, Ph.D.
Professor, Biological Sciences, Eastern Kentucky University, Richmond, Kentucky

James I. Salter, M.D.
Richmond, Kentucky

Dr. Cronin assisted with the chapter on antineoplastic drugs; Ms. McPhetridge assisted with the chapter on antidiabetic drugs; Dr. Otero assisted with several chapters related to antimicrobial drugs; and Dr. Salter assisted with the two chapters related to female sex hormones and drugs affecting uterine motility. The author feels fortunate to be acquainted with these well-qualified people who exemplify high standards in their fields.

Finally, the author wishes to recognize the contributions of Joyce Mkitarian, an editor at J. B. Lippincott Company. As with the first edition, Joyce has improved both content and format by her efforts. In addition, she has encouraged and assisted the author to complete the task of revision in a timely manner.

CONTENTS

I

INTRODUCTION TO DRUG THERAPY

1

INTRODUCTION TO PHARMACOLOGY

Pharmacology is the study of drugs. Drugs are chemicals that alter functions of living organisms. Drugs are generally given to prevent, diagnose, or cure disease processes or to provide palliation (relief of signs and symptoms without cure of the underlying disease). They may be given for local or systemic effects. Drugs that have local effects, such as creams, ointments, and local anesthetics, act mainly at the site of application. Those that have systemic effects are absorbed into the bloodstream and circulated to various parts of the body. Most drugs are given for their systemic effects.

Sources of drugs

Drugs are obtained from plant, animal, and mineral sources and are also made synthetically. Plants yield pharmacologically active substances such as alkaloids. An alkaloid is an alkaline substance that reacts with an acid to form a salt. For example, morphine is an alkaloid, and morphine sulfate is a salt. The salt forms are more often used as drugs because they are more soluble. Drugs obtained from animal sources include hormones extracted from animal endocrine glands. Insulin, for example, is extracted from pork and beef pancreas. Mineral sources provide iron and potassium preparations, among others. Synthetic drugs are artificially prepared from chemical substances in laboratories. Semisynthetic drugs are naturally occurring substances that have been chemically altered.

Drug nomenclature

Drugs are classified or grouped according to their effects on particular body systems, their therapeutic uses, and their chemical characteristics. For example, morphine can be classified as a central nervous system (CNS) depressant, a narcotic analgesic, and an opium derivative. Individual drugs that represent classifications or groups of drugs are called *prototypes.* Morphine is the prototype of narcotic analgesics and is the standard with which other narcotic analgesics are compared. Drug classifications and prototypes are extremely stable, and most new drugs can be assigned to a group and compared with an established prototype.

Individual drugs may have several different names. The two most commonly used are the generic name and the trade name. The generic name is related to the chemical or official name and is independent of the manufacturer. The trade or brand name is designated and patented by the manufacturer. For example, ampicillin is the generic name of an antibiotic. Ampicillin is manufactured by several pharmaceutical companies, each of which assigns a specific trade name such as Amcill, Penbriten, and Omnipen. (Trade names are capitalized; generic names are lower case.) Drugs may be prescribed and sold by generic or trade name.

Sources of drug information

There are many sources of drug data. Among the most useful are pharmacology textbooks, drug reference books, and journal articles. For the beginning student of pharmacology, a textbook is usually the best source of information because it describes groups of drugs in relation to therapeutic uses. Thus, an overview of the major drug classifications and their effects on the human body can be obtained.

Drug reference books are usually most helpful in relation to individual drugs. Two authoritative sources are the *American Hospital Formulary Service* and the *AMA Drug Evaluations.* The former is published by the American Society of Hospital Pharmacists and kept current by the periodic addition of revisions and updated monographs. The latter is prepared by the American Medical Association Department of Drugs. New editions are published every 3 to 5 years. A widely available but less authoritative source is the *Physicians' Desk Reference* (PDR). The PDR is simply a compilation of manufacturers' package inserts for selected drugs.

Many pharmacologic, medical, and nursing journals contain information on drugs. Journal articles often describe drug usage in specific disease processes. Some helpful journals include the *Journal of the American Medical Association, The New England Journal of Medicine, Drug Therapy,* and the *American Journal of Nursing.*

Drug laws and standards

Two major drug laws are important in nursing practice. One is the *Federal Food, Drug and Cosmetics Act of 1938* and its amendments. This law regulates the manufacture, distribution, advertising, and labeling of drugs in an attempt to ensure safety and effectiveness. It confers official status on drugs listed in *The Pharmacopeia of the United States* and *The National Formulary.* The names of these drugs may be followed by the letters *USP* or *NF.* Official drugs must meet standards of purity and strength as determined by chemical analysis or animal response to specified doses (bioassay). The law also requires extensive testing of new drugs before they are marketed for general use. The Food and Drug Administration (FDA) is charged with enforcing the law. In addition, the Public Health Service regulates vaccines and other biologic products, and the Federal Trade Commission (FTC) can suppress misleading advertisements of nonprescription drugs.

The second law important in nursing practice is the *Comprehensive Drug Abuse Prevention and Control Act of 1970.* Title II of this law, called the *Controlled Substances Act,* regulates distribution of narcotics and other drugs of abuse. It categorizes these drugs according to therapeutic usefulness and potential for abuse. These categories are listed as follows:

Schedule I. Drugs that are not approved for medical use and that have high abuse potentials are included in this category (heroin, LSD, peyote, mescaline, tetrahydrocannibols, marihuana).

Schedule II. These drugs are used medically and have high abuse potentials; abuse may lead to severe psychologic or physical dependence. Included in this group are morphine, opium, codeine, hydromorphone (Dilaudid), methadone, meperidine (Demerol), oxycodone (Percodan), oxymorphone (Numorphan), cocaine, dextroamphetamine (Dexedrine), methamphetamine (Desoxyn), phenmetrazine (Preludin), methylphenidate (Ritalin), amobarbital (Tuinal), secobarbital (Seconal), and pentobarbital (Nembutal).

Schedule III. These drugs have less potential for abuse than those listed in Schedules I and II. Abuse may lead to high psychologic or low to moderate physical dependence. Included are mixtures containing small amounts of controlled substances such as codeine, glutethimide (Doriden), methyprylon (Noludar), barbiturates not listed in other schedules, benzphetamine (Didrex), phendimetrazine (Plegine), and paregoric.

Schedule IV. Drugs included in this category are those with some potential for abuse, such as phenobarbital, chloral hydrate, ethchlorvynol (Placidyl), ethinamate (Valmid), meprobamate (Equanil), paraldehyde, fenfluramine (Pondimin), diethylpropion (Tenuate), phentermine (Fastin), mazindol (Mazanor, Sanorex), chlordiazepoxide (Librium), diazepam (Valium), clorazepate (Tranxene), flurazepam (Dalmane), oxazepam (Serax), clonazepam (Klonopin), prazepam (Centrax), lorazepam (Ativan), and propoxyphene (Darvon).

Schedule V. These products contain moderate amounts of controlled substances. They may be dispensed by the pharmacist without a physician's prescription but with some restrictions regarding amount, record keeping, and other safeguards. Included are antidiarrheal drugs such as diphenoxylate and atropine (Lomotil).

In addition to federal laws, state laws regulate the sale and distribution of drugs.

Mechanisms of drug action and movement

How do drugs act in the human body? It is thought that most drug actions occur at the cellular level, either on the cell surface or within the cell. Drug action is relatively selective; that is, not all cells respond to a given drug. The most widely accepted explanation for selective action is that responsive cells contain receptor sites for particular drugs. Receptors are thought to be chemical groups that participate in some aspect of cell metabolism, such as enzyme activity. Drug molecules must connect or interact with receptors for drug action to occur. Additional elements of the receptor theory of drug action include the following:

1. Only drugs with an affinity for the affected tissue are able to interact with receptors and exert pharmacologic effects. Thus, molecules of other drugs may be present in tissue fluids surrounding the cell, but they do not influence cell function.
2. When a drug molecule chemically binds with a cell receptor, two types of pharmacologic effects may occur. One type, called *agonism* or *agonist effects,* involves stimulation of cell function. The other type, called *antagonism* or *antagonist effects,* prevents stimulation of cell function by natural body substances (*e.g.,* neurotransmitters, hormones) or molecules of other drugs. The antagonist drug occupies cell receptor sites and prevents their interaction with other substances.
3. The number of receptor sites available to interact with drug molecules largely determines the extent of drug action. If many receptors are available but only a few are occupied by drug molecules, few drug effects will occur. If a few receptors are available for many drug molecules, receptors may be saturated. In the first instance, increasing drug dose increases a drug's effects. In the second instance, if most or all receptor sites are occupied, increasing drug dose produces no additional pharmacologic effect.

In order to act, drugs must be able to reach tissue fluids surrounding responsive cells in adequate concentrations. Specific mechanisms of drug movement are passive diffusion, facilitated diffusion, and active transport.

Passive diffusion is the most common of these mechanisms. It involves movement of a drug from an area of higher concentration to one of lower concentration. For example, when an orally administered drug reaches the upper small intestine, its relatively high concentration promotes movement of its molecules into the bloodstream. The blood carries the molecules to other parts of the body; thus, drug concentration in the blood is low compared with that in the intestinal tract. When the drug molecules reach responsive cells, their greater concentration in the blood promotes movement of the drug into the fluids surrounding the cells or into the cells themselves. Passive diffusion continues until a state of equilibrium is reached between the amount of drug in the tissues and the amount in the blood. Facilitated diffusion is a similar process, except that drug molecules combine with a carrier substance such as an enzyme or other protein. In active transport, drug molecules are moved from an area of lower concentration to one of higher concentration. This process requires both a carrier substance and the release of cellular energy.

Drug movement and therefore drug action are affected by a drug's ability to cross cell membranes. For example, a drug given orally must pass through the cell membranes that line the intestinal tract, lymphatic vessels, and capillary walls to reach the bloodstream and circulate through the body. Cell membranes are complex structures composed of lipid and protein. Lipid-soluble drugs cross cell membranes by dissolving in the lipid layer; water-soluble drugs cross cell membranes through pores or openings. Lipid-soluble drugs are able to cross cell membranes more easily than water-soluble ones. Most drugs are lipid soluble.

Pharmacokinetics

Pharmacokinetics includes the four processes a drug undergoes after entering the body: absorption, distribution, metabolism, and excretion.

ABSORPTION

Absorption is the process occurring between the time a drug enters the body and the time it enters the bloodstream to be circulated. The rate and extent of absorption are affected by the dosage form of the drug, its route of administration, gastrointestinal function, and other variables. Dosage form is a major determinant of a drug's bioavailability (the amount of drug absorbed into the bloodstream).

Most oral drugs must be swallowed, dissolved in gastric fluid, and reach the small intestine before they are absorbed. Liquid medications are usually absorbed faster than tablets or capsules because they do not have to be dissolved in gastrointestinal fluids. Injected drugs are generally absorbed more rapidly than oral drugs. Increases in gastric emptying time and in intestinal motility usually lead to increases in drug absorption by promoting contact with absorptive mucous membrane. (However, increased gastric emptying time may result in less absorption, because of degradation of the drug in the stomach. Also, excessive peristalsis may move a drug through the intestinal tract too rapidly for it to be absorbed.) The presence of food in the stomach tends to slow the rate of absorption and generally decreases the amount of drug absorbed. When factors related to increased absorption are present, drug actions are usually rapid and of short duration. Factors related to decreased absorption may prevent a drug from reaching adequate concentrations at cellular receptor sites.

DISTRIBUTION

The term *distribution* refers to the transport of drug molecules within the body. Once a drug is injected or absorbed into the bloodstream, it is carried by the blood and tissue fluids to its sites of pharmacologic action, metabolism, and excretion. Distribution depends largely on the adequacy of the blood circulation. Drugs are distributed rapidly to those organs receiving a large blood supply, such as the heart, liver, and kidneys. Distribution to other internal organs, muscle, fat, and skin is usually slower. Most drugs are transported in combination with plasma proteins, especially albumin, which act as carriers. Drug molecules bound to plasma proteins are pharmacologically inactive because the large size of the complex keeps them in the bloodstream and prevents their reaching sites of action, metabolism and excretion. Only the free or unbound portion of a drug acts on body cells. As the free drug acts on cells, the decrease in serum drug levels causes some of the bound drug to be released. Thus, plasma protein binding can be viewed as a method by which the body stores drugs. Some drugs are also stored in muscle, fat, or other body tissues and released gradually into the bloodstream when serum drug levels fall. Drugs that are tightly bound to plasma proteins or stored extensively in other tissues tend to have a long duration of action.

Drug distribution in the CNS is unique. Many drugs do not enter the brain and cerebrospinal fluid, at least in therapeutic concentrations, because they cannot pass the blood–brain barrier. The blood–brain barrier is a group of cells that acts as a selectively permeable membrane to protect the CNS. However, its presence can also make drug therapy of CNS disorders more difficult.

Drug distribution during pregnancy and lactation is also distinctive. During pregnancy, despite the so-called placental barrier, most drugs cross the placenta and affect the developing fetus. During lactation, many drugs enter breast milk and thus affect the nursing infant.

METABOLISM

The term *metabolism,* also called *biotransformation,* refers to the way in which drugs are inactivated by the body. Drugs are metabolized by the body in several ways. Most often, an active drug is changed into one or more inactive metabolites, which are then excreted. Some active drugs yield metabolites that are also active and that continue to exert their effects on body cells until they are metabolized further or excreted. Other drugs are initially inactive and exert no pharmacologic effects until they are metabolized.

Most drugs are lipid soluble. This characteristic aids their movement across cell membranes. However, the kidneys, which are the primary excretory organs, can excrete only water-soluble substances. Therefore, one function of metabolism is to convert fat-soluble drugs into water-soluble metabolites.

Most drugs are metabolized by enzymes in the liver; plasma, the kidneys, and the intestinal mucosa also contain drug-metabolizing enzymes. These enzymes catalyze the chemical reactions of oxidation, reduction, hydrolysis, and synthesis, by which drugs are biotransformed. With chronic administration, some drugs activate the hepatic enzymes, thereby accelerating drug metabolism. The rate of drug metabolism is reduced in infants, owing to immaturity of the hepatic enzyme system, and in people with severe hepatic or cardiovascular disease. Factors that increase the rate of drug metabolism decrease the intensity and duration of drug action. Factors that slow or prolong metabolism cause drug accumulation and increased incidence of adverse reactions.

When drugs are given orally, they are absorbed from the gastrointestinal tract and carried to the liver through the portal circulation. Some drugs are extensively metabolized in the liver, with only a portion of a drug dose reaching the systemic circulation for distribution to sites of action. This phenomenon is called the *first-pass effect.*

EXCRETION

The term *excretion* refers to elimination of a drug from the body. Effective excretion requires adequate functioning of the circulatory system and of the organs of excretion (kidneys, bowel, lungs, and skin). Most drugs are excreted by the kidneys and eliminated unchanged or as metabolites in the urine. Some drugs are excreted in bile, then eliminated in feces or reabsorbed, metabolized, and eventually excreted in urine. Some oral drugs are not absorbed and are excreted in the feces. The lungs mainly remove volatile substances such as anesthetic gases. The skin has minimal excretory function. Factors impairing excretion, especially severe

renal disease, lead to drug accumulation and potentially severe adverse reactions.

SERUM HALF-LIFE

Serum half-life, also called *elimination half-time,* is the time required for the serum concentration of a drug to decrease by 50%. It is determined by the drug's rates of absorption, metabolism, and excretion. A drug with a short half-life requires more frequent administration than one with a long half-life.

When a drug is given at a stable dose, about four or five half-lives are required to achieve steady-state concentrations and develop equilibrium between tissue and serum concentrations. Since maximal therapeutic effects do not occur until equilibrium is established, some drugs are not fully effective for days or weeks. Maintenance of equilibrium requires that the amount of drug given daily equal the amount eliminated from the body.

Variables that affect drug actions

Expected responses to drugs, desired and undesired, are largely based on those occurring when a particular drug is given to healthy adults (18 to 65 years old) of average weight (150 lb or 70 kg). These responses may be altered by drug-related as well as client-related variables.

DOSAGE

A *dose* of a drug is the amount to be given at one time. The term *dosage* refers to regulation of the frequency, size, and number of doses. Dosage is a major determinant of drug actions and responses, both therapeutic and adverse. If a dose is too small, no pharmacologic action occurs because the drug does not reach an adequate concentration at cellular receptor sites. If a dose is too large, toxicity (poisoning) may occur. Because dosage includes both the amount of the drug and the frequency of administration, overdosage may occur with a single large dose or with chronic ingestion of smaller amounts. Doses that produce signs and symptoms of toxicity are called *toxic doses.* Doses that cause death are called *lethal doses.*

Dosages recommended in drug literature are usually those that produce particular responses in 50% of the people tested, usually healthy adults of average weight. These dosages usually produce a mixture of therapeutic and adverse effects. Dosage of a particular drug depends on many characteristics of the drug (purpose for use, potency, pharmacokinetics, route of administration, dosage form, and others) and of the recipient (age, weight, state of health or illness, function of cardiovascular, renal, and hepatic systems). Thus, the recommended dosages are intended as guidelines for individualizing dosages.

ROUTE OF ADMINISTRATION

Routes of administration affect drug actions and responses largely by influencing absorption and distribution. For rapid drug action and response, the intravenous route is most effective because the drug is injected into the bloodstream and thus bypasses barriers to absorption. For many drugs, the intramuscular route also produces drug action within a few minutes because muscles have an abundant blood supply. The oral route generally produces slower drug action than parenteral routes. Absorption and action of topical drugs vary according to the specific method of administration.

DRUG–DIET INTERACTIONS

Food slows absorption of oral drugs by slowing gastric emptying time and altering gastrointestinal secretions and motility. When tablets or capsules are taken with or soon after food, they dissolve more slowly; therefore, drug molecules are delivered to absorptive sites in the intestine more slowly. Food may also decrease absorption by combining with a drug to form an insoluble drug–food complex.

In addition, some foods contain substances that react with certain drugs. One such interaction occurs between tyramine-containing foods and monoamine oxidase (MAO) inhibitor drugs. Tyramine causes release of norepinephrine, a potent vasoconstrictive agent, from the adrenal medulla and sympathetic neurons. Normally, norepinephrine is active for only a few milliseconds before it is inactivated by MAO. MAO inhibitor drugs prevent inactivation of norepinephrine and may produce severe hypertension or intracranial hemorrhage. MAO inhibitor drugs include isocarboxazid (Marplan) and phenelzine (Nardil), which are antidepressants, and procarbazine (Matulane), an antineoplastic drug. Tyramine-rich foods to be avoided by persons taking MAO inhibitor drugs include beer, wine, aged cheeses, yeast products, chicken livers, and pickled herring.

An interaction may occur between oral anticoagulants such as warfarin (Coumadin) and foods containing vitamin K. Since vitamin K antagonizes the action of oral anticoagulants, large amounts of green leafy vegetables such as spinach and other greens may offset anticoagulant effects and predispose the person to thromboembolic disorders.

A third interaction occurs between tetracycline, an antibiotic, and dairy products such as milk and cheese. The drug combines with the calcium in milk products to form an insoluble, unabsorbable compound that is excreted in the feces.

DRUG–DRUG INTERACTIONS

The action of a particular drug may be increased or decreased by its interaction with another drug in the body. Most interactions occur whenever the interacting drugs are present in the body; some, especially those affecting absorption, occur when the interacting drugs are given at or near the same time.

Interactions that can increase the therapeutic or adverse effects of drugs are described in the following list:

1. *Additive effects* occur when two drugs with similar pharmacologic actions are taken.
   Example: alcohol + sedative drug → increased sedation
2. *Synergism* or *potentiation* occurs when two drugs with different sites or mechanisms of action produce greater effects when taken together than either does when taken alone.
   Example: codeine + aspirin → increased analgesia
3. *Interference* by one drug with the metabolism or elimination of a second drug may result in intensification of the second drug.
   Examples: isoniazid (an antituberculosis drug) + phenytoin (an anticonvulsant) → potentiation of the effects of phenytoin on the CNS. In this instance, isoniazid inhibits enzymatic breakdown of phenytoin. Probenecid (a uricosuric drug) + penicillin (an antibiotic) → increased antibacterial effect of penicillin. Probenecid inhibits excretion of penicillin by kidney tubules.
4. *Displacement* of one drug from plasma protein binding sites by a second drug increases the effects of the displaced drug. This increase occurs because the molecules of the displaced drug, freed from their bound form, become pharmacologically active.
   Example: aspirin (an anti-inflammatory–analgesic–antipyretic agent) + warfarin (an anticoagulant) → increased anticoagulant effect

Interactions in which drug effects are decreased are grouped under the term *antagonism*. Examples of such interactions are given in the following list:

1. In some situations, a drug that is a specific antidote is given to antagonize the toxic effects of another drug.
   Example: naloxone (a narcotic antagonist) + morphine (a narcotic analgesic) → relief of narcotic-induced respiratory depression
   In the above example, naloxone molecules displace morphine molecules from their receptor sites on nerve cells so that the morphine molecules cannot continue to exert their depressant effects.
2. Decreased intestinal absorption of oral drugs occurs when drugs combine to produce nonabsorbable compounds.
   Example: aluminum hydroxide (an antacid) + tetracycline (an antibiotic) → binding of tetracycline to aluminum, causing decreased absorption and decreased antibiotic effect of tetracycline.
3. Activation of drug-metabolizing enzymes in the liver increases the metabolism rate of any drug metabolized primarily in the liver. Some anticonvulsants, barbiturates, and antihistamines are known "enzyme inducers."
   Example: phenobarbital (a barbiturate) + warfarin (an anticoagulant) → decreased effects of warfarin
4. Increased excretion occurs when urinary *p*H is changed and renal reabsorption is blocked.
   Example: sodium bicarbonate + phenobarbital → increased excretion of phenobarbital
   In the above example, the sodium bicarbonate alkalinizes the urine, raising the number of barbiturate ions in the renal filtrate. The ionized particles cannot pass easily through renal tubular membranes. Therefore, less drug is reabsorbed into the blood, and more is excreted by the kidneys.

AGE

The effects of age on drug action are most pronounced in young children and elderly people. In children, drug action depends largely on age and developmental stage. During pregnancy, many drugs cross the placenta and may adversely affect the fetus. The fetus has no effective mechanisms for metabolizing or eliminating drugs because liver and kidney function are immature. The newborn infant generally handles drugs less efficiently than the older child or adult. Patterns of drug distribution, metabolism, and excretion differ markedly in the neonate because organ systems are not fully developed. Older children tend to metabolize drugs very rapidly; otherwise, older children handle drugs similarly to healthy adults.

In elderly adults, physiologic changes may alter all pharmacokinetic processes. Changes in the gastrointestinal tract include decreased gastric acidity, decreased blood flow, and decreased motility. Despite these changes, however, there is relatively little difference in absorption. Changes in the cardiovascular system include decreased cardiac output and therefore slower distribution of drug molecules to their sites of action, metabolism, and excretion. In the liver, there is decreased blood flow and probably a decreased number of metabolizing enzymes. Thus, many drugs are metabolized more slowly, have a longer action, and are more likely to accumulate with chronic administration. In the kidneys, there is decreased blood flow, decreased glomerular filtration rate, and decreased tubular secretion of drugs. All these changes tend to slow excretion and promote accumulation of drugs in the body. Impaired kidney and liver function greatly increase the risks of adverse drug effects.

In addition, elderly people are more likely to have acute and chronic illnesses that require multiple drugs or long-term drug therapy. Thus, possibilities for interactions among drugs and between drugs and diseased organs are greatly multiplied.

BODY WEIGHT

Body weight affects drug action mainly in relation to dosage. The ratio between the amount of drug given and body weight influences drug distribution and concentration at sites of action. Generally, people of greater-than-average weight need larger doses, provided that renal, hepatic, and cardiovascular functions are adequate. Recommended dosage for many drugs is listed in terms of grams or milligrams per kilogram of body weight. Most pediatric dosages are calculated with formulas that use body weight to determine the fraction of an adult dose to be given to a child.

SEX

The influence of sex on drug action is most pronounced during pregnancy, when drugs are generally contraindicated because of possible adverse effects on the fetus and, if the mother breast-feeds, on the newborn.

PATHOLOGIC CONDITIONS

Pathologic conditions or disease processes are capable of altering pharmacokinetic processes. All such processes are decreased in cardiovascular disorders characterized by decreased blood flow to tissues, such as hypotension, shock, low plasma volume, and congestive heart failure. In addition, absorption of oral drugs is decreased with vomiting, diarrhea, intestinal malabsorption, and other gastrointestinal disorders. Distribution is altered in malnutrition, liver or kidney disease, and other conditions that decrease the number of plasma proteins providing drug-binding sites. Metabolism is decreased with severe liver disease; it may be increased in conditions that generally increase body metabolism, such as hyperthyroidism and fever. Excretion is decreased with severe kidney disease.

PSYCHOLOGIC CONSIDERATIONS

Psychologic considerations influence individual responses to drug administration, although specific mechanisms are not known. An example is the "placebo response." A placebo is a pharmacologically inactive substance such as sugar or sodium chloride solution. Placebos are sometimes given to a client without his knowledge to satisfy a demand for medication. They are also used in clinical drug trials to compare the medication being tested with a "dummy" medication. Interestingly, recipients often report both therapeutic and adverse effects from placebos.

Attitudes and expectations related to drugs in general, a particular drug, or a placebo influence client response. They also influence compliance or willingness to carry out the prescribed drug regimen, especially with long-term drug therapy.

Adverse effects of drugs

As used in this book, the term *adverse effects* refers to any undesired responses to drug administration, as opposed to *therapeutic effects,* which are desired responses. Most drugs produce a mixture of therapeutic and adverse effects; all drugs are capable of producing adverse effects. Adverse effects may be common or rare, mild or severe and life threatening, localized or widespread, depending on the drug and the person receiving it.

Some adverse effects occur with usual therapeutic doses of drugs; others are more likely to occur and to be more severe with high doses. Many factors influence the incidence and severity of adverse effects; some of these are indicated in the following list:

1. Gastrointestinal effects—anorexia, nausea, vomiting, constipation, diarrhea—are among the most common adverse reactions to drugs. These occur with many oral drugs owing to local irritation of the gastrointestinal tract and with drugs that stimulate the vomiting center in the medulla oblongata, whatever the route of administration. Some drugs also cause bleeding or ulceration, notably aspirin and nonsteroidal anti-inflammatory agents.
2. Hematologic effects—blood coagulation disorders, bleeding disorders, bone marrow depression, ane-

mias, leukopenia, agranulocytosis, thrombocytopenia—are relatively common and potentially life threatening. They are especially associated with antineoplastic drugs but may occur with others as well.

3. Hepatotoxicity—hepatitis, hepatic necrosis, biliary tract obstruction—is relatively rare but potentially life threatening. Since most drugs are metabolized by the liver, the liver is especially susceptible to drug-induced injury. Commonly used hepatotoxic drugs include acetaminophen (Tylenol), chlorpromazine (Thorazine), halothane (Fluothane), isoniazid (INH), methotrexate (Mexate), methyldopa (Aldomet), nitrofurantoin (Macrodantin), oxymetholone (Anadrol), phenelzine (Nardil) and other MAO inhibitors, phenytoin (Dilantin), aspirin and other salicylates, and tetracycline (Achromycin). In the presence of drug-induced or disease-induced liver damage, the metabolism of many drugs is impaired. Consequently, drugs metabolized by the liver tend to accumulate in the body and cause adverse effects. Besides actual hepatotoxicity, many drugs cause asymptomatic increases in liver function tests.
4. Nephrotoxicity—renal insufficiency or failure—occurs with several antimicrobial agents (*e.g.*, gentamicin and other aminoglycosides) and some other drug classes. It is potentially serious because it may interfere with drug excretion, thereby causing drug accumulation and increased adverse effects.
5. Hypersensitivity or allergy may occur with almost any drug in susceptible persons. It is largely unpredictable and unrelated to dose. It occurs in persons who have previously been exposed to the drug or a similar substance (antigen) and who have developed antibodies. When readministered, the drug reacts with the antibodies to cause cell damage and release of histamine and other intracellular substances. These substances produce reactions ranging from mild skin rashes to anaphylactic shock. Anaphylactic shock is a life-threatening hypersensitivity reaction characterized by respiratory distress and cardiovascular collapse. It occurs within a few minutes after drug administration and requires emergency treatment with epinephrine, antihistamines, and bronchodilator drugs. Some allergic reactions occur 1 to 2 weeks after the drug was administered.
6. Idiosyncrasy refers to an unexpected reaction to a drug that occurs the first time the drug is administered. These reactions are usually attributed to genetic characteristics that alter the person's drug-metabolizing enzymes. For example, some people rapidly metabolize isoniazid (INH), an antituberculosis drug, while others metabolize it slowly; others lack the cholinesterase enzyme that normally inactivates succinylcholine (Anectine), a potent muscle relaxant used in major surgical procedures, and have prolonged paralysis and apnea. Some people have deficient glucose-6-phosphate dehydrogenase (G6PD), an enzyme normally found in red blood cells and other body tissues. These people may develop hemolytic anemia with administration of antimalarial drugs, sulfonamides, analgesics, antipyretics, and other drugs. The term *hypersensitivity* (see No. 5, above) is sometimes used to refer to unusually great sensitivity to a drug.
7. Drug dependence may occur with mind-altering drugs such as narcotic analgesics, sedative-hypnotic agents, antianxiety agents, and amphetamines. Dependence may be physiologic or psychologic. Physiologic dependence produces unpleasant physical symptoms when the drug is withdrawn. Psychologic dependence leads to drug-seeking behavior. Drug dependence is discussed in detail in Chapter 15.
8. Carcinogenicity is the ability of a substance to cause cancer. Several drugs are carcinogens, including some hormones and anticancer drugs. Carcinogenicity apparently results from drug-induced alterations in cellular deoxyribonucleic acid (DNA).
9. Teratogenicity is the ability of a substance to cause abnormal fetal development when given to pregnant women. Drug groups considered teratogenic include analgesics, diuretics, antihistamines, antibiotics, antiemetics, and others.

Tolerance and cross tolerance

Drug tolerance is a situation in which the body becomes accustomed to a particular drug over time so that larger doses must be given to produce the same effects. Tolerance may be acquired to the pharmacologic action of many drugs, especially narcotic analgesics, barbiturates, alcohol, and other CNS depressants. Tolerance to pharmacologically related drugs is called *cross tolerance*. For example, a person who regularly ingests large amounts of alcohol becomes able to ingest even larger amounts before becoming intoxicated. This is tolerance to alcohol. If the person is then given sedative-type drugs or a general anesthetic, larger than normal doses are usually required to produce a pharmacologic effect. This is referred to as cross tolerance. Tolerance and cross tolerance are usually attributed to activation of drug-metabolizing enzymes in the liver, which accelerate metabolism and excretion of the drug. They are also attributed to a decrease in the sensitivity of drug receptor sites to the drug and to a decrease in the number of receptor sites. Rapid development of tolerance after only a few doses of a drug is called *tachyphylaxis.*

Selected References

American Medical Association (AMA) Division of Drugs: AMA Drug Evaluations, 5th ed. New York, John Wiley & Sons, 1983

Benet LZ, Massoud N, Gambertoglio JG (eds): Pharmacokinetic Basis for Drug Treatment. New York, Raven Press, 1984

Benet LZ, Sheiner LB: Pharmacokinetics: The dynamics of drug absorption, distribution, and elimination. In Gilman AG, Goodman LS, Rall TW, Murad F (eds): The Pharmacological Basis of Therapeutics, 7th ed, pp 3–34. New York, Macmillan, 1985

Butler RN, Bearn AG: The Aging Process: Therapeutic Implications. New York, Raven Press, 1985

Carey KW (ed.): Drug Interactions. Springhouse, PA, Springhouse Corporation, 1984

Cefalo RC: Drugs in pregnancy—which to use and which to avoid. Drug Ther 13:167–175, April 1985

Chow MP, Durand BA, Feldman MN, Mills MA: Handbook of Pediatric Primary Care, 2nd ed, pp 589–600. New York, John Wiley & Sons, 1984

Cohen MR: Action Stat! Drug-induced anaphylaxis. Nursing 15:43, February 1985

Dickerson JK, Simkover RA: Adverse drug reactions. In Wiener MB, Pepper GA (eds): Clinical Pharmacology and Therapeutics in Nursing, 2nd ed, pp 87–106. New York, McGraw-Hill, 1985

Fielo S, Rizzolo MA: The effects of age on pharmacokinetics. Geriatric Nursing 6:328–331, November–December 1985

Giovannetti C, Schwinghammer T: Food and drugs: Managing the right mix for your patient. Nursing 11:26–31, July 1981

Hansten PD: Drug Interactions: Clinical Significance of Drug–Drug Interactions, 5th ed. Philadelphia, Lea & Febiger, 1985

Herfindal ET, Hirschman JL (eds): Clinical Pharmacy and Therapeutics, 3rd ed. Baltimore, Williams & Wilkins, 1984

MacLeod SM, Radde IC (eds): Textbook of Pediatric Clinical Pharmacology. Littleton, MA, PSG Publishing, 1985

Manzo M: A drug by any other name: Your guide to generic and brand names. Nursing 13:97–111, November 1983

Mar DD: Drug-induced hepatotoxicity. Am J Nurs 82:124–126, January 1982

Murad F, Gilman AG: Appendix III. Drug interactions. In Gilman AG, Goodman LS, Rall TW, Murad F (eds): The Pharmacological Basis of Therapeutics, 7th ed., pp 1734–1750. New York, Macmillan, 1985

Parker WA: Effects of pregnancy on pharmacokinetics. In Benet LZ, Massoud N, Gambertoglio JG (eds): Pharmacokinetic Basis for Drug Treatment, pp 249–268. New York, Raven Press, 1984

Rodman MJ, Karch AM, Boyd EH, Smith DW: Pharmacology and Drug Therapy in Nursing, 3rd ed. Philadelphia, J B Lippincott, 1985

Stewart CM, Stewart LB: Pediatric Medications: An Emergency and Critical Care Reference. Rockville, MD, Aspen Systems Corp., 1984

2

ADMINISTERING MEDICATIONS

Drugs given for therapeutic purposes are usually called *medications.* Giving medications to clients is an important nursing responsibility, especially in agencies such as hospitals and extended-care facilities. The goal of medication administration is often stated as the "five rights"; that is, giving the right *drug,* in the right *dose,* to the right *client,* by the right *route,* at the right *time.* To meet this goal, the nurse must be able to function within the agency medication system, interpret drug orders accurately, select correct drug preparations, calculate drug dosages accurately, and use different routes of administration safely and accurately.

Medication systems

Each agency has a system for dispensing drugs. A widely used method is the unit-dose system, in which most drugs are dispensed in single or unit-dose packages containing one tablet or capsule, for example. Drug orders are checked by pharmacy personnel who then place the indicated number of doses in the client's medication drawer at scheduled intervals. When a dose is due, the nurse places the medication in a medication container to be carried to the client. Unit-dose wrappings should be left in place until the medication is administered at the client's bedside.

One advantage of the unit-dose system is that nurses spend less time preparing drugs for administration. Another advantage is that each drug is always readily identifiable because the label remains intact until the drug reaches the client. Whatever dispensing system is used, each dose of a drug must be recorded on a medication sheet after administration.

Controlled drugs, such as narcotic analgesics, are usually kept as a stock supply in a locked drawer or cabinet and replaced as needed. Each dose is signed out on a special narcotic sheet as well as recorded on the client's medication sheet. Two nurses count narcotics and other controlled substances, usually at the end of each 8-hour working shift. Each nurse must comply with legal regulations for dispensing and recording controlled drugs.

Medication orders

Nurses administer medications from orders by licensed physicians and dentists. Drug orders should include the full name of the client; location (*e.g.,* room number); generic or trade name of the drug; dosage, route, and frequency of administration; and date, time, and signature of the prescribing physician. Written orders are safer and much preferred. Occasionally, verbal or telephone orders are acceptable. These are written on the order sheet, signed by the person taking the order, and later countersigned by the physician.

Once written on the client's order sheet, drug

orders are usually transcribed to medication sheets or computer terminals to facilitate administration. Transcription is usually done by a ward secretary or clerk, checked for accuracy, and countersigned by a registered nurse.

To interpret medication orders accurately, the nurse must know some commonly used abbreviations for routes, dosages, and times of drug administration. These are listed in Table 2-1. If the nurse is unable to read the physician's order or if the order seems erroneous, she must question the order before giving the drug.

Drug preparations and dosage forms

Drug preparations and dosage forms vary according to chemical characteristics, purposes, and routes of administration. Some drugs are available in only one preparation or dosage form; others are available in several forms.

Dosage forms of systemic drugs include liquids, tablets, capsules, and transdermal and pump delivery systems. Systemic liquids are given orally or parenterally. Those given by injection must be sterile.

Tablets and capsules are given orally. Tablets contain an active drug plus various amounts of inactive substances, such as binders. They are available in many shapes, sizes, and colors. Capsules usually contain a powder or liquid form of active drug enclosed in a gelatin capsule. Most tablets and capsules dissolve in the acid fluids of the stomach and are absorbed in the alkaline fluids of the upper small intestine. Some—called *enteric-coated tablets and capsules*—are coated with a substance that is insoluble in stomach acids. This is done to delay dissolution until the medications reach the intestine, usually to avoid gastric irritation or to keep the drug from being destroyed by gastric acid. Their absorption may be delayed or incomplete. Tablets for sublingual or buccal administration must be specifically formulated for such use.

Several "controlled-release" dosage forms or drug delivery systems have been developed to allow less frequent administration and more consistent serum drug levels. Although sustained-release tablets and capsules have been available for some years, newer formulations and mechanisms of release continue to be developed. Transdermal formulations include systemically absorbed nitroglycerin (*e.g.,* NitroDur, Nitrodisc) and scopolamine. Pump delivery systems may be external or implanted under the skin and refillable or long acting without refills. Pumps have been used to administer narcotic analgesics, insulin, and antineoplastic and other drugs.

Ointments, creams, and suppositories are applied topically to skin or mucous membranes. They are usually specifically formulated for the intended route of administration.

TABLE 2-1. COMMON ABBREVIATIONS

I. Routes of drug administration	IM	intramuscular
	IV	intravenous
	OD	right eye
	OS	left eye
	OU	both eyes
	PO	by mouth, oral
	SC	subcutaneous
II. Drug dosages	cc	cubic centimeter
	g	gram
	gr	grain
	gt	drop*
	mg	milligram
	ml	milliliter
	oz	ounce
	tbsp	tablespoon
	tsp	teaspoon
III. Times of drug administration	a.c.	before meals
	ad lib	as desired
	b.i.d.	twice daily
	h.s.	bedtime
	p.c.	after meals
	PRN	when needed
	q.d.	every day, daily
	q4h	every four hours
	q.i.d.	four times daily
	q.o.d.	every other day
	stat	immediately
	t.i.d.	three times daily

* drops = gtt.

Calculating drug dosages

To give the "right dose" of a medication, the nurse must be able to calculate drug dosages. In addition to basic skills in arithmetic, especially those using fractions and decimals, the nurse must know common units of measurement, equivalents among systems, and methods of using these data.

The most commonly used system of measurement is the *metric system,* in which the meter is used for linear measure, the gram for weight, and the liter for volume. These units are interrelated in that one milliliter (ml) equals one cubic centimeter (cc), and both equal one gram (g) of water. An older system is the *apothecary system,* with units of measurement called grains, minims, drams, ounces, pounds, pints, and quarts. The *household system,* with units of drops, teaspoons, tablespoons, and cups, is infrequently used in health-care agencies but may be used at home. Table 2-2 lists equivalent measurements within and among these systems. Equivalents are approximate.

TABLE 2-2. COMMONLY USED EQUIVALENTS

Metric	Apothecary	Household
1 ml = 1 cc	= 15 or 16 minims	= 15 or 16 drops
4 or 5 ml	= 1 fluid dram	= 1 tsp
60 or 65 mg	= 1 gr	
30 or 32 mg	= ½ gr	
30 g = 30 ml	= 1 oz	= 2 tbsp
250 ml	= 8 oz	= 1 cup
454 g	= 1 lb	
500 ml = 500 cc	= 16 oz = 1 pint	= 1 pint
1 liter = 1000 ml	= 32 oz = 1 quart	= 1 quart
1000 g = 1 kg	= 2.2 lb	= 2.2 lb
0.6 g = 600 mg or 650 mg	= 10 gr	

A few drugs are ordered and measured in terms of units or milliequivalents. Units express biologic activity in animal tests (*i.e.,* the amount of drug required to produce a particular response). Units are unique for each drug. Concentrations of insulin, heparin, and penicillin are expressed in units. There is *no* relationship or correspondence between a unit of insulin, for example, and a unit of heparin. These drugs are usually ordered in the number of units per dose (*e.g.,* NPH insulin 30 units SC every morning or heparin 3000 units SC ql2h) and labeled in number of units per milliliter (U 100 insulin contains 100 units/ml; heparin may have 1,000, 5,000, or 10,000 units/ml). Milliequivalents express ionic activity of a drug. Drugs such as potassium chloride are ordered in the number of milliequivalents per dose and labeled in terms of milliequivalents per dosage form.

Most physicians' drug orders and most drug labels are expressed in metric units of measurement. If the amount specified in the order is the same as that on the drug label, no calculations are required, and preparing the "right dose" is a simple matter. For example, if the order reads "aspirin 300 mg PO" and the drug label reads "aspirin 300-mg tablets," it is clear that one tablet is to be given.

What happens if the order calls for a 600-mg dose and 300-mg tablets are available? Then calculations are necessary to determine how many 300-mg tablets are needed to give a dose of 600 mg. This can be done with the following formula:

$$\frac{D}{H} = \frac{X}{V}$$

D = desired dose (dose ordered by the physician)
H = on-hand or available dose (dose on the drug label)
X = unknown (tablets, in this example)
V = unit (one tablet, here)

$$\frac{600 \text{ mg}}{300 \text{ mg}} = \frac{X \text{ tablets}}{1 \text{ tablet}}$$

Cross multiply

$$300 X = 600$$

$$X = \frac{600}{300} = 2 \text{ tablets}$$

What happens if the order and the label are written in different systems? The usual dose of aspirin may be ordered as 600 mg, 650 mg, 10 gr, or gr x. The label may read 300-mg, 325-mg, or 5-gr tablets. For example, assume that the order reads "aspirin gr x" and the drug label reads "aspirin 300-mg tablets." The first step in solving this problem is knowing that x is the roman numeral for 10. The second step is to convert the order and the label to the same units. It does not matter which one is converted. Using the equivalent of 60 mg = 1 gr, an equation can be set up as follows:

$$\frac{60 \text{ mg}}{1 \text{ gr}} = \frac{X \text{ mg}}{10 \text{ gr}}$$

Cross multiply

$$X = 60 \times 10 \text{ or } 600 \text{ mg}$$

The third step is to use the new information in the formula, which then becomes

$$\frac{D}{H} = \frac{X}{V}$$

$$\frac{600 \text{ mg}}{300 \text{ mg}} = \frac{X \text{ tablets}}{1 \text{ tablet}}$$

$$300 X = 600 \text{ mg}$$

$$X = 2 \text{ tablets}$$

Note that the desired or ordered dose and the available or label dose *must* be in the same units of measurement.

The same procedure and formula can be used to calculate portions of tablets or dosages of liquids. These are illustrated in the following problems:

1. Order: 25 mg PO
   Label: 50-mg tablet

$$\frac{25 \text{ mg}}{50 \text{ mg}} = \frac{X \text{ tablet}}{1 \text{ tablet}}$$

$$50 X = 25$$

$$X = \frac{25}{50} = \tfrac{1}{2} \text{ tablet}$$

2. Order: 25 mg IM
   Label: 50 mg in 1 cc

$$\frac{25 \text{ mg}}{50 \text{ mg}} = \frac{X \text{ cc}}{1 \text{ cc}}$$

$$50 X = 25$$

$$X = 0.5 \text{ cc}$$

3. Order: 50 mg PO
   Label: 10 mg/cc

$$\frac{50 \text{ mg}}{10 \text{ mg}} = \frac{X \text{ cc}}{1 \text{ cc}}$$

$$10 X = 50$$

$$X = 5 \text{ cc}$$

4. Order: Heparin 3,000 U
   Label: Heparin 10,000 units/ml

$$\frac{3{,}000 \text{ U}}{10{,}000 \text{ U}} = \frac{X \text{ ml}}{1 \text{ ml}}$$

$$10{,}000 X = 3{,}000$$

$$X = \frac{3{,}000}{10{,}000} \text{ or } 0.3 \text{ ml}$$

5. Order: KCl 20 mEq
   Label: KCl 10 mEq/5 ml

$$\frac{20 \text{ mEq}}{10 \text{ mEq}} = \frac{x \text{ ml}}{5 \text{ ml}}$$

$$10 X = 100$$

$$X = 10 \text{ ml}$$

Routes of administration

Routes of administration depend largely on drug characteristics, client characteristics, and desired responses. The major routes are oral, parenteral, and topical. Each has advantages, disadvantages, indications for use, and specific techniques of administration.

ORAL ROUTE

The oral route of drug administration is the one most commonly used. It is simple, convenient, and relatively inexpensive, and it can be used by most people. The main disadvantages are rather slow drug action and possible irritation of gastrointestinal mucosa, which may produce adverse effects such as anorexia, nausea, vomiting, diarrhea, and ulcerations.

Drugs may also be given through tubes placed into the gastrointestinal tract, such as nasogastric or gastrostomy tubes. In people who cannot take drugs orally for prolonged periods, this route is usually preferable to injections.

PARENTERAL ROUTES

The term *parenteral route* refers to any route other than gastrointestinal (enteral) but is commonly used to indicate subcutaneous, intramuscular, and intravenous injections. Injections require special drug preparations and equipment.

Drugs for injection

Parenteral drugs must be prepared, packaged, and administered in such a way as to maintain sterility. Vials are closed glass or plastic containers with rubber stoppers through which a sterile needle can be inserted for withdrawing medication. Multiple-dose vials can be reused if sterility is maintained. Ampules are sealed glass containers, the tops of which must be broken off to allow insertion of a needle and withdrawal of the medication. Broken ampules and remaining medication are discarded; they are no longer sterile and cannot be reused. When vials or ampules contain a powder form of the drug, a sterile solution must be added and the drug dissolved before withdrawal. Tubexes are a brand of glass tubes of medication solutions with attached needles. They are inserted into specially designed holders and used like other needle–syringe units. Most injectable narcotic analgesics and several other drugs are available in ready-to-use Tubexes. Figure 2-1 illustrates a vial, an ampule, and a Tubex.

Equipment for injections

Sterile needles and syringes are used to contain, measure, and administer parenteral medications. They may be packaged together or separately. Needles are available in various gauges and lengths. The term *gauge* refers to lumen size, with larger numbers indicating smaller lumen sizes. For example, a 25-gauge needle is smaller than an 18-gauge needle. Choice of needle gauge and length depends on route of administration, viscosity of the solution to be given, and size of the client. Usually, a 25-gauge, $\frac{5}{8}$-inch needle is used for SC injections, and a 22- or 20-gauge, $1\frac{1}{2}$-inch needle is used for IM injections. Other needle sizes are available for special uses, such as intradermal injections. Figure 2-2 compares the gauge and length of several needles.

Syringes are also available in various sizes, such as 1, 3, 5, 10, 20, and 50 ml. The 3-ml size is probably used most often. It is usually plastic and is available

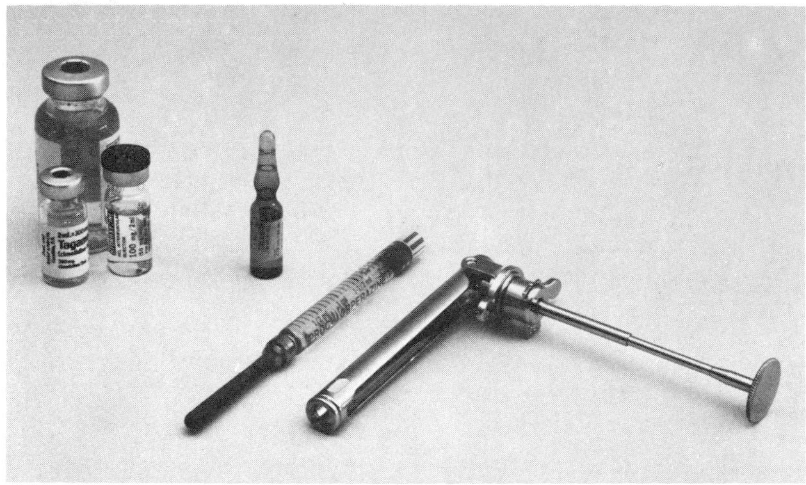

Figure 2-1. *Vials* (left), *an ampule* (center), *and a Tubex* (right).

with or without an attached needle. Syringes are calibrated so that drug doses can be accurately measured. However, the calibrations vary according to the size and type of syringe.

Insulin and tuberculin syringes are used for specific purposes. Insulin syringes are calibrated to measure up to 100 units of insulin. Safe practice requires that *only* insulin syringes be used to measure insulin and that they be used for no other drugs. Tuberculin syringes have a capacity of 1 ml (16 minims). They should be used for small doses of any drug because measurements are more accurate than with larger syringes. Figure 2-3 depicts sizes and calibrations on some commonly used syringes.

Subcutaneous route

The subcutaneous (SC) route involves injection of drugs under the skin. This route is used for a small volume (approximately 1 ml or less) of drug. Absorption is slower, and drug action is generally longer with subcutaneous injections than with intravenous or intramuscular injections. The subcutaneous route is commonly used for only a few drugs. Many drugs cannot be given subcutaneously because they are too irritating to subcutaneous tissues and may cause tissue necrosis and abscess formation. Insulin is a major drug that is given subcutaneously. Common sites for subcutaneous injections are the upper arms, abdomen, back, and thighs (Fig. 2-4).

Intramuscular route

The intramuscular (IM) route involves injection of drugs into certain muscles. This route is used for several drugs, usually in doses of 3 ml or less. Absorption is more rapid than from subcutaneous injections because muscle tissue has a greater blood supply. Site

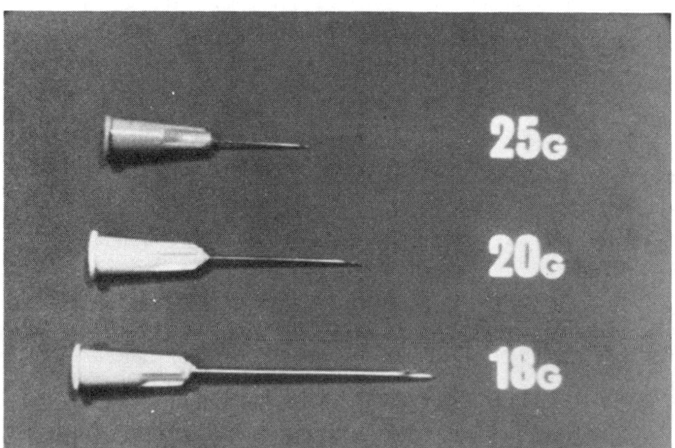

Figure 2-2. *Needles of various gauges and lengths:* (top) *25 gauge, 5/8 inch;* (center) *20 gauge, 1 inch;* (bottom) *18 gauge, 1½ inch.*

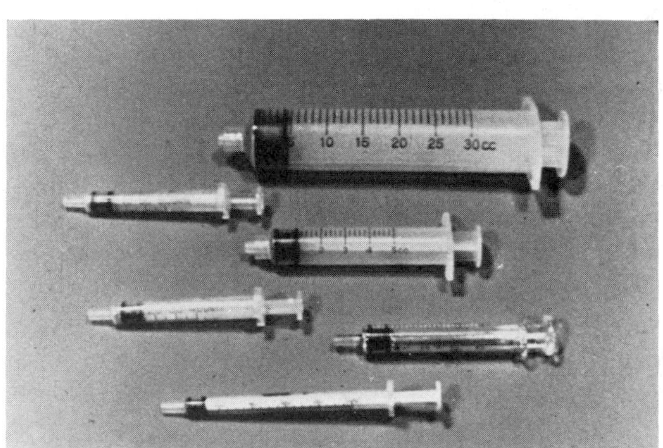

Figure 2-3. *Syringes of various sizes and calibrations.*

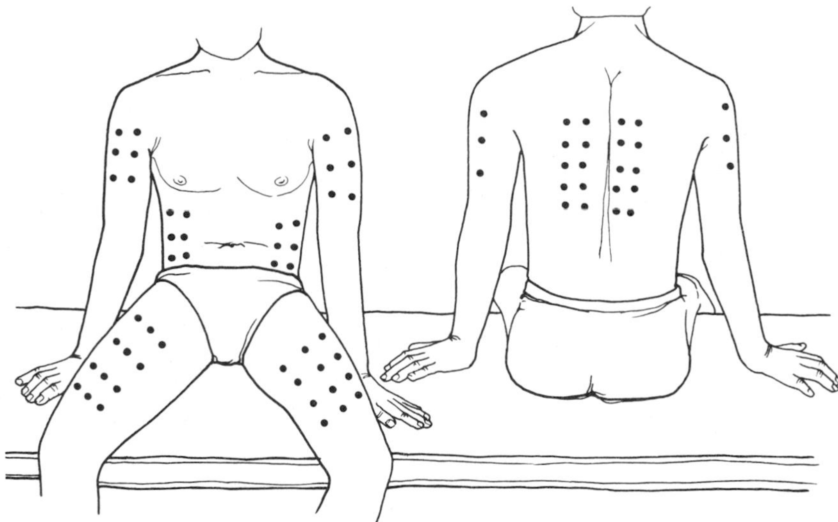

Figure 2-4. *Subcutaneous injection sites.*

selection is especially important with intramuscular injections because incorrect placement of the needle may damage blood vessels or nerves. Commonly used sites are the deltoid, dorsogluteal, ventrogluteal, and vastus lateralis. These sites must be selected by first identifying anatomic landmarks. The sites and anatomic landmarks are illustrated in Figures 2-5 through 2-8.

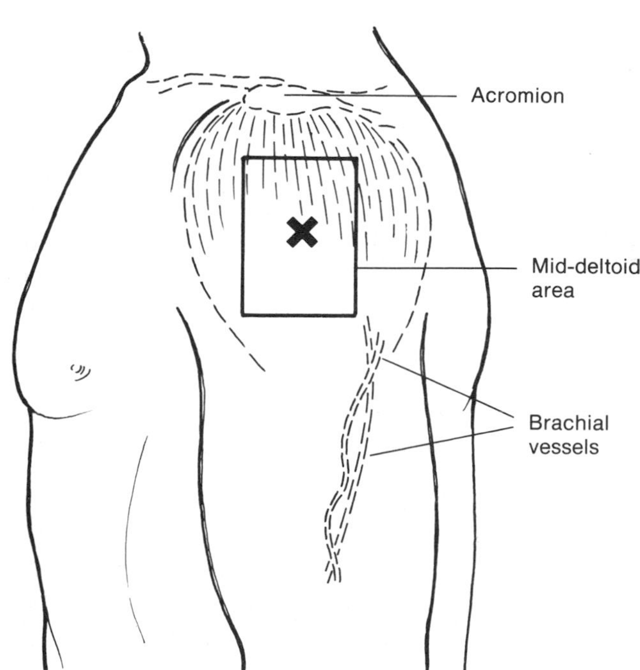

Figure 2-5. *Placement of the needle for insertion into the deltoid muscle. The area of injection is bounded by the lower edge of the acromion on the top to a point on the side of the arm opposite the axilla on the bottom. The side boundaries of the rectangular site are parallel to the arm and one third and two thirds of the way around the side of the arm.*

Intravenous route

The intravenous (IV) route involves injection of a drug into the bloodstream. Drugs given intravenously act

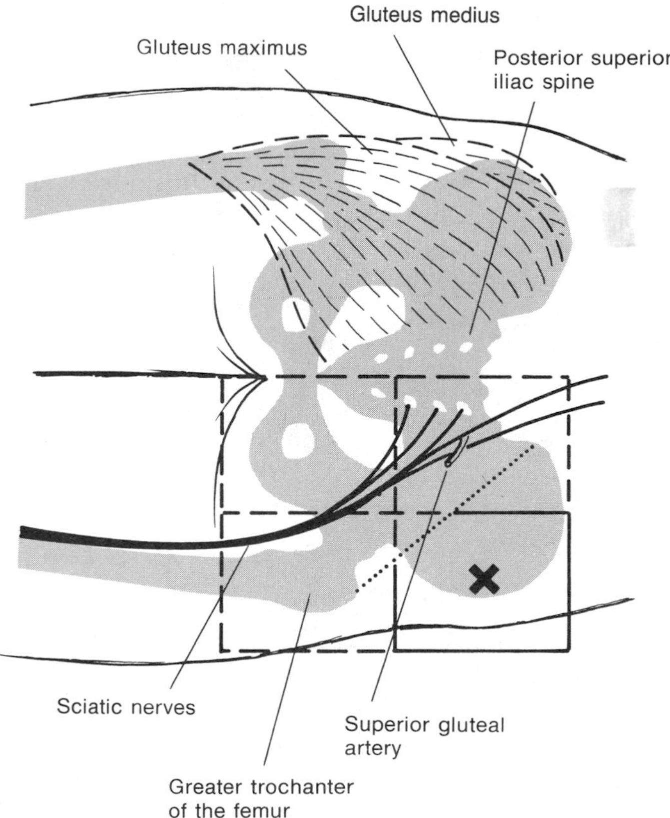

Figure 2-6. *Proper placement of the needle for an IM injection into the dorsogluteal site. It is above and outside a diagonal line drawn from the greater trochanter of the femur to the posterior superior iliac spine. Notice how this site allows the nurse to avoid entering an area near the sciatic nerve and the superior gluteal artery.*

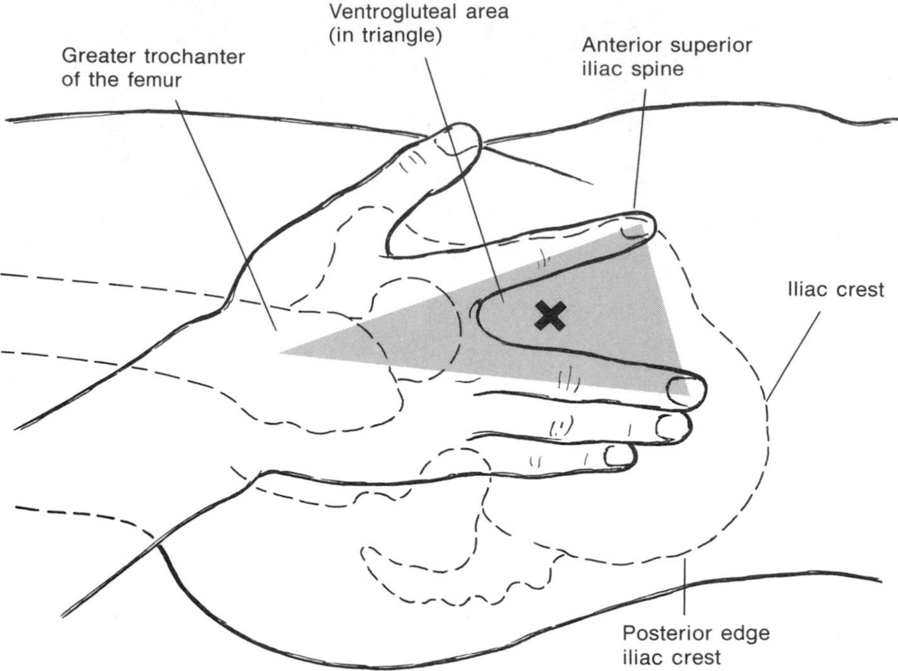

Figure 2-7. Placement of the needle for insertion into the ventrogluteal area. Notice how the nurse's palm is placed on the greater trochanter, and the index finger on the anterior superior iliac spine. The middle finger is spread posteriorly as far as possible along the iliac crest. The injection is made in the middle of the triangle formed by the nurse's fingers and the iliac crest.

rapidly, and larger amounts can be given than by subcutaneous or intramuscular injection. One way of giving drugs intravenously is to prepare the drug with a needle and syringe, insert the needle into a vein, and inject the drug. More often, however, drugs are given through an established intravenous line, intermittently or continuously.

Direct injection is useful for emergency drugs, intermittent infusion is often used for antibiotics, and continuous infusion is used for potassium chloride and a few other drugs. Drug administration is usually more comfortable and convenient for the client when he has an intravenous line. Disadvantages of this route include not only the time and skill required for venipuncture but also the difficulty of maintaining intravenous lines and the problem of increased adverse reactions from the rapid drug action.

Other parenteral routes

In addition to the ones discussed, other parenteral routes include injection into layers of the skin (intradermal), injection into arteries (intra-arterial), injection into joints (intra-articular), and injection into cerebrospinal fluid (intrathecal). The latter three routes are used only by physicians.

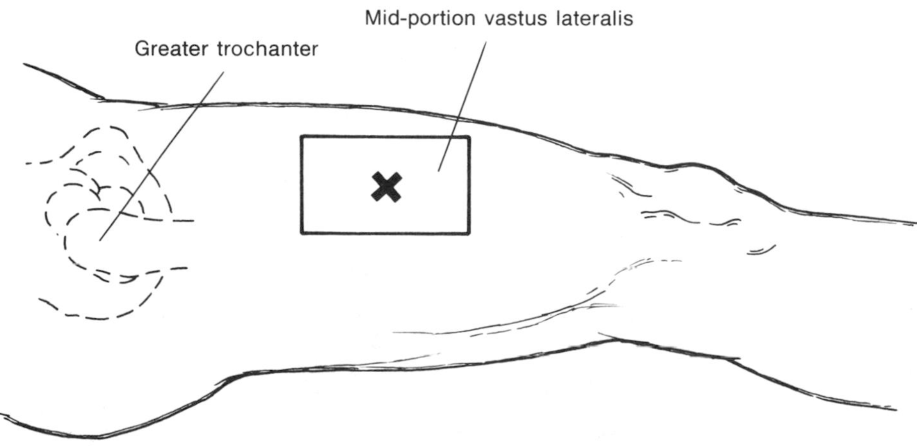

Figure 2-8. Placement of the needle for insertion into the vastus lateralis. It is generally easier to have the client lying on his back. However, the client may be sitting when using this site for IM injections. It is a suitable site for children when the nurse grasps the muscle in her hand to concentrate the muscle mass for injection.

TOPICAL ROUTES

Topical administration involves application of drugs to skin or mucous membranes. Application to mucous membranes includes drugs given by inhalation into the lungs, instillation into the eyes, nose, and ears, insertion under the tongue (sublingual), insertion into the cheek (buccal), and insertion into the vagina or rectum. An advantage of topical administration is that many of the drugs act locally where applied; therefore, the possibility of systemic adverse reactions is decreased. (Some topical drugs are given for systemic effects, however.) A disadvantage is that specific drug preparations must be used for the various routes. Thus, only dermatologic preparations are safe to use on skin, only ophthalmic drugs are used in the eyes, only a few drugs are given sublingually or bucally, and only vaginal or rectal preparations are given by those respective routes.

NURSING ACTIONS: DRUG ADMINISTRATION

Nursing Actions	*Rationale/Explanation*
1. Follow general rules for administering medications safely and effectively	
a. Prepare and give drugs in well-lighted areas, as free of interruptions and distractions as possible.	To prevent errors in selecting ordered drugs, calculating dosages, and identifying clients
b. Wash hands before preparing medications and, if needed, during administration.	To prevent infection and cross contamination
c. Use sterile technique in preparing and administering injections.	To prevent infection. Sterile technique involves using sterile needles and syringes, using sterile drug solutions, not touching sterile objects to any unsterile objects, and cleansing injection sites with an antiseptic.
d. Read medication sheets carefully and repeatedly. Read the label on the drug container and compare with the medication sheet in terms of drug, dosage or concentration, and route of administration.	For accurate drug administration. Most nursing texts instruct the nurse to read a drug label three times: when removing the container, while measuring the dose, and before returning the container.
e. Do not leave medications unattended.	To prevent accidental or deliberate ingestion by anyone other than the intended person. Also, to prevent contamination or spilling of medications.
f. Identify the client, preferably by comparing the identification wrist band to the medication sheet.	This is the best way to verify identity. Calling by name, relying on the name on a door or bed, and asking someone else are unreliable methods, although they must be used occasionally when the client lacks a name band.
g. Identify yourself, if indicated, and state your reason for approaching the client. For example, "I'm . . . I have your medication for you."	Explaining actions helps to decrease client anxiety and increase cooperation in taking prescribed medication.
h. Position the client appropriately for the intended route of administration.	To prevent complications such as aspiration of oral drugs into the lungs
i. Provide water or other supplies as needed.	To promote comfort of the client as well as to ensure drug administration
j. Do not leave medications at the bedside as a general rule. Possible exceptions are antacids, nitroglycerin, and eye medications.	To prevent omitting or losing the drug or hoarding of the drug by the client
k. Do not give a drug when signs and symptoms of toxicity are present. Notify the physician and record that the drug was omitted and why.	Additional doses of a drug increase toxicity. However, drugs are not omitted without a careful assessment of the client's condition and a valid reason.

Nursing Actions	***Rationale/Explanation***
l. Record drug administration (or omission) as soon as possible and according to agency policies.	To maintain an accurate record of drugs received by the client
m. If it is necessary to omit a scheduled dose for some reason, the decision to give the dose later or omit it completely depends largely on the drug and frequency of administration. Generally, give drugs ordered once or twice daily at a later time. For others, omit the one dose and give the drug at the next scheduled time.	Clients may be unable to take the drug at the scheduled time because of diagnostic tests or many other reasons. A temporary change in the time of administration—usually for one dose only—may be necessary to maintain therapeutic effects.
n. For medications ordered as needed (PRN), assess the client's condition, check the physician's orders or medication sheets for the name, dose, and frequency of administration, and determine the time of the most recently administered dose.	Administration of PRN medications is somewhat different from that of regularly scheduled drugs. Analgesics, antiemetics, and antipyretics are often ordered PRN.
o. For narcotics and other controlled substances, sign drugs out on separate narcotic records according to agency policies.	To meet legal requirements for dispensing controlled substances
p. If, at any time during drug preparation or administration, any question arises regarding the drug, the dose, or whether the client is supposed to receive it, check the original physician's order. If the order is not clear, call the physician for clarification before giving the drug.	To promote safety and prevent errors. The same procedure applies when the client questions drug orders at the bedside. For example, the client may state he has been receiving different drugs or different doses.
2. For oral medications	
a. Without touching the medication, place it in a medicine cup and give it to the client. For oral liquids, hold the cup at eye level and measure the dosage at the bottom of the meniscus.	To maintain clean technique and administer drugs accurately
b. Have the client in a sitting position when not contraindicated.	To decrease risks of aspirating medication into lungs. Aspiration may lead to difficulty in breathing and aspiration pneumonia.
c. Give before, with, or after meals as indicated by the specific drug.	Food in the stomach usually delays drug absorption and action. It also decreases gastric irritation, a common side-effect of oral drugs. Giving drugs at appropriate times in relation to food intake can both increase therapeutic effects and decrease adverse effects.
d. Give most oral drugs with a full glass (8 oz) of water or other fluid.	To promote dissolution and absorption of tablets and capsules. Also, to decrease gastric irritation by diluting drug concentration.
e. Do not give oral drugs if the client is	
(1) NPO (receiving nothing by mouth)	Oral drugs and fluids may interfere with diagnostic tests or be otherwise contraindicated. Most drugs can be given after diagnostic tests are completed. If the client is having surgery, preoperative drug orders are cancelled. New orders are written postoperatively.
(2) Vomiting	Oral drugs and fluids increase vomiting. Thus, no benefit results from the drug. Also, fluid and electrolyte problems may result from loss of gastric acid.
(3) Excessively sedated or unconscious	To avoid aspiration of drugs into the lungs owing to impaired ability to swallow

Nursing Actions	***Rationale/Explanation***
3. For medications given by nasogastric tube	
a. Use a liquid preparation when possible. If necessary, crush a tablet or empty a capsule into about 30 ml of water and mix well. Do not crush or empty sustained-release products.	Particles of tablets or powders from capsules may obstruct the tube lumen. Altering sustained-release products increases risks of overdosage and adverse effects.
b. Use a clean bulb syringe or other catheter-tipped syringe.	The syringe allows aspiration and serves as a funnel for instillation of medication and fluids into the stomach.
c. Before instilling medication, aspirate the stomach contents or instill 10 to 20 cc of air while listening with a stethoscope over the stomach.	To be sure the tube is in the stomach
d. Instill medication by gravity flow and follow it with at least 50 ml of water. Do not allow the syringe to empty completely between additions.	Gravity flow is safer than applying pressure. Water "pushes" the drug into the stomach and rinses the tube, thereby maintaining tube patency. Additional water or other fluids may be given according to fluid needs of the client. Add fluids to avoid instilling air into the stomach unnecessarily with possible client discomfort.
e. Clamp off the tube from suction or drainage for at least 30 minutes.	To avoid removing the medication from the stomach
4. For SC injections	
a. Use only sterile drug preparations labeled or commonly used for SC injections.	Many parenteral drugs are too irritating to subcutaneous tissue for use by this route.
b. Use a 25-gauge, $\frac{5}{8}$-inch needle for most SC injections.	This size needle is effective for most clients and drugs.
c. Select an appropriate injection site, based on client preferences, drug characteristics, and visual inspection of possible sites. In long-term therapy, such as with insulin, rotate the injection sites. Avoid areas with lumps, bruises, or other lesions.	These techniques allow the client to participate in his or her care; avoid tissue damage and unpredictable absorption, which occur with repeated injections in the same location; and increase client comfort and cooperation.
d. Cleanse the site with an alcohol sponge.	To prevent infection
e. Tighten the skin or pinch a fold of skin and tissue between thumb and fingers.	Either is acceptable for most clients. If the client is obese, tightening the skin may be easier. If the client is very thin, the tissue fold may keep the needle from hitting bone.
f. Hold the syringe like a pencil and insert the needle quickly at a 45° angle. Use enough force to penetrate the skin and subcutaneous tissue in one smooth movement.	To give the drug correctly with minimal client discomfort
g. Release the skin so that both hands are free to manipulate the syringe. Pull back gently on the plunger (aspirate). If no blood enters the syringe, inject the drug. If blood is aspirated into the syringe, remove the needle and reprepare the medication.	To prevent accidental injection into the bloodstream. Blood return in the syringe is an uncommon occurrence.
h. Remove the needle quickly and apply gentle pressure for a few seconds.	To prevent bleeding
5. For IM injections	
a. Use only drug preparations labeled or commonly used for IM injections. Check label instructions for mixing drugs in powder form.	Some parenteral drug preparations cannot be given safely by the IM route.

Nursing Actions	Rationale/Explanation
b. Use a $1\frac{1}{2}$-inch needle for most adults and a $\frac{5}{8}$-inch to $1\frac{1}{2}$-inch needle for children, depending on the size of the client.	A long needle is necessary to reach muscle tissue, which underlies subcutaneous fat.
c. Use the smallest gauge needle that will accommodate the medication. A 22 gauge is satisfactory for most drugs; a 20 gauge may be used for viscous medications.	To decrease tissue damage and client discomfort
d. Select an appropriate injection site, based on client preferences, drug characteristics, anatomic landmarks, and visual inspection of possible sites. Rotate sites if frequent injections are being given and avoid areas with lumps, bruises, or other lesions.	To increase client comfort and participation and to avoid tissue damage. Identification of anatomic landmarks is mandatory for safe administration of IM drugs.
e. Cleanse the site with an alcohol sponge.	To prevent infection
f. Tighten the skin, hold the syringe like a pencil, and insert the needle quickly at a 90° angle. Use enough force to penetrate the skin and subcutaneous tissue into the muscle in one smooth motion.	To give the drug correctly with minimal client discomfort
g. Aspirate (see 4g, SC Injections).	
h. Remove the needle quickly and apply pressure for several seconds.	To prevent bleeding
6. For IV injections	
a. Use only drug preparations that are labeled for IV use.	Others are not likely to be pure enough for safe injection into the bloodstream or are not compatible with the blood *p*H (7.35–7.45).
b. Check label instructions for the type and amount of fluid to use for dissolving or diluting the drug.	Some drugs require special preparation techniques to maintain solubility or pharmacologic activity. Most drugs in powder form can be dissolved in sterile water or sodium chloride for injection. Most drug solutions can be given with dextrose or dextrose and sodium chloride IV solutions.
c. Prepare drugs just before use, as a general rule. Also, add drugs to IV fluids just before use.	Some drugs are unstable in solution. In some agencies, drugs are mixed and added to IV fluids in the pharmacy. This is the preferred method because sterility can be better maintained.
d. For venipuncture and direct injection into a vein, apply a tourniquet, select a site in the arm, cleanse the skin with an antiseptic (*e.g.*, povidone-iodine or alcohol), insert the needle, and aspirate a small amount of blood into the syringe to be sure that the needle is in the vein. Remove the tourniquet and inject the drug slowly. Remove the needle and apply pressure until there is no evidence of bleeding.	For safe and accurate drug administration with minimal risk to the client. The length of time required to give the drug depends on the specific drug and the amount. Slow administration, over several minutes, allows immediate discontinuation if adverse effects occur.
e. For administration by an established IV line:	
(1) Check the infusion for patency and flow rate. Check the venipuncture site for signs of infiltration and phlebitis before each drug dose.	The solution must be flowing freely for accurate drug administration. If infiltration or phlebitis is present, do not give the drug until a new IV line is begun.
(2) For direct injection, cleanse an injection site on the IV tubing, insert the needle, and inject the drug slowly.	Most tubings have injection sites to facilitate drug administration.
(3) To use a volume control set, fill it with 50 to 100 ml of IV fluid and clamp it so that no further fluid enters the chamber and dilutes the drug. Inject the drug into an injection site after cleansing the site with	This method is often used for administration of antibiotics on an intermittent schedule. Dilution of the drug decreases adverse effects.

Nursing Actions	***Rationale/Explanation***
an alcohol sponge and infuse, usually in 1 hour or less. Once the drug is infused, add solution to maintain the infusion.	
(4) To use a "piggyback" method, add the drug to 50 to 100 ml of IV solution in a separate container. Attach the IV tubing and a needle. Insert the needle in an injection site on the main IV tubing after cleansing the site. Infuse the drug over 15 to 60 minutes, depending on the drug.	This method is also used for intermittent administration of antibiotics and other drugs. Whether a volume control or piggyback apparatus is used depends on hospital policy and equipment available.
f. When more than one drug is to be given, flush the line between drugs. Do not mix drugs in syringes or in IV fluids unless the drug literature states that the drugs are compatible.	Physical and chemical interactions between the drugs may occur and cause precipitation, inactivation, or increased toxicity. Most nursing units have charts depicting drug compatibility, or information may be obtained from the pharmacy.
7. For application to skin	
Use drug preparations labeled for dermatologic use. Cleanse the skin, remove any previously applied medication, and apply the drug in a thin layer. For broken skin or open lesions, use sterile gloves, tongue blade, or cotton-tipped applicator to apply the drug.	To promote therapeutic effects and minimize adverse effects
8. For instillation of eye drops	
Use drug preparations labeled for ophthalmic use. Wash your hands, open the eye to expose the conjunctival sac, and drop the medication into the sac, not on the eyeball, without touching the dropper tip to anything. Provide a tissue for blotting any excess drug. If two or more eye drops are scheduled at the same time, wait 1 to 5 minutes between instillations.	Ophthalmic preparations must be sterile to avoid infection. Blot any excess drug from the inner canthus near the nose to decrease systemic absorption of the drug.
9. For instillation of nose drops and nasal sprays	
Have the client hold his head back, and drop the medication into the nostrils. Give only as ordered.	When nose drops are used for rhinitis and nasal congestion accompanying the common cold, overuse results in a rebound congestion that may be worse than the original symptom.
10. For instillation of ear medications	
Open the ear canal by pulling the ear up and back for adults, down and back for children, and drop the medication on the side of the canal.	To straighten the canal and promote maximal contact between medication and tissue
11. For rectal suppositories	
Lubricate the end with a water-soluble lubricant, wear a glove or finger cot, and insert into the rectum the length of the finger. Place the suppository next to the mucosal wall. If the client prefers and is able, provide supplies for self-administration.	To promote absorption. Allowing self-administration may prevent embarrassment to the client. The nurse must be sure that the client knows the correct procedure.
12. For vaginal medications	
Use gloves or an applicator for insertion. If an applicator is used, wash thoroughly with soap and water after each use. If the client prefers and is able, provide supplies for self-administration.	Some women may be embarrassed and prefer self-administration. The nurse must be sure that the client knows the correct procedure.

Selected References

Brill EL, Kilts DF: Foundations for Nursing. New York, Appleton-Century-Crofts, 1980

Chaplin G, Shull, II, Welk PC, III: How safe is the air-bubble technique for IM injections? Nursing 15:59, September 1985

Giving medication through a nasogastric tube. Nursing 10:71–73, May 1980

Hermann CS: Performing intradermal skin tests—the right way. Nursing 13:50–53, October 1983

Langer RS: New drug delivery systems. Drug Ther 13:217–231, April 1983

Lenz CL: Make your needle selection right to the point. Nursing 13:50–51, February 1983.

Malseed RT: Pharmacology: Drug Therapy and Nursing Considerations, 2d ed. Philadelphia, J B Lippincott, 1985

Morris ME: Intravenous drug incompatibilities. Am J Nurs 79:1288–1295, July 1979

Newton DW, Newton M: Route, site and technique: Three key decisions in giving parenteral medication. Nursing 9:18–25, July 1979

Pierce ME: Reporting and following up on medication errors. Nursing 14:77–81, January 1984

Richardson LI, Richardson JK: The Mathematics of Drugs and Solutions with Clinical Applications, 3rd ed. New York, McGraw–Hill, 1985

Rodman MJ, Karch AM, Boyd EH, Smith DW: Pharmacology and Drug Therapy in Nursing, 3rd ed. Philadelphia, J B Lippincott, 1985

Sager DP, Bomar SK: Intravenous Medications: A Guide to Preparation, Administration, and Nursing Management. Philadelphia, J B Lippincott, 1980

Sorenson KC, Luckmann J: Basic Nursing: A Psychophysiologic Approach. Philadelphia, W B Saunders, 1979

3

THE ROLE OF THE NURSE IN DRUG THERAPY

Drug therapy involves the use of drugs to prevent or treat disease processes and manifestations. The goal of drug therapy is to maximize the beneficial effects of the drugs administered and to minimize their harmful or adverse effects. To meet this goal, the nurse must be knowledgable about pharmacology (drugs and their effects on the body), physiology (normal body functions), and pathophysiology (alterations in body functions due to disease processes). More specifically, effective drug therapy requires knowledge of the particular drug and the person receiving it.

Chapter 1 included general information about drugs and human responses to drugs. Chapter 2 emphasized techniques of preparing and administering drugs safely and effectively. Although the importance of safe and accurate administration cannot be overemphasized, this is only one aspect of the nursing role in drug therapy. The nurse must also observe individual responses to drug therapy, both therapeutic and adverse, and teach the client about prescribed drugs.

Even though medication administration is usually described as a dependent function because a physician's order is required, it involves independent functions and judgments as well. One of these is deciding when to give PRN medications. Another involves choosing between two or more PRN drugs. A third may be deciding to omit one or more drug doses. These decisions and others must be based on knowledge of the drug, knowledge of the client, and continuing assessment of the client's responses. Specific assessment data are individualized. For example, the responsible and conscientious nurse will measure, record, and evaluate blood pressure for clients receiving antihypertensive drugs, apical and radial pulse rate and rhythm for clients receiving antiarrhythmic drugs, and serum potassium reports for clients receiving potassium-losing diuretics or potassium supplements, whether or not these procedures are ordered by the physician. Many safety and comfort measures are independent judgments as well. Among these are using siderails, maintaining bed rest, or assisting in ambulation when a client has received a sedative-type drug. To help the nurse gain knowledge and skills related to drug therapy, this chapter includes suggestions for studying pharmacology, legal responsibilities of the nurse, general principles of drug therapy, and general nursing actions. The remainder of this book is devoted to more specific aspects of drug therapy with particular drug groups and individual drugs.

A rational approach to pharmacology

The beginning student of pharmacology is faced with a bewildering number and variety of drugs. This number can be greatly reduced by concentrating initial study on therapeutic classifications or groups of drugs and prototypes of those groups. For example, narcotic analgesics is one classification or group, and morphine is the prototype of that group. Morphine and other narcotic analgesics have many common characteristics, including the following:

1. They are used primarily to relieve pain.
2. They produce central nervous system (CNS) depression ranging from slight drowsiness to unconsciousness, depending on dose.
3. A major adverse reaction is respiratory depression (depression of the respiratory center in the medulla oblongata as part of the CNS depression). Thus, the nurse must check rate and depth of respiration.
4. They have a high potential for abuse and dependence. Therefore, their use is regulated by narcotic laws and requires special records and procedures.
5. They must be used with caution in people who already have respiratory depression or an impaired level of consciousness.

If these and other characteristics are clearly understood, study of all other narcotic analgesics is facilitated because they are compared to morphine, especially in ability to relieve pain and likelihood of causing respiratory depression.

Once the characteristics of the major drug groups are known, continued study is necessary to add depth and scope to drug knowledge. Almost all new or unfamiliar drugs fit into an established classification. For example, you may know that the unfamiliar drug is a thiazide diuretic. By recalling your knowledge of this drug classification, you have a base of information on which to build as you study the unfamiliar drug.

When one is learning about an individual drug, a large amount of data must be assimilated. Although some people attempt to memorize drug information, this is not an effective way to learn, retain, and apply drug knowledge. Some guidelines for effective study include the following:

1. Attempt to understand how the drug acts in the body. This allows the nurse to predict therapeutic effects and to predict, prevent, or minimize adverse effects by early detection and treatment.
2. Concentrate study efforts on major characteristics. These include the main indications for use, common and potentially serious adverse effects, conditions in which the drug is relatively or absolutely contraindicated, usual dosage ranges, and related nursing actions.
3. Compare the drug with a prototype when possible. Relating the unknown to the known aids learning and retention of knowledge.
4. Keep an authoritative drug reference readily available, preferably at both work and home. This is a much more reliable source of drug information than the nurse's memory. Use the reference freely whenever an unfamiliar drug is encountered or when a question arises about a relatively familiar one.
5. When you are taking notes or writing drug information cards, use your own words when possible. Copying word for word promotes memorizing but does not aid learning.
6. Mentally practice applying drug knowledge in nursing care by asking yourself, "What if I have a client who is receiving this drug? What must I do? What must I observe for? What if my client is an elderly person or child?"

Legal responsibilities of the nurse

The registered nurse is legally empowered, under state nurse practice acts, to give medications from the orders of licensed physicians and dentists. The nurse cannot legally prescribe medications, except in a few exceptional circumstances, because that is practicing medicine. The nurse cannot legally dispense medications, because that is practicing pharmacy.

When giving medications, the nurse is legally responsible for safe and accurate administration (right drug, right dose, right client, right route, and right time). This means the nurse may be held liable for *not* giving a drug or for giving a wrong drug or a wrong dose. Also, the nurse is expected to have sufficient drug knowledge to recognize and question erroneous orders. If, after questioning the prescribing physician and seeking information from other authoritative sources, the nurse considers that administering the drug is unsafe, the nurse must refuse to give the drug. The fact that a physician wrote an erroneous order does not excuse the nurse from legal liability if he or she carries out that order. The nurse is also legally responsible for actions delegated to people known to be inadequately prepared or legally barred from performing the act of administering medications, such as allowing a nurse's aide to do so.

The nurse is responsible for storing narcotics and other controlled substances in locked containers, administering them only to people for whom they are prescribed, recording each dose given on appropriate narcotic sheets as well as on the client's medication sheet, counting the amounts of each drug at the end of a working shift, and reporting any discrepancies to the proper authorities.

The nurse who follows safe practices in giving medications does not need to be excessively concerned about legal liability. The basic techniques and guidelines listed in Chapter 2 are aimed toward safe and accurate preparation and administration; most errors result when these practices are not followed consistently.

Legal responsibilities in other aspects of drug therapy—observing for therapeutic and adverse effects, teaching clients—are less tangible and clear-cut. Probably the major responsibility is to recognize, record, and report adverse reactions.

General principles of drug therapy

GENERAL ASSESSMENT GUIDELINES

Drug therapy should be client centered, not physician or nurse or drug centered. The first step in individualizing drug therapy is assessing the client's condition. General assessment factors—age, disease, and others—that influence drug therapy were discussed in Chapter 1. Additional information is needed regarding the person's experiences with and attitudes toward drug therapy. Most of this information can be obtained during the nursing history interview. In addition, a medication history (Fig. 3-1) can provide useful information. Some specific questions and areas of assessment include the following:

1. What are current drug orders?
2. What does the client know about current drugs? Is teaching needed?
3. What drugs has the client taken before? Include any drugs taken regularly, such as those taken for chronic illnesses (hypertension, diabetes mellitus, arthritis, and others). It may be helpful to ask specifically about corticosteroids, oral contraceptive pills, and other hormonal drugs because they may have long-lasting effects. It may also be helpful to ask about nonprescription (over-the-counter, or OTC) drugs for headache, colds, indigestion, or constipation because some people do not consider OTC preparations to be drugs.
4. Has the client ever had an allergic reaction to a drug? If so, what specific signs and symptoms occurred? This information is necessary because many people describe minor nausea and other symptoms as allergic reactions. Unless the reaction is further explored, the client may have therapy withheld inappropriately.
5. What are the client's attitudes about drugs? Try to obtain information to help assess whether the client takes drugs freely or reluctantly, is likely to comply with a prescribed drug regimen, and is likely to abuse drugs.
6. If long-term drug therapy is likely, will the client be financially able to purchase medications?
7. Is the client able to communicate his needs, such as requesting medication? Is he able to swallow oral medications? Are any other conditions present that influence drug therapy?
8. In addition to the nursing history, use progress notes, laboratory reports, and other sources of assessment data as they are available and relevant. As part of the initial assessment, obtain baseline data on measurements to be used in monitoring therapeutic or adverse effects. Specific data to be acquired depend on the medication and the client's condition. Laboratory tests of liver, kidney, and bone marrow function are often helpful because some drugs may damage these organs. Also, if liver or kidney damage exists, drug metabolism or excretion may be altered. More specific laboratory tests include serum potassium levels before diuretic therapy, culture and susceptibility studies before antimicrobial therapy, and blood clotting tests before anticoagulant therapy. Nonlaboratory data that may be relevant include vital signs, weight, and urine output.
9. Continue to assess the client's condition throughout drug therapy.

USE OF NURSING INTERVENTIONS

Drug therapy should be integrated with other aspects of care, and nondrug measures should be used when appropriate to decrease the need for drugs, to enhance therapeutic effects, or to decrease adverse effects. General nursing measures include positioning, assisting to cough and deep breathe, ambulating, applying heat or cold, increasing or decreasing sensory stimulation, scheduling activities to allow rest periods, and recording vital signs, fluid intake, urine output, and other assessment data whether or not they are ordered by the physician. Specific nursing measures depend on the medication and the client's condition.

GENERAL DRUG SELECTION AND DOSAGE CONSIDERATIONS

Although many factors influence the physician's prescription and the nurse's administration of drugs, general guidelines include the following:

MEDICATION HISTORY

Name ______________________________ Age __________

Health problems, acute and chronic

Are you allergic to any medications?

If yes, describe specific effects or symptoms.

Part 1: Prescription Medications

1. Do you take any prescription medications on a regular basis?

2. If yes, ask the following about each medication.
   Name — Dose
   Frequency — Specific times
   How long taken — Reason for use

3. Are you able to take this medicine pretty much as described?

4. Does anyone else help you take your medications?

5. What information or instructions were you given when the medications were first prescribed?

6. Do you think the medication is doing what it was prescribed to do?

7. Have you had any problems that you attribute to the medication?

8. Do you take any prescription medications on an irregular basis?
   If yes, ask the following about each medication.
   Name — Reason
   Dose — How long taken
   Frequency

Part 2: Nonprescription Medications

1. Do you take OTC medications?

	Medication			
Problem	*Yes/No*	*Name*	*Amount*	*Frequency*
Pain				
Headache				
Sleep				
Cold				
Indigestion				
Heartburn				
Diarrhea				
Constipation				
Other				

Part 3: Social Drugs

	Yes/No	*Amount*
Coffee		
Tea		
Cola drinks		
Alcohol		
Tobacco		

Figure 3-1. *Medication history.*

1. For the most part, as few drugs in as few doses as possible should be used. Minimizing the number of drugs and the frequency of administration increases client compliance with the prescribed drug regimen and decreases risks of serious adverse effects, including hazardous drug interactions.

   There are some notable exceptions to this basic rule. For example, multiple drugs are recommended for the treatment of moderate-to-severe hypertension and for tuberculosis and other severe infections.
2. Individual drugs are generally preferred over fixed-dose combinations of drugs because they allow greater flexibility and individualization of dosage. However, fixed-dose combination products are commonly used because they are convenient and may promote compliance. Separate drugs should be given initially. Then, if established dosages are similar to those in a combination product, the combination product may be given.
3. The least amount of the least potent drug that will yield therapeutic benefit should be given, in order to decrease adverse reactions. For example, if a mild, nonnarcotic and a strong, narcotic analgesic are both ordered, the nonnarcotic drug should be given if it is effective in relieving pain.
4. Recommended dosages are listed in amounts likely to be effective for most people, but they are only guidelines to be interpreted according to the client's condition. A seriously ill client may require larger doses than one with a milder illness. Clients with severe kidney disease often need much smaller than usual doses of renally excreted drugs.
5. Treatment with a particular drug can be started rapidly or slowly. If a drug has a long half-life and maximal therapeutic effects do not usually occur for several days or weeks, the physician may give a limited number of relatively large (loading) doses followed by a regular schedule of smaller (maintenance) doses. When drug actions are not urgent, therapy may be initiated with a maintenance dose.
6. Different salts of the same drug rarely differ pharmacologically. Hydrochloride, sulfate, and sodium salts are often used. Pharmacists and chemists choose salts on the basis of cost, convenience, solubility, and stability. For example, solubility is especially important with parenteral drugs, while taste is a factor with oral drugs.

DRUG USE IN PREGNANCY AND LACTATION

Drug therapy during pregnancy and lactation requires special consideration because of the potential effects of drugs on the fetus or nursing infant. During pregnancy, medications given to the mother reach the fetus by placental transfer, which begins at approximately the fifth week of embryonic life. Fetal organogenesis occurs during the first trimester of pregnancy. Consequently, drugs administered during early pregnancy may cause teratogenic effects. Drug teratogenicity is difficult to establish, partly because genetic disorders may also cause fetal malformations and partly because animal tests may not accurately indicate the effects of drugs on the human fetus. Once organogenesis is complete, adverse effects of drugs are usually manifested in the newborn infant as growth retardation, respiratory problems, infection, or bleeding. During lactation, many drugs given to the mother reach the infant by way of the breast milk. For most drugs, the amount found in breast milk is too small to cause significant effects.

For many drugs, safety and effectiveness of use during pregnancy and lactation have not been established. All drugs are relatively contraindicated during pregnancy, and drug therapy during pregnancy and lactation should be cautious and minimal. Specific guidelines include the following:

1. Medications should be given only when clearly indicated. Anticipated benefits of drug therapy for the mother must be carefully weighed against the risks of harm to the infant. When feasible, nondrug measures should be used rather than drug therapy.
2. When drug therapy is required, the choice of drug should be based on the stage of pregnancy and the available drug information. During the first trimester, for example, an older drug that has not been associated with teratogenic effects may be preferable to a newer drug of unknown teratogenicity.
3. Any drugs used during pregnancy and lactation should be administered in the lowest effective doses and for the shortest effective time.
4. Nontherapeutic drugs may also harm the developing fetus. Alcohol ingestion and cigarette smoking are contraindicated during pregnancy; no "safe" level of either has been established. Heavy ingestion of alcohol may cause fetal alcohol syndrome, a condition characterized by multiple congenital defects and mental retardation. Cigarette smoking (nicotine and carbon monoxide ingestion) decreases infant birth weight and increases the incidence of premature delivery, abortion, and neonatal death.
5. Drugs should be used cautiously by women of reproductive age who are sexually active and not using contraceptive measures. Otherwise, poten-

tially harmful agents may be ingested before pregnancy is suspected or confirmed.

GENERAL PEDIATRIC CONSIDERATIONS

In pediatric drug therapy, most general principles and techniques of drug administration are applicable. Additional guidelines include the following:

1. All aspects of pediatric drug therapy must be guided by the child's age, weight, and level of growth and development.
2. Choice of drug is often restricted because many drugs commonly used in adult drug therapy have not been sufficiently investigated to ensure safety and effectiveness in children.
3. Safe dosage ranges are less well defined for children than for adults. Some drugs are not recommended for use in children, and therefore dosages have not been established. Other drugs have recommended dosage ranges expressed in amount of drug to be given per kilogram of body weight or square meter of body surface area. When dosage ranges for children are listed in drug literature, these should be used. Many times, however, the dosage must be calculated as a fraction of the adult dose. The following methods are used for these calculations:

   (a) Clark's rule is based on weight and is used for children at least 2 years old.

   $$\frac{\text{Weight (in pounds)}}{150} \times \text{adult dose} = \text{child's dose}$$

   (b) Young's rule is based on age, which is considered a less desirable basis than weight or body surface area. If followed, it is used for children at least 2 years old.

   $$\frac{\text{Age (in years)}}{\text{Age (in years)} + 12} \times \text{adult dose} = \text{child's dose}$$

   (c) Fried's rule is used for children less than 2 years old.

   $$\frac{\text{Age (in months)}}{150} \times \text{adult dose} = \text{child's dose}$$

   (d) Calculations based on body surface area are considered more accurate than those based on age or weight. Body surface area is, in turn, based on height and weight. The nomogram (Fig. 3-2) is a device used for rapid estimation of body surface area.

   $$\frac{\text{Body surface area (in square meters)}}{\text{1.73 square meters (m}^2\text{)}} \times \text{adult dose} = \text{child's dose}$$

   Dosages obtained from these calculations are approximate and *must* be individualized. These doses can be used initially and then increased or decreased according to the child's response.
4. The oral route of drug administration should be used when possible. Children under approximately 5 years of age may be unable to swallow tablets and capsules, but they can usually take liquids or chewable tablets. If necessary, medication can be added to fluids or foods such as applesauce to increase acceptability to the child. If this is done, use a small amount and be sure the child takes all of it. Otherwise, less than the ordered dose is given. Try to obtain the child's cooperation; *never* force oral medications. Forcing may lead to aspiration.
5. If intramuscular injections are required in infants, the thigh muscles should be used because the deltoid muscles are quite small, and the gluteal muscles do not develop until the child is walking. Adverse effects with thigh injections may include nerve damage or quadriceps contracture. Quadriceps contracture leads to prolonged difficulty in walking. If intravenous injections are required, give a drug very slowly to avoid high serum drug levels and toxicity.
6. For safety, all medications must be kept out of reach of children and never referred to as "candy."
7. In the newborn, any drug is used very cautiously. Drugs usually must be given less often because they are handled more slowly. Immature liver and kidney function prolong drug action and increase risks of toxicity. Also, it is safer to initiate drug therapy with low doses, especially of drugs that are highly bound to plasma proteins. Neonates have few binding proteins, which leads to increased amounts of free, active drug and increased toxicity even at lower doses. Finally, in assessing the neonate's condition, drugs received by the mother before birth or during lactation must be considered.

GENERAL GERIATRIC CONSIDERATIONS

In geriatric drug therapy, general principles and techniques of administration apply. In addition, adverse drug effects are especially likely to occur in elderly people because of physiologic changes associated with aging, pathologic changes due to disease processes, multiple drug therapy for acute and chronic disorders, poor memory, and difficulty in complying with drug

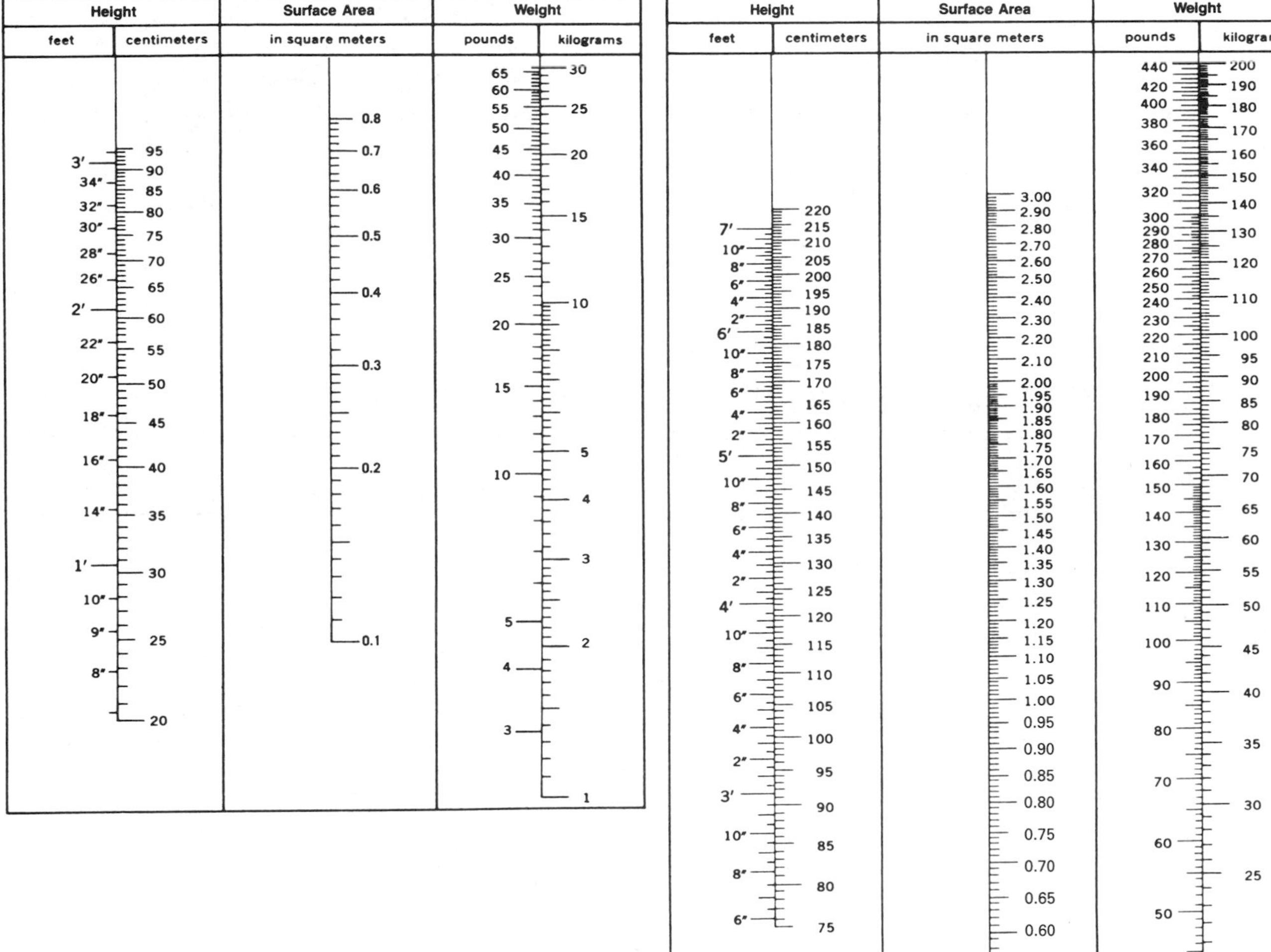

Figure 3-2. Body-surface nomograms. To determine the surface area of the client, draw a straight line between the point representing his height on the left vertical scale to the point representing his weight on the right vertical scale. The point at which this line intersects the middle vertical scale represents the client's surface area in square meters. (Courtesy of Abbott Laboratories)

orders. Guidelines to help increase safety and effectiveness while reducing adverse reactions include the following:

1. When the elderly client's condition is assessed, it is often difficult to separate the effects of aging from those of disease processes or drug therapy, especially long-term drug therapy. It is very possible that symptoms attributed to aging or disease are in fact caused by medications. To minimize assessment errors and improve care, a reasonable approach would be periodic reevaluation of the client's needs for particular drugs. Some physicians discontinue all drugs, evaluate the client's condition, then reorder necessary drugs while discontinuing those that are no longer needed.
2. The basic principle of giving the smallest effective number of drugs applies especially to the elderly client. A regimen consisting of several drugs increases the incidence of adverse reactions and potentially hazardous drug interactions, and some studies have demonstrated that three or four drugs are all that can be self-administered effectively. Beyond three or four drugs, many elderly persons are unable or unwilling to follow instructions regarding their drug therapy.
3. To increase compliance, the smallest number of effective doses should be prescribed.
4. When any drug is started, the dosage generally should be smaller than for younger adults. Then, dosage can be increased or decreased according to response. This conservative approach is indicated because decreased liver and kidney function may lead to slowed metabolism and excretion of drugs.

5. Nondrug measures should be used to decrease the need for drugs and to increase their effectiveness or decrease their adverse effects. For example, constipation is common in the elderly. When feasible, increasing dietary fiber, fluid intake, and activity is a healthier way of handling constipation than taking laxatives or enemas.
6. For people receiving long-term drug therapy at home, use measures to help them take drugs as prescribed.
   a. If necessary, label drug containers with large lettering for easier readability.
   b. Be sure the client can open drug containers.
   c. Write a schedule and devise reminders of which drug is to be taken and when. For example, doses can be marked on a calendar or chart when taken. This helps prevent omitting or repeating drug doses.
   d. Enlist family members or friends when necessary.

NURSING ACTIONS: MONITORING DRUG THERAPY

Nursing Actions	*Rationale/Explanation*
1. Prepare and administer drugs accurately (see Chap. 2)	
a. Practice the five rights of drug administration (right *drug,* right *client,* right *dose,* right *route,* and right *time*).	These rights are ensured if the techniques described in Chapter 2 are consistently followed. The time may vary by about 30 minutes. For example, a drug ordered for 9 AM can be given between 8:30 AM and 9:30 AM. No variation is allowed in the other "rights."
b. Use correct techniques for different routes of administration.	For example, sterile equipment and techniques are required for injection of any drug.
c. Follow label instructions regarding mixing or other aspects of giving specific drugs.	Some drugs require specific techniques of preparation and administration.
2. Observe for therapeutic effects	Generally, the nurse should know the expected effects and when they are likely to occur. Specific observations depend on the specific drug or drugs being given.
3. Observe for adverse effects	All drugs are potentially harmful, although the incidence and severity of adverse reactions vary among drugs and clients. People most likely to suffer adverse reactions are those with severe liver or kidney disease, those who are very young or very old, those receiving several drugs, and those receiving large doses of any drug. Specific adverse effects to be observed for depend on the drugs being given.
4. Observe for drug interactions	The nurse must be knowledgeable about common and potentially significant drug interactions. Also, since interactions may occur anytime the client is receiving two or more drugs concurrently, they should be considered as a possible cause of unexpected responses to drug therapy.
5. Teach clients about their drug therapy	
a. General instructions	
(1) Take medications as directed.	Therapeutic effect greatly depends on taking medications correctly. Altering the dose or time may cause underdosage or overdosage.
(2) Do not start or stop drugs without consulting the physician.	Drug therapy is often a state of delicate balance. Altering this balance greatly increases risks of drug interactions, adverse effects, and loss of therapeutic effectiveness.

Nursing Actions	***Rationale/Explanation***
(3) Do not keep drugs for long periods.	The chemical composition of drugs tends to become altered over a period of time. Manufacturers' drug labels often include a date after which the drug should be discarded. This information is not ordinarily included with prescription drugs dispensed to clients. Outdated drugs at best do no good and at worst may be harmful.
(4) Do not take medications prescribed for others even if problems seem similar.	The chance of having the right drug in the right dose is extremely remote and the risk of adverse reactions extremely high under such circumstances. So many factors influence a person's response to drugs that outcome is not predictable when do-it-yourself drug therapy is instituted.
(5) Develop a routine for taking medications. For example, take them at the same time and place each day.	Having a routine helps clients remember to take medications as directed.
(6) Do not keep medications in the bathroom medicine cabinet.	Medications may deteriorate more rapidly owing to warmth and moisture.
(7) Never put several medications, such as different tablets, in one container.	This is never a safe practice. The risk of taking the wrong medication or wrong dose is greatly increased if this is done. In addition, the drugs may interact chemically, altering drug composition.
(8) Take medication in a well-lighted area.	To allow reading the label to ensure that the drug taken is the one intended
(9) Keep all medications out of reach of children and never refer to medications as "candy."	To prevent accidental ingestion and poisoning
b. Instructions related to specific drugs	Many drugs are self-administered, and information is required to do this correctly, safely, and effectively.
(1) Name of the drug(s)	Knowledge of the drug name can be a safety measure, especially if the person has an allergic or other potentially serious adverse reaction or an overdose. It may also give the person a greater sense of control and responsibility regarding drug therapy.
(2) Purpose of the drug	People vary in the amount of drug information they want and need. For most, the purpose can be simply stated in terms of symptoms to be relieved or other expected benefits.
(3) Dosage schedule	This should be specific and as convenient as possible within the limitations imposed by the particular drugs. Working with the client to individualize drug therapy may help increase compliance with the prescribed regimen.
(4) Method of administration	Most people are accustomed to taking drugs orally, although they may need information about the amount or type of fluids to take with a particular drug or other instructions. For other routes of administration, instructions may need to be more specific and complete. Rectal suppositories and topical application of drugs to the eyes or skin are examples in which correct administration is essential to therapeutic effect.
(5) Adverse reactions or side-effects to be reported	The goal is to provide needed information without causing unnecessary anxiety. Most drugs produce undesirable effects; some of these are minor, and others are potentially serious. Many people stop taking a drug rather than report adverse reactions. If reactions are reported, it may be possible to allow continued drug therapy by reducing dosage or by implementing other measures. The occurrence of severe reactions indicates that the drug should be stopped. In such cases the prescribing physician should be notified.
(6) Miscellaneous instructions such as safety measures for taking certain drugs, storage, and others as indicated	

Selected References

Alford DM, Moll JA: Helping elderly patients in ambulatory settings cope with drug therapy. Nurs Clin North Am 17:275–282, June 1982

American Medical Association (AMA) Division of Drugs: AMA Drug Evaluations, 5th ed. New York, John Wiley & Sons, 1983

Bressler R: Geriatric prescribing: Adverse drug reactions in the elderly. Drug Ther 11:71–80, February 1981

Brill EL, Kilts DF: Foundations for Nursing. New York, Appleton-Century-Crofts, 1980

Butler RN, Bearn AG: The Aging Process: Therapeutic Implications. New York, Raven Press, 1985

Cefalo RC: Drugs in pregnancy—which to use and which to avoid. Drug Ther (Hosp. Ed.), 8:30–41, May 1983

Covington TR, Walker JI (eds): Current Geriatric Therapy. Philadelphia, W B Saunders, 1984

Ebert NJ: The nursing process applied to the aged person receiving medication. In Yurick AG, Spier BE, Robb SS, Ebert NJ: The Aged Person and the Nursing Process, 2d ed., pp 509–523. Norwalk, CT, Appleton-Century-Crofts, 1984

Fielo S, Rizzolo MA: The effects of age on pharmacokinetics. Geriatric Nurs 6:328–331, November–December 1985

Hansten PD: Drug Interactions: Clinical Significance of Drug–Drug Interactions, 5th ed. Philadelphia, Lea & Febiger, 1985

Hayes JE: Normal changes of aging and nursing implications of drug therapy. Nurs Clin North Am 17:253–262, June 1982

Hudson MF: Drugs and the older adult: Take special care. Nursing 14:46–51, August 1984

Jennings B, Tourville JF, Pepper GA: Pharmacotherapeutics through the life span. In Wiener MB, Pepper GA (eds): Clinical Pharmacology and Therapeutics in Nursing, 2d ed, pp 107–133. New York, McGraw–Hill, 1985

Kenny AD: Geriatric prescribing: How to avoid pitfalls with commonly used drugs. Drug Ther 10:96–107, September 1980

Lamy PP: Modifying drug dosage in elderly patients. In Covington TR, Walker JI (eds): Current Geriatric Therapy, pp 35–72. Philadelphia, W B Saunders, 1984

MacLeod SM, Radde IC (eds): Textbook of Pediatric Clinical Pharmacology. Littleton, MA, PSG Publishing, 1985

Malseed RT: Pharmacology: Drug Therapy and Nursing Considerations, 2d ed. Philadelphia, J B Lippincott, 1985

Pagliaro LA, Pagliaro AM (eds): Pharmacologic Aspects of Aging. St. Louis, C V Mosby, 1983

Poe WD, Holloway DA: Drugs and the Aged. New York, McGraw–Hill, 1980

Pulliam JP, Bennett WM: Using drugs safely in the patient with failing kidneys. Drug Ther 14:99–110, September 1984

Roberts RJ: Drug Therapy in Infants: Pharmacologic Principles and Experience. Philadelphia, W B Saunders, 1984

Rodman MJ, Karch AM, Boyd EH, Smith DW: Pharmacology and Drug Therapy in Nursing, 3rd ed. Philadelphia, J B Lippincott, 1985

Roe DA (ed): Drugs and Nutrition in the Geriatric Patient. New York, Churchill Livingstone, 1984

Sahu S: Drugs and the nursing mother. Am Fam Physician 24:137–138, December 1981

Shimp LA, Ascione FJ, Glazer HM, Atwood BF: Potential medication-related problems in noninstitutionalized elderly. Drug Intell Clin Pharmacol 19:766–772, October 1985

Silvester L, Fletcher J: Assisting the elderly with drug therapy in the home. Nurs Clin North Am 17:293–301, June 1982

Simonson W: Medications and the Elderly: A Guide for Promoting Proper Use. Rockville, MD: Aspen Systems Corp, 1984

Stewart CM, Stewart LB: Pediatric Medications: An Emergency and Critical Care Reference. Rockville, MD, Aspen Systems Corp, 1984

Szigeti E, Sagraves R: Women's health care. In Wiener MB, Pepper GA (eds.): Clinical Pharmacology and Therapeutics in Nursing, 2d ed., pp 891–933. New York, McGraw-Hill, 1985

II

DRUGS AFFECTING THE CENTRAL NERVOUS SYSTEM

4

PHYSIOLOGY OF THE CENTRAL NERVOUS SYSTEM

The central nervous system (CNS), composed of the brain and spinal cord, is mainly concerned with higher intellectual functions such as thought, learning, reasoning, and memory as well as with muscle function, both skeletal and smooth. It coordinates a person's reactions to a constantly changing internal and external environment. Information on blood levels of oxygen and carbon dioxide, body temperature, and sensory stimuli is constantly fed into the CNS. The CNS processes the information and sends messages to various parts of the body to adjust the environment toward homeostasis.

The basic functional unit of the CNS is the nerve cell or neuron. *Neurons* are specialized cells that exhibit excitability (the ability to be stimulated) and conductivity (the ability to convey electrical impulses). Neurons in a chain do not touch each other; they are separated by a microscopic gap called a *synapse.* The electrical impulse arriving at the end of the first neuron (presynaptic fiber) causes blisterlike granules (*synaptic vesicles*) to release a chemical substance called a *neurotransmitter.* Molecules of neurotransmitter apparently float across the synapse to receptors on the postsynaptic fiber and produce a new wave of electric current. Neurotransmitter substances include acetylcholine, catecholamines (dopamine, epinephrine, norepinephrine), histamine, serotonin, endorphins, and enkephalins.

Characteristics and functions of the central nervous system

The following paragraphs contain a brief review of some of the structures and functions of the CNS. This discussion is included to help orient the reader to the following chapters of this section, which cover drugs that act by altering the function of the nerve cells of the brain and spinal cord.

CEREBRAL CORTEX

The cerebral cortex is involved in all conscious processes, such as learning, memory, reasoning, verbalization, and voluntary body movements. Some parts of the cortex receive incoming nerve impulses and are called *sensory areas;* other parts send out impulses to peripheral structures and are called *motor areas.* Around the sensory and motor areas are the "association" areas, which occupy the greater portion of the cortex. These areas analyze the information received by the sensory areas and decide on the appropriate response. In some instances, the response may be to store the perception in memory; in others, it may involve stimulation of motor centers to produce movement or speech.

THALAMUS

The thalamus receives impulses carrying sensations such as heat, cold, pain, and muscle position sense. These sensations produce only a crude awareness at the thalamic level. They are relayed to the cerebral cortex, where they are interpreted regarding location, quality, intensity, and significance.

HYPOTHALAMUS

The hypothalamus has extensive neuronal connections with higher and lower levels of the CNS and the posterior pituitary gland and regulates activity of the anterior pituitary. It constantly collects information about the internal environment of the body and helps to maintain homeostasis by making continuous adjustments in water balance, body temperature, hormone levels, arterial blood pressure, heart rate, gastrointestinal motility, and other body functions. The hypothalamus is stimulated or inhibited by nerve impulses from different portions of the nervous system as well as by concentrations of nutrients, electrolytes, water, and hormones in the blood. Specific functions include the following:

1. Production of oxytocin and antidiuretic hormone (ADH), which are then stored in the posterior pituitary gland and released in response to nerve impulses from the hypothalamus. Oxytocin helps to deliver milk from the glands of the breast to the nipples during breast feeding and helps initiate uterine contractions to begin the process of labor and delivery at the end of gestation. ADH helps to maintain fluid balance by controlling water excretion. ADH secretion is controlled by the osmolarity of the extracellular fluid. When osmolarity is high, more ADH is secreted. This means that water is retained in the body to dilute the extracellular fluid and return it toward normal or homeostatic levels. When osmolarity is low, less ADH is secreted and more water is excreted in the urine.
2. Regulation of body temperature. When body temperature is elevated, sweating and dilation of blood vessels in the skin lower the temperature. When body temperature is low, sweating ceases and vasoconstriction occurs. When heat loss is decreased, the temperature is raised.
3. Assisting in regulation of arterial blood pressure by its effects on the vasomotor center. The vasomotor center in the medulla oblongata and pons maintains a state of partial contraction in blood vessels, a state called *vasomotor tone.* The hypothalamus can exert excitatory or inhibitory effects on the vasomotor center, depending on which portions of the hypothalamus are stimulated. When nerve impulses from the hypothalamus excite the vasomotor center, vasomotor tone or vasoconstriction is increased and blood pressure is raised. When the impulses from the hypothalamus inhibit the vasomotor center, vasomotor tone or vasoconstriction is decreased, with the overall effect of relative vasodilation and lowering of arterial blood pressure.
4. Regulation of anterior pituitary hormones. These hormones include thyroid-stimulating hormone (TSH), adrenocorticotropic hormone (ACTH or corticotropin), and growth hormone, among others. The hypothalamus secretes "releasing factors," which cause the anterior pituitary to secrete these hormones. There is a hypothalamic releasing factor for each hormone. The hypothalamic factor prolactin-inhibiting factor (PIF) inhibits secretion of prolactin, another anterior pituitary hormone.
5. Regulation of food and water intake by the hypothalamic thirst, appetite, hunger, and satiety centers.

MEDULLA OBLONGATA

The medulla oblongata contains groups of neurons that form the vital cardiac, respiratory, and vasomotor centers. For example, if the respiratory center is stimulated, respiratory rate and depth are increased. If the respiratory center is depressed, respiratory rate and depth are decreased. The medulla also contains reflex centers for coughing, vomiting, sneezing, swallowing, and salivating.

The medulla and pons varolii also contain groups of neurons from which originate cranial nerves 5 through 12. Together with the midbrain, these structures form the brain stem.

RETICULAR FORMATION

The reticular formation is a network of neurons that extends from the spinal cord through the medulla and pons to the thalamus and hypothalamus. It receives impulses from all parts of the body, evaluates the significance of the impulses, and decides which impulses to transmit to the cerebral cortex. It also excites or inhibits motor nerves that control both reflex and voluntary movement. Stimulation of the reticular formation produces wakefulness and mental alertness, while depression causes sedation and loss of consciousness.

LIMBIC SYSTEM

The limbic system is an area of the brain that involves several structures, including the thalamus, hypothalamus, basal ganglia, hippocampus, amygdala, and septum. The function of the limbic system is to regulate emotions (*e.g.*, pleasure, fear, anger, sadness) and behavior (*e.g.*, laughing, crying). Many nerve impulses from the limbic system are transmitted through the hypothalamus; thus, physiologic changes in blood pressure, heart rate, respiration, and hormone secretion occur in response to the emotions.

CEREBELLUM

The cerebellum is connected with motor centers in the cerebral cortex and basal ganglia. It coordinates muscular activity. When several skeletal muscles are involved, some are contracted and some are relaxed for smooth, purposeful movements. It also helps to maintain balance and posture by receiving nerve impulses from the inner ear that produce appropriate reflex responses.

BASAL GANGLIA

The basal ganglia are concerned with skeletal muscle tone and orderly activity. Normal function is influenced by dopamine, a neurotransmitter produced in the midbrain by a specific group of nerve cells called the *substantia nigra.* Degenerative changes in these cells cause dopamine to be released in decreased amounts. This process is a factor in the development of Parkinson's disease, which is characterized by rigidity and increased muscle tone.

PYRAMIDAL AND EXTRAPYRAMIDAL SYSTEMS

The pyramidal and extrapyramidal systems are tracts or pathways out of the cerebral cortex. In the pyramidal or corticospinal tract, nerve fibers originate in the cerebral cortex, go down the brain stem to the medulla, where the fibers cross, and continue down the spinal cord, where they end at various levels. Impulses are then carried from the spinal cord to skeletal muscle. Since the fibers cross in the medulla, impulses from the right side of the cerebral cortex control skeletal muscle movement of the left side of the body, and impulses from the left control muscle movements of the right side. In the extrapyramidal system, fibers originate mainly in the premotor area of the cerebral cortex and travel to the basal ganglia and brain stem. The fibers are called extrapyramidal because they do not enter the medullary pyramids and cross over. Pyramidal and extrapyramidal systems intermingle in the spinal cord; disease processes affecting higher levels of the CNS involve both tracts.

BRAIN METABOLISM

To function correctly, the brain must have an adequate and continuous supply of nutrients, especially oxygen, glucose, and thiamine. Oxygen is carried to the brain by the carotid and vertebral arteries. The brain requires more oxygen than any other organ of the body. Cerebral cortex cells are very sensitive to oxygen lack (hypoxia), and interruption of blood supply causes immediate loss of consciousness. Brain stem cells are less sensitive to hypoxia. People in whom hypoxia is relatively prolonged may survive, although they may have irreversible brain damage. Glucose is required as an energy source for brain cell metabolism. Hypoglycemia (low blood sugar) may cause mental confusion, dizziness, convulsions, loss of consciousness, and permanent damage to the cerebral cortex. Thiamine is required for production and utilization of glucose. Thiamine deficiency can reduce glucose utilization by about half and can cause degeneration of the myelin sheaths of nerve cells. Such degeneration in central neurons leads to a form of encephalopathy known as Wernicke–Korsakoff's syndrome. Degeneration in peripheral nerves leads to polyneuritis and muscle atrophy, weakness, and paralysis.

SPINAL CORD

The spinal cord is continuous with the medulla oblongata and extends downward through the vertebral column to the sacral area. The cord is made up of 31 segments, each of which is the point of origin for a pair of spinal nerves. The cord functions as a pathway for conduction of impulses to and from the brain and as a center for reflex actions. Reflexes are involuntary responses to certain nerve impulses received by the spinal cord. Examples are the knee-jerk and pupillary reflexes.

Classifications of central nervous system drugs

Drugs affecting the CNS, sometimes called centrally active drugs, are broadly classified as depressants or stimulants. Some drugs, such as general anesthetics and narcotic analgesics, produce a general depression of the CNS. Mild CNS depression is characterized by lack of interest in surroundings and inability to focus on a topic (short attention span). As depression progresses, there is drowsiness or sleep, decreased muscle tone, decreased ability to move, and decreased perception of sensations such as pain, heat, and cold. Severe CNS depression produces unconsciousness or coma, loss of reflexes, respiratory failure, and death.

Some of these drugs produce somewhat selective depression, at least in recommended doses. Anticonvulsants, for example, can reduce seizure activity without excessive interference with mental and physical functions. Similarly, analgesics such as morphine can reduce pain without producing unconsciousness, and antipsychotic drugs can calm an emotionally upset person without inducing sleep.

CNS stimulants produce a variety of effects. Mild stimulation is characterized by wakefulness, mental alertness, and decreased fatigue. Increasing stimulation produces hyperactivity, excessive talking, nervousness, and insomnia. Excessive stimulation can cause convulsive seizures, cardiac arrhythmias, and death. Excessive, harmful CNS stimulation by these drugs is difficult to avoid. Therefore, CNS stimulants are less useful for therapeutic purposes than are CNS depressants.

Selected References

Anderson PD: Basic Human Anatomy and Physiology: Clinical Implications for the Health Professions. Monterey, CA, Wadsworth, 1984

Bloom FE: Neurohumoral transmission and the central nervous system. In Gilman AG, Goodman LS, Rall TW, Murad F (eds): The Pharmacological Basis of Therapeutics, 7th ed. pp 236–260. New York, Macmillan, 1985

Guyton AC: Textbook of Medical Physiology, 7th ed. Philadelphia, W B Saunders, 1986

Hahn AB, Oestreich SJK, Barkin RB: Mosby's Pharmacology in Nursing, 16th ed. St Louis, C V Mosby, 1986

Rodman MJ, Karch AM, Boyd EH, Smith DW: Pharmacology and Drug Therapy in Nursing, 3rd ed. Philadelphia, J B Lippincott, 1985

Watson JE: Medical–Surgical Nursing and Related Physiology. Philadelphia, W B Saunders, 1979

5

NARCOTIC ANALGESICS AND NARCOTIC ANTAGONISTS

Description and uses

Narcotic analgesics are drugs that relieve moderate-to-severe pain by reducing perception of pain sensation, producing sedation, and decreasing the emotional upsets often associated with pain. Most of these analgesics are Schedule II drugs under federal narcotics laws and may lead to drug abuse and dependence. Morphine, obtained from the seeds of the opium poppy, is the prototype of these analgesics and the standard by which others are measured. These drugs are often called *opiates* or *opioids,* terms indicating drugs that act like morphine in the body. Opioids relieve pain by binding to opioid receptors located on the cell membranes of specific neurons in discrete regions of the brain. Opioid receptors also bind with endogenous (produced by the body) pain-relieving substances called *enkephalins* and *endorphins.* These substances act like opioid drugs in the body. The word "endorphin" was coined from "endogenous morphine."

Morphine and other opioids exert widespread pharmacologic effects, especially in the central nervous system (CNS) and in nerve fibers in the gastrointestinal system. These effects occur with usual doses and may be therapeutic or adverse, depending on the reason for use. CNS effects include analgesia, CNS depression varying from drowsiness to sleep, decreased mental and physical activity, respiratory depression, nausea and vomiting, and pupil constriction. Sedation and respiratory depression are major adverse effects and are potentially life threatening. Most newer narcotic analgesics have been developed in an effort to find drugs as effective as morphine in relieving pain while causing less sedation, less respiratory depression, and less dependence liability. This effort has not been successful because equianalgesic doses of these drugs produce sedative and respiratory depressant effects comparable to those of morphine.

In the gastrointestinal system, narcotic analgesics slow motility. They may also cause smooth muscle spasm in the bowel, biliary tract, and urinary tract.

The main clinical use of morphine and other opioids is to prevent or relieve acute pain of moderate-to-severe intensity. Pain is one of the most common symptoms prompting persons to seek health care. It is an unpleasant sensation that occurs following stimulation of nerve endings. The sensation is carried to the CNS by sensory nerve fibers. If possible, reflex action from the spinal cord causes rapid withdrawal from the painful stimulus; sometimes the impulse travels to the brain for analysis and determination of action needed.

Painful stimuli may be physical (such as heat or pressure) or chemical (such as pain related to products of inflammation, including histamine and bradykinin). Pain receptors or free nerve endings are widespread in the skin, joint surfaces, arterial walls, and periosteum. Most internal organs, such as the lung parenchyma and uterus, have few pain receptors.

The lowest intensity of a stimulus that will produce a sensation of pain is called the *pain threshold.* Differences in individual reactions to painful stimuli were formerly explained as differences in pain thresholds; that is, some people were thought to have high thresholds and less sensitivity to pain, while others had low thresholds and more sensitivity. However, recent studies have demonstrated no significant differences in pain thresholds among persons. Differences in pain perception may result from psychologic components, especially when fatigue, anxiety, and other stressors are present along with the pain.

Generally, pain is a protective mechanism because it indicates that tissue damage is occurring and impels the person to remove the painful stimulus. This relationship is not consistent, however, since extensive tissue damage may occur in malignant disease before pain develops. Also, pain does not indicate the extent of tissue damage, and it may be reported when there is no evident cause.

Pain is often described as acute or chronic, superficial or deep. Acute pain demands the attention of the person experiencing it and compels behavior to seek relief. It is often accompanied by objective signs of discomfort, such as sweating, facial grimacing, or assuming a position to protect the affected body part as well as by anxiety. Chronic pain less urgently demands attention, may not be characterized by visible signs, and is more likely to be accompanied by depression than by anxiety. Superficial pain originates in the skin or closely underlying structures and is readily localized by the person experiencing it. Deep pain originates in bones, abdominal viscera, or thoracic viscera and produces a dull, aching sensation that is difficult to localize.

Specific conditions in which opioid drugs are used for analgesic effects include acute myocardial infarction, biliary colic, renal colic, burns and other traumatic injuries, and postoperative states. These drugs are usually given for chronic pain only when other measures and milder drugs are ineffective, as in terminal malignancy. Other clinical uses include the following:

1. Before and during surgery to promote sedation, decrease anxiety, facilitate induction of anesthesia, and decrease the amount of anesthesia required.
2. Before and during invasive diagnostic procedures such as angiograms and endoscopic examinations.
3. During labor and delivery (obstetric analgesia).
4. Treating gastrointestinal disorders such as abdominal cramping and diarrhea.
5. Treating acute pulmonary edema. Morphine is used.
6. Treating severe, unproductive cough. Codeine is generally used.

These drugs are contraindicated or must be used very cautiously in people with respiratory depression, chronic lung disease, liver or kidney disease, prostatic hypertrophy, increased intracranial pressure, or hypersensitivity reactions to opiates and related drugs.

Narcotic antagonists are drugs that reverse the depressant effects of narcotics. They act by displacing narcotics from their cellular receptor sites. When an opiate is unable to bind to receptor sites, it is "neutralized" and unable to exert its depressant effects on body cells. Narcotic antagonists do not relieve depressant effects of other drugs, such as sedative–hypnotics, antianxiety agents, and antipsychotic agents. The chief clinical use of these drugs is to relieve the severe CNS and respiratory depression that occurs with narcotic overdose. They produce withdrawal symptoms when given to narcotic-dependent persons and are sometimes used to diagnose narcotic drug dependence.

Individual drugs

MORPHINE AND RELATED DRUGS

Morphine sulfate is a naturally occurring opium alkaloid. As the prototype of the strong analgesics, morphine has the characteristics and effects described earlier for the drug group. It is used mainly to relieve acute, severe pain. It is a Schedule II narcotic.

Morphine is usually given parenterally. Client response depends on both route and dosage. After intravenous injection, maximal analgesia and respiratory depression usually occur within 10 to 20 minutes. After intramuscular injection, these effects occur in about 30 minutes. With subcutaneous injection, effects may be delayed up to 60 to 90 minutes. Oral administration of morphine is increasing, usually for chronic pain associated with cancer. When it is given orally on a long-term basis, higher doses are required, because a portion of the oral drug dose is metabolized in the liver before it reaches the systemic circulation. Concentrated solutions (*e.g.,* Roxanol, which contains 20 mg morphine/ml) and controlled-release tablets (*e.g.,* MS Contin, which contains 30 mg/tablet) have been developed for oral administration of these high doses. In some instances of severe pain that cannot be controlled by other methods, morphine is administered as a continuous intravenous infusion.

Morphine is primarily metabolized in the liver and excreted by the kidneys. Consequently, impaired liver and kidney function may cause prolonged drug action and accumulation with subsequent increased incidence and severity of adverse effects.

Routes and dosage ranges

Adults: PO 10–20 mg q4h PRN
PO controlled-release tablets 30 mg q8–12h
IM, SC 5–15 mg q4h PRN
IV 2.5–10 mg, injected slowly PRN
Infants and children: IM, SC 0.1–0.2 mg/kg. Maximal dose, 15 mg

Camphorated opium tincture (Paregoric) contains opium and other substances. It is indicated only in diarrhea. Usual adult dose is equivalent to 2 to 4 mg of morphine. This drug is not likely to produce dependence unless used for chronic diarrhea. It has been used infrequently since diphenoxylate and loperamide became available.

Route and dosage range

Adults: PO 5–10 ml q4h PRN
Children: PO 0.25–0.5 ml/kg 1–4 times daily PRN

Hydromorphone hydrochloride (Dilaudid) is a semisynthetic derivative of morphine that has the same actions, uses, contraindications, and adverse effects as morphine. Hydromorphone is more potent on a milligram basis and is relatively more effective orally than morphine. Effects occur in 15 to 30 minutes, peak in 30 to 90 minutes, and last 4 to 5 hours.

Routes and dosage ranges

Adults: PO 2 mg q4h PRN
IM, SC, IV 1–1.5 mg q4–6h PRN, may be increased to 4 mg for severe pain
Rectal suppository 3 mg q6–8h

Levorphanol tartrate (Levo-Dromoran) is a synthetic drug that is chemically and pharmacologically related to morphine. It has the same uses and produces the same adverse effects, although some reports indicate a lower occurrence of nausea and vomiting. The average dose is probably equianalgesic with 10 mg of morphine. Maximal analgesia occurs 60 to 90 minutes after subcutaneous injection. Effects last 4 to 8 hours.

Routes and dosage range

Adults: PO, SC 2–3 mg q4–6h PRN

Methadone hydrochloride (Dolophine) is a synthetic drug that has essentially the same pharmacologic actions as morphine. Compared to morphine, methadone has a longer duration of action and is relatively more effective when given orally. Analgesia occurs within 10 to 20 minutes after injection and 30 to 60 minutes after oral administration. Methadone is used for severe pain and in the detoxification and maintenance treatment of opiate addicts.

Routes and dosage ranges

Adults: IM, SC 2.5–10 mg q3–4h PRN
PO 5–20 mg q6–8h PRN

Oxymorphone hydrochloride (Numorphan) is a semisynthetic derivative of morphine. Its actions, uses, and adverse effects are very similar to those of morphine, except that it has little antitussive effect.

Routes and dosage ranges

Adults: IM, SC 1–1.5 mg q4–6h PRN
IV 0.5 mg q4–6h PRN
Rectal suppository 5 mg q4–6h PRN
Obstetric analgesia, IM 0.5–1 mg

MEPERIDINE AND RELATED DRUGS

Meperidine hydrochloride (Demerol) is a synthetic drug that is very similar to morphine in pharmacologic actions. It is one of the most frequently prescribed narcotic analgesics. A parenteral dose of 80 to 100 mg is approximately equivalent to 10 mg of morphine. Oral meperidine is only half as effective as a parenteral dose because about half is metabolized in the liver and never reaches the systemic circulation. Meperidine produces sedation and respiratory depression comparable to that occurring with morphine. Meperidine differs from morphine as follows:

1. It has a shorter duration of action and requires more frequent administration. After parenteral administration, analgesia occurs in about 10 to 20 minutes, peaks in about 1 hour, and lasts about 2 to 4 hours.
2. It has little antitussive effect. However, excessive sedation with meperidine reduces ability to cough effectively.
3. It causes less respiratory depression in the newborn when used for obstetric analgesia.
4. It causes less smooth muscle spasm and is preferred in renal and biliary colic.
5. With chronic use or toxic doses, meperidine may cause CNS stimulation, characterized by tremors, hallucinations, and seizures. These effects are attributed to accumulation of a metabolite.

Routes and dosage ranges

Adults: IM, IV, SC, PO 50–100 mg q2–4h
Obstetric analgesia, IM, SC 50–100 mg q2–4h for three or four doses

Children: PO, SC, IM 1–1.5 mg/kg q3–4h PRN, maximal dose, 100 mg

Alphaprodine (Nisentil) is chemically and pharmacologically related to meperidine and produces similar adverse effects. It is more potent and has a more rapid onset and shorter duration of action than meperidine. When given intravenously, analgesic effects occur in 1 to 2 minutes and last 30 to 90 minutes; when given subcutaneously, effects occur within 10 minutes and last 1 to 2 hours. Intramuscular administration is not recommended because absorption is unpredictable. Alphaprodine may be used for preoperative analgesia and short procedures such as obstetrics and minor urologic, orthopedic, and ophthalmic procedures. In children, it is used only for dental procedures and given only by the submucosal route. Alphaprodine is a Schedule II drug under federal narcotic law.

Route and dosage ranges

Adults: IV 0.4–0.6 mg/kg, injected over 3–4 minutes. Maximal single dose, 30 mg; maximal daily (24 hours) dose, 240 mg
SC 0.4–1.2 mg/kg. Maximal single dose, 60 mg; maximal daily dose, 240 mg
Children: Submucosal route only, 0.3–0.6 mg/kg

Diphenoxylate hydrochloride is a meperidine derivative indicated only for treating diarrhea. It is usually combined with atropine sulfate. It is a Schedule V drug under federal narcotic law. The combination drug (Lomotil, others) contains 2.5 mg of diphenoxylate and 25 μg of atropine per tablet or 5 ml of oral liquid preparation.

Route and dosage range

Adults: PO 1–2 tablets or 5–10 ml 4 times daily
Children: PO age 2–12 years, 0.3–0.4 mg/kg, given in divided doses (2 mg or 4 ml 3–5 times daily). Do not give to children under 2 years

Loperamide (Imodium) is a meperidine derivative indicated only for treatment of diarrhea. It is available in tablet and liquid form.

Route and dosage ranges

Adults: PO 4–8 mg daily, maximal daily dose, 16 mg
Children: 8–12 years (weighing more than 30 kg), PO 2 mg 3 times daily; 5–8 years (20–30 kg), 2 mg twice daily; 2–5 years (13–20 kg), 1 mg 3 times daily. Not recommended for children under 2 years

OTHER STRONG ANALGESICS

Butorphanol tartrate (Stadol) is a potent analgesic that is not classified as a narcotic drug. It is reportedly less potent than morphine and meperidine. It is used in moderate-to-severe pain and is given only parenterally. After intramuscular administration, analgesia occurs within 30 minutes and peaks in about 60 minutes. After intravenous use, analgesia occurs rapidly and peaks within 30 minutes. It also has narcotic antagonist activity and therefore should not be given to people who have been receiving narcotic analgesics or who have narcotic dependence. Other adverse reactions are drowsiness, weakness, and sweating. Butorphanol has not been established as a safe and effective drug for use in pregnancy, labor, delivery, or lactation or in children under 18 years of age.

Routes and dosage range

Adults: IM, IV, SC 1–4 mg q3–4h
Children: not recommended

Nalbuphine hydrochloride (Nubain) is similar to butorphanol in being a potent analgesic, currently classified as a nonnarcotic, used for moderate-to-severe pain, and given parenterally. Onset, duration, and extent of analgesia and respiratory depression are comparable to those produced by morphine. Other adverse effects include sedation, sweating, headache, and psychotic symptoms, but these are reportedly minimal at doses of 10 mg or less. Nalbuphine also has narcotic antagonist activity and may precipitate withdrawal symptoms in people who have been taking narcotic analgesics.

Routes and dosage range

Adults: IM, IV, SC 10 mg/70 kg of body weight q3–h

Pentazocine lactate or hydrochloride (Talwin) is a synthetic potent analgesic initially thought to be nonaddicting. However, it has been determined that pentazocine is a drug of abuse and may produce physical and psychic drug dependence. It is a Schedule IV drug under federal narcotic law. It has narcotic antagonist activity and may produce withdrawal symptoms in people taking narcotics. Generally, pentazocine is used for the same clinical indications as other strong analgesics and causes similar adverse effects. Recommended doses for analgesia are less effective than usual doses of morphine or meperidine. Some people may tolerate pentazocine better than morphine or meperidine, however. Parenteral pentazocine usually produces analgesia within 10 to 30 minutes and lasts 2 to 3 hours. Relatively unique characteristics of pentazocine include production of psychologic effects that may include hallucinations, bizarre dreams or nightmares, depression, nervousness, feelings of depersonalization, extreme euphoria, tissue damage with ulceration and necrosis or fibrosis at injection sites with long-term use, and respiratory depression, which can be reversed by naloxone (Narcan) but not by other antagonists.

One method of abuse involved dissolving oral tablets of pentazocine and tripelennamine, an antihistamine, and injecting the resultant mixture, called "Ts and Blues," intravenously. Potentially lethal adverse effects include pulmonary emboli and stroke (from obstruction of blood vessels by talc and other insoluble ingredients in the tablets). As a result, the manufacturer added 0.5 mg of naloxone to the 50-mg pentazocine tablet. This product is called Talwin NX. Naloxone, a narcotic antagonist, prevents the effects of pentazocine if the oral tablet is injected. It has no pharmacologic action if taken orally.

Routes and dosage ranges

Adults: PO 50–100 mg q3–4h (do not exceed 600 mg daily)
IM, SC, IV 30–60 mg q3–4h (do not exceed 360 mg daily)
Children: Not recommended for children under 12 years

CODEINE AND RELATED DRUGS

Codeine sulfate or phosphate is a naturally occurring opium alkaloid used for analgesic and antitussive effects. Codeine is similar to morphine but generally produces weaker analgesic and antitussive effects and milder adverse effects. Compared with other narcotic analgesics, codeine is more effective when given orally and is less likely to lead to abuse and dependence. Parenteral administration is more effective in relieving pain than oral administration, but onset (15 to 30 minutes) and duration of action (4 to 6 hours) are about the same. Larger doses are required for analgesic than for antitussive effects. Codeine is frequently given with aspirin or acetaminophen (Tylenol) for additive analgesic effects.

Routes and dosage ranges

Adults: PO, SC, IM 15–60 mg 4–6 times daily PRN
Cough, PO 10–20 mg q4h
Children: PO, SC, IM 0.5 mg/kg 4–6 times daily PRN
Cough, 1–1.5 mg/kg/day in 6 doses

Hydrocodone bitartrate (Codone) is very similar to codeine. It is combined with other ingredients in several antitussive and analgesic–antipyretic mixtures.

Route and dosage ranges

Adults: PO 5–10 mg 3–4 times daily
Children: PO 0.6 mg/kg/day in 3–4 divided doses

Oxycodone hydrochloride is a semisynthetic derivative of codeine used to relieve moderate pain. It is reportedly less potent and less likely to produce dependence than morphine but more potent and more likely to produce dependence than codeine. It is a drug of abuse. Pharmacologic actions are similar to those of other narcotic analgesics. Oxycodone is available only in combination with other drugs. Percodan contains oxycodone and aspirin. Percocet-5 and Tylox contain oxycodone and acetaminophen.

Route and dosage range

Adults: PO 5 mg (1 tablet) q6h PRN
Children: Not recommended for children under 12 years

Propoxyphene (Darvon) is a synthetic drug chemically related to methadone. It is used for mild-to-moderate pain but is considered less effective than codeine and no more effective than 650 mg of aspirin or acetaminophen. It is usually administered with aspirin or acetaminophen. Propoxyphene is apparently widely abused (alone and with alcohol or other CNS-depressant drugs) and is responsible for a large number of deaths from drug overdose. An overdose causes respiratory depression, excessive sedation, and circulatory failure. Propoxyphene is a Schedule IV drug, and physicians are requested to omit or limit prescription refills if they must prescribe the drug at all.

Routes and dosage ranges

Propoxyphene hydrochloride

Adults: PO 65 mg q4h PRN; maximal daily dose, 390 mg
Children: Not recommended

Propoxyphene napsylate

Adults: PO 100 mg q4h PRN; maximal daily dose, 600 mg
Children: Not recommended

NARCOTIC ANTAGONISTS

Naloxone hydrochloride (Narcan) injection is the drug of choice in respiratory depression known or thought to be caused by a narcotic. Therapeutic effects occur within minutes after parenteral injection and last 1 to 2 hours. Naloxone has a shorter duration of action than narcotics, and repeated injections are usually needed. For a long-acting drug such as methadone, injections may be needed for 2 to 3 days. Naloxone produces few adverse effects, and repeated injections can be given safely.

Naloxone is newer than the other narcotic antagonists, levallorphan (Lorfan) and nalorphine (Nalline). Naloxone is preferred because it is a pure narcotic antagonist, whereas the others have both agonist and antagonist effects. That is, in the absence of narcotics, levallorphan and nalorphine exert agonist activity and may cause or deepen respiratory depression and other adverse effects, while naloxone does not exert any pharmacologic action of its own.

Routes and dosage ranges

Adults: IV, IM, SC 0.1–0.4 mg, repeated intravenously q2–3 minutes as necessary

Children: IV, IM, SC 0.01 mg/kg of body weight initially, repeated intravenously q2–3 minutes as necessary

Naltrexone (Trexan) is a newer narcotic antagonist that is structurally and pharmacologically similar to naloxone. It competes with narcotics for opioid receptor sites in the brain to prevent narcotic binding with receptors or displaces narcotics already occupying receptor sites. This action blocks euphoria, analgesia, and other physiologic effects of narcotics. Naltrexone is used in the maintenance of opiate-free states in opiate addicts. It is apparently effective in highly motivated, detoxified persons. If given before the client is detoxified, acute withdrawal symptoms occur. Clients receiving naltrexone will not respond to analgesics if pain control is needed. The drug is recommended for use in conjunction with psychologic and social counseling.

Route and dosage range

Adults: PO 50 mg daily

Principles of therapy: narcotic analgesics

ASSESSMENT GUIDELINES

Assess the client's condition in relation to pain, initially to determine appropriate action and later to determine response to drug administration. Specific assessment data usually include the following:

1. *Location.* Determining location may assist in relieving pain and in determining its underlying cause. Ask the person to show you "where it hurts," if possible, and whether the pain stays in one place or radiates to other parts of the body. The term *referred pain* is used when pain arising from tissue damage in one area of the body is felt in another area. Patterns of referred pain may be helpful in diagnosis. For example, pain of cardiac origin may radiate to the neck, shoulders, chest muscles, and down the arms, more often on the left side. This form of pain usually results from myocardial ischemia due to atherosclerosis of coronary arteries. Stomach pain is usually referred to the epigastrium and may indicate gastritis or peptic ulcer. Gallbladder and bile duct pain is usually localized in the midepigastrium or right upper quadrant of the abdomen. Uterine pain is usually felt as abdominal cramping or low back pain.
2. *Intensity or severity.* Since pain is a subjective experience, assessment of severity is based on the client's description and the nurse's observations. It may be helpful to ask the client to rank the pain as mild, moderate, or severe or on a number scale such as 0 to 10.

   Signs and symptoms of pain vary greatly, depending on characteristics of the pain and the client, but they often include facial expressions of distress; moaning or crying; positioning to protect the affected part; tenderness, edema, skin color, or temperature changes in the affected part; and either restlessness and excessive movement or limited movement if movement increases pain. Superficial pain or pain of low-to-moderate intensity usually stimulates the sympathetic nervous system and produces increased blood pressure, pulse, and respiration, dilated pupils, and increased skeletal muscle tension such as rigid posture or clenched fists. Deep pain or severe pain stimulates the parasympathetic nervous system and produces decreased blood pressure and pulse, nausea and vomiting, weakness, syncope, and possibly loss of consciousness.
3. *Relationship to time, activities, and other signs and symptoms.* Specific questions include the following:
   When did the pain start?
   What activities were going on when the pain started?
   Does the pain occur with exercise or when at rest?
   Do other signs and symptoms occur before, during, or after the pain?
   Is this the first episode of this particular type of pain or a repeated occurrence?
   How long does the pain last?
   What, if anything, decreases or relieves the pain?
   What, if anything, aggravates the pain?
4. *Other data* as indicated by the client's condition and treatment regimen. For example, do not assume that postoperative pain is incisional and requires narcotic analgesics for relief. A person who has had abdominal surgery may have headache, muscle discomfort, or "gas pains." Also, restlessness may be caused by hypoxia rather than pain.

NURSING INTERVENTIONS

Use measures to prevent, relieve, or decrease pain when possible. General measures include those that promote optimal body functioning and those that prevent trauma, inflammation, infection, and other sources of painful stimuli. Specific measures include the following:

1. Encourage pulmonary hygiene techniques such as coughing, deep breathing, and activity to promote respiration and prevent pulmonary complications such as pneumonia and atelectasis
2. Use sterile technique when caring for wounds, urinary catheters, or intravenous lines
3. Use exercises, ambulation, and position changes to promote circulation
4. Handle any injured tissue very gently to avoid further trauma
5. Prevent bowel or bladder distention
6. Apply heat or cold
7. Use relaxation or distraction techniques

DRUG SELECTION

1. When more than one analgesic drug is ordered, use the least potent drug that is effective in relieving pain. For example, use nonnarcotic analgesics such as aspirin or acetaminophen (Tylenol) rather than a narcotic analgesic, when feasible.
2. Nonnarcotic analgesics may be alternated with the narcotic analgesics, especially in chronic pain. This increases client comfort, reduces the likelihood of drug abuse and dependence, and decreases tolerance to pain-relieving effects of the narcotic analgesics.

DOSAGE AND SCHEDULING

Dosage of narcotic analgesics must be individualized because people vary in their responses to drugs. Guidelines to assist in individualizing dosage include the following:

1. Small to moderate doses relieve constant, dull pain; moderate to large doses relieve intermittent, sharp pain caused by trauma or conditions affecting the viscera.
2. When a narcotic analgesic is ordered in variable amounts, such as 8 to 10 mg of morphine, give the smaller amount as long as it is effective in relieving pain.
3. Dosages of narcotic analgesics should be reduced for people who are also receiving other CNS depressants, such as antipsychotic or antianxiety agents, barbiturates, or other sedative–hypnotic drugs.

Narcotic analgesics are usually ordered as needed or PRN within prescribed dosage and time limitations. Some guidelines for giving PRN drugs include the following:

1. Have a clear-cut system by which the client reports pain or requests medication. The client should know that analgesic drugs have been ordered and will be given promptly when needed. If a drug cannot be given or if administration must be delayed, explain this to the client.
2. Offer or administer the drug when indicated by the client's condition rather than waiting for the client to request medication.

Additional guidelines include the following:

1. In acute pain, narcotic analgesics are most effective when given parenterally and at the onset of pain. In chronic, severe pain, narcotic analgesics are most effective when given on a regular schedule.
2. When needed, analgesics should be administered before coughing and deep breathing exercises, dressing changes, and other therapeutic and diagnostic procedures.
3. Evaluate increased need for analgesics to determine if it is caused by increased severity of pain resulting from progression of pathologic processes or by development of drug tolerance.
4. Narcotics should not be used for longer than 24 to 48 hours at a time except for advanced malignant disease. Hospitals usually have an "automatic stop order" for narcotics after 48 to 72 hours. This means that the drug is either reordered by the physician or discontinued when the time limit expires.

USE IN SPECIFIC SITUATIONS

Malignant disease

When narcotic analgesics are required in the chronic pain associated with malignancy, the main consideration is client comfort, not preventing drug addiction. Antianxiety or antidepressant drugs may increase comfort and allow reduced dosage of analgesics.

Biliary, renal, or ureteral colic

When narcotic analgesics are used to relieve the acute, severe pain associated with various types of colic, an antispasmodic drug such as atropine may be needed as well. Narcotic analgesics may increase smooth muscle tone and cause spasm. Atropine does not have strong antispasmodic properties of its own in usual doses, but it apparently reduces the spasm-producing effects of narcotic analgesics.

Postoperative use

When analgesics are used postoperatively, the goal is to relieve pain without excessive sedation so that clients can do deep breathing exercises, cough, ambulate, and implement other measures to promote recovery.

Burns

In severely burned persons, use narcotic analgesics very cautiously. A common cause of respiratory arrest in burned clients is excessive administration of analgesic drugs. Generally, agitation in a burned person should be interpreted as hypoxia or hypovolemia, rather than pain, until proved otherwise. When narcotic analgesics are necessary, they are usually given intravenously in small doses. Drugs administered by other routes are absorbed erratically in the presence of shock and hypovolemia.

Obstetrics

When narcotic analgesics are given to women in labor, two special factors must be considered. One factor involves the effects of drugs on the labor process. Because these analgesics depress the CNS, large doses or frequent administration may decrease uterine contractility and slow or stop progress toward delivery. A second factor involves the effects of drugs on the fetus. These analgesics cross the placenta and may cause respiratory depression in the newborn. Meperidine reportedly causes less respiratory depression than morphine and is usually preferred for obstetric analgesia. Also, respiratory depression in the neonate can be avoided or minimized by giving these analgesics intramuscularly rather than intravenously and by giving them 2 to 3 hours before delivery. Respiratory depression may be treated by administration of naloxone (Narcan), a narcotic antagonist.

MANAGEMENT OF TOXICITY OR OVERDOSE

Acute toxicity or narcotic overdose can occur from therapeutic use or from abuse by drug-dependent persons (see Chap. 15). The main goal of treatment is to restore and maintain adequate respiratory function. This can be accomplished by inserting an artificial airway such as an endotracheal tube and starting mechanical ventilation or by administering a narcotic antagonist.

GERIATRIC CONSIDERATIONS

For elderly clients, use narcotic analgesics very cautiously, if at all. As a general rule, these drugs should be used only for acute, severe pain or for terminal cancer pain. When they are prescribed, smaller doses are given than those for other adults. Elderly people are especially sensitive to respiratory depression and other adverse effects.

NURSING ACTIONS: NARCOTIC ANALGESICS

Nursing Actions	*Rationale/Explanation*
1. Administer accurately	
a. Check the rate, depth, and rhythm of respirations before each dose. If the rate is below 12 per minute, delay or omit the dose and report to the physician.	Respiratory depression is a major adverse reaction to strong analgesics. Assessing respirations before each dose can help prevent or minimize potentially life-threatening respiratory depression.
b. Have the client lie down to receive injections of narcotic analgesics and for at least a few minutes afterward.	To prevent or minimize hypotension, nausea, and vomiting. These side-effects are more likely to occur in the ambulatory client. Also, the client may be sedated enough to make ambulation hazardous without help.
c. When injecting narcotic analgesics intravenously, give small doses; inject slowly, over several minutes; and have narcotic antagonist drugs, artificial airways, and equipment for artificial ventilation readily available.	Large doses or rapid intravenous injection may cause severe respiratory depression and hypotension.
d. Give meperidine and pentazocine intramuscularly rather than subcutaneously.	Subcutaneous injections of these drugs may cause pain, tissue irritation, and possible abscess. This reaction is more likely with long-term use.

Nursing Actions	***Rationale/Explanation***
e. Put siderails up; instruct the client not to smoke or try to ambulate without help. Keep the call light within reach.	These are safety measures to prevent falls or other injuries.
2. Observe for therapeutic effects	Therapeutic effects depend on the reason for use, usually for analgesic effects, sometimes for antitussive or antidiarrheal effects.
a. A verbal statement of pain relief	
b. Decreased behavioral manifestations of pain or discomfort	
c. Sleeping	
d. Increased participation in usual activities of daily living, including social interactions with other people in the environment	
e. Fewer and shorter episodes of nonproductive coughing when used for antitussive effects	Narcotic analgesics relieve cough by depressing the cough center in the medulla oblongata.
f. Lowered blood pressure, decreased pulse rate, slower and deeper respirations, and less dyspnea when morphine is given for pulmonary edema	Morphine may relieve pulmonary edema by causing vasodilation, which in turn decreases venous return to the heart and decreases cardiac work.
g. Decreased diarrhea when given for constipating effects	These drugs slow secretions and motility of the gastrointestinal tract. Constipation is usually an adverse effect. However, in severe diarrhea or with ileostomy, the drugs decrease the number of bowel movements and make the consistency more pastelike than liquid.
3. Observe for adverse effects	
a. Respiratory depression—hypoxemia, restlessness, dyspnea, slow, shallow breathing, changes in blood pressure and pulse, decreased ability to cough	Respiratory depression is a major adverse effect of narcotic analgesics and results from depression of the respiratory center in the medulla oblongata. Respiratory depression occurs with usual therapeutic doses and increases in incidence and severity with large doses or frequent administration.
b. Hypotension	Hypotension stems from drug effects on the vasomotor center in the medulla oblongata that cause peripheral vasodilation and lowering of blood pressure. This is a therapeutic effect with pulmonary edema.
c. Excessive sedation—drowsiness, slurred speech, impaired mobility and coordination, stupor, coma	This is caused by depression of the CNS and is potentially life threatening.
d. Nausea and vomiting	Narcotic analgesics stimulate the chemoreceptor trigger zone in the brain. Consequently, nausea and vomiting may occur with oral or parenteral routes of administration. They are more likely to occur with ambulation than with recumbency.
e. Constipation	This is caused by the drug's slowing effects on the gastrointestinal tract. Constipation may be alleviated by activity, adequate food and fluid intake, and regular administration of mild laxatives.
4. Observe for drug interactions	
a. Drugs that *increase* effects of narcotic analgesics	
(1) CNS depressants—alcohol, general anesthetics, antianxiety agents, tricyclic antidepressants,	All these drugs alone, as well as the narcotic analgesics, produce CNS depression. When combined, additive CNS de-

Nursing Actions	Rationale/Explanation
antihistamines, antipsychotic agents, barbiturates, and other sedative–hypnotic drugs	pression results. If dosage of one or more interacting drugs is high, severe respiratory depression, coma, and death may ensue.
(2) Diuretics	Orthostatic hypotension, an adverse effect of both strong analgesics and diuretics, may be increased if the two drug groups are given concurrently.
(3) Monoamine oxidase (MAO) inhibitors	These drugs interfere with detoxification of some narcotic analgesics, especially meperidine. They may cause additive CNS depression with hypotension and respiratory depression or CNS stimulation with hyperexcitability and convulsions. If an MAO inhibitor is necessary, dosage should be reduced because the combination is potentially life threatening.
(4) *Rauwolfia* alkaloids	Additive CNS depression occurs
b. Drugs that *decrease* effects of narcotic analgesics	
(1) Narcotic antagonists	These drugs reverse respiratory depression produced by narcotic analgesics. This is their only clinical use, and they should not be given unless severe respiratory depression is present. They do not reverse respiratory depression caused by other CNS depressants.
(2) Butorphanol, nalbuphine, and pentazocine	These analgesics are weak antagonists of narcotic analgesics, and they may cause withdrawal symptoms in people who have been receiving opiates or who are physically dependent on narcotic analgesics.
5. Teach clients	
a. Take only as prescribed. If desired effects are not achieved, report to the physician. Do not increase the dose and do not take medication more often than prescribed.	Although these principles apply to all medications, they are especially important with analgesics because of potentially serious adverse reactions, including drug dependence, and because analgesics may mask or enable the client to tolerate pain for which medical attention is needed.
b. Do not drink alcohol or take other drugs without the physician's knowledge.	Both alcohol and pain-relieving narcotics depress the nervous system; combining them can cause serious, even life-threatening, problems. Numerous other drugs have depressant effects as well, and additive effects leading to excessive adverse reactions can result. For example, tranquilizers, sleeping pills, antihistamines, and cold remedies can all increase the risks of drug-induced problems that could be worse than the initial problem.
c. Do not drive a car or operate machinery when drowsy or dizzy or when vision is blurred from medication.	Automobiles and machinery should be operated only by fully alert persons with good vision.
d. Do not smoke when drowsy from medication.	Smoking when less than alert is clearly unsafe.
e. Stay in bed at least 30 to 60 minutes after receiving injection of an analgesic.	To prevent or minimize hypotension, nausea, and vomiting, which often occur with ambulation. Also, a sedated person is risking falls and traumatic injuries. An exception may be the person who has been receiving the drug for some time and who has developed tolerance to its sedative effects.
f. Do not object to having side rails up on the bed after an injection of analgesic.	Side rails promote safety by serving as a reminder to stay in bed or to call for assistance.
g. If not contraindicated, eat high fiber foods such as whole-grain cereals, fruits, and vegetables, drink 2 to 3 quarts of fluid daily, and be as active as tolerated.	To prevent or minimize constipation

Selected References

Atkinson JH: Current perspectives in the management of chronic pain. Drug Ther 13:72–88, June 1983

American Medical Association (AMA) Division of Drugs: AMA Drug Evaluations, 5th ed. New York, John Wiley & Sons, 1983

Burgess KE: Cerebral depressants: Their effects and safe administration. Nursing 15:46–53, August 1985

Citron ML et al: Safety and efficacy of continuous intravenous morphine for severe cancer pain. Am J Med 77:199–204, August 1984

Cummings D: Stopping chronic pain before it starts. Nursing 11:60–62, January 1981

Facts and Comparisons. St. Louis, J B Lippincott (Updated monthly)

Foley KM: The practical use of narcotic analgesics. Med Clin North Am 66:1091–1104, September 1982

Fraulini KE, Gorski DW: Don't let perioperative medications put you in a spin. Nursing 13:26–30, December 1983

Friedman FB (ed.): PRN analgesics: Controlling the pain or controlling the patient? RN 46:67–78, March 1983

Groer MW, Shekleton ME: Basic Pathophysiology: A Conceptual Approach, 2d ed. St. Louis, C V Mosby, 1983

Guyton AC: Textbook of Medical Physiology, 7th ed. Philadelphia, W B Saunders, 1986

Hansten PD: Drug Interactions: Clinical Significance of Drug–Drug Interactions, 5th ed. Philadelphia, Lea & Febiger, 1985

Heidrich G, Perry S: Helping the patient in pain. Am J Nurs 82:1828–1833, December 1982

Hershey LA: Meperidine and central neurotoxicity. Ann Intern Med 98:548–549, April 1983

Hollister LE: Neurologic disorders. In Melmon KL, Morelli HF (eds): Clinical Pharmacology: Basic Principles in Therapeutics, 2d ed, pp 874–912. New York, Macmillan, 1978

Inturrisi CE: Narcotic drugs. Med Clin North Am 66:1061–1071, September 1982

Jaffe JH, Martin WR: Opioid analgesics and antagonists. In Gilman AG, Goodman LS, Rall TW, Murad F (eds): The Pharmacological Basis of Therapeutics, 7th ed, pp 491–531. New York, Macmillan, 1985

Kaiks RF et al: Narcotics in the elderly. Med Clin North Am 66:1079–1089, September 1982

Kenney AD: Geriatric prescribing: How to avoid pitfalls with commonly used drugs. Drug Ther 10:96–107, September 1980

Korberly BH: Pharmacologic treatment of children's pain. Pediatr Nurs 11:292–294, July–August 1985

Lipman AG, Mooney K: Pain. In Wiener MB, Pepper GA (eds): Clinical Pharmacology and Therapeutics in Nursing, 2d ed., pp 219–244. New York, McGraw-Hill, 1985

Malseed RT: Pharmacology: Drug Therapy and Nursing Considerations, 2d ed. Philadelphia, J B Lippincott, 1985

McGuire L: 7 myths about pain relief. RN 46:30–31, December 1983

McGuire L, Dizard S, Panayotoff K: Managing pain . . . in the young patient . . . in the elderly patient. Nursing 12:52–57, August 1982

McGuire L, Wright A: Continuous narcotic infusion: It's not just for cancer patients. Nursing 14:50–55, December 1984

Rodman MJ, Karch AM, Boyd EH, Smith DW: Pharmacology and Drug Therapy in Nursing, 3rd ed. Philadelphia, J B Lippincott, 1985

Taddeini L, Rotschafer JC: Pain syndromes associated with cancer: Achieving effective relief. Postgrad Med 75:101–108, January 1984

West BA: Understanding endorphins: Our natural pain relief system. Nursing 11:50–53, February 1981

6

ANALGESIC–ANTIPYRETIC–ANTI-INFLAMMATORY AND RELATED DRUGS

Description and uses

The analgesic–antipyretic–anti-inflammatory drugs relieve pain, fever, and inflammation. Acetylsalicylic acid (ASA, aspirin) is the prototype of the group. The other drugs in this group are often called aspirinlike or nonsteroidal anti-inflammatory drugs (NSAIDs). Several of these are used primarily for their anti-inflammatory effects in rheumatic diseases such as rheumatoid arthritis and gout. The other drugs included in this chapter are those used in the prevention and treatment of gout attacks and those used in the treatment of migraine. The adrenocorticosteroids, which are the most potent anti-inflammatory drugs, are discussed in Chapter 24. Most of these drugs inhibit the synthesis of prostaglandins, and both therapeutic and adverse effects are attributed primarily to this action. To understand the effects of these drugs, therefore, an understanding of prostaglandins, as well as of pain, fever, and inflammation, is needed.

Prostaglandins are substances synthesized in the body from arachidonic acid, a free fatty acid released from the phospholipids in cell membranes in response to various physical, chemical, hormonal, bacterial, and other stimuli. Nine groups of prostaglandins have been identified and are arbitrarily labeled by letters A through I (*e.g.*, PGA, PGB). They are further identified by subscripts that describe the chemical structure (*e.g.*, PGE_2). Prostaglandins regulate many cell functions, including the following:

1. In the inflammatory process, prostaglandins potentiate the pain and edema caused by bradykinin, histamine, and other substances released in areas of tissue damage.
2. They regulate smooth muscle in blood vessels, the gastrointestinal tract, respiratory system, and reproductive system.
3. They protect gastrointestinal mucosa from the erosive effects of gastric acid.
4. They regulate renal blood flow and distribution.
5. They control platelet function.
6. They maintain a patent ductus arteriosus in the fetus.

Prostaglandins are produced in specific body tissues, where they exert their effects and are then rapidly inactivated. The specific type of prostaglandin produced depends on the tissue involved, the stimulus, the hormonal environment, and other factors. Once a prostaglandin is produced, its actions are cell specific and may be different or even opposing in various cells. For example, PGE_2 relaxes arterial and bronchial smooth muscle, contracts longitudinal but relaxes circular smooth muscle in the gastrointestinal tract, contracts or relaxes uterine smooth muscle depending on concentration, stimulates renin release in the kidneys, and activates the hypothalamic thermoregulatory center to cause fever.

Pain is the sensation of discomfort, hurt, or distress. It may be mild or severe, acute or chronic (see Chap. 5).

Fever is an elevation of body temperature above the normal range. Body temperature is controlled by a regulating center in the hypothalamus. Normally, there is a balance between heat production and heat loss so that a constant body temperature is maintained. When there is excessive heat production, mechanisms to increase heat loss are activated. As a result, blood vessels dilate, more blood flows through the skin, sweating occurs, and body temperature usually stays within normal range. When fever occurs, the heat-regulating center in the hypothalamus is reset so that it tolerates a higher body temperature. Fever may be produced by dehydration, inflammatory and infectious processes, some drugs, brain injury, or disease involving the hypothalamus. Prostaglandin formation is stimulated by such circumstances, and, along with bacterial toxins and other substances, prostaglandins act as pyrogens (fever-producing agents).

Inflammation is the normal body response to tissue damage or injury from chemicals, microorganisms, trauma, foreign bodies, surgery, and ionizing radiation. It may occur in any tissue or organ. It is an attempt by the body to remove the damaging agent and repair the damaged tissue. The local manifestations of inflammation are redness, heat, edema, and pain. Redness and heat result from vasodilation and increased blood supply; edema results from leakage of blood plasma into the area; and pain is produced by pressure of edema and secretions on nerve endings and by chemical irritation of bradykinin, histamine, and other substances released by the damaged cells. Prostaglandins are also released and increase the pain and edema caused by other substances. Systemic manifestations of inflammation include leukocytosis, increased erythrocyte sedimentation rate (ESR), fever, headache, loss of appetite, lethargy or malaise, and weakness. Both local and systemic manifestations vary according to the cause and extent of tissue damage. Like pain, inflammation may be acute or chronic.

In relieving pain, the analgesic–antipyretic–anti-inflammatory drugs are thought to act peripherally to prevent sensitization of pain receptors to various chemical substances released by damaged cells. In relieving fever the drugs apparently act on the hypothalamus to decrease its response to pyrogens and reset the "thermostat" at a lower level. In inflammation they prevent prostaglandins from increasing the pain and edema produced by bradykinin and other substances released by damaged cells. Although these drugs relieve symptoms and contribute greatly to the client's comfort and quality of life, they do not cure the underlying disorders that cause the symptoms.

In addition to analgesic–antipyretic–anti-inflammatory activity, aspirin and NSAIDs exert other pharmacologic actions, including inhibition of platelet aggregation, irritation and ulceration of gastric mucosa, and production of gastrointestinal bleeding. Most of the newer drugs in this group have been developed in an effort to retain the analgesic and anti-inflammatory properties of aspirin while decreasing the adverse effects. These efforts have been only partly successful.

Despite their many similarities, these drugs vary in chemical groups, indications for use, and incidence and severity of adverse effects. Aspirin, a salicylate, has long been the drug of choice in many disorders characterized by pain, fever, or inflammation, and it may be used for one, two, or all three of these symptoms. Acetaminophen, which differs chemically from aspirin, is commonly used as an aspirin substitute for pain and fever, but it lacks anti-inflammatory effects. Ibuprofen (Motrin) and other propionic acid derivatives were initially used as anti-inflammatory agents, but they are gaining acceptance as analgesics as well. Most of the other NSAIDs are considered too toxic to use as analgesics and antipyretics. They are used primarily in rheumatoid arthritis and other musculoskeletal disorders that do not respond to safer drugs.

Contraindications to clinical use of these drugs include peptic ulcer disease, gastrointestinal or other bleeding disorders, and history of hypersensitivity reactions.

Individual drugs

ASPIRIN AND NSAIDs

Aspirin, also called acetylsalicylic acid or ASA, is the prototype of the analgesic–antipyretic–anti-inflammatory drugs and by far the most commonly used salicylate. It also has antiplatelet effects. Aspirin is effective in pain of low to moderate intensity, especially that involving the skin, muscles, joints, and other connective tissue. It is especially useful in disorders in which inflammation contributes to pain, such as rheumatoid arthritis. However, it does not relieve the underlying disease process that produces those symptoms.

Because aspirin is a nonprescription drug, it is a frequently used home remedy for headaches, colds, influenza and other respiratory infections, muscular aches, and fever. It is also prescribed by physicians for a variety of clinical conditions, often with codeine for additive analgesic effects. Other common conditions in which aspirin is used are dysmenorrhea, acute rheumatic fever, rheumatoid arthritis, and other musculoskeletal disorders. Aspirin may also be given for its antiplatelet effect in certain cardiovascular disorders.

Aspirin can be purchased in the form of plain or chewable tablets, enteric-coated tablets, effervescent tablets, and rectal suppositories. It is not marketed in liquid form because it is not stable in solution. It is also available in combination with other analgesics, antacids, and antihistamines and is an ingredient in many nonprescription cold and allergy remedies.

Routes and dosage ranges

Adults: Analgesia and antipyresis, PO 325–650 mg q4h PRN. Usual single dose is 650 mg
Anti-inflammatory effect, PO, rectal suppository 2.6–5.2 g daily
Rheumatic fever, PO, up to 7.8 g daily in divided doses

Children: Analgesia and antipyresis, PO, rectal suppository 11 mg/kg 6 times daily or 16 mg/kg 4 times daily
Anti-inflammatory effect, PO, rectal suppository 100–125 mg/kg/day in divided doses q4–6h. Reduce amount for long-term use
Rheumatic fever, PO, rectal suppository 3 g daily in divided doses

Acetaminophen, USP (Tylenol and others), is equal to aspirin in analgesic and antipyretic effects, but it lacks anti-inflammatory activity. Acetaminophen is a nonprescription drug commonly used as an aspirin substitute because it produces fewer adverse reactions than aspirin. More specifically, acetaminophen in usual therapeutic doses does not cause nausea, vomiting, or gastrointestinal bleeding, and it does not interfere with blood clotting. However, toxic doses produce potentially fatal liver necrosis and usual therapeutic doses may cause liver damage in alcoholics. Acetaminophen is available in tablet, liquid, and rectal suppository forms and is in numerous combination products marketed as analgesics and cold remedies. It is often prescribed with codeine or oxycodone (Percocet-5) for additive analgesic effects.

Routes and dosage ranges

Adults: PO, rectal suppository 325–650 mg q4–6h, or 1000 mg 3–4 times daily. Maximum daily dose, 4 g

Children: PO, rectal suppository 10 mg/kg or according to age, as follows: 0–3 months, 40 mg; 4–11 months, 80 mg; 1–2 years, 120 mg; 2–3 years, 160 mg; 4–5 years, 240 mg; 6–8 years, 320 mg; 9–10 years, 400 mg; 11 years, 480 mg. Doses may be given q4h–6h to a maximum of 5 doses in 24 hours.

Diflunisal (Dolobid), a derivative of salicylic acid, is reportedly equal or superior to aspirin in analgesic effectiveness in mild to moderate pain or osteoarthritis. It differs from aspirin in that it has less antipyretic effect and causes less gastric irritation; its longer duration of action allows for twice-daily administration.

Route and dosage ranges

Adults: Pain, PO 500–1000 mg initially, then 250–500 mg q8–12h
Osteoarthritis, PO 500–1000 mg q12h, increased to a maximum daily dose of 1500 mg if necessary

Fenoprofen (Nalfon), **ibuprofen** (Motrin), and **naproxen** (Naprosyn) are propionic acid derivatives that are chemically and pharmacologically very similar. In addition to their use as anti-inflammatory agents in rheumatoid arthritis, osteoarthritis, gout, tendonitis, and bursitis, they are used as analgesics in conditions not necessarily related to inflammation (*e.g.,* dysmenorrhea, episiotomy, minor trauma), and as antipyretics. Ibuprofen (Advil, Nuprin) is available without prescription. Although these drugs are usually better tolerated than aspirin, they are much more expensive and may cause all the adverse effects associated with aspirin and other prostaglandin inhibitors.

Route and dosage ranges

Fenoprofen

Adults: Rheumatoid arthritis, osteoarthritis, PO 300–600 mg 3–4 times daily. Maximum daily dose, 3200 mg
Mild to moderate pain, PO 200 mg q4–6h PRN

Ibuprofen

Adults: Rheumatoid arthritis, osteoarthritis, PO 300–600 mg 3–4 times daily. Maximum daily dose, 2400 mg
Mild to moderate pain, PO 200–400 mg q4–6h PRN
Primary dysmenorrhea, PO 400 mg q4h PRN

Naproxen

Adults: Rheumatoid arthritis, osteoarthritis, ankylosing spondylitis, PO 250–375 mg twice daily
Acute gout, PO 750 mg initially, then 250 mg q8h until the attack subsides

Mild to moderate pain, primary dysmenorrhea, acute tendonitis and bursitis, PO 500 mg initially, then 250 mg q6–8h

Naproxen sodium (Anaprox)

Adults: Rheumatoid arthritis, osteoarthritis, ankylosing spondylitis, PO 275 mg twice daily
Acute gout, PO 825 mg initially, then 275 mg q8h until the attack subsides
Mild to moderate pain, primary dysmenorrhea, acute tendonitis and bursitis, PO 550 mg initially, then 275 mg q6–8h

Indomethacin (Indocin), **sulindac** (Clinoril), and **tolmetin** (Tolectin) are indole derivatives used for moderate-to-severe rheumatoid arthritis, osteoarthritis, ankylosing spondylitis, acute gouty arthritis, and acute, painful shoulder (bursitis, tendonitis). These drugs have potent anti-inflammatory effects but are associated with greater incidence and severity of adverse effects than aspirin and the propionic acid derivatives. Thus, they are not recommended for general use as analgesics or antipyretics. Uncommon but potentially serious adverse effects include gastrointestinal ulceration, bone marrow depression, hemolytic anemia, mental confusion, depression, and psychosis. These adverse effects are especially associated with indomethacin; the other drugs were developed in an effort to find equally effective but less toxic derivatives of indomethacin. Although adverse reactions occur less often with sulindac and tolmetin, they are still common.

In addition to their above uses, tolmetin is approved for treatment of juvenile rheumatoid arthritis and intravenous indomethacin is approved for treatment of patent ductus arteriosus in premature infants. The ductus arteriosus joins the pulmonary artery to the aorta in the fetal circulation. When it fails to close, blood is shunted from the aorta to the pulmonary artery, causing severe cardiopulmonary problems.

Routes and dosage ranges

Indomethacin

Adults: PO, rectal suppository 75 mg daily initially, increased by 25 mg daily at weekly intervals to a maximum of 150–200 mg daily
Acute gouty arthritis, acute painful shoulder, PO 75–150 mg daily in 3–4 divided doses until pain and inflammation are controlled (approximately 3–5 days for gout, 7–14 days for painful shoulder), then discontinued

Children: Premature infants with patent ductus arteriosus, IV 0.2–0.3 mg/kg q12–24h for a total of 3 doses

Sulindac

Adults: PO 150–200 mg twice daily. Maximum daily dose 400 mg
Acute gouty arthritis, acute painful shoulder, PO 200 mg twice daily until pain and inflammation are controlled (about 7–14 days), then discontinued

Tolmetin

Adults: PO 400 mg 3 times daily initially, increased to 1600 mg daily for osteoarthritis or 2000 mg daily for rheumatoid arthritis if necessary.

Children: Rheumatoid arthritis, PO 20 mg/kg/day in 3–4 divided doses

Meclofenamate (Meclomen) and **mefenamic acid** (Ponstel) are fenamate NSAIDs that are used less frequently than most other agents because of frequent gastrointestinal and neurologic adverse effects.

Route and dosage ranges

Meclofenamate

Adults: Rheumatoid arthritis, osteoarthritis, PO 200–400 mg daily in 3–4 divided doses

Mefenamic acid

Adults: Acute pain, PO 500 mg initially, then 250 mg q6h PRN for no longer than 1 week
Primary dysmenorrhea, PO 500 mg at start of menses, then 250 mg q6h PRN for 2–3 days

Children over 14 years: Acute pain, PO 500 mg initially, then 250 mg q6h PRN for no longer than 1 week

Phenylbutazone (Butazolidin) is a pyrazolone NSAID with pharmacologic activity similar to aspirin. However, its potentially severe adverse effects (*e.g.,* bone marrow depression, gastrointestinal ulceration, congestive heart failure, hepatitis, nephritis, hypersensitivity reactions) limit its clinical usefulness. It is recommended for short-term treatment of acute attacks of rheumatoid arthritis or gout.

Route and dosage range

Adults: PO 100 mg 3–4 times daily for 1 week

Piroxicam (Feldene) is an oxicam NSAID that differs chemically from other agents but has similar pharmacologic properties. Approved for treatment of rheumatoid arthritis and osteoarthritis, it reportedly causes less gastrointestinal irritation than aspirin. Its long half-life allows for once-daily dosing, but optimal efficacy may not occur for 1 to 2 weeks.

Route and dosage range

Adults: PO 20 mg daily

DRUGS USED IN GOUT AND HYPERURICEMIA

Allopurinol (Zyloprim) is a unique drug used to prevent or treat hyperuricemia (high levels of uric acid in the blood), which occurs with gout and with antineoplastic drug therapy. Uric acid is formed by purine metabolism and an enzyme called xanthine oxidase. Allopurinol prevents formation of uric acid by inhibiting xanthine oxidase. It is especially useful in chronic gout characterized by tophi (deposits of uric acid crystals in the joints, kidneys, and soft tissues) and impaired renal function. The drug promotes resorption of urate deposits and prevents their further development. Acute attacks of gout may result when urate deposits are mobilized. These may be prevented by concomitant administration of colchicine until serum uric acid levels are lowered.

Route and dosage ranges

Adults: Mild gout, PO 200–400 mg daily
Severe gout, PO 400–600 mg daily
Hyperuricemia in clients with renal insufficiency, PO 100–200 mg daily
Secondary hyperuricemia from anticancer drugs, PO 100–200 mg daily to a maximum of 800 mg/day

Children: Secondary hyperuricemia from anticancer drugs; under 6 years, PO 150 mg daily; 6–10 years, PO 300 mg daily

Colchicine is an anti-inflammatory drug that is effective only in gout. It has no analgesic or antipyretic effects. It is given to prevent or treat acute attacks of gout. In acute attacks, it is the drug of choice for relieving joint pain and edema.

Routes and dosage ranges

Adults: Acute attacks, PO 0.5 mg q1h until pain is relieved or toxicity (nausea, vomiting, diarrhea) occurs; 3-day interval between courses of therapy
IV, 1–2 mg initially, then 0.5 mg q3–6h until response is obtained, to a maximum total dose of 4 mg
Prophylaxis, PO 0.5–1 mg daily

Probenecid (Benemid) increases urinary excretion of uric acid. This uricosuric action is used therapeutically to treat hyperuricemia and gout. It is not effective in acute attacks of gouty arthritis but prevents hyperuricemia and tophi associated with chronic gout. Probenecid may precipitate acute gout until serum uric acid levels are within normal range. Concomitant administration of colchicine prevents this effect. (Probenecid is also used with penicillin, most often in treating sexually transmitted diseases. It increases blood levels and prolongs the action of penicillin by decreasing the rate of urinary excretion.)

Route and dosage ranges

Adults: PO 250 mg twice daily for 1 week, then 500 mg twice daily

Children over 2 years: PO 40 mg/kg/day in divided doses

Sulfinpyrazone (Anturane) is a uricosuric agent similar to probenecid. It is not effective in acute gout but prevents or decreases tissue changes of chronic gout. Colchicine is usually given during initial sulfinpyrazone therapy to prevent acute gout. This drug is chemically related to phenylbutazone and produces similar adverse reactions.

Route and dosage range

Adults: PO 100–200 mg twice daily, gradually increased over 1 week to a maximum daily dose of 400–800 mg

DRUGS USED IN MIGRAINE

Ergotamine tartrate (Ergomar) is an ergot alkaloid (see Chap. 67) used only in the treatment of migraine. Migraine, which involves paroxysmal attacks of severe headache, vomiting, and increased sensitivity to light and sound, is attributed to dilation of the extracerebral cranial arteries. Ergot preparations relieve migraine by constricting the vascular smooth muscle of blood vessels in the brain. Ergotamine is most effective when given sublingually or by inhalation at the onset of headache. When given orally, ergotamine is erratically absorbed, and therapeutic effects may be delayed for 20 to 30 minutes.

Ergotamine is contraindicated during pregnancy and in the presence of severe hypertension, peripheral vascular disease, coronary artery disease, renal or hepatic disease, and severe infections.

Routes and dosage ranges

Adults: PO 1–2 mg at onset of acute migraine attack, then 2 mg every 30 minutes, if necessary, to a maximal amount of 6 mg/24 hours or 10 mg/week
SL 2 mg at onset of acute migraine, then 2 mg every 30 minutes, if necessary, to a maximal amount of 6 mg/24 hours or 10 mg/week
Inhalation 0.36 mg (one inhalation) at onset of acute migraine, repeated in 5 minutes if necessary, to a maximal dose of 6 inhalations/24 hours

Ergotamine tartrate and caffeine (Cafergot) is a commonly used antimigraine preparation. Caffeine reportedly increases absorption and vasoconstrictive effects of ergotamine. The combination product is available in oral tablets containing ergotamine 1 mg and caffeine 100 mg, and in rectal suppositories containing ergotamine 2 mg and caffeine 100 mg.

Routes and dosage ranges

Adults: PO 2 tablets at the onset of acute migraine, then 1 tablet every 30 minutes, if necessary, up to 6 tablets per attack or 10 tablets/week
Rectal suppository $\frac{1}{2}$–1 suppository at the onset of acute migraine, repeated in 1 hour, if necessary, up to 2 suppositories per attack or 5 suppositories/week

Children: PO $\frac{1}{2}$–1 tablet initially, then $\frac{1}{2}$ tablet every 30 minutes, if necessary, up to a maximal amount of 3 tablets

Dihydroergotamine mesylate (DHE 45) is a semisynthetic derivative of ergotamine that is less toxic and less effective than the parent drug

Routes and dosage ranges

Adults: IM 1 mg at onset of acute migraine, repeated hourly, if necessary, to a total of 3 mg
IV 1 mg, repeated if necessary, after 1 hour. Maximal dose, 2 mg. Do not exeed 6 mg/week

Methysergide maleate (Sansert) is an ergot derivative used only for prophylaxis of migraine; it is ineffective in acute migraine attacks. Methysergide is thought to block serotonin receptors. Serotonin is a substance that may be involved in the etiology of vascular headache. The drug is indicated only when migraine attacks are frequent or severe.

Route and dosage range

Adults: PO, 4–8 mg daily in divided doses.

Principles of therapy: analgesic–antipyretic–anti-inflammatory and related drugs

ASSESSMENT OF PAIN, FEVER, AND INFLAMMATION

General assessment factors for pain include location, intensity, duration, and precipitating factors (see Chap. 5). Fever is simple to verify with a thermometer. Readings above 99.6° F or 37.3° C are usually considered fever. Hot, dry skin, flushed face, reduced urine output, and concentrated urine may accompany fever if the person is also dehydrated. Local signs of inflammation are redness, heat, edema, and pain or tenderness. Systemic signs include fever, leukocytosis, and weakness.

NURSING INTERVENTIONS

Implement measures to prevent or minimize pain, fever and inflammation.

1. Diagnosis and treatment of the underlying condition are very important. Measures aimed at relief of the disorder, such as prevention or treatment of infections and improvement of the blood supply, may be helpful in alleviating symptoms.
2. Institute treatment measures as soon as they seem indicated. Timing depends on thorough assessment and the ability to recognize early signs and symptoms. When drug therapy seems indicated, it generally should not be delayed any longer than necessary. With pain, for example, early treatment may prevent severe pain and allow usage of milder analgesic drugs. Other measures that may be used instead of or along with drug therapy include positioning, hygienic care, heat or cold applications, rest or exercise, and distraction or relaxation techniques. Assess response to various therapeutic approaches as carefully as initial signs and symptoms.

GUIDELINES FOR THERAPY WITH ASPIRIN

When pain, fever, or inflammation is present, aspirin is often the drug of choice, and its usefulness extends across a wide range of clinical conditions. Because it is a nonprescription drug and widely available, people tend to underestimate its effectiveness. Like any other drug, aspirin must be used appropriately to maximize therapeutic benefits and minimize adverse reactions. Some guidelines to correct usage include the following:

1. In pain, aspirin is useful alone when the discomfort is of low-to-moderate intensity. For more severe pain, aspirin may be combined with a narcotic or given between narcotic doses for better analgesia or to allow lower doses of the narcotic. Aspirin and narcotic analgesics act by different mechanisms, so such usage is rational. Aspirin with codeine is especially effective. Aspirin may be used with other narcotics in clients who can take oral medications. In acute pain, aspirin is taken when the pain occurs and is often effective within a few minutes. In chronic pain, a regular schedule of administration, such as every 4 to 6 hours, is more effective.

2. In fever, aspirin is usually the drug of choice if drug therapy is indicated. However, aspirin may delay diagnosis of conditions in which fever and its patterns of occurrence are significant.
3. In inflammation, aspirin is useful in both short-term and long-term therapy. It is especially useful in conditions characterized by both pain and inflammation, such as rheumatoid arthritis.
4. Aspirin is usually the drug of choice when salicylate therapy is indicated. Sodium salicylate may be used for people who are hypersensitive to aspirin, but it is less effective, produces similar adverse reactions, and may be contraindicated because of its sodium content. Choline salicylate and a few other preparations are advertised as producing fewer gastrointestinal adverse reactions but seem to offer no particular advantage over aspirin.
5. For most purposes, plain aspirin tablets are preferred. Enteric-coated tablets are more slowly absorbed and therefore take longer to exert their therapeutic effects. They may be better tolerated for long-term use of high doses in rheumatoid arthritis, however. Rectal suppositories are sometimes used when oral administration is contraindicated.
6. Aspirin dosage depends mainly on the condition in question. Larger doses are needed for anti-inflammatory effects than for analgesic and antipyretic effects. Lower doses are needed when there is a low serum albumin level because a larger proportion of the dose is free to exert pharmacologic activity.
7. Aspirin and related drugs should be used cautiously during perioperative periods, and they are contraindicated during anticoagulant therapy (see Chap. 57). Because they inhibit platelet aggregation and cause hypoprothrombinemia, they interfere with blood coagulation and increase the risk of bleeding.
8. Salicylate intoxication may occur. In mild salicylism, stopping the drug or reducing the dose is usually sufficient. In severe salicylate overdose, treatment is symptomatic and aimed toward preventing further absorption from the gastrointestinal tract, increasing urinary excretion, and correcting fluid, electrolyte, and acid–base imbalances. When the drug is still thought to be in the gastrointestinal tract, emesis, gastric lavage, and activated charcoal, or a combination of these, helps to reduce absorption. Intravenous sodium bicarbonate produces an alkaline urine in which salicylates are more rapidly excreted. Intravenous fluids are indicated when hyperthermia or dehydration is present. The specific content of intravenous fluids depends on serum electrolyte and acid base status. In children, metabolic acidosis develops rapidly and is likely to be present on initial contact. In adults, metabolic acidosis develops more slowly and with severe overdosage.

GUIDELINES FOR THERAPY WITH ACETAMINOPHEN

Acetaminophen is an effective aspirin substitute for treatment of pain and fever when aspirin is contraindicated or not tolerated. It may be the drug of choice for children with febrile illness (because of the association of aspirin with Reye's syndrome), elderly adults with impaired renal function (because aspirin may cause further impairment), and pregnant women (because aspirin is associated with several maternal and fetal disorders).

Probably the major drawback to acetaminophen is liver damage. Factors related to identification and treatment of hepatotoxicity include the following:

1. Acute hepatic failure may occur with a single large dose, usually about 10 to 15 g, but it has been reported with 6 g. Acute acetaminophen poisoning may be characterized by cyanosis, anemia, pancytopenia, jaundice, fever, vomiting, and central nervous system stimulation with excitement and delirium followed by vascular collapse, convulsions, coma, and death. Early symptoms, within 24 hours after ingestion, are nonspecific (*e.g.,* anorexia, nausea, vomiting). Peak hepatotoxicity occurs in 3 to 4 days and recovery occurs in 7 to 8 days.
2. If overdose is detected soon after ingestion, activated charcoal can be given to inhibit absorption. However, the specific antidote is acetylcysteine (Mucomyst), a mucolytic agent given by inhalation in respiratory disorders (see Chap. 49). For acetaminophen poisoning, it is given orally. It combines with a toxic metabolite and prevents hepatotoxicity if given within 24 hours of acetaminophen ingestion.
3. Hepatotoxicity also occurs with chronic ingestion of acetaminophen (5 to 8 g daily for several weeks or 3 to 4 g daily for a year) and short-term ingestion of usual therapeutic doses in alcoholics.

NONSALICYLATE NSAIDs

Nonsalicylate NSAIDs are used primarily for anti-inflammatory effects in rheumatoid arthritis and other musculoskeletal disorders. Although none has been proved more effective than aspirin, one of these drugs may be better tolerated by some clients. They are much more expensive than aspirin and are being increasingly associated with nephrotoxicity, especially in clients with preexisting renal impairment.

GUIDELINES RELATED TO PREGNANCY AND LACTATION

1. During pregnancy, acetaminophen is apparently the safest one of these drugs, especially for short-term use of therapeutic doses. Aspirin is generally contraindicated because of potential adverse effects on both the mother and fetus. Maternal effects include prolonged gestation, prolonged labor, and antepartal and postpartal hemorrhage. Fetal effects include constriction of the ductus arteriosus, low birth weight, and increased incidence of stillbirth and neonatal death. However, for the pregnant client with rheumatoid arthritis, aspirin is considered the drug of choice. The lowest possible doses should be given. Nonsalicylate NSAIDs are contraindicated. None has been studied adequately for use during pregnancy. Since these drugs also inhibit prostaglandin synthesis, they would likely produce the same effects as aspirin.
2. During lactation, all these drugs are excreted in breast milk. Acetaminophen and aspirin are considered safe for occasional use; NSAIDs are contraindicated.

PEDIATRIC CONSIDERATIONS

In pediatric drug therapy, acetaminophen or aspirin may be given for pain, but acetaminophen is probably the drug of choice for fever. Although aspirin has long been used for fever, some studies have indicated an association with Reye's syndrome, a life-threatening illness characterized by encephalopathy, hepatic damage, and other serious problems. Reye's syndrome usually occurs after a viral illness, such as influenza B or chickenpox, during which aspirin was administered for fever. For juvenile rheumatoid arthritis, aspirin is the drug of choice. With the exception of tolmetin (see p. 55), other NSAIDs are not approved for use in children and do not have established pediatric doses.

GERIATRIC CONSIDERATIONS

Elderly clients have a high incidence of inflammatory musculoskeletal disorders, and aspirin or a nonsalicylate NSAID is frequently prescribed. The elderly adult is more likely to have adverse reactions to these drugs. Small doses, gradual increments, and careful monitoring of response may minimize adverse effects.

GUIDELINES FOR TREATING RHEUMATOID ARTHRITIS AND RELATED DISORDERS

1. The primary goals of treatment are to control pain and inflammation and to minimize immobilization and disability. Rest, exercise, physical therapy, and drugs are used to attain these goals. None of these measures prevents joint destruction or related pathologic conditions.
2. Aspirin is the initial drug of choice for most adults and children because it is effective in relieving both pain and inflammation. It is also inexpensive, an important factor in the long-term treatment of these chronic disorders. Generally, the dosage of aspirin required for anti-inflammatory effects is large but must be individualized. One way of individualizing dosage is by starting with small doses and increasing them. Salicylate blood levels are helpful in establishing dose and frequency of administration. Regular administration of aspirin every 4 to 6 hours will usually produce a serum salicylate level of 15 to 25 mg/100 ml, which is considered to be in the therapeutic range. The optimal dosage schedule is that which produces most relief of symptoms without toxicity.
3. For people who cannot take aspirin because of peptic ulcer disease, bleeding disorders, and other contraindications, nonsteroidal anti-inflammatory drugs are usually ordered. The choice of a specific drug is largely empirical; a given person may respond better to one aspirinlike drug than another. A drug may be given for 2 or 3 weeks on a trial basis. If therapeutic benefits occur, the drug may be continued; if no benefits seem evident or toxicity occurs, then another drug may be tried. Fenoprofen, ibuprofen, and naproxen are often used because they are associated with gastrointestinal intolerance less often than other NSAIDs. However, they do cause significant toxicity in some cases and are quite expensive for long-term use. Indomethacin is effective, but its usage is limited because of toxicity. Phenylbutazone is recommended only for short-term use in acute flare-ups of rheumatoid arthritis, gouty arthritis, and other disorders because of potentially severe toxicity. Frequent blood counts are necessary during therapy with phenylbutazone. Other drugs that may be used include corticosteroids, gold, hydroxychloroquine (Plaquenil) and immunosuppressant drugs such as azathioprine (Imuran), cyclophosphamide (Cytoxan), and methotrexate. These drugs may cause significant toxicity and are used mainly in clients who do not respond to the NSAIDs. Several weeks are required for therapeutic effects.

4. For people who are allergic to aspirin, NSAIDs are contraindicated. People who are hypersensitive to aspirin may also be hypersensitive to other drugs that inhibit prostaglandin synthesis.
5. In children, aspirin or tolmetin is preferred because these drugs have been tested more extensively in children. Pediatric dosages have not been established for most of the other drugs.

GUIDELINES FOR TREATING HYPERURICEMIA AND GOUT

Opinions differ regarding treatment of asymptomatic hyperuricemia. Some authorities do not think drug therapy is indicated, while others think that lowering serum uric acid levels may prevent both joint inflammation and renal calculi. Allopurinol, probenecid, or sulfinpyrazone may be given for this purpose. Colchicine should also be given for several weeks to prevent acute attacks of gout while serum uric acid levels are being lowered. During initial administration of these drugs, a high fluid intake (to produce about 2000 ml of urine per day) and alkaline urine are recommended to prevent renal calculi. Urate crystals are more likely to precipitate in acid urine.

GUIDELINES FOR TREATING MIGRAINE

For treatment of migraine and similar disorders, give ergot preparations at the onset of headache and have the client lie down in a quiet, darkened room. Assist the client to identify and avoid precipitating factors, when possible.

NURSING ACTIONS: ANALGESIC–ANTIPYRETIC–ANTI-INFLAMMATORY AND RELATED DRUGS

Nursing Actions	*Rationale/Explanation*
1. Administer accurately	
a. Give aspirin, indomethacin, phenylbutazone, sulindac, and tolmetin with a full glass of water or other fluid and with or just after meals.	To decrease gastric irritation
b. Give fenoprofen, ibuprofen, naproxen, diflunisal, and piroxicam when the stomach is empty if tolerated. Give with or after food if necessary.	Food in the stomach delays absorption and decreases peak plasma levels of the drugs. However, the drugs may be given with food if manifestations of gastric irritation occur.
c. Give antimigraine preparations at the onset of headache.	To prevent development of more severe symptoms.
d. Give methysergide with meals.	To decrease nausea and vomiting.
2. Observe for therapeutic effects	
a. When drugs are given for pain, observe for decreased or absent manifestations of pain.	Pain relief is usually evident within 30–60 minutes.
b. When drugs are given for fever, record temperature every 2–4 hours and observe for a decrease.	
c. When drugs are given for arthritis and other inflammatory disorders, observe for decreased pain, edema, redness, heat, and stiffness of joints. Also observe for increased joint mobility and exercise tolerance.	With aspirin, improvement is usually noted within 24–48 hours. With most of the nonsteroidal anti-inflammatory drugs, 1–2 weeks may be required before beneficial effects become evident.
d. When colchicine is given for acute gouty arthritis, observe for decreased pain and inflammation in involved joints.	Therapeutic effects occur within 4–12 hours after intravenous colchicine administration and 24–48 hours after oral administration. Edema may not decrease for several days.
e. When allopurinol, probenecid, or sulfinpyrazone is given for hyperuricemia, observe for normal serum uric acid level (about 2–8 mg/100 ml).	Serum uric acid levels usually decrease to normal range within 1–3 weeks.
f. When the above drugs are given for chronic gout, observe for decreased size of tophi, absence of new	

Nursing Actions	***Rationale/Explanation***
tophi, decreased joint pain and increased joint mobility, and normal serum uric acid levels.	
g. When ergot preparations are given in migraine headache, observe for relief of symptoms.	Therapeutic effects are usually evident within 15–30 minutes.
3. Observe for adverse effects	
a. With analgesic–antipyretic–anti-inflammatory and antigout agents, observe for	
(1) Gastrointestinal problems—anorexia, nausea, vomiting, diarrhea, bleeding, ulceration	These are common reactions, more likely with aspirin, indomethacin, phenylbutazone, piroxicam, sulindac, tolmetin, colchicine, and sulfinpyrazone and less likely with acetaminophen, diflunisal, fenoprofen, ibuprofen, and naproxen.
(2) Hematologic problems—petechiae, bruises, hematuria, melena, epistaxis, and bone marrow depression (leukopenia, thrombocytopenia, anemia)	Bone marrow depression is more likely to occur with phenylbutazone and with colchicine.
(3) Central nervous system effects—headache, dizziness, fainting, ataxia, insomnia, confusion, drowsiness	These effects are relatively common with indomethacin and may occur with most of the other drugs, especially with high dosages.
(4) Skin rashes, dermatitis	
(5) Hypersensitivity reactions with dyspnea, bronchospasm, skin rashes	These effects may simulate asthma in people who are allergic to aspirin and aspirinlike drugs.
(6) Tinnitus, blurred vision	Tinnitus (ringing or roaring in the ears) is a classic sign of aspirin overdose (salicylate intoxication). It occurs with NSAIDs as well, especially with overdosage.
(7) Nephrotoxicity—decreased urine output, increased blood urea nitrogen (BUN), increased serum creatinine, hyperkalemia	More likely to occur in people with preexisting renal impairment, especially when fluid intake is decreased or fluid loss is increased. Elderly adults are at greater risk because of decreased renal blood flow and increased incidence of congestive heart failure and diuretic therapy. Renal damage is usually reversible when the drug is discontinued.
(8) Cardiovascular and hepatic effects	These are not common with usual therapeutic doses, but all vital organs may be adversely affected with overdoses.
b. With antimigraine preparations, observe for	
(1) Nausea, vomiting, diarrhea	These drugs have a direct effect on the vomiting center of the brain and stimulate contraction of gastrointestinal smooth muscle.
(2) Symptoms of ergot poisoning (ergotism)—coolness, numbness and tingling of the extremities, headache, vomiting, dizziness, thirst, convulsions, weak pulse, confusion, anginalike chest pain, transient tachycardia or bradycardia, muscle weakness and pain, cyanosis, gangrene of the extremities.	The ergot alkaloids are highly toxic; poisoning may be acute or chronic. Acute poisoning is rare; chronic poisoning is usually a result of overdosage. Circulatory impairments may result from vasoconstriction and vascular insufficiency. Large doses also damage capillary endothelium and may cause thrombosis and occlusion. Gangrene of extremities rarely occurs with usual doses unless peripheral vascular disease or other contraindications are also present.
(3) Hypertension	Blood pressure may rise as a result of generalized vasoconstriction induced by the ergot preparation.
(4) Hypersensitivity reactions—local edema and pruritus, anaphylactic shock	Allergic reactions are relatively uncommon.
(5) With methysergide—inflammation followed by fibrosis in some body tissues. Retroperitoneal fibrosis can lead to urinary tract obstruction; fibrosis of lung tissue can lead to pulmonary complications. Cardiac valves and major arteries may also be affected by fibrotic thickening.	These growths usually regress if symptoms are detected and the drug discontinued. The client is examined frequently during long-term therapy. A drug-free interval of several weeks is recommended between courses of therapy.
4. Observe for drug interactions	
a. Drugs that *increase* effects of aspirin and other NSAIDs	

Nursing Actions	***Rationale/Explanation***
(1) Acidifying agents (*e.g.,* ascorbic acid)	Acidify urine and thereby decrease the urinary excretion rate of salicylates.
(2) Alcohol	Increases gastric irritation and occult blood loss
(3) Anticoagulants, oral	Increase risk of bleeding substantially. People taking anticoagulants should not take aspirin or aspirin-containing products.
(4) Codeine, other narcotic analgesics and some related analgesics such as methotrimeprazine (Levoprome) and pentazocine (Talwin)	Additive analgesic effects because of different mechanisms of action. Aspirin can be used with these drugs to provide adequate pain relief without excessive doses and sedation, in many cases.
(5) Corticosteroids (*e.g.,* prednisone)	Additive gastric irritating and ulcerogenic effects.
b. Drugs that *decrease* effects of aspirin and other NSAIDs	
Alkalinizing agents (*e.g.,* sodium bicarbonate)	Increase rate of renal excretion
c. Drugs that *increase* effects of indomethacin	
(1) Anticoagulants, oral	Increase risk of gastrointestinal bleeding. Indomethacin causes gastric irritation and is considered an ulcerogenic drug.
(2) Corticosteroids	Increase ulcerogenic effects
(3) Salicylates	Increase ulcerogenic effects
(4) Heparin	Increase risk of bleeding. These drugs should not be used concurrently.
d. Drugs that *decrease* effects of indomethacin	
Antacids	Delay absorption from the gastrointestinal tract.
e. Drugs that *increase* effects of phenylbutazone	Phenylbutazone is recommended only for short-term use (about 1 week). For clients who are taking the listed interacting drugs on a long-term basis, another nonsteroidal anti-inflammatory drug is preferred. The combination of phenylbutazone and oral anticoagulants is particularly hazardous.
Acidifying agents, androgens, oral anticoagulants, corticosteroids	Increase risk of gastrointestinal bleeding; probably increase ulcerogenic effects
f. Drugs that *decrease* effects of allopurinol, probenecid and sulfinpyrazone	
(1) Alkalinizing agents (*e.g.,* sodium bicarbonate)	Decrease risks of renal calculi from precipitation of uric acid crystals. Alkalinizing agents are recommended until serum uric acid levels return to normal.
(2) Colchicine	Decreases attacks of acute gout. Recommended for concurrent use until serum uric acid levels return to normal.
(3) Diuretics	Decrease uricosuric effects
(4) Salicylates	Mainly at salicylate doses less than 2 g/day, decrease uricosuric effects of probenecid and sulfinpyrazone but do not interfere with the action of allopurinol. Salicylates are uricosuric at doses greater than 5 g/day.
g. Drugs that *increase* effects of ergot preparations	
Vasoconstrictors (*e.g.,* ephedrine, epinephrine, phenylephrine)	Additive vasoconstriction with risks of severe, persistent hypertension and intracranial hemorrhage
5. Teach clients	
a. With analgesic–antipyretic–anti-inflammatory and antigout agents	
(1) Take the drugs with a full glass of liquid.	To decrease stomach irritation and upset
(2) Drink $2\frac{1}{2}$–3 quarts of fluid daily if not contraindicated.	To decrease gastric irritation. With long-term use of aspirin, an adequate fluid intake is also needed to prevent precipitation of salicylate crystals in the urinary tract. With allopurinol, probenecid, and sulfinpyrazone, fluids are needed to help prevent precipitation of urate crystals and formation of urate

Nursing Actions	***Rationale/Explanation***
	kidney stones. Fluid intake is especially important initially when serum uric acid levels are high and large amounts of uric acid are being excreted in the urine.
(3) Report signs of bleeding (nosebleed, vomiting blood, bruising, blood in urine or stools), difficulty in breathing, skin rash or hives, ringing in ears, dizziness, or severe stomach upset.	
(4) Store aspirin in a closed child-proof container and keep out of reach of children. *Never* call aspirin ''candy.''	A closed container reduces exposure of the drug to moisture and air, which cause chemical breakdown. Aspirin that is deteriorating smells like vinegar (acetic acid). Special precautions are needed with children because aspirin ingestion is a common cause of drug poisoning in children.
(5) With phenylbutazone, report sore throat, fever, or other problems.	These signs and symptoms may indicate a serious blood disorder (agranulocytosis) and require stopping the drug.
(6) With colchicine for chronic gout, carry the drug and start taking as directed (usually one pill every hour for several hours until relief is obtained or nausea, vomiting, and diarrhea occur) when joint pain starts.	To prevent or minimize an attack of gouty arthritis
b. With ergot preparations, report signs of vascular insufficiency such as tingling sensation or coldness, numbness, or weakness of the extremities. Do not exceed recommended doses.	These are symptoms of ergot toxicity. To avoid potentially serious adverse reactions, do not exceed recommended doses.

Selected References

American Medical Association (AMA) Division of Drugs: AMA Drug Evaluations, 5th ed. New York, John Wiley & Sons, 1983

Auranofin (Ridaura). Med Lett Drugs Ther 27:89–90, October 25, 1985

Blackshear JL, Napier JS, Davidman M, et al: NSAID-induced nephrotoxicity: Avoidance, detection and treatment. Drug Ther 14:199–210, May 1984

Blackshear JL, Davidman M, Stillman MT: Identification of risk for renal insufficiency from nonsteroidal anti-inflammatory drugs. Arch Intern Med 143:1130–1134, June 1983

Carter MA, Evens RP, Small RE: Immune and inflammatory disorders. In Wiener MB, Pepper GA (eds.): Clinical Pharmacology and Therapeutics in Nursing, 2nd ed., pp 389–419. New York, McGraw-Hill, 1985

Drugs for rheumatoid arthritis. Med Lett Drugs Ther 27:25–28, March 15, 1985

Facts and Comparisons. St Louis, J B Lippincott (Updated monthly)

Flower RG, Moncada S, Vane JR: Analgesic-antipyretics and anti-inflammatory agents; drugs employed in the treatment of gout. In Gilman AG, Goodman LS, Rall TW, Murad F (eds): The Pharmacological Basis of Therapeutics, 7th ed, pp 674–715. New York, Macmillan, 1985

Friedman A: Migraine: New approaches to an old problem. Drug Ther 14:143–146, February 1984

Groer MW, Shekleton ME: Basic Pathophysiology: A Conceptual Approach, 2d ed. St. Louis, C V Mosby, 1983

Hansten PD: Drug Interactions: Clinical Significance of Drug–Drug Interactions, 5th ed. Philadelphia, Lea & Febiger, 1985

Ibuprofen without a prescription. Med Lett Drugs Ther 26:63–65, July 6, 1984

Kantor TG: Selecting the appropriate NSAID. Drug Ther 14:59–66, February 1984

Kaysen GA, Pond SM, Roper MH, et al: Combined hepatic and renal injury in alcoholics during therapeutic use of acetaminophen. Arch Intern Med 145:2019–2023, November 1985

Malseed RT: Pharmacology: Drug Therapy and Nursing Considerations, 2d ed. Philadelphia, J B Lippincott, 1985

McCaffery M: Newer uses of NSAIDs. Am J Nurs 85:781–782, July 1985

Neuberger GB: The role of the nurse with arthritis patients on drug therapy. Nurs Clin North Am 19:593–604, December 1984

Reeves WB, Foley RJ, Weinman EJ: Renal dysfunction from nonsteroidal anti-inflammatory drugs (editorial). Arch Intern Med 144:1943–1944, October 1984

Rodman MJ, Karch AM, Boyd EH, Smith DW: Pharmacology and Drug Therapy in Nursing, 3rd ed. Philadelphia, J B Lippincott, 1985

Stillman MT, Napier J, Blackshear JL: Adverse effects of nonsteroidal anti-inflammatory drugs on the kidney. Med Clin North Am 68:371–385, March 1984

Strand CV, Clark SR: Adult arthritis: Drugs and remedies. Am J Nurs 83:266–270, February 1983

7

SEDATIVE–HYPNOTICS

Description and uses

Sedative drugs produce relaxation and decrease anxiety; hypnotic drugs produce sleep. The difference between the two types of drugs is one of degree and depends largely on dosage. Since these drugs generally depress the central nervous system (CNS), some of them are used as antianxiety, anticonvulsant, and anesthetic agents. The drugs discussed in this chapter are those used primarily to induce sleep.

Sleep is a recurrent period of decreased mental and physical activity during which the person is relatively unresponsive to sensory and environmental stimuli. Normal sleep allows rest, renewal of energy for performing activities of daily living, and alertness upon awakening. When a person retires for sleep, there is an initial period of drowsiness or sleep latency, which lasts about 30 minutes. Once the person is asleep, cycles occur approximately every 90 minutes during the sleep period. During each cycle, the individual progresses from drowsiness (stage I) to deep sleep (stage IV). These stages are characterized by depressed body functions, nonrapid eye movements (nonREM), and nondreaming and are thought to be physically restorative. Stage IV is followed by a period of 5 to 20 minutes during which rapid eye movements (REM), dreaming, and increased physiologic activity occur. REM sleep is thought to be mentally and emotionally restorative.

Insomnia, a prolonged inability to sleep, is the most common sleep disorder. *Initial insomnia* is the inability to go to sleep when desired (prolonged latency period). *Intermittent insomnia* is the inability to stay asleep (frequent awakening). In *terminal insomnia,* the person awakens early and is unable to return to sleep. Insomnia has many causes, including such stressors as pain, anxiety, illness, changes in lifestyle or environment, and various drugs. Occasional sleeplessness is a normal response to many stimuli and is not usually harmful.

Sedative–hypnotic drugs produce varying degrees of CNS depression ranging from drowsiness and mild sedation to sleep, anesthesia, respiratory depression, and death. The mechanism by which these drugs induce sleep is probably depression of the reticular formation in the brain. Sedative–hypnotic drugs given in hypnotic doses for insomnia alter normal sleep patterns by decreasing REM sleep and increasing nonREM sleep. The clinical significance of these alterations is not completely understood. Upon discontinuation of drug use, however, decreased REM sleep is followed by compensatory REM sleep, as though the mind needs to make up the lost dreaming time. This REM rebound effect can occur when sleeping pills are used for only 3 or 4 days. With longer drug use, REM rebound may be severe and accompanied by vivid dreams, nightmares, restlessness, and frequent awakenings.

After drugs that alter sleep patterns are taken, normal patterns may not return for several weeks after the drug is discontinued. Some authorities think that the altered patterns promote dependence on and abuse of hypnotic drugs because people continue taking the drugs to avoid REM rebound and the prolonged changes in sleep patterns that occur on discontinuation of drug use. In fact, unless these effects are explained, people may attribute their continued sleeping difficulties to physical, emotional, or environmental problems rather than to drug use.

Sedative–hypnotic drugs are usually subclassified as barbiturates and nonbarbiturates. Barbiturates are considered prototype drugs, although their use has declined with the development of newer agents. All barbiturates have similar pharmacologic actions and differ primarily in onset and duration of action. They are usually described as ultrashort, short, intermediate, and long acting. The ultrashort-acting barbiturates are used mainly for anesthesia and are discussed in Chapter 14. Barbiturates are metabolized into water-soluble, inactive metabolites in the liver; the metabolites are excreted by the kidneys. They are also "enzyme inducers" and activate drug-metabolizing enzymes in the liver. As a result, their own rate of metabolism is increased. This enzyme induction mechanism partially accounts for the development of tolerance to their sedative–hypnotic effects and of cross tolerance with other CNS depressant drugs. In addition, they increase the metabolism rate of several other drug groups, including oral anticoagulants and corticosteroids. Barbiturates do not relieve pain or insomnia caused by pain. If given in these circumstances without an analgesic drug, they may cause increased perception of pain (hyperalgesia), excitement, confusion, and delirium.

Nonbarbiturate sedative–hypnotics include several drugs from different chemical groups. With the exception of the benzodiazepine group, these drugs offer no significant advantage over the barbiturates. The benzodiazepines include diazepam (Valium) and related drugs (see Chap. 8), some of which are used only as hypnotics.

Clinical indications for use of sedative–hypnotic drugs include short-term treatment of insomnia and sedation prior to surgery or invasive diagnostic tests (*e.g.*, angiograms and endoscopies). Barbiturates are also used for their general anesthetic and anticonvulsant effects.

Contraindications to sedative–hypnotic drugs include severe respiratory disorders, hypersensitivity reactions, a history of alcohol or drug abuse, and severe liver or kidney disease. In addition, barbiturates are contraindicated in acute intermittent porphyria (a rare hereditary metabolic disorder characterized by recurrent attacks of physical and mental disturbances).

Individual sedative–hypnotic drugs

BARBITURATES (Table 7-1)

BENZODIAZEPINES

Flurazepam (Dalmane), **temazepam** (Restoril), and **triazolam** (Halcion) are benzodiazepines promoted by manufacturers as oral hypnotics. They have become the primary drugs of choice for treatment of insomnia. Compared to other hypnotics, the benzodiazepines are safer, less likely to cause abuse and dependence, and less likely to be lethal in overdose. In addition, they apparently do not suppress REM sleep or cause drug interactions as other hypnotics do. They are Schedule IV drugs and may cause abuse and dependence, especially with large doses or long-term use or both. The drugs should not be stopped abruptly after long-term use.

Flurazepam has been available and widely prescribed for several years. It decreases sleep induction time, decreases the number of awakenings and time spent awake, and increases duration or total amount of sleep time. Thus, it is effective in initial, intermittent, and terminal insomnia. Hypnotic effectiveness lasts about 1 month when taken nightly; it is not recommended for longer use. Flurazepam is converted to an active metabolite with a long half-life. This accounts for its greater effectiveness on the second or third night of administration and for the occurrence of residual sedation ("morning hangover"), which may last for several days after the drug is discontinued.

Temazepam and triazolam are newer drugs with shorter half-lives and inactive metabolites. Therefore, they are less likely to cause daytime sedation or accumulation.

Route and dosage ranges

Flurazepam and temazepam

Adults: PO 15–30 mg at bedtime
Elderly or debilitated adults: PO 15 mg at bedtime
Children: Not recommended

Triazolam

Adults: PO 0.25–0.5 mg at bedtime
Elderly or debilitated adults: PO 0.125–0.25 mg at bedtime
Children: Not recommended

Nonbarbiturates, Nonbenzodiazepines

Chloral hydrate, the oldest sedative–hypnotic drug, is relatively safe, effective, and inexpensive in usual ther-

TABLE 7-1. BARBITURATES

	Generic name	Trade name	Major clinical use	Routes and dosage ranges: Adults	Routes and dosage ranges: Children	Remarks
Short-acting barbiturates	Hexobarbital	Sombulex	Hypnotic, pre- and post-operative sedation	*Hypnotic:* PO 250–500 mg		Schedule III drug
	Pentobarbital sodium	Nembutal	Hypnotic, pre-operative sedation	*Sedative:* PO 30 mg 3–4 times daily; rectal 120–200 mg *Hypnotic:* PO 100 mg; rectal 120–200 mg; IM 150–200 mg; IV 100 mg	*Sedative:* PO, rectal 2 mg/kg/day in 4 divided doses *Hypnotic:* IM 25–80 mg	Pentobarbital and secobarbital are Schedule II controlled substances. They lose effectiveness as hypnotics in about 2 weeks of continuous administration.
	Secobarbital sodium	Seconal	Hypnotic, pre-operative sedation	*Sedative:* rectal 120–200 mg *Hypnotic:* PO 100 mg; rectal 120–200 mg; IV 50–250 mg; IM 100–200 mg	*Sedative:* PO, rectal 6 mg/kg/day in 3 divided doses *Hypnotic:* IM 3–5 mg/kg; maximum dose, 100 mg	See pentobarbital
Intermediate-acting barbiturates	Amobarbital sodium	Amytal	Hypnotic	*Sedative:* PO 50–300 mg daily in divided doses *Hypnotic:* PO 65–200 mg; IM, IV 65–500 mg	*Sedative:* over 12 years, same as adult dosage; under 12 years, PO 2 mg/kg/day in 4 divided doses *Hypnotic:* over 12 years, same as adult dosage	Schedule II drug
	Aprobarbital	Alurate	Sedative, hypnotic	*Sedative:* PO 40 mg 3 times daily *Hypnotic:* PO 40–160 mg		Schedule III drug
	Butabarbital sodium	Butisol	Sedative	*Sedative:* PO 50–120 mg/day in 3–4 divided doses *Hypnotic:* PO 50–100 mg	*Sedative:* PO 2 mg/kg/day in 3 divided doses	Schedule IV drug
	Talbutal	Lotusate	Hypnotic	PO 120 mg 15–30 minutes before bedtime		Schedule III drug
Long-acting barbiturates	Mephobarbital	Mebaral	Anticonvulsant	PO 200 mg at bedtime to 600 mg daily in divided doses	*Over 5 years:* PO 32–64 mg 3–4 times daily *Under 5 years:* PO 16–32 mg 3–4 times daily	Serum levels of phenobarbital can be used as guidelines for adjusting dosage because mephobarbital is metabolized to phenobarbital.
	Metharbital	Gemonil	Anticonvulsant	PO 100 mg at bedtime to 300 mg daily in divided doses; maximum dose, 800 mg daily	PO 5–15 mg/kg/day in divided doses	
	Phenobarbital	Luminal, others	Sedative, anticonvulsant	*Sedative:* PO, IM, IV 30–120 mg daily in 2–3 divided doses *Hypnotic:* PO, IM, IV 100–300 mg *Anticonvulsant:* PO 100–300 mg daily in 2–3 divided doses	*Sedative:* PO, rectal 1–2 mg/kg/day in 2–3 divided doses *Hypnotic:* PO 2–4 mg/kg *Anticonvulsant:* PO 5 mg/kg/day in 2–3 divided doses	Schedule IV drug. Not likely to produce abuse or dependence with chronic administration of anticonvulsant doses. Therapeutic plasma levels in seizure disorders are usually 10–25 μg/ml.

apeutic doses. It reportedly does not suppress REM sleep. When given as a hypnotic, it reduces initial insomnia (latency) and the number of awakenings. It produces drowsiness in about 15 minutes, and effects last up to 8 hours. Tolerance develops after about 2 weeks of continual use. It is a drug of abuse and may cause physical dependence.

Routes and dosage ranges

Adults: Sedative, PO, rectal suppository 250 mg 3 times daily after meals
Hypnotic, PO, rectal suppository 500–1000 mg at bedtime
Maximum daily dose, 2 g
Children: Sedative, PO, rectal suppository 25 mg/kg/day in 3–4 divided doses
Hypnotic, PO, rectal suppository 50 mg/kg
Maximum *single* dose, 1 g

Ethchlorvynol (Placidyl) is indicated only as an oral hypnotic for short-term use. It has a rapid onset—15 to 30 minutes—and a short duration of action. It suppresses REM sleep and may produce REM rebound when it is discontinued. It is a drug of abuse and produces tolerance and dependence. It induces drug-metabolizing enzymes in the liver and thereby accelerates biotransformation of drugs metabolized by those enzymes.

Route and dosage range

Adults: PO 500–1000 mg at bedtime
Children: Contraindicated

Ethinamate (Valmid) is an oral hypnotic with a rapid onset and brief duration of action. Its effects on REM sleep are unknown. Chronic use may produce psychologic and physical dependence.

Route and dosage range

Adults: PO 500–1000 mg at bedtime
Children: No dosage established

Glutethimide (Doriden) has been used as an oral hypnotic, but it is becoming obsolete because of significant abuse, physical and psychologic dependence, and tolerance. Also, both acute intoxication and chronic abuse are very difficult to treat.

Route and dosage range

Adults: PO 250–500 mg at bedtime
Children: No dosage established

Methyprylon (Noludar) is an oral hypnotic with potential for abuse, tolerance, and physical and psychologic dependence. It is similar to other sedative–hypnotic drugs in other characteristics.

Route and dosage ranges

Adults: PO 200–400 mg at bedtime
Children: PO 50 mg initially, up to 200 mg if necessary
Do not use in children under 3 months

Principles of therapy: sedative–hypnotic drugs

ASSESSMENT GUIDELINES

Assess the client's need for and response to sedative–hypnotic drugs. Initially, try to identify factors contributing to anxiety or insomnia and usual mechanisms for coping with stress. Also, assess the likelihood of drug abuse and dependence. People who abuse other drugs, including alcohol, are likely to abuse sedative–hypnotics. Once drug therapy is begun, assess the client's condition before each dose so that excessive sedation can be avoided.

NURSING INTERVENTIONS

Implement measures to decrease need for or increase effectiveness of sedative–hypnotic drugs, such as the following:

1. Modify the environment to promote rest and sleep by reducing noise and light or by changing ventilation and temperature.
2. Plan care to allow uninterrupted periods of rest and sleep when possible.
3. Relieve symptoms that interfere with rest and sleep. Drugs such as analgesics for pain or antitussives for cough are usually safer and more effective than sedative–hypnotic drugs. Nondrug measures such as positioning, exercise, and backrubs may be helpful in relieving muscle tension and other discomforts. Allowing the client to verbalize concerns, providing information so that the client knows what to expect, or consulting other personnel (*e.g.*, social worker, chaplain) may be useful in decreasing anxiety.
4. Assist the client to modify lifestyle when indicated. Some changes that may help in promoting sleep include avoiding or limiting intake of caffeine-containing beverages, limiting intake of fluids during evening hours if nocturia interferes with sleep, avoiding daytime naps, having a regular schedule of rest and sleep periods, increasing phys-

ical activity, and not trying to sleep unless tired or drowsy.

DRUG SELECTION AND SCHEDULING TO ACHIEVE TREATMENT GOALS

The goal of treatment with sedative–hypnotic drugs is to relieve anxiety or sleeplessness without permitting sensory perception, responsiveness to the environment, or alertness to drop below safe levels. Guidelines to help meet this goal include the following:

1. Give the least amount of the least potent drug for the shortest time that will be effective. This basic principle applies especially to sedative–hypnotic drug therapy because abuse, dependence, overdose, and suicide are more likely to occur with large doses and prolonged use.
2. As a general rule, start with small doses and increase them only if necessary. Low doses are often adequate in people who are elderly or debilitated or have liver or kidney disease.
3. Do not give sedative–hypnotic drugs every night unless really necessary. Intermittent administration helps maintain drug effectiveness and decreases risks of drug abuse and dependence. It also decreases disturbances of normal sleep patterns and REM rebound.
4. When sedative–hypnotic drugs are prescribed for outpatients, the prescription should limit the number of doses dispensed and the number of refills. This is one way of decreasing abuse, suicide, and other problems.

In chronic insomnia, no hypnotic drug has any real advantage over the others. They all lose their effectiveness in producing sleep after 1 to 2 weeks of daily use, except for the benzodiazepines, which last about 4 weeks. It is not helpful to switch from one drug to another because cross tolerance develops. To restore the sleep-producing effect, administration of the hypnotic drug must be interrupted for 1 to 2 weeks.

PEDIATRIC CONSIDERATIONS

In pediatric drug therapy, sedative–hypnotic drugs are rarely indicated except for phenobarbital in seizure disorders. If used, these drugs must be selected and given very cautiously because most of them have not been established as safe and effective for children.

GERIATRIC CONSIDERATIONS

In geriatric drug therapy, sedative–hypnotic drugs should be avoided or minimized despite frequent complaints of insomnia. Elderly people are likely to experience adverse effects and toxicity. Intensive efforts to find and treat the cause of insomnia are much safer. Physical discomfort and excessive sleep during daytime hours are common causes. Also, depression may cause insomnia, and depression is better treated with antidepressant drugs than with sedative–hypnotics.

NURSING ACTIONS: SEDATIVE-HYPNOTIC DRUGS

Nursing Actions	*Rationale/Explanation*
1. Administer accurately	
a. Give oral sedative–hypnotic drugs with a glass of water or other fluid.	The fluid enhances dissolution and absorption of the drug for a quicker onset of action.
b. Prepare the client for sleep before giving hypnotic doses of any drug.	Most of these drugs cause drowsiness within 15 to 30 minutes. The client should be in bed when he becomes drowsy to increase the therapeutic effectiveness of the sedative–hypnotic as well as to decrease the likelihood of falls or other injuries.
c. Do not leave a dose of sedative–hypnotic drugs at the client's bedside.	There is a risk that the client will save the drugs and use them to commit suicide or inadvertently take an overdose.
d. Use the following special precautions when giving barbiturates parenterally:	
(1) Do not use any parenteral solutions that are cloudy or contain a precipitate.	
(2) Do not mix with any other drugs in the same syringe.	Many drugs form precipitates if mixed with barbiturates.

Nursing Actions	***Rationale/Explanation***
(3) For intramuscular administration, inject deeply into a large muscle mass.	To minimize tissue irritation
(4) For intravenous injection, inject *slowly,* and have equipment available for artificial ventilation.	The intravenous route is usually used only for anesthesia or to terminate acute convulsions. Check agency policy regarding administration of intravenous medications by nurses.
(5) When giving barbiturates parenterally, be very careful to avoid extravasation of the drug into surrounding tissues and accidental intra-arterial injection.	Parenteral barbiturate solutions are highly alkaline and irritating to tissues. Accidental injection into an artery causes severe vasoconstriction and ischemia and can cause gangrene of the extremity. Acute, severe pain, edema, redness, and obliteration of pulses beyond the injection site occur rapidly in the affected limb.
2. Observe for therapeutic effects	Therapeutic effects depend largely on the reason for use.
a. When a drug is given for mild sedation and antianxiety effects, the recipient appears relaxed, perhaps drowsy, but is easily aroused.	The degree of drowsiness desired or tolerated could be different in a hospitalized person as compared with someone continuing work or other usual activities.
b. When a drug is given for hypnotic effects, the recipient goes to sleep within about 30 minutes, does not awaken more than once or twice, and sleeps several hours. During this time, the person can be easily aroused if necessary.	
c. When a drug is given for anticonvulsant effect, lack of seizure activity is a therapeutic effect.	
3. Observe for adverse effects	
a. Excessive sedation—drowsiness, stupor, slurred speech, impaired mobility, impaired mental processes, coma	This is due to depressant effects on the CNS. The severity depends mostly on drug dosage and the degree of drug tolerance that has developed. It is more likely to occur when drug therapy is begun and it usually decreases within a week.
b. Respiratory depression—hypoxemia, restlessness, dyspnea, shallow breathing	This stems from depression of the respiratory center in the medulla oblongata. Respiratory failure is the usual cause of death in acute drug intoxication. If death is delayed, it is likely to be caused by hypostatic pneumonia or pulmonary edema.
c. Shock—hypotension, tachycardia	Shock probably results from hypoxia and depression of the vasomotor center in the brain
d. Chronic intoxication—sedation, confusion, emotional lability, muscular incoordination, impaired mental processes, mental depression, gastrointestinal problems, weight loss	This is similar to chronic alcohol abuse.
e. Withdrawal or abstinence syndrome—anxiety, insomnia, restlessness, irritability, tremulousness, postural hypotension, seizures	This syndrome develops when the drugs are suddenly withdrawn in dependent persons. These symptoms progressively increase in severity. They can be prevented or minimized by using a long-acting agent (*i.e.,* phenobarbital) and gradually tapering the dose.
4. Observe for drug interactions	
a. Drugs that *increase* effects of sedative–hypnotics	
(1) CNS depressants—alcohol, narcotic analgesics, antidepressants, antihistamines, phenothiazine and other antipsychotic agents	All these drugs produce CNS depression when given alone. Any combination initially increases CNS depression and is potentially serious or even fatal. With long-term use, tolerance develops and CNS depression becomes less apparent. As a general rule, these drugs should not be given concurrently.
(2) Cimetidine	Prolongs elimination half-life and increases plasma concentrations of diazepam

Nursing Actions	***Rationale/Explanation***
b. Drugs that *decrease* effects of sedative–hypnotics Enzyme inducers (*e.g.,* barbiturates)	With chronic use these drugs antagonize their own actions and the actions of other drugs metabolized in the liver. They increase the rate of drug metabolism and elimination from the body.
c. Drugs that *increase* effects of barbiturates (in addition to those that increase effects of sedative–hypnotics in general)	
(1) Acidifying agents (*e.g.,* ascorbic acid)	These agents increase absorption of barbiturates in the gastrointestinal tract and increase drug reabsorption in renal tubules (except for phenobarbital).
(2) Benzodiazepines (*e.g.,* diazepam)	May potentiate sedative and respiratory effects of barbiturates.
d. Drugs that *decrease* barbiturate effects Alkalinizing agents (*e.g.,* sodium bicarbonate)	Increase renal excretion of phenobarbital
5. Teach clients	
a. Take sedative–hypnotic drugs as prescribed—do not increase the amount or frequency of administration.	This is especially important in view of drug dependence and other serious or life-threatening adverse reactions that can occur with these drugs. Risks of adverse reactions and habituation increase with prolonged use.
b. Do not take other drugs without the physician's knowledge.	Sedative–hypnotic drugs may interact with other drugs, including nonprescription cold remedies.
c. Avoid alcohol.	Alcohol depresses the CNS, as do the sedative–hypnotics. Combining the depressants can cause excessive drowsiness, which may progress to respiratory depression and death.
d. Use nondrug measures to relax or go to sleep when possible.	Individuals vary greatly in what they find relaxing or sleep inducing. For one person, it may be reading; for another, it may be watching television. It is advantageous for anyone to identify and use relaxation techniques rather than drugs.
e. Store sedative–hypnotic drugs safely.	
(1) Never keep at the bedside.	A person sedated by a previous dose may take additional doses if the drugs are within reach.
(2) Keep the drugs away from children and from adults who are confused or less than alert.	
f. Do not smoke, ambulate without help, drive a car, or operate machinery after taking a sedative–hypnotic drug.	All these activities may be hazardous if undertaken while the client is sedated. Clients who are taking relatively small doses are more drowsy at the beginning of drug therapy than later because they develop a tolerance for the drug. Clients who take large doses, such as a hypnotic dose at bedtime, are at high risk for injury.
g. Do not take "sleeping pills" evey night.	These drugs lose their effectiveness in inducing sleep within 2 weeks if taken every night. The exceptions are the benzodiazepines, which are effective for about 4 weeks with nightly administration.
h. When "sleeping pills" are discontinued, there may be increased dreaming or more frequent awakenings temporarily.	These effects are caused by withdrawal of the medication. They are *not* caused by the sleeping problem for which the medication was originally prescribed. Continuing the drug to avoid these effects aggravates the situation. This reaction is less likely with benzodiazepines.
i. As a general rule, take these drugs in the smallest effective dose for the shortest possible time.	To avoid occurrence of abuse and dependence

Selected References

American Medical Association (AMA) Division of Drugs: AMA Drug Evaluations, 5th ed. New York, John Wiley & Sons, 1983

Anderson PD: Basic Human Anatomy and Physiology: Clinical Implications for the Health Professions. Monterey, CA, Wadsworth, 1984

Burgess KE: Cerebral depressants: Their effects and safe administration. Nursing 15:46–53, August 1985

Byerley B, Gillin JC: Diagnosis and management of insomnia. Psychiatric Clin North Am 7:773–789, December 1984

Erman MK: Insomnia: Treatment approaches. Drug Ther 14:43–58, August 1984

Facts and Comparisons. St Louis, J B Lippincott (Updated monthly)

Guyton AC: Textbook of Medical Physiology, 7th ed. Philadelphia, W B Saunders, 1986

Hansten PD: Drug Interactions: Clinical Significance of Drug–Drug Interactions, 5th ed. Philadelphia, Lea & Febiger, 1985

Harris E: Sedative–hypnotic drugs. Am J Nurs 81:1329–1334, July 1981

Harvey SC: Hypnotics and sedatives. In Gilman AG, Goodman LS, Rall TW, Murad F (eds): The Pharmacological Basis of Therapeutics, 7th ed, pp 339–371. New York, Macmillan, 1985

Meyer R: Benzodiazepines in the elderly. Med Clin North Am 66:1017–1035, September 1982

Rodman MJ, Karch AM, Boyd EH, Smith DW: Pharmacology and Drug Therapy in Nursing, 3rd ed. Philadelphia, J B Lippincott, 1985

Simon C: Benzodiazepine hypnotics for insomnia. Am J Nurs 83:1330–1332, September, 1983

8

ANTIANXIETY DRUGS

Description and uses

Antianxiety agents are among the most frequently prescribed drugs. Central nervous system (CNS) depressants with sedative–hypnotic properties, they are used to relieve anxiety associated with emotional disorders, physical disorders, and situations of unusual environmental stress. Anxiety is difficult to define because it is primarily subjective, and related terminology is inconsistent. It may be described as worry, fear, tension, or nervousness that occurs when a person perceives a situation as threatening to physical, emotional, social, or economic well being. Behavioral manifestations may include a wide range of nonspecific problems, such as nausea, vomiting, diarrhea, frequent urination, tremors, hyperactivity, and insomnia. The perceived threat may be real, imaginary, or subconscious and outside the client's level of awareness. It is a nearly universal experience.

Types or degrees of anxiety are usually described as mild, moderate, or severe. Mild anxiety is also called "normal" anxiety when it occurs in response to a real problem or situation that can be validated by other people, such as a test, job interview, or performance evaluation. Thus, anxiety is part of everyday life and can be beneficial when it motivates the person toward constructive, problem-solving activities. Moderate anxiety occurs as an exaggerated response to the perceived problem or when there is no real reason to feel anxious. Moderate anxiety interferes with a client's ability to solve problems and reach goals; failure to solve problems and reach goals creates more anxiety. Thus, a cycle of self-perpetuating anxiety may develop. Severe anxiety or panic decreases a client's ability to function and may indicate the presence of a more serious emotional disorder such as depression or schizophrenia.

Causes of anxiety vary among persons and even in the same person at different times. Many of them occur with everyday events associated with home, work, social activities and chronic illness. Others occur episodically, such as an acute illness, death, divorce, loss of a job, starting a new job, or moving to a new location. A person who experiences several anxiety-provoking life events or stimuli close together, even when they are not especially severe or prolonged, may feel greater anxiety than a person who experiences the same events over a longer period. People in whom anxiety develops in response to indiscernible or seemingly mild stimuli are most likely to require psychotherapy or drug therapy.

The benzodiazepines are, by far, the most commonly used antianxiety agents. Chlordiazepoxide (Librium) is the prototype of the group, although diazepam (Valium) is more often prescribed. When first developed, the drugs were thought to be effective in relieving emotional distress with minimal adverse effects. Compared to the barbiturates, the benzodiazepines had a wider margin of safety between therapeutic and toxic doses and caused few significant drug interactions. They were also thought to be nonaddictive. Consequently, they were widely prescribed and popular with both physicians and clients. Within a few years, however, it became evident that the drugs were being abused and were causing physical and psychologic dependence. Although still widely used, the current trend is to prescribe the drugs more selectively and for shorter periods.

Pharmacologically, all the benzodiazepines have similar characteristics and produce the same effects. They apparently exert their therapeutic effects by binding with receptor sites in the brain and increasing the effects of gamma-aminobutyric acid (GABA), which inhibits transmission of nerve impulses in the brain. They are highly lipid soluble, widely distributed in body tissues, and extensively bound to plasma proteins. Most are metabolized in the liver and excreted in the urine. They are Schedule IV drugs under the Controlled Substances Act. They are well absorbed with oral administration. Chlordiazepoxide, diazepam, and lorazepam (Ativan) are available for parenteral use. Chlordiazepoxide and diazepam are usually painful, erratically absorbed, and produce lower serum levels when given intramuscularly; lorazepam is well absorbed with intramuscular use. Diazepam is frequently given intravenously.

The benzodiazepines differ in clinical indications for use because the manufacturers developed and promoted them for particular purposes. For example, clonazepam (Klonopin) is approved for use as an anticonvulsant; flurazepam (Dalmane), temazepam (Restoril), and triazolam (Halcion) are approved as hypnotics. Actually, a sufficient dose of any benzodiazepine would produce hypnotic effects. Diazepam (Valium) has been extensively studied and has more approved uses than other benzodiazepines.

The drugs also differ in duration of action. Several (*e.g.*, chlordiazepoxide, diazepam, clorazepate [Tranxene], and flurazepam) have long half-lives and produce pharmacologically active metabolites that also have long half-lives. As a result, these drugs require about 5 to 7 days to reach steady-state serum levels. Therapeutic effects (*e.g.*, decreased anxiety) and adverse effects (*e.g.*, sedation, ataxia) are more likely to occur after 2 or 3 days of therapy than initially. Such effects accumulate with chronic usage and persist for several days after the drugs are discontinued. The other drugs have short half-lives and produce inactive metabolites; thus their durations of action are much shorter, and they do not accumulate.

In addition to uses as antianxiety, hypnotic, and anticonvulsant agents, the drugs are also used for preoperative sedation, sedation before or during invasive diagnostic tests such as endoscopy and angiography, and prevention of delirium tremens in acute alcohol withdrawal. Contraindications include severe respiratory disorders, severe liver or kidney disease, hypersensitivity reactions, and a history of drug abuse.

Individual antianxiety drugs

BENZODIAZEPINES (Table 8-1)

NONBENZODIAZEPINE ANTIANXIETY AGENTS

Hydroxyzine (Vistaril) is chemically different from the benzodiazepines but shares a number of their clinical indications, such as treatment of anxiety and preoperative sedation. When hydroxyzine is combined with narcotic analgesics, dosage of the analgesics must be reduced because hydroxyzine potentiates their sedative effects. In contrast to the benzodiazepines, hydroxyzine has antiemetic and antihistaminic effects that account for a large portion of its clinical usefulness. It is often used, for example, to relieve nausea and vomiting that occur after surgery and with motion sickness. Its antihistaminic effects have been useful in treating urticaria and other manifestations of allergic dermatoses. Hydroxyzine is not a controlled drug.

Routes and dosage ranges

Adults: PO 75–400 mg daily in 3–4 divided doses
Preoperative and postoperative and prepartum and postpartum sedation, IM 25–100 mg in a single dose

Children: PO 2 mg/kg/day in 4 divided doses
Preoperative and postoperative sedation, IM 1 mg/kg in a single dose

Meprobamate (Equanil, Miltown) is an antianxiety agent that is chemically different from the benzodiazepines and hydroxyzine. It is also used as a muscle relaxant, but its effectiveness for that purpose is questionable. Meprobamate is a Schedule IV drug. Drug tolerance, abuse, dependence, and withdrawal symptoms occur with long-term use.

Route and dosage range

Adults: PO 1.2–1.6 g daily in 3–4 divided doses, maximum daily dose of 2.4 g

Children over 6 years: PO 25 mg/kg/day in 2–3 divided doses.

Children under 6 years: Not recommended

TABLE 8-1. BENZODIAZEPINES

Generic name	Brand name	Clinical indications	Half-life (hr)	Metabolite(s)	Routes and dosage ranges
Alprazolam	Xanax	Anxiety	Short (7–15)	Active	Adults: PO 0.25–0.5 mg 3 times daily; maximal dose, 4 mg daily in divided doses Elderly or debilitated adults: 0.25 mg 2–3 times daily, increased gradually if necessary
Chlordiazepoxide	Librium	Anxiety Acute alcohol withdrawal	Long (5–30)	Active	Adults: PO 15–100 mg daily, once at bedtime or in 3–4 divided doses. IM, IV 50–100 mg, maximal daily dose 300 mg; for short-term use Elderly or debilitated adults: PO 5–10 mg 2–4 times daily Children over 6 years: PO, IM 0.5 mg/kg/day in 3–4 divided doses Children under 6 years: Not recommended
Clonazepam	Klonopin	Seizure disorders	Long (20–40)	Inactive	Adults: PO 0.5 mg 3 times daily, increased by 0.5–1 mg every 3 days until seizures are controlled or adverse effects occur. Maximal daily dose, 20 mg
Clorazepate	Tranxene	Anxiety Seizure disorders	Long (30–100)	Active	Adults: PO 7.5 mg 3 times daily, increased by no more than 7.5 mg/week. Maximal daily dose, 90 mg Children 9–12 years: PO 7.5 mg 2 times daily, increased by no more than 7.5 mg/week. Maximal daily dose, 60 mg Children under 9 years: Not recommended
Diazepam	Valium	Anxiety Seizure disorders Acute alcohol withdrawal Muscle spasm Preoperative sedation Hypnotic	Long (20–50)	Active	Adults: PO 2–10 mg 2–4 times daily; sustained release, PO 15–30 mg once daily IM, IV 5–10 mg, repeated in 3–4 hours if necessary Elderly or debilitated adults: PO 2–5 mg once or twice daily, increased gradually if needed and tolerated. Children: PO 1–2.5 mg 3–4 times daily increased gradually if needed and tolerated Children > 30 days and <5 years of age: Seizures IM, IV 0.2–0.5 mg/2–5 minutes to a maximum of 5 mg Children 5 years or older: Seizures IM, IV 1 mg/2–5 minutes to a maximum of 10 mg
Flurazepam	Dalmane	Insomnia	Long (47–100)	Active	Adults: PO 15–30 mg at bedtime Elderly or debilitated adults: PO 15 mg at bedtime
Halazepam	Paxipam	Anxiety	Short (5–15)	Active	Adults: PO 20–40 mg 3–4 times daily
Lorazepam	Ativan	Anxiety Preoperative sedation	Short (8–15)	Inactive	Adults: PO 2–6 mg/day in 2–3 divided doses IM 0.05 mg/kg to a maximum of 4 mg IV 2 mg, diluted with 2 ml of sterile water, sodium chloride, or 5% dextrose injection, injected over 1 minute or longer Elderly or debilitated adults: PO 1–2 mg/day in divided doses
Oxazepam	Serax	Anxiety Acute alcohol withdrawal	Short (5–15)	Inactive	Adults: PO 30–120 mg daily in 3–4 divided doses Elderly or debilitated adults: PO 30 mg daily in 3 divided doses, gradually increased to 45–60 mg daily if necessary
Prazepam	Centrax	Anxiety	Long (30–100)	Active	Adults: PO 20–40 mg daily in divided doses Elderly or debilitated adults: PO 10–15 mg daily in divided doses
Temazepam	Restoril	Insomnia	Short (9–12)	Inactive	Adults: PO 15–30 mg at bedtime Elderly or debilitated adults: PO 15 mg at bedtime
Triazolam	Halcion	Insomnia	Ultrashort (1–5)	Inactive	Adults: PO 0.25–0.5 mg at bedtime Elderly or debilitated adults: PO 0.125–0.25 mg at bedtime

Principles of therapy: antianxiety drugs

ASSESSMENT GUIDELINES

Assess the client's need for antianxiety drugs. Manifestations of anxiety are more obvious with moderate or severe anxiety. Some guidelines for assessing anxiety include the following:

1. What is the client's statement of the situation? Does he dwell on physical problems or symptoms as a cause of distress? Does he describe himself as being worried, tense, or nervous? Is distress attributed to situational factors such as illness, death of a friend or family member, divorce, or job stress? All these may indicate anxiety, but additional information is needed for verification.
2. How does the stated problem affect the client's ability to function? Both interview and observation are needed to answer this question. Generally, try to determine to what extent the client is able to carry out his usual activities of daily living. If he is overactive and agitated or underactive and withdrawn, ability to function and productivity are likely to be impaired.
3. Obtain a careful history of drugs taken previously and currently, paying particular attention to alcohol ingestion and sedative–hypnotic drugs.
4. Try to identify factors that precipitate anxiety. For example, what does the client see as anxiety-provoking events? Is misinformation or lack of information a source of anxiety?
5. Observe for behavioral manifestations of anxiety such as facial grimaces, tense posture, and crying.
6. Observe for physiologic manifestations of anxiety. These may include increased blood pressure and pulse rate, increased rate and depth of respiration, increased muscle tension, and pale, cool skin.
7. If behavioral or physiologic manifestations seem to indicate anxiety, try to determine whether this is actually the case. Since similar manifestations may indicate pain or other problems rather than anxiety, the observer's perceptions must be validated by the client before appropriate action can be taken.
8. Identify coping mechanisms and support systems used in handling previous situations of stress and anxiety. These are very individualized. Reading, watching television, listening to music, or talking to a friend are examples. Some people are quiet and inactive, while others participate in strenuous activity. Some prefer to be alone, while others prefer being with a "significant other" or a group.

NURSING INTERVENTIONS

Use nondrug measures to relieve anxiety or to enhance the effectiveness of antianxiety drugs.

1. Support the client's usual coping mechanisms when feasible. That is, provide the opportunity for reading, exercising, or watching television, promote contact with significant others, or simply allow the client to be alone and uninterrupted for a while.
2. Use interpersonal and communication techniques to assist the client in handling anxiety. The degree of anxiety and the clinical situation largely determine which techniques are appropriate. For example, staying with the client, showing interest, listening, and allowing him to verbalize his concerns may be sufficient to decrease anxiety.

   Providing information may be a therapeutic technique when anxiety is related to medical conditions. Persons vary in the amount and kind of information desired. Generally, however, the following topics should be included:
   a. The overall treatment plan, including medical or surgical treatment, choice of outpatient care or hospitalization, expected length of treatment, and expected outcomes in terms of health and ability to function in activities of daily living.
   b. Specific diagnostic tests, including preparation, after-effects if any, and the way in which the client will be informed of results.
   c. Specific medication and treatment measures, including expected therapeutic results.
   d. What the client must do in carrying out the plan of treatment. When offering information and explanations to clients, keep in mind that anxiety interferes with intellectual functioning. Thus, communication should be brief, clear, and repeated as necessary because clients may misunderstand or forget what is said.
3. Modify the environment to decrease anxiety-provoking stimuli. Modifications may involve altering temperature, light, and noise levels or changing roommates.
4. Use measures to increase physical comfort. These may include a wide variety of activities, such as positioning, assisting to bathe or ambulate, giving backrubs, or providing fluids of the client's choice.
5. Consult with other services and departments in the client's behalf. For example, if financial problems

were identified as causes of anxiety, social services may be able to help.

GUIDELINES FOR RATIONAL USE OF ANTIANXIETY DRUGS

There are few clear-cut guidelines for using antianxiety drugs. Although still widely used, they are declining in popularity. One reason for their decreased use is their potential for producing drug abuse as well as physiologic and psychologic dependence. These drugs have been extensively abused, often in combination with alcohol. A second reason regards the advisability of drug therapy for everyday stresses and anxiety. Some authorities believe such usage promotes reliance on drugs and decreases development of more healthful coping mechanisms.

Few problems develop with short-term use of antianxiety drugs unless an overdose is taken or other CNS-depressant drugs are taken concurrently. Most problems occur with long-term use, especially of larger-than-usual doses. To minimize these problems, some recommendations include the following:

1. As a general rule, use antianxiety drugs only for those people whose anxiety causes disability and interference with job performance, interpersonal relationships, and other activities of daily living.
2. Give the drugs for short periods, at the lowest effective dose.
3. Chronic anxiety states are probably more effectively treated with psychotherapy.
4. Chronic physical disorders such as angina pectoris, hypertension, and peptic ulcer disease are more effectively treated with drugs specifically indicated in those conditions. The secondary effects claimed for antianxiety agents, such as muscle relaxant or antispasmodic effects, occur with any drug that depresses the CNS and are rarely significant with recommended doses.
5. Since anxiety often accompanies pain, antianxiety agents are sometimes used in the management of pain. In the management of chronic pain, antianxiety drugs have not demonstrated a definite benefit. Anxiety about recurrence of pain is probably better controlled by adequate analgesia than by antianxiety drugs.

DOSAGE AND SCHEDULING

Dosage requirements of antianxiety agents vary among clients. The goal of drug therapy is to find the lowest effective dose that does not cause excessive daytime drowsiness. One way of doing this is to start with the smallest dose that is likely to be effective, then evaluating the client's response and increasing the dose only if necessary. Additional guidelines include the following:

1. Generally, smaller-than-usual doses are adequate for elderly or debilitated clients. In the elderly, most benzodiazepines are metabolized more slowly and half-lives are longer than in younger adults. Exceptions are oxazepam and lorazepam, whose half-lives and dosages are the same for elderly adults as for younger ones.
2. Larger-than-usual doses may be needed for clients who are severely anxious or agitated. Also, large doses are usually required to relax skeletal muscle, control muscle spasm, control seizures, and provide sedation before surgery, cardioversion, endoscopy, and angiography.
3. The benzodiazepines are usually given in three or four daily doses. This is necessary for the short-acting agents, but there is no pharmacologic basis for multiple daily doses of the long-acting drugs. Because of their prolonged actions, all or most of the daily dose can be given at bedtime. This schedule promotes sleep, and there is usually enough residual sedation to maintain antianxiety effects throughout the next day. If necessary, one or two small supplemental doses may be given during the day.
4. When antianxiety drugs are used with narcotic analgesics, the analgesic dose should be reduced initially and increased gradually to avoid excessive CNS depression.
5. The withdrawal syndrome that indicates physical dependence on benzodiazepines is more likely to occur if the drug is short acting, has been taken regularly for more than 4 months, if higher doses have been taken, and if the drug is abruptly discontinued. Common manifestations include increased anxiety, insomnia, irritability, headache, tremor, and palpitations. Less common but more serious manifestations include confusion, abnormal perception of movement, depersonalization, psychosis, and seizures. Although the drugs have not been proved effective for more than 4 months of regular use, this period is probably exceeded quite frequently in clinical practice. The dose should be tapered and gradually discontinued following long-term use.

USE IN PREGNANCY AND LACTATION

Antianxiety drugs should generally be avoided during pregnancy and lactation. If taken during the first trimester, they may cause physical deformities in the fetus. If taken during labor, they may cause sedation and respiratory depression in the newborn. If taken during lactation, most of the drugs are excreted in breast milk and may cause lethargy and weight loss in infants.

PEDIATRIC CONSIDERATIONS

In pediatric drug therapy with benzodiazepines, only chlordiazepoxide and diazepam have been extensively used. Others do not have established dosages and are not recommended for use in children.

GERIATRIC CONSIDERATIONS

In geriatric drug therapy, the short-acting benzodiazepines are the drugs of choice. The dose should generally be small, at least initially, and increased only if necessary.

USE IN LIVER DISEASE

In the presence of liver disease (*e.g.,* cirrhosis, hepatitis), there is slowed metabolism of most benzodiazepines with resultant accumulation and increased risk of adverse effects. If a benzodiazepine is deemed necessary, oxazepam or lorazepam is preferred because liver disease does not significantly affect drug elimination.

NURSING ACTIONS: ANTIANXIETY DRUGS

Nursing Actions	*Rationale/Explanation*
1. Administer accurately	
a. When feasible, give larger proportions of the ordered daily dose at bedtime.	To promote sleep, minimize adverse reactions, and allow more nearly normal daytime activities
b. If given a choice, administer antianxiety agents orally when feasible.	These drugs are well absorbed from the gastrointestinal tract, and onset of action occurs within a few minutes. Chlordiazepoxide and diazepam are better absorbed with oral than with intramuscular administration. When injected intramuscularly, these drugs crystallize in muscle tissue and are slowly absorbed so that many hours may be required to achieve therapeutic concentrations in the blood.
c. Give intramuscular antianxiety agents deeply, into large muscle masses such as the gluteus muscle of the hip. If repeated intramuscular injections are necessary, rotate injection sites.	These drugs are irritating to tissues and may cause pain at the injection site.
d. To give chlordiazepoxide parenterally, follow manufacturer's instructions for preparation of the solution.	This drug is dispensed in powder form because it is unstable in solution. Preparation and administration differ with intramuscular and intravenous routes.
e. To give diazepam intravenously (1) Inject slowly, at least 1 minute for each 5 mg (1 ml) (2) Do not use small veins such as wrist veins or those on the dorsum of the hand. (3) Be very careful to avoid intra-arterial administration or extravasation into surrounding tissues. (4) If not feasible to inject directly into a vein, it may be injected slowly through infusion tubing as close as possible to the venipuncture site.	These precautions are necessary to prevent apnea and minimize venous thrombosis, phlebitis, local irritation, edema and vascular impairment due to the highly irritating effect of diazepam on body tissues.
(5) Have equipment available for respiratory assistance.	Apnea may occur.
f. Do not mix chlordiazepoxide or diazepam with any other drug in a syringe or add to intravenous fluids.	Chlordiazepoxide is unstable in solution, and diazepam is physically incompatible with other drugs and solutions.
g. Hydroxyzine can be mixed in the same syringe with atropine, meperidine, and most other narcotic analgesics	Hydroxyzine is also very irritating to body tissues and causes pain with intramuscular injection. It is not given subcutan-

Nursing Actions	***Rationale/Explanation***
that are likely to be ordered at the same time for preoperative sedation. Give hydroxyzine orally and intramuscularly only.	eously because of tissue irritation with pain, induration and possible thrombus formation.
2. Observe for therapeutic effects	As with most other drugs, therapeutic effects depend on the reason for use. Observations of individual recipients of antianxiety drugs can be more accurate if the same nurse assesses the person before and after the drug is given.
a. When a drug is given for anxiety, observe for (1) Verbal statements such as "less worried," "more relaxed," "resting better" (2) Decrease or absence of behavioral manifestations of anxiety such as rigid posture, facial grimaces, and crying (3) Decrease or absence of physiologic manifestations of anxiety such as elevated blood pressure, pulse, and respiration	
b. When a drug is given for sedation or sleep, drowsiness should be apparent within a few minutes.	
c. When diazepam is given intravenously for control of acute convulsive disorders, seizure activity should decrease or stop almost immediately.	
d. When hydroxyzine is given for nausea and vomiting, absence of vomiting and verbal statements of relief indicate therapeutic effect.	
e. When hydroxyzine is given for antihistaminic effects in skin disorders, observe for decreased itching and fewer statements of discomfort.	
3. Observe for adverse effects	Most adverse reactions are caused by CNS depression.
a. Oversedation—drowsiness, ataxia, fatigue, dizziness, respiratory depression	Drowsiness is the most common adverse effect, although the others also occur relatively often. They are more likely to occur with large doses or if the recipient is elderly, debilitated, or has liver disease that slows drug metabolism. Respiratory depression and apnea are most likely to occur with rapid intravenous administration of diazepam or chlordiazepoxide.
b. Hypotension	More likely to occur with rapid intravenous administration of diazepam or chlordiazepoxide.
c. Pain and induration at injection site	These symptoms are caused by local irritation of tissues. They can be minimized by deep intramuscular injection into the large gluteal muscles or intravenous injection into a large vein.
d. Paradoxic excitement, anger, aggression, and hallucinations	This reaction is difficult to predict but may occur more often in clients who are more than 50 years of age and in those who are psychotic.
e. Skin rashes	
4. Observe for drug interactions	
a. Drugs that *increase* effects of antianxiety agents (1) CNS depressants—alcohol, antidepressants, barbiturates and other sedative–hypnotics, narcotic analgesics, phenothiazines and other antipsychotics	All these drugs cause additive CNS depression, sedation, and respiratory depression. Combinations of these drugs are hazardous and should be avoided. Alcohol with antianxiety drugs may cause respiratory depression, coma, and convulsive seizures.

Nursing Actions	***Rationale/Explanation***
(2) Cimetidine, disulfiram, isoniazid	These drugs interfere with the hepatic metabolism of diazepam and other benzodiazepines. They do not affect elimination of oxazepam or lorazepam.
b. Drugs that *decrease* effects of antianxiety agents (1) CNS stimulants—adrenergic drugs (*e.g.*, ephedrine, pseudoephedrine, phenylpropanolamine), theophylline, caffeine	Adrenergic drugs are frequent components of over-the-counter cold remedies, decongestants, and appetite suppressants.
5. Teach clients **a.** Use the drugs only when necessary—do not increase dosage, do not increase frequency of administration, and do not take for prolonged periods.	These drugs are frequently misused and abused. They can produce psychologic and physiologic dependence, which may eventually cause worse problems than the original anxiety.
b. These drugs produce more beneficial effects and fewer adverse reactions when used in the smallest effective doses and for the shortest duration feasible in particular circumstances.	
c. Do not drive a car or operate machinery.	All these drugs can produce drowsiness and staggering gait, which interfere with both mental and physical functioning. The risk of serious injury is great unless precautions are taken.
d. Do not take other drugs without the physician's knowledge, including alcohol or nonprescription sleeping medications.	These drugs also cause drowsiness and sedation and the additive effects of the combination can result in serious respiratory depression and coma. Alcohol is especially hazardous in this regard and should generally be avoided while antianxiety drugs are being taken.
e. Large amounts of coffee can cancel or decrease the sedative and antianxiety effects of these drugs.	Coffee contains caffeine, which is a stimulant. Cola beverages and tea also contain caffeine, although in lesser amounts. Other stimulant drugs, such as appetite suppressants, can also decrease the effects of these drugs.

Selected References

American Medical Association (AMA) Division of Drugs: AMA Drug Evaluations, 5th ed. New York, John Wiley & Sons, 1983

Baldessarini RJ: Drugs and the treatment of psychiatric disorders. In Gilman AG, Goodman LS, Rall TW, Murad F (eds): The Pharmacological Basis of Therapeutics, 7th ed. pp 387–445. New York, Macmillan, 1985

Burgess KE: Cerebral depressants: Their effects and safe administration. Nursing 15:46–53, August 1985

Evans RL, Richart NA: Psychiatric disorders. In Wiener MB, Pepper GA (eds): Clinical Pharmacology and Therapeutics in Nursing, 2d ed, pp 622–654. New York, McGraw-Hill, 1985

Facts and Comparisons. St. Louis, J B Lippincott (Updated monthly)

Hansten PD: Drug Interactions: Clinical Significance of Drug–Drug Interactions, 5th ed. Philadelphia, Lea & Febiger, 1985

Harris E: Sedative–hypnotic drugs. Am J Nurs 81:1329–1334, July 1981

Harvey SL: Hypnotics and sedatives. In Gilman AG, Goodman LS, Rall TW, Murad F (eds): The Pharmacological Basis of Therapeutics. 7th ed, pp 339–371. New York, Macmillan, 1985

Lader M: The efficiency and safety of drugs to treat anxiety. In Stancer HC, Garfunkel PE, Rakoff VM (eds): Guidelines for the Use of Psychotropic Drugs: A Clinical Handbook, pp 303–313. Jamaica, NY, Spectrum Publications, 1984

Malseed RT: Pharmacology: Drug Therapy and Nursing Considerations, 2d ed. Philadelphia, J B Lippincott, 1985

Rodman MJ, Karch AM, Boyd EH, Smith DW: Pharmacology and Drug Therapy in Nursing, 3rd ed. Philadelphia, J B Lippincott, 1985

Sellers EM: Summary of the guidelines for the use of psychotropic drugs in the treatment of anxiety. In Stancer HC, Garfunkel PE, Rakoff VM (eds): Guidelines for the Use of Psychotropic Drugs: A Clinical Handbook, pp 297–301. Jamaica, NY, Spectrum Publications, 1984

Tallman JF, Paul SM, Skolnick P, Gallager DW: Receptors for the age of anxiety: Pharmacology of the benzodiazepines. Science 207:274–281, January 1980

9

ANTIPSYCHOTIC DRUGS

Description and uses

Antipsychotic drugs are used mainly for treatment of severe mental illnesses such as schizophrenia and other psychotic disorders. These drugs come from several different chemical groups and are broadly categorized as phenothiazines and nonphenothiazines. Despite chemical differences, pharmacologic actions of the antipsychotic drugs are very similar. These drugs antagonize the action of dopamine in the brain. Dopamine is a catecholamine neurotransmitter. Antipsychotic drugs are also called *major tranquilizers* and *neuroleptics.* The first term is misleading because it implies that the drugs' antipsychotic effects result from their sedative or tranquilizing actions; actually, additional actions are involved. The second term indicates drug effects such as psychomotor slowing, emotional quieting, and extrapyramidal reactions.

The largest and most frequently used group of antipsychotic drugs is the phenothiazines, of which chlorpromazine (Thorazine) is the prototype. The phenothiazines are well absorbed after oral and parenteral administration. They are distributed to most body tissues and reach high concentrations in the brain. They are metabolized in the liver and excreted in urine. Some metabolites have pharmacologic activity similar to that of the parent compound. These drugs cross the placenta and appear in the fetus as well as in the milk of nursing mothers. They do not cause physical or psychologic drug dependence.

Phenothiazines exert many pharmacologic effects in the body. These include central nervous system (CNS) depression, autonomic nervous system depression (antiadrenergic and anticholinergic effects), antiemetic effect, lowering of body temperature, hypersensitivity reactions, and others. All phenothiazines are similar in pharmacologic actions and antipsychotic effectiveness. They differ mainly in potency and adverse effects. Differences in potency are demonstrated by the fact that some phenothiazines (piperazine subgroup) are as effective in doses of a few milligrams as others (aliphatic and piperadine subgroups) are in doses of several hundred milligrams. All phenothiazines produce the same kinds of adverse effects, but the subgroups differ in incidence and severity of particular adverse effects.

Nonphenothiazine antipsychotic drugs represent several different chemical groups but are few in number. These drugs have pharmacologic actions, clinical uses, and adverse effects very similar to those of the phenothiazines.

The major clinical indication for use of antipsychotic drugs is psychosis. Psychotic persons are unable to distinguish reality. They react to internal stimuli rather than to the real world. Consequently, their inaccurate perceptions of reality lead them to behave in disorganized, bizarre ways. Some have hallucinations (hearing or seeing people or objects that are not present in the external environment). Some have delusions (false beliefs, such as the conviction that they are being poisoned or otherwise harmed) that they adhere to in the absence of reason or evidence.

Most psychoses are functional rather than organic. *Organic psychoses* are caused by a physical disorder such as brain damage related to cerebrovascular disease or head injury. In *functional psychoses,* no organic cause for the symptoms is evident.

Schizophrenia is the most common functional psychosis. It is not a single disease; rather, it includes a variety of conditions or groups of symptoms. Subgroups of schizophrenia are called simple, hebephrenic, catatonic, and paranoid types; symptoms and drug therapy are similar for all types. Major symptoms include disturbed thinking, abnormal emotional responses such as inappropriate laughter, autism (self-absorption in which the person pays no attention to the environment or to other people), and behavior ranging from complete inactivity to hyperactivity, agitation, aggressiveness, and combativeness. These symptoms may begin gradually or suddenly at almost any age. They are more likely to start during adolescence or early adulthood when a stressful situation is encountered. The cause of schizophrenia is unknown.

Antipsychotic drugs are used in other psychiatric disorders as well as schizophrenia, but the indications for use are less clear-cut. Thus, they are probably useful in chronic brain syndromes (relatively permanent organic impairments of cerebral function related to various disorders, such as brain tumor) to control hyperactivity, delusions, agitation, and other psychotic symptoms. They may be useful in the manic phase of manic–depressive disorder to control manic behavior until lithium, the drug of choice, becomes effective. They are not generally used for mental depression but may occasionally be used to treat agitated depression.

Clinical indications not associated with psychiatric illness include prevention and treatment of nausea and vomiting, potentiation of pain-relieving effects of narcotic analgesics, and treatment of intractable hiccups. These drugs are occasionally used to prevent shivering during hypothermia. Antipsychotic agents relieve nausea and vomiting by depressing the function of the chemoreceptor trigger zone (CTZ). The CTZ is a group of neurons in the medulla oblongata that, when activated by physical or psychologic stimuli, causes nausea and vomiting. The pain-relieving effects of antipsychotic agents probably result from their sedative properties. The mechanisms by which antipsychotic agents relieve hiccups and prevent shivering associated with hypothermia are unclear.

Antipsychotic drugs are generally not indicated in acute organic brain syndromes (severe mental symptoms caused by head injury, infection, or other pathologic conditions in a previously normal person) or toxic psychosis (psychosis due to ingestion of poisonous agents such as alcohol). They may precipitate seizures during drug-withdrawal reactions and increase symptoms associated with abuse of hallucinogenic drugs. An exception is their use to treat amphetamine-induced psychosis. Toxic delirium caused by excessive dosage of atropine or other anticholinergic drugs may be intensified and prolonged by antipsychotic drugs because these drugs also have anticholinergic properties. Antipsychotic drugs are not indicated in treatment of symptoms resulting from alcohol abuse, including acute and chronic alcoholism as well as alcohol withdrawal. Other contraindications include CNS depression, coma, hypersensitivity reactions, blood dyscrasias, and severe liver disease.

Individual antipsychotic drugs

PHENOTHIAZINES

Commonly used phenothiazine antipsychotic drugs are listed in Table 9-1. Promethazine (Phenergan) is a phenothiazine that is not used clinically for antipsychotic effects but is often used for sedative, antiemetic, and antihistaminic effects.

NONPHENOTHIAZINES

Chlorprothixene (Taractan) and **thiothixene** (Navane) are chemically similar to phenothiazines. They are potent and effective antipsychotic drugs used clinically only for their antipsychotic effects, although they produce other effects similar to those of the phenothiazines. A 100-mg dose of chloroprothixene is therapeutically equivalent to 100 mg of chlorpromazine. A 4-mg dose of thiothixene is equivalent to 100 mg of chlorpromazine.

Routes and dosage ranges

Chlorprothixene

Adults: Acute psychosis, PO, IM 75–200 mg daily in divided doses, increased to a maximal oral dose of 600 mg daily, if necessary

Elderly or debilitated adults: PO, IM 30–100 mg daily in divided doses, reduced when symptoms have been controlled

Children over 12 years: PO, IM same as adults

Children 6–12 years: PO 30–100 mg daily in divided doses. IM dosage not established

Children under 6 years: dosage not established

Thiothixene

Adults: PO 6–10 mg daily in divided doses. Maximal daily dose, 60 mg
Acute psychosis, IM 8–16 mg daily in divided doses. Maximal daily dose, 30 mg

Elderly or debilitated adults: PO, IM one third to one half the usual adult dosage

Children over 12 years: same as adults

Children under 12 years: dosage not established

(Text continues on p. 84.)

TABLE 9-1. PHENOTHIAZINE ANTIPSYCHOTIC DRUGS

Generic name	Trade name	Routes of administration and dosage ranges	Major side-effects (incidence)			Remarks
			Sedation	*Extra-pyramidal reactions*	*Hypotension*	
Chlorpromazine	Thorazine	Adults: PO 200–600 mg daily in divided doses Dose may be increased by 100 mg daily q2–3 days until symptoms are controlled, adverse effects occur, or a maximum daily dose of 2 g is reached. IM 25–100 mg initially for acute psychotic symptoms, repeated in 1–4 hours PRN until control is achieved Elderly or debilitated adults: PO one third to one half usual adult dose, increased by 25 mg daily q2–3 days if necessary IM 10 mg q6–8h until acute symptoms are controlled Children: PO IM 0.5 mg/kg q4–8h. Maximum IM dose, 40 mg daily in children below 5 years of age and 75 mg for older children	High	Moderate	Moderate to high	Sustained-release capsules and liquid concentrates are available
Acetophenazine	Tindal	Adults: PO 60 mg daily in divided doses, may be gradually increased by 20 mg daily until therapeutic or adverse effects occur Usual optimal dosage is 80–120 mg daily. Elderly or debilitated adults: one third to one half usual adult dose Children: 0.8–1.6 mg/kg/day in 3 divided doses (maximum, 80 mg daily)	Moderate	High	Low	20 mg is equivalent to 100 mg of chlorpromazine
Fluphenazine decanoate and enanthate	Prolixin decanoate; Prolixin enanthate	Adults under 50 years: IM, SC 12.5 mg initially followed by 25 mg every 2 weeks Dosage requirements rarely exceed 100 mg q2–6 weeks. Adults over 50, debilitated clients or clients with a history of extrapyramidal reactions: 2.5 mg initially followed by 2.5–5 mg q10–14 days Children: No dosage established	Low to moderate	High	Low	
Fluphenazine hydrochloride	Prolixin, Permitil	Adults: PO 2.5–10 mg initially, gradually reduced to maintenance dose of 1–5 mg (doses above 3 mg are rarely necessary) Acute psychosis: IM 1.25 mg initially, increased gradually to 2.5–10 mg daily in 3–4 divided doses Elderly or debilitated adults: PO 1–2.5 mg daily IM one third to one half the usual adult dose	Low to moderate	High	Low	2 mg of the oral hydrochloride salt is equivalent to 100 mg of chlorpromazine

TABLE 9-1. PHENOTHIAZINE ANTIPSYCHOTIC DRUGS (*Continued*)

Generic name	Trade name	Routes of administration and dosage ranges	Major side-effects (incidence)			Remarks
			Sedation	*Extra-pyramidal reactions*	*Hypotension*	
		Children: PO 0.75–10 mg daily in children 5 to 12 years IM no dosage established				
Mesoridazine	Serentil	Adults and children over 12 years: PO 150 mg daily in divided doses initially, increased gradually in 50-mg increments until symptoms are controlled. Usual dose range, 100–400 mg IM 25–175 mg daily in divided doses Elderly and debilitated adults: one third to one half usual adult dose Children under 12 years: No dosage established	High	Low	Moderate	50 mg is equivalent to 100 mg of chlorpromazine
Perphenazine	Trilafon	Adults: PO 16–64 mg daily in divided doses Acute psychoses: IM 5–10 mg initially, then 5 mg q6h if necessary. Maximum daily dose, 15 mg for ambulatory clients and 30 mg for hospitalized clients Elderly or debilitated adults: PO, IM one third to one half usual adult dose Children: PO dosages not established, but the following amounts have been given in divided doses: Ages 1–6 years, 4–6 mg daily; 6–12 years, 6 mg daily; over 12 years, 6–12 mg daily	Low to moderate	High	Low	8 mg is equivalent to 100 mg of chlorpromazine
Prochlorperazine	Compazine	Adults: PO 10 mg 3–4 times daily, increased gradually (usual daily dose, 100–150 mg) IM 10–20 mg; may be repeated in 2–4 hours. Switch to oral form as soon as possible Children over age 2 years: PO, rectal 2.5 mg 2–3 times daily IM 0.06 mg/lb	Moderate	High	Low	10 mg is equivalent to 100 mg of chlorpromazine
Promazine	Sparine	Adults: initially, 50–150 mg IM; maintenance, PO, IM 10–200 mg q4–6h Children over 12 years: 10–25 mg q4–6h	Moderate	Moderate	Moderate	200 mg is equivalent to 100 mg of chlorpromazine
Thioridazine	Mellaril	Adults: PO 150–300 mg daily in divided doses, gradually increased if necessary to a maximum daily dose of 800 mg Elderly or debilitated adults: PO one third to one half the usual adult dose Children 2 years and over: 1	High	Low	Moderate	Thioridazine is probably the most frequently used antipsychotic drug. It differs from other phenothiazines by lacking antiemetic effects. It also has little, if any, effect

TABLE 9-1. PHENOTHIAZINE ANTIPSYCHOTIC DRUGS *(Continued)*

Generic name	Trade name	Routes of administration and dosage ranges	Major side-effects (incidence)			Remarks
			Sedation	*Extra-pyramidal reactions*	*Hypotension*	
		mg/kg/day in divided doses. Maximum dose, 3 mg/kg/day Children under 2 years: no dosage established				on seizure threshold; 100 mg is equivalent to 100 mg of chlorpromazine
Trifluoperazine	Stelazine	Adults: Outpatients PO 2–4 mg daily in divided doses Hospitalized clients, PO 4–10 mg daily in divided doses Acute psychoses: IM 1–2 mg q4–5h, maximum of 10 mg daily Elderly or debilitated adults: PO, IM one third to one half usual adult dose If given IM, give at less frequent intervals than above. Children 6 years or over: PO, IM 1–2 mg daily, maximum daily dose 15 mg Children under 6 years: No dosage established	Moderate	High	Low	5 mg is equivalent to 100 mg of chlorpromazine
Triflupromazine	Vesprin	Adults: PO, IM 50–150 mg daily Elderly or debilitated adults: Acute psychosis: IM 10–75 mg daily; PO 20–30 mg daily in divided doses Children: PO 2 mg/kg/day in divided doses. Maximum daily dose, 150 mg. IM (children over 2½ years) 0.2–0.25 mg/kg/day to a maximum of 10 mg daily	High	Moderate	Moderate to high	25 mg is equivalent to 100 mg of chlorpromazine

Haloperidol (Haldol) is a butyrophenone compound and the only drug of this group available for use in psychiatric disorders. A related drug, droperidol (Inapsine), is used in anesthesia and as an antiemetic. Haloperidol is a frequently used antipsychotic agent that is chemically different but pharmacologically similar to the phenothiazines. It is a potent, long-acting drug that is readily absorbed following oral or intramuscular administration, metabolized in the liver, and excreted in urine and bile. Haloperidol may cause adverse effects similar to those of other antipsychotic drugs. Usually, it produces a relatively low incidence of hypotension and sedation and a high incidence of extrapyramidal effects.

Haloperidol is used as the initial drug in treating psychotic disorders or as a substitute in clients who are hypersensitive or refractory to the phenothiazines. It is also used for some conditions in which other antipsychotic drugs are not used. These include mental retardation with hyperkinesia (abnormally increased motor activity), Tourette's syndrome (a rare disorder characterized by involuntary movements and vocalizations), and Huntington's disease (a rare genetic disorder that involves progressive psychiatric symptoms and involuntary movements). A 2-mg dose is therapeutically equivalent to 100 mg of chlorpromazine.

Routes and dosage ranges

Adults: Acute psychosis, PO 1–15 mg daily initially in divided doses, gradually increased to 100 mg daily if necessary. Usual maintenance dose, 2–8 mg daily

IM 2–10 mg q1–8h until symptoms are controlled (usually within 72 hours)

Chronic refractory schizophrenia, PO 6–15 mg daily to a maximum of 100 mg daily. Dosage is

produced by each drug, response to antipsychotic drugs in the past, subjective response to the drugs, such as the adverse reactions a person is willing to tolerate, supervision available, and the physician's experience with a particular drug. Some specific factors include the following:

1. Antipsychotic drugs are apparently equally effective regardless of the client's symptoms. Drugs producing greater sedation are often prescribed for agitated, overactive persons, and drugs producing less sedation are prescribed for those who are apathetic and withdrawn.
2. Despite the similarities of antipsychotic drugs in both therapeutic benefits and adverse effects, some persons who do not respond well to one type of antipsychotic drug may respond to another. Unfortunately, there is no way of predicting which drug is likely to be most effective for a particular client.
3. There is no logical basis for giving more than one antipsychotic agent at a time. There is no therapeutic advantage, and the risk of serious adverse reactions is increased.
4. If lack of therapeutic response requires that another antipsychotic drug be substituted for the one a client is currently receiving, this substitution must be done gradually. Abrupt substitution may cause reappearance of symptoms. This can be avoided by gradually decreasing doses of the old drug while substituting equivalent doses of the new one.
5. Nonphenothiazine antipsychotic drugs are probably best used for clients with chronic schizophrenia whose symptoms have not been controlled by the phenothiazines and for clients with hypersensitivity reactions to the phenothiazines. Although adverse reactions to these agents are very similar to those caused by phenothiazines, clients who are allergic to the phenothiazines can usually tolerate one of the other antipsychotic drugs.
6. Unless choice of a drug is dictated by the client's previous favorable response to a particular drug, the preferred drug should be available in both parenteral and oral forms for flexibility of administration.
7. Clients who are unable or unwilling to take daily doses of a maintenance antipsychotic drug may be given periodic injections of a long-acting form of fluphenazine.
8. Any person who has had an allergic or hypersensitivity reaction to an antipsychotic drug should generally not be given that particular drug again or any drug in the same chemical subgroup. Cross sensitivity apparently occurs, and the likelihood of another allergic reaction is high.

DOSAGE AND ADMINISTRATION

Dosage and route of administration must be individualized. Initial drug therapy for acute psychotic episodes usually requires high dosage, intramuscular administration, divided doses, and hospitalization. Symptoms are usually controlled within 48 to 72 hours, after which oral drugs can be given and dosage gradually reduced to the lowest effective amount. For maintenance therapy, drug dosages are usually much smaller, oral drugs are preferred, and a single bedtime dose is effective for most people. This schedule increases compliance with prescribed drug therapy, allows better nighttime sleep, and decreases hypotension and daytime sedation. Effective maintenance therapy requires close supervision and contact with the client and family members.

ADDITIONAL GUIDELINES

Duration of therapy

Antipsychotic drugs are usually given for months or years. There are no clear guidelines on duration of drug therapy. Drug-free periods of 1 to 3 days are recommended once or twice yearly to decrease the total amount of drug given, decrease adverse effects, allow earlier detection of adverse effects such as tardive dyskinesia, and reevaluate the client's need for the drug.

Management of extrapyramidal symptoms

For most people receiving antipsychotic drugs, concurrent antiparkinson drug therapy should be given only after extrapyramidal symptoms (*e.g.*, abnormal rigidity and muscle movements) occur. Such neuromuscular symptoms appear in fewer than half the clients taking antipsychotic drugs and are better handled by reducing dosage if this does not cause recurrence of psychotic symptoms. If antiparkinson drugs are given, they should be gradually discontinued in about 3 months. Extrapyramidal symptoms do not usually recur despite continued administration of the same antipsychotic drug and the same dosage.

Temporary discontinuation of therapy

Antipsychotic drugs should be discontinued in persons receiving spinal or epidural anesthesia or adrenergic blocking agents because of the increased risk of hypotension. They should also be discontinued at least 48 hours before surgery because they potentiate other

CNS-depressant drugs that are often used before, during, and after surgery.

USE IN PREGNANCY, LABOR, DELIVERY, LACTATION

Antipsychotic drugs are not recommended for use during pregnancy, labor, delivery, or lactation because of potential adverse effects on the fetus and newborn.

PEDIATRIC CONSIDERATIONS

In pediatric drug therapy, many of the antipsychotic drugs have not been established as safe and effective.

GERIATRIC CONSIDERATIONS

In geriatric drug therapy, antipsychotic drugs should be used very cautiously. Before these drugs are started, a thorough assessment is needed because psychiatric illness in elderly people is often a result of other drugs or of organic disease. If this is the case, stopping the offending drug or treating the medical condition may cancel the need for antipsychotic drugs. When antipsychotic drugs are necessary, adverse effects can be minimized by giving small, divided doses (one third to one half the usual adult dosage), increasing dosage gradually, and reducing dosage to the lowest effective level as soon as possible. Adverse effects are likely to occur in elderly people because of slowed drug metabolism.

NURSING ACTIONS: ANTIPSYCHOTIC DRUGS

Nursing Actions	*Rationale/Explanation*
1. Administer accurately	
a. When feasible, give oral antipsychotic drugs once daily, within 1 to 2 hours of bedtime.	Peak sedation occurs about 2 hours after administration and aids sleep. Hypotension, dry mouth, and other adverse reactions are less bothersome with this schedule. Although antipsychotic drugs are probably more often prescribed in two or three daily doses, their long duration of action usually allows once daily dosage.
b. When preparing oral concentrated solutions or parenteral solutions, try to avoid contact with the solution. If contact is made, wash the area immediately.	These solutions are irritating to the skin and may cause contact dermatitis.
c. Mix liquid concentrates with at least 60 ml of fruit juice or water just before administration.	To mask the taste. If the client does not like juice or water, check the package insert for other diluents. Some of the drugs may be mixed with coffee, tea, milk, or carbonated beverages.
d. For intramuscular injections	
(1) Give only those preparations labeled for intramuscular use.	
(2) Do not mix any other drugs in the same syringe with antipsychotic drugs.	These drugs are physically incompatible with many other drugs, and a precipitate may occur.
(3) Change the needle after filling the syringe for injection.	Parenteral solutions of these drugs are highly irritating to body tissues. Changing needles helps to protect the tissues of the injection tract from unnecessary contact with the drug.
(4) Inject slowly and deeply into gluteal muscles.	Using a large muscle mass for the injection site decreases tissue irritation.
(5) Have the client lie down for 30 to 60 minutes after the injection.	To observe for adverse reactions. Orthostatic hypotension is likely if the client tries to ambulate.
e. Do not give antipsychotic drugs subcutaneously, except for fluphenazine decanoate and fluphenazine enanthate	More tissue irritation occurs with subcutaneous administration than with intramuscular administration.
f. When parenteral fluphenazine is ordered, check the drug preparations very closely.	The hydrochloride solution of fluphenazine is given intramuscularly only. The decanoate and enanthate preparations

Nursing Actions	***Rationale/Explanation***
	(long-acting, sesame oil preparations) can be given intramuscularly or subcutaneously.
2. Observe for therapeutic effects	
a. When drug is given for acute psychotic episodes, observe for decreased agitation, combativeness, and psychomotor activity.	The sedative effects of antipsychotic drugs are exerted within 48 to 72 hours. Sedation that occurs with treatment of acute psychotic episodes is a therapeutic effect. Sedation that occurs with treatment of nonacute psychotic disorders, or excessive sedation at any time, is an adverse reaction.
b. When drug is given for acute or chronic psychosis, observe for decreased psychotic behavior, such as (1) Decreased auditory and visual hallucinations (2) Decreased delusions (3) Continued decrease in or absence of agitation, hostility, hyperactivity, and other behavior associated with acute psychosis (4) Increased socialization (5) Increased ability in self-care activities (6) Increased ability to participate in other therapeutic modalities along with drug therapy.	These therapeutic effects may not be evident for 3 to 6 weeks after drug therapy is begun.
c. When drug is given for antiemetic effects, observe for decreased or absent nausea or vomiting.	
3. Observe for adverse effects	
a. Excessive sedation—drowsiness, lethargy, fatigue, slurred speech, impaired mobility, and impaired mental processes	Excessive sedation is most likely to occur during the first few days of treatment of an acute psychotic episode, when large doses are usually given. Psychotics also seem sedated because the drug lets them catch up on psychosis-induced sleep deprivation. Sedation is more likely to occur in elderly or debilitated persons. Tolerance to the drugs' sedative effects develops, and sedation tends to decrease with continued drug therapy.
b. Extrapyramidal reactions	
(1) Akathisia—compulsive, involuntary restlessness and body movements	Akathisia is the most common extrapyramidal reaction, and it may occur about 5 to 60 days after the start of antipsychotic drug therapy. The motor restlessness may be erroneously interpreted as psychotic agitation necessitating increased drug dosage. This condition can sometimes be controlled by substituting an antipsychotic drug that is less likely to cause extrapyramidal effects or by giving an anticholinergic antiparkinson drug.
(2) Parkinsonism—loss of muscle movement (akinesia), muscular rigidity and tremors, shuffling gait, postural abnormalities, masklike facial expression, hypersalivation and drooling	These symptoms are the same as those occurring with idiopathic Parkinson's disease. They can be controlled with anticholinergic antiparkinson drugs, given along with the antipsychotic drug for about three months, then discontinued. This reaction may occur about 5 to 30 days after antipsychotic drug therapy is begun.
(3) Dyskinesias (involuntary, rhythmic body movements) and dystonias (uncoordinated, bizarre movements of the neck, face, eyes, tongue, trunk, or extremities)	These are less common extrapyramidal reactions, but they may occur suddenly, about 1 to 5 days after drug therapy is started, and be very frightening to affected persons and health care personnel. The movements are caused by muscle spasms and result in exaggerated posture and facial distortions. These symptoms are sometimes misinterpreted as seizures, hysteria, or other disorders. Antiparkinson drugs are given parenterally during acute dystonic reactions, but con-

Nursing Actions	**Rationale/Explanation**
	tinued administration is not usually required. These reactions occur most often in younger persons.
(4) Tardive dyskinesia—hyperkinetic movements of the face (sucking and smacking of lips, tongue protrusion, and facial grimaces) and choreiform movements of the trunk and limbs	This syndrome occurs after months or years of high-dose antipsychotic drug therapy. The drugs may mask the symptoms so that the syndrome is more likely to be diagnosed when dosage is decreased or the drug is discontinued for a few days. It occurs gradually and at any age but is more common in older people, women, and persons with organic brain disorders. The condition is usually irreversible, and there is no effective treatment. Symptoms are not controlled and may be worsened by antiparkinson drugs. Low dosage and short-term use of antipsychotic drugs help prevent tardive dyskinesia; drug-free periods may aid early detection.
c. Antiadrenergic effects—hypotension, tachycardia, dizziness, faintness, and fatigue	Hypotension is potentially one of the most serious adverse reactions to the antipsychotic drugs. It is most likely to occur when the client assumes an upright position after sitting or lying down (orthostatic or postural hypotension), but it does occur in the recumbent position. It is caused by peripheral vasodilation. Orthostatic hypotension can be assessed by comparing blood pressure readings taken with the client in supine and standing positions. Tachycardia occurs as a compensatory mechanism in response to hypotension and also as an anticholinergic effect in which the normal vagus nerve action of slowing the heart rate is blocked.
d. Anticholinergic effects—dry mouth, dental caries, blurred vision, constipation, paralytic ileus, urinary retention	These atropinelike effects are common with therapeutic doses and increased with large doses of phenothiazines.
e. Respiratory depression—slow, shallow breathing and decreased ability to breathe deeply, cough, and remove secretions from the respiratory tract	This stems from general CNS depression, which causes drowsiness and decreased movement. It may cause pneumonia or other respiratory problems, especially in people with hypercarbia and chronic lung disease.
f. Endocrine effects—menstrual irregularities, possibly impotence and decreased libido in the male, weight gain	These apparently result from drug-induced changes in pituitary and hypothalamic functions.
g. Hypothermia or hyperthermia	Antipsychotic drugs may impair the temperature-regulating center in the hypothalamus. Hypothermia is more likely to occur. Hyperthermia occurs with high doses and warm environmental temperatures.
h. Hypersensitivity reactions	
(1) Cholestatic hepatitis—may begin with fever and influenzalike symptoms followed in about 1 week by jaundice	Cholestatic hepatitis results from drug-induced edema of the bile ducts and obstruction of bile flow. It occurs most often in women and after 2 to 4 weeks of receiving the drug. It is usually reversible if the drug is discontinued.
(2) Blood dyscrasias—leukopenia, agranulocytosis (fever, sore throat, weakness)	Some degree of leukopenia occurs rather often and does not seem to be serious. Agranulocytosis, on the other hand, occurs rarely but is life threatening. Agranulocytosis is most likely to occur during the first 4 to 10 weeks of drug therapy, in women, and in older people.
(3) Skin reactions—photosensitivity, dermatoses	Skin pigmentation and discoloration may occur with exposure to sunlight.
i. Electrocardiogram (ECG) changes	The mechanism and clinical significance of ECG changes are not completely clear. However, some antipsychotic drugs, especially thioridazine, alter normal impulse conduction

Nursing Actions	***Rationale/Explanation***
	through the ventricles. There is probably increased risk of cardiac arrhythmias, which may be serious in a person with cardiovascular disease.
4. Observe for drug interactions	
a. Drugs that *increase* effects of antipsychotic drugs	
(1) Anticholinergic drugs (*e.g.,* atropine)	Additive anticholinergic effects, especially with thioridazine
(2) Antidepressants, tricyclic	Potentiation of sedative and anticholinergic effects. Additive CNS depression, sedation, orthostatic hypotension, urinary retention, and glaucoma may occur unless dosages are decreased. Apparently these two drug groups inhibit the metabolism of each other, thus prolonging the actions of both groups if they are given concomitantly.
(3) Antihistamines	Additive CNS depression and sedation
(4) CNS depressants—alcohol, narcotic analgesics, antianxiety agents, barbiturates, and other sedative–hypnotics.	Additive CNS depression. Also, severe hypotension, urinary retention, seizures, severe atropinelike reactions, and others may occur, depending on which group of CNS depressant drugs is given.
(5) Propranolol (Inderal)	Additive hypotensive and electrocardiographic effects
(6) Thiazide diuretics such as hydrochlorothiazide (HydroDIURIL)	Additive hypotension
(7) Lithium	Acute encephalopathy, including irreversible brain damage and dyskinesias, has been reported.
b. Drugs that *decrease* effects of antipsychotic drugs	
(1) Antacids	Oral antacids, especially aluminum hydroxide and magnesium trisilicate, may inhibit gastrointestinal absorption of antipsychotic drugs.
(2) Barbiturates	By induction of drug-metabolizing enzymes in the liver
(3) Levarterenol (Levophed), phenylephrine (Neo-Synephrine)	Antagonize the hypotensive effects of antipsychotic drugs
5. Teach clients	
a. About the planned drug therapy regimen, including the desired therapeutic results and the length of time it takes before therapeutic results can be expected.	This is especially necessary to improve compliance in long-term drug therapy. Failure to take prescribed medications is a frequent reason for recurring episodes of acute illness and hospitalization.
b. Possible side-effects of drug therapy. Emphasize those related to safety; for example, warn the client not to drive a car or operate machinery.	Providing a detailed list of side-effects is not necessary and may confuse the client or increase anxiety. It may be helpful to note that drowsiness and impaired mental and motor activity are especially evident during the first 2 weeks of drug therapy but tend to decrease over time.
c. Report unusual side-effects and all physical illnesses.	Changes in drug therapy may be indicated.
d. Avoid using *any* nonprescribed drugs such as those available without prescription or those prescribed for another person.	To avoid undesirable drug interactions. Alcohol and sleeping pills should be avoided because they may cause excessive drowsiness and decreased awareness of safety hazards in the environment.
e. Consult the physician who prescribed the medication before taking any drug prescribed by another physician.	Again, to avoid undesirable drug interactions
f. Do not take antacids with these drugs. If an antacid is needed, take it 1 hour before or 2 hours after the antipyschotic drug.	Antacids may decrease absorption of these drugs from the intestine.
g. Lie down for about an hour after receiving medication when drug therapy is started or after any injection.	To avoid low blood pressure, dizziness, and faintness, which may occur with standing

Nursing Actions	Rationale/Explanation
h. If dizziness and faintness occur on standing, they can be minimized by changing positions slowly and sitting on the bedside a few minutes before standing. Do not try to stand or walk when feeling dizzy.	To avoid falls or other injuries
i. Practice good oral hygiene measures, including dental checkups, thorough and frequent toothbrushing, drinking fluids, and frequent mouth rinsing.	Mouth dryness is a common side-effect of these drugs. Although more annoying than serious for the most part, it can predispose to mouth infections, dental cavities, and ill-fitting dentures.
j. If skin reactions occur, stay out of sunlight or wear protective clothing and use sunscreen lotions.	Sensitivity to sunlight is an adverse reaction of these drugs.
k. Avoid exposure to excessive heat.	Fever (hyperthermia) and heat prostration may occur with high environmental temperatures.

Selected References

American Medical Association (AMA) Division of Drugs: AMA Drug Evaluations, 5th ed. New York, John Wiley & Sons, 1983

Baldessarini RJ: Drugs and the treatment of psychiatric disorders. In Gilman AG, Goodman LS, Rall TW, Murad F (eds): The Pharmacological Basis of Therapeutics, 7th ed, pp 387–445. New York, Macmillan, 1985

Bernstein JG: Handbook of Drug Therapy in Psychiatry. Boston, John Wright, 1983

Black JL, Richelson E, Richardson JW: Antipsychotic agents: A clinical update. Mayo Clin Proc 60:777–789, November 1985

Coyle JT: The clinical use of antipsychotic medications. Med Clin North Am 66:993–1009, September 1982

Davidhizar R, McBride A: Teaching the client with schizophrenia about medication. Patient Ed Counsel 7:137–145, June 1985

Drugs that cause psychiatric symptoms. Med Lett Drugs Ther 26:75–78, August 17, 1984

Evans RL, Richart NA: Psychiatric disorders. In Wiener MB, Pepper GA (eds): Clinical Pharmacology and Therapeutics in Nursing, 2d ed, pp 622–654. New York, McGraw-Hill, 1985

Facts and Comparisons. St. Louis, J B Lippincott (Updated monthly)

Hansten PD: Drug Interactions: Clinical Significance of Drug–Drug Interactions, 5th ed. Philadelphia, Lea & Febiger, 1985

Harris E: Antipsychotic medications and extrapyramidal side effects of antipsychotic medications. Am J Nurs 81:1316–1328, July 1981

Malseed RT: Pharmacology: Drug Therapy and Nursing Considerations, 2d ed. Philadelphia, J B Lippincott, 1985

Rodman MJ, Karch AM, Boyd EH, Smith DW: Pharmacology and Drug Therapy in Nursing, 3rd ed. Philadelphia, J B Lippincott, 1985

Stancer HC, Garfunkel PE, Rakoff VM (eds): Guidelines for the Use of Psychotropic Drugs: A Clinical Handbook. Jamaica, NY, Spectrum Publications, 1984.

Walker JI, Covington TR: Psychiatric disorders. In Covington TR, Walker JI (eds): Current Geriatric Therapy, pp 75–102. Philadelphia, W B Saunders, 1984

10
ANTIDEPRESSANTS

Description and uses

Antidepressant agents are used in the pharmacologic management of depressive disorders. Mental depression is a common disorder characterized by depressed mood, sadness, or emotional upset. Depression may be mild or severe, primary or secondary. Mild depression, in the absence of specific depressive symptoms, occurs in most people at one time or another and usually does not require treatment. Severe depression, however, is a psychiatric disorder and does require treatment. Depression as a psychiatric disorder consists of depressed mood plus at least five of the following depressive symptoms:

1. Loss of energy, fatigue
2. Indecisiveness
3. Difficulty thinking and concentrating
4. Loss of interest in appearance, work, leisure-time activities, and sexual activities
5. Inappropriate feelings of guilt and worthlessness
6. Loss of appetite and weight loss or excessive eating and weight gain
7. Sleep disorders (hypersomnia or insomnia)
8. Somatic symptoms (*e.g.,* constipation, headache, atypical pain)
9. Obsession with death, thoughts of suicide

Primary depression is depression that cannot be related to an identifiable cause. The etiologic basis of primary depression is uncertain. The biogenic amine hypothesis states that depression results from a relative deficiency of neurotransmitters (*i.e.,* dopamine, norepinephrine, serotonin) at postsynaptic adrenergic receptors in the brain. Secondary depression may be precipitated by *environmental stress* (*e.g.,* job loss or dissatisfaction, financial worries), by *adverse life events* (*e.g.,* divorce, death of a family member or friend), by *drugs* (alcohol; antihypertensive drugs such as clonidine, guanethidine, and reserpine; corticosteroids; propranolol and metoprolol; opiates; and oral contraceptive agents), or by *concurrent disease states* (*e.g.,* Parkinson's disease, hypothyroidism, pancreatic disease, mastectomy, amputation of any body part, and loss of health in general).

Serious depressive illness is frequently a recurrent disorder. Patterns of recurrence may be unipolar or bipolar. Unipolar depression is more common. In this disorder, periods of depression are interspersed with periods of normal mood. In bipolar depression (formerly called manic–depressive illness), periods of depression are interspersed with periods of mania or hypomania. Mania is defined as a mood state characterized by hyperactivity, talkativeness, racing thoughts, decreased need for sleep, distractibility, impulsive behavior, and delusions of grandeur.

Antidepressant drugs exert therapeutic effects by enhancing the activity of neurotransmitter substances (*i.e.,* norepinephrine, serotonin, dopamine) in the brain. The tricyclic antidepressants (TCAs) and newer agents, maprotiline and trazodone, prevent reuptake of one or more neurotransmitters by presynaptic nerve fibers, thereby increasing the amounts of these substances available to postsynaptic nerve fibers. The monoamine oxidase (MAO) inhibitors inactivate MAO, an enzyme that normally metabolizes the neurotransmitters norepinephrine, serotonin, and dopamine. Thus, although the mechanisms of action differ, both groups of drugs increase neurotransmitter availability.

Other characteristics of these drugs and lithium, an antimanic agent used for bipolar depressive disorder, are described in the following section.

TRICYCLIC AND RELATED ANTIDEPRESSANTS

Tricyclic antidepressants comprise a group of eight chemically and pharmacologically similar drugs. These compounds contain a triple-ring nucleus from which their name is derived. The drugs are structurally similar to phenothiazine antipsychotic agents (see Chap. 9) and have similar antiadrenergic and anticholinergic properties. They produce a relatively high incidence of sedation, orthostatic hypotension, cardiac arrhythmias, and other adverse effects in addition to dry mouth and anticholinergic effects. TCAs are well absorbed after oral administration. However, first-pass metabolism by the liver results in blood-level variations of 10- to 30-fold among persons given identical doses. Once absorbed, these drugs are widely distributed throughout body tissues and metabolized by the liver to active and inactive metabolites. Amitriptyline (Elavil) and imipramine (Tofranil) are commonly used TCAs.

Newer antidepressants are both similar to and different than TCAs. *Maprotiline* (Ludiomil) is a tetracyclic antidepressant that also has anxiolytic properties. It causes adverse effects similar to the TCAs and seems to have few, if any, advantages over the TCAs. *Trazodone* (Desyrel) is a triazolopyridine derivative and represents a different chemical class of antidepressants. Oral trazodone is well absorbed, and peak plasma concentrations are obtained within 30 minutes to 2 hours. Trazodone is metabolized by the liver and excreted primarily by the kidneys. Although trazodone reportedly produces less anticholinergic activity than the TCAs, it causes a number of other adverse effects including sedation, dizziness, edema, cardiac dysrhythmias, and priapism (prolonged and painful penile erection).

MONOAMINE OXIDASE INHIBITOR ANTIDEPRESSANTS

Monoamine oxidase inhibitors are drugs that block the metabolism of norepinephrine, serotonin, and dopamine in the brain. This action is thought to relieve depression by increasing the amount and normalizing the balance of the centrally active monoamine neurotransmitters.

MAO inhibitors are well absorbed following oral administration. These agents produce maximal inhibition of MAO within 5 to 10 days. However, clinical improvement in depression may require 2 to 3 weeks.

MAO inhibitors may interact with numerous foods and drugs to produce hypertensive crisis (*i.e.*, severe hypertension, severe headache, fever, possible myocardial infarction, or intracranial hemorrhage). Foods that interact with MAO inhibitor drugs are those containing tyramine, a monoamine precursor of norepinephrine. Normally, tyramine is deactivated in the gastrointestinal tract and liver so that large amounts do not reach the systemic circulation. However, when deactivation of tyramine is blocked by MAO inhibitor drugs, tyramine is absorbed systemically and transported to adrenergic nerve terminals, where it causes a sudden release of large amounts of norepinephrine. Hypertensive crisis may result. Several drugs may also interact with MAO inhibitors to cause hypertensive crisis. Foods and drugs to be avoided during (and 2 to 3 weeks after) drug therapy with MAO inhibiting agents are listed in Table 10-1.

ANTIMANIC AGENT

Lithium carbonate (Eskalith) is a naturally occurring metallic salt that is used in the management of bipolar

TABLE 10-1. FOODS AND DRUGS TO BE AVOIDED DURING THERAPY WITH MAO INHIBITOR DRUGS

Foods to avoid	Drugs to avoid
Aged cheeses (*e.g.*, cheddar, Camembert, Stilton, Gruyere)	Amphetamines
Alcoholic beverages (beer, Chianti and other red wines)	Antiallergy and antiasthmatic drugs (*e.g.*, ephedrine, epinephrine, phenylpropanolamine, pseudoephedrine)
Avocados and guacamole dip	Antihistamines (including over-the-counter cough and cold remedies)
Bananas	Antihypertensive drugs (*i.e.*, guanethidine, methyldopa)
Caffeine-containing beverages (coffee, tea, cola drinks)	Levodopa
Chicken livers	Meperidine
Chocolate (in large amounts)	
Fava bean pods	
Figs (canned)	
Meat tenderizers	
Pickled herring	
Raisins	
Sour cream	
Soy sauce	
Yeast supplements	
Yogurt	

disorders. In clients with bipolar disorders, lithium is most effective in the treatment and prevention of mania or hypomania. The drug is considered less effective in preventing depressive illness. Lithium is sometimes described as a "mood stabilizing" agent.

The mechanism by which lithium exerts therapeutic effects is unknown. The drug is well absorbed after oral administration. Peak serum levels occur in 1 to 3 hours after a dose of lithium, and steady-state concentrations are reached in 5 to 7 days. There is wide interclient variation in serum concentrations of lithium with comparable doses. Therefore, frequent monitoring of serum lithium concentration is required (see Principles of Therapy).

Lithium is not metabolized by the body; it is entirely excreted by the kidney. Adequate renal function is a prerequisite for lithium therapy. Approximately 80% of a lithium dose is reabsorbed in the proximal renal tubules. The amount of reabsorption depends on the concentration of sodium in the proximal tubules. A deficiency of sodium causes more lithium to be reabsorbed and increases risks of lithium toxicity; excessive sodium intake causes more lithium to be excreted (*i.e.*, "lithium diuresis") and may lower serum lithium levels to nontherapeutic ranges.

Before lithium therapy is begun, baseline studies of renal, cardiac, and thyroid status should be obtained because adverse drug effects involve these organ systems. Baseline electrolyte studies are also necessary.

INDICATIONS

Antidepressant drug therapy may be indicated if depressive symptoms persist at least 2 weeks, impair social relationships or work performance, and occur independently of life events. In addition, tricyclic antidepressants may be used in the management of enuresis in children and adolescents. Enuresis is involuntary urination ("bed wetting") resulting from a physical or psychologic disorder. A tricyclic antidepressant drug may be given after physical causes (*e.g.*, urethral irritation, excessive intake of fluids) have been ruled out.

CONTRAINDICATIONS

Antidepressant drugs are contraindicated or must be used with caution in clients with acute schizophrenia, mixed mania and depression, suicidal tendencies, severe renal, hepatic, or cardiovascular disease, narrow-angle glaucoma, and seizure disorders.

Individual antidepressants

Individual antidepressants are listed in Table 10-2.

Principles of therapy: antidepressants

ASSESSMENT IN DEPRESSIVE DISORDERS

Assess the client's condition in relation to depressive disorders.

1. Identify clients at risk for current or potential depression. Areas to assess include health–illness status, family–social relationships, and work status. Severe or prolonged illness, impaired interpersonal relationships, inability to work, and job dissatisfaction may precipitate mental depression. Depression also occurs without a specific, discernible cause.
2. Observe for the signs and symptoms of depression listed earlier in this chapter. Manifestations may occur in any client, not just those who have or are suspected of having psychiatric illness. It is important to remember that clinical manifestations are nonspecific and vary in severity. For example, fatigue and insomnia may be caused by a variety of disorders and range from mild to severe. When symptoms are present, try to determine their frequency, duration, and severity.
3. Identify the client's usual coping mechanisms for stressful situations. Coping mechanisms vary widely among people, and behavior that may be helpful to one client may not be helpful to another. For example, one person may prefer being alone or having decreased contact with family and friends, whereas another may find increased contact desirable.

NURSING INTERVENTIONS

Use measures to prevent or decrease severity of depression. General measures include supportive psychotherapy and reduction of environmental stress. Specific measures include the following:

1. Support the client's usual mechanism for handling stressful situations, when feasible. Helpful actions may involve relieving pain or insomnia, schedul-

TABLE 10-2. ANTIDEPRESSANT AGENTS

	Generic name	Trade name	Routes and dosage ranges: Adults	Routes and dosage ranges: Children
Tricyclic antidepressants	Amitriptyline	Elavil, Endep, others	PO 75–100 mg daily in divided doses, gradually increased to 150–300 mg daily if necessary. Maintenance dose, 50–100 mg once daily at bedtime. IM 80–120 mg daily in 4 divided doses *Elderly adults,* PO 10 mg 3 times daily and 20 mg at bedtime	Adolescents, PO 10 mg 3 times daily and 20 mg at bedtime Enuresis in children aged 5–14 years, PO 25 mg once daily at bedtime
	Amoxapine	Asendin	PO 50 mg 3 times daily, increased to 100 mg 3 times daily on the third day. Maintenance dose may be given in a single dose at bedtime	Not recommended for children under age 16 years
	Desipramine	Pertofrane, Norpramin	PO 75 mg daily in divided doses, gradually increased to a maximum of 200–300 mg daily if necessary *Elderly adults,* PO 25–50 mg daily in divided doses, gradually increased to 100 mg daily if necessary	Not recommended
	Doxepin	Sinequan, Adapin	PO 75–150 mg daily, gradually increased to a maximum of 300 mg daily if necessary	Not recommended
	Imipramine	Tofranil	PO 75 mg daily in 3 divided doses, gradually increased to a maximum of 300 mg daily if necessary. Maintenance dose, 75–150 mg daily *Elderly adults,* PO 30–40 mg daily in divided doses, increased to 100 mg daily if necessary	Enuresis, PO 25–50 mg 1 hour before bedtime
	Nortriptyline	Aventyl, Pamelor	PO 40 mg daily in divided doses, gradually increased to 100–150 mg daily if necessary	Enuresis, PO 25 mg once daily at bedtime
	Protriptyline	Vivactil	PO 15 mg daily in divided doses, increased to 60 mg daily if necessary	
	Trimipramine maleate	Surmontil	PO 75–100 mg daily, gradually increased to 300 mg daily if necessary	
Tricyclic-related antidepressants	Maprotiline	Ludiomil	PO 75 mg daily in single or divided doses, increased to a maximum dose of 300 mg daily if necessary	Not recommended for children under age 18 years
	Trazodone	Desyrel	PO 100–300 mg daily, increased to a maximum dose of 600 mg daily if necessary	
Monoamine oxidase inhibitor antidepressants	Isocarboxazid	Marplan	PO 30 mg daily in divided doses. Maintenance dose, up to 20 mg daily	Dosage not established
	Phenelzine	Nardil	PO 60 mg daily in 3 divided doses, increased to 90 mg daily if necessary	Dosage not established
	Tranylcypromine	Parnate	PO 20 mg daily in 2 divided doses in the morning and afternoon for 2 weeks, then adjusted according to client's response. Maximal daily dose, 30 mg	Dosage not established
Antimanic agent	Lithium carbonate	Eskalith	Bipolar disorder (formerly called manic–depressive disorder), PO 900–1200 mg daily in divided doses, gradually increased in 300-mg increments if necessary, according to serum lithium levels and client's response	Dosage not established in children under 12 years

ing rest periods, and increasing or decreasing socialization with other people.

2. Call the client by name, encourage self-care activities, allow him or her to participate in goal setting and decision making, and praise efforts to accomplish tasks. These actions help to promote a positive self-image.
3. When signs and symptoms of depression are observed, report them to the physician so that treatment can be initiated before depression becomes severe.

DRUG SELECTION

The choice of an antidepressant drug depends largely on the type of depression present and its severity. Guidelines for choosing a drug include the following:

1. A TCA agent is the primary drug of choice for most clients experiencing mental depression. There is relatively little basis for choosing one TCA over another. However, some clients may tolerate or respond better to one TCA than to another.
   a. Initial selection of a specific TCA may be based on the client's previous response or susceptibility to adverse effects. For example, if a client (or a close family member) responded well to a particular drug in the past, that drug is probably the drug of choice for repeated episodes of depression. The response of family members to individual drugs may be significant because there is a strong genetic component to depression and drug response. In relation to adverse effects, a TCA with strong sedative properties (amitriptyline, doxepin, maprotiline, trimipramine) may be preferred for a client with agitated depression; a TCA with minimal anticholinergic effect (desipramine, trazodone) is probably the drug of choice for a client with prostatic hypertrophy or narrow-angle glaucoma.
   b. The two first TCAs to be developed, imipramine and amitriptyline, are the most commonly prescribed agents. If therapeutic effects do not occur within 4 weeks, the TCA probably should be discontinued or changed.
2. MAO inhibitors are considered second-line drugs for treatment of depression because of their potential interactions with other drugs and certain foods. An MAO inhibitor is most likely to be prescribed when the client does not respond to a tricyclic antidepressant and when electroconvulsive therapy (ECT) is refused or contraindicated.
3. Lithium is the primary drug of choice in clients with bipolar disorder. When used therapeutically, lithium is effective in controlling mania in approximately 80% of clients. When used prophylactically, the drug decreases frequency and intensity of manic cycles.

DOSAGE AND ADMINISTRATION

Dosage of antidepressant drugs should be individualized according to clinical response. Antidepressant drug therapy is usually initiated with small, divided doses that are gradually increased (every 2 to 3 days) until therapeutic or adverse effects occur. Specific guidelines for dosage include the following:

1. With TCAs, therapy is begun with small doses, which are increased to the desired dose over 1 to 2 weeks. Minimal effective doses are approximately 150 mg of imipramine or its equivalent daily. TCAs can be administered once or twice daily because they have long elimination half-lives. Once dosage is established, TCAs are often given once daily at bedtime. This regimen is effective and well tolerated by most clients. Elderly clients may experience fewer adverse reactions if divided doses are continued. After recovery from acute depression, a maintenance dose of smaller amounts is usually continued for approximately 3 to 6 months, then gradually tapered and discontinued.
2. With lithium therapy, dosage should be based on serum lithium levels, control of symptoms, and occurrence of adverse effects. Serum levels are required because therapeutic doses are only slightly lower than toxic doses and because clients vary widely in rates of lithium absorption and excretion. Consequently, a dose that is therapeutic in one client may be toxic or lethal in another.

   When lithium therapy is being initiated, serum drug concentration should be measured two or three times weekly, in the morning, 12 hours after the last dose of lithium. For most clients, the therapeutic range of serum levels is 0.8 to 1.2 mEq/liter. For clients in an acute manic state, serum level of lithium may need to be higher (1.2 to 1.4 mEq/liter). Serum lithium levels should not exceed 1.5 mEq/liter because the risk of serious toxicity is increased at higher levels. Once symptoms of mania are controlled, lithium doses should be lowered to maintain serum levels of approximately 0.7 mEq to 1 mEq/liter. During long-term maintenance therapy, serum lithium levels should be measured at least every 3 months.

USE IN PREGNANCY AND LACTATION

TCAs and MAO inhibitors have not been established as safe and effective for use during pregnancy and lactation. Usage of these agents, especially during the first trimester of pregnancy, must be carefully considered in terms of expected benefits versus potential risks. Lithium is usually contraindicated during pregnancy because there is evidence of a greater incidence of cardiac abnormalities and neurologic depression in infants whose mothers took lithium during pregnancy. If lithium must be used, small divided doses are given throughout the day, serum levels are maintained at the lowest effective range, and serum levels are measured frequently. Lithium is also contraindicated during lactation because the drug is excreted in breast milk. If lithium must be used, breast feeding should be avoided.

PEDIATRIC CONSIDERATIONS

In pediatric drug therapy, antidepressant agents have not generally been established as safe and effective for children under 12 years of age. An exception is the use of a tricyclic agent, usually imipramine or amitriptyline, to treat enuresis. The drug is often effective for short-term therapy. However, effectiveness in controlling bed wetting may decrease with continued drug therapy, and no residual benefits continue once drug therapy is stopped.

GERIATRIC CONSIDERATIONS

In geriatric drug therapy, antidepressant agents are usually given in small doses, and doses are increased gradually. Thus, both initial and maintenance doses are smaller in elderly clients than in younger adults. Doses of tricyclic antidepressants should be decreased by 30% to 50% because the rate of drug metabolism and excretion is decreased in elderly clients.

ASSESSMENT AND MANAGEMENT OF TOXICITY

Antidepressant drugs are highly toxic and potentially lethal when taken in large doses. Toxicity is most likely to occur in depressed clients who intentionally ingest large amounts of drug in suicide attempts and in young children who accidentally gain access to improperly stored medication containers. Measures to prevent acute poisoning from drug overdose include dispensing only a few days' supply (*i.e.*, 5 to 7 days) to clients with suicidal tendencies and storing the drugs in places that are inaccessible to young children. General measures to treat acute poisoning include early detection of signs and symptoms, stopping the drug, and instituting treatment if indicated. Specific measures include the following:

1. With overdosage of tricyclic antidepressants, symptoms occur approximately 1 to 4 hours after drug ingestion and consist primarily of anticholinergic and cardiovascular effects (*e.g.*, nystagmus, tremor, restlessness, decreased bowel sounds, dilated pupils, hypotension, arrhythmias, and myocardial depression). Death usually results from cardiac, respiratory, and circulatory failure.

   Management of TCA toxicity consists of gastric lavage and administration of activated charcoal to reduce drug absorption, administration of cathartics to increase drug excretion, establishing and maintaining a patent airway, continuous electrocardiographic monitoring of comatose clients or those with respiratory insufficiency or wide QRS intervals, administration of intravenous fluids and vasopressors for severe hypotension, and administration of phenytoin or diazepam if seizures occur. Physostigmine (Antilirium), 1 to 3 mg administered intravenously, has been used to reverse anticholinergic effects, but severe bradycardia, asystole, and seizures may occur.
2. With overdosage of MAO inhibitors, symptoms occur 12 hours or longer after drug ingestion and consist primarily of adrenergic effects (*e.g.*, tachycardia, increased rate of respiration, agitation, tremors, convulsive seizures, sweating, heart block, hypotension, delirium, and coma). Management measures consist of forced diuresis, acidification of urine, or hemodialysis to remove the drug from the body.
3. With lithium overdose, toxic manifestations occur with serum lithium levels above 2.5 mEq/liter and include nystagmus, tremors, oliguria, confusion, impaired consciousness, visual or tactile hallucinations, choreiform movements, convulsions, coma, and death. Management measures include administration of intravenous fluids and electrolytes to replace nutrients and administration of osmotic diuretics (*e.g.*, mannitol) and sodium lactate to facilitate excretion of lithium. Sodium lactate increases excretion of lithium by alkalinizing the urine. In addition, anticonvulsant drugs may be needed if seizures occur, and peritoneal dialysis or hemodialysis may be indicated if renal function is impaired.

NURSING ACTIONS: ANTIDEPRESSANTS

Nursing Actions	*Rationale/Explanation*
1. Administer accurately	
a. Give lithium with or just after meals.	To decrease gastric irritation
2. Observe for therapeutic effects	
a. With tricyclic antidepressants and MAO inhibitors, observe for statements of feeling better or being less depressed; increased appetite, physical activity, and interest in surroundings; improved sleep patterns; improved appearance; decreased anxiety; decreased somatic complaints.	Therapeutic effects usually do not occur for 2 to 3 weeks after drug therapy is started.
b. With lithium, observe for decreases in manic behavior and mood swings.	Therapeutic effects do not occur until approximately 7 to 10 days after therapeutic serum drug levels are attained. In severe mania, an antipsychotic drug is usually given to control behavior until the lithium takes effect.
3. Observe for adverse effects	
a. With TCAs, observe for (1) Dry mouth, constipation, blurred vision, tachycardia, orthostatic hypotension, drowsiness, dizziness, excessive sweating (2) Urinary retention, fainting, tremor, nausea, cardiac arrhythmias (3) Confusion, delirium, seizures, skin rash, agranulocytosis, cholestatic jaundice, impotence, transition to mania in clients with bipolar disorder	Most adverse effects result from anticholinergic or antiadrenergic activity. Symptoms listed in (1) commonly occur, especially when TCA therapy is initiated. Symptoms listed in (2) occur less frequently and those listed in (3) rarely occur.
b. With MAO inhibitors, observe for hypotension, dizziness, increased incidence of angina, dry mouth, blurred vision, constipation, urinary retention, hypoglycemia	Anticholinergic effects are common. Hypoglycemia results from a drug-induced reduction in blood sugar.
c. With lithium, observe for (1) Metallic taste, hand tremors, nausea, polyuria, polydipsia, diarrhea, muscular weakness, fatigue, edema, and weight gain (2) More severe nausea and diarrhea, vomiting, ataxia, incoordination, dizziness, slurred speech, blurred vision, tinnitus, muscle twitching and tremors, increased muscle tone	Most clients who take lithium experience adverse effects. Symptoms listed in (1) are common, occur at therapeutic serum drug levels (0.8 to 1.2 mEq/liter) and usually subside during the first few weeks of drug therapy. Symptoms listed in (2) occur at higher serum drug levels (1.5 to 2.5 mEq/liter). Nausea may be decreased by giving lithium with meals. Propranolol (Inderal), 20 to 120 mg daily, may be given to control tremors. Severe or persistent adverse effects may be managed by decreasing lithium dosage, omitting a few doses, or discontinuing the drug temporarily. Toxic symptoms occur at serum drug levels above 2.5 mEq/liter.
4. Observe for drug interactions	
a. Drugs that *increase* effects of TCAs	
(1) Antihistamines, atropine, and other drugs with anticholinergic effects	Additive anticholinergic effects (*e.g.,* dry mouth, blurred vision, urinary retention, constipation)
(2) Alcohol, antihistamines, benzodiazepines (*e.g.,* diazepam [Valium]), narcotic analgesics	Additive sedation
(3) Urinary alkalizers (*e.g.,* sodium bicarbonate)	Decrease excretion of TCAs
b. Drugs that *decrease* effects of TCAs	
(1) Barbiturates, chloral hydrate, nicotine (cigarette smoking)	These drugs decrease blood levels of TCAs by increasing the rate of hepatic metabolism of the antidepressant agent.
(2) Urinary acidifiers (*e.g.,* ascorbic acid)	Increase excretion of TCAs

Nursing Actions	Rationale/Explanation
c. Drugs that *increase* effects of MAO inhibitors	
(1) Anticholinergic drugs (*e.g.,* atropine, antipsychotic agents, tricyclic antidepressants)	Additive anticholinergic effects
(2) Adrenergic agents (*e.g.,* epinephrine, isoproterenol, phenylephrine), alcohol (some beers and wines), guanethidine, levodopa, meperidine, reserpine	Hypertensive crisis may occur.
d. Drugs that *increase* effects of lithium	
(1) Diuretics (*e.g.,* ethacrynic acid, furosemide, hydrochlorothiazide)	Increase neurotoxicity and cardiotoxicity of lithium by increasing excretion of sodium and potassium and thereby decreasing excretion of lithium
(2) Phenothiazines	Increased risk of hyperglycemia
(3) Potassium iodide, tricyclic antidepressants	Increased risk of hypothyroidism
(4) Tricyclic antidepressants	May increase antidepressant effects of lithium and are sometimes given in combination with lithium for this purpose. These drugs may also precipitate a manic episode.
e. Drugs that *decrease* effects of lithium	
(1) Acetazolamide (Diamox), sodium bicarbonate, sodium chloride (in excessive amounts), drugs with a high sodium content (*e.g.,* carbenicillin, ticarcillin), theophylline compounds	Increase excretion of lithium
5. Teach clients	
a. Take antidepressant drugs as directed. Do not alter doses when symptoms subside.	To maximize therapeutic benefits and minimize adverse effects. TCAs and MAO inhibitors are usually given for several months; lithium therapy may be lifelong.
b. Do not take any other drugs without the physician's knowledge, including over-the-counter cold remedies.	Potentially serious drug interactions may occur with prescription or nonprescription drugs.
c. Therapeutic effects (*i.e.,* relief of symptoms) may not occur for 2 or 3 weeks after drug therapy is started.	If clients do not know that therapeutic effects are delayed, they may think the drug is ineffective and stop taking it prematurely.
d. If another physician, surgeon, or dentist is consulted, inform him or her about the antidepressant drugs being taken.	Potentially serious adverse effects or drug interactions may occur if certain other drugs are prescribed.
e. With TCAs, report urinary retention, fainting, irregular heart beat, seizures, restlessness, and mental confusion.	These are potentially serious adverse drug effects. The physician may be able to alter drug therapy and decrease adverse effects.
f. With MAO inhibitors	
(1) Report severe headache to the physician.	Severe headache may be a symptom of a serious adverse effect.
(2) Avoid the foods and drugs listed in Table 10-1.	Severe hypertension and intracranial hemorrhage may occur.
g. With lithium	
(1) Do not decrease dietary salt intake.	Decreased salt intake (*e.g.,* low-salt diet) increases risk of adverse effects from lithium.
(2) Minimize activities that cause excessive perspiration.	Loss of salt in sweat increases risk of adverse effects from lithium.
(3) Report for measurements of lithium blood levels as instructed, and do not take the morning dose of lithium until the blood sample has been obtained.	Regular measurements of blood lithium levels are necessary for safe and effective lithium therapy. Accurate measurement of serum drug levels requires that blood be drawn 12 hours after the previous dose of lithium.

Selected References

American Medical Association (AMA) Division of Drugs: AMA Drug Evaluations, 5th ed. New York, John Wiley & Sons, 1983

Baldessarini RJ: Drugs and the treatment of psychiatric disorders. In Gilman AG, Goodman LS, Rall TW, Murad F (eds): The Pharmacological Basis of Therapeutics, 7th ed. pp 387–445. New York, Macmillan, 1985

Bernstein JG: Handbook of Drug Therapy in Psychiatry. Boston, John Wright, 1983

Bernstein JG: Kids and drugs. II. Therapeutic uses. Drug Ther 14:115–121, April 1984

Bressler R: Treating geriatric depression: Current options. Drug Ther 14:129–1144, September 1984

Davidson J: When and how to use MAO inhibitors. Drug Ther 13:197–202, January 1983

DeGennaro MD, Hymen R, Crannell AM, Mansky PA: Antidepressant drug therapy. Am J Nurs 81:1304–1310, July 1981

Drugs that cause psychiatric symptoms. Med Lett Drugs Ther 26:75–78, August 17, 1984

Facts and Comparisons. St. Louis, J B Lippincott (Updated monthly)

Feinberg SS, Halbreich U: Treatment-resistant depression. II. Conventional therapies. Drug Ther 15:113–125, February 1985

Glassman AH, Bigger JT: Cardiovascular effects of therapeutic doses of tricyclic antidepressants. Arch Gen Psych 38:815–820, July 1981

Grof P, O'Sullivan K: Somatic side effects of long-term lithium treatment. In Stancer HC, Garfunkel PE, Rakoff VM (eds): Guidelines for the Use of Psychotropic Drugs: A Clinical Handbook, pp 105–108. Jamaica, NY, Spectrum Publications, 1984

Hansen HE: Renal toxicity of lithium. Drugs 22:461–476, 1981

Hansten PD: Drug Interactions: Clinical Significance of Drug–Drug Interactions, 5th ed. Philadelphia, Lea & Febiger, 1985

Harris E: Lithium. Am J Nurs 81:1310–1315, July 1981

Kuehnle JC: The safe and effective use of lithium. Drug Ther 10:96–100, March 1980

Malseed RT: Pharmacology: Drug Therapy and Nursing Considerations, 2d ed. Philadelphia, J B Lippincott, 1985

Marshall JB, Forker AD: Cardiovascular effects of tricyclic antidepressant drugs: Therapeutic usage, overdose, and management of complications. Am Heart J 103:401–414, March 1982

McDermott J: Ready or not: Here comes your patient on lithium. Nursing 13:44–48, August 1983

Rodman MJ, Karch AM, Boyd EH, Smith DW: Pharmacology and Drug Therapy in Nursing, 3rd ed. Philadelphia, J B Lippincott, 1985

11 ANTICONVULSANTS

Description and uses

Anticonvulsant drugs are used to treat seizure disorders. The terms *seizure disorders, convulsions,* and *epilepsy* are often used interchangeably, although they are not the same. *Convulsions* are involuntary spasmodic contractions of muscles. Most people probably think that a convulsion is the generalized tonic–clonic reaction that occurs with grand mal or major motor epilepsy, although it occurs in other situations as well. A *seizure* is a sudden attack of epilepsy or another disorder and may or may not involve a generalized convulsion. For example, with absence seizures (petit mal seizures), there may be no abnormal movements at all; in some other types of seizures, only a part of the body may be affected by abnormal movements. A convulsion or seizure may occur as an isolated incident, such as one associated with fever in a young child. When convulsions or seizures are recurrent, the term *epilepsy* is used.

Anticonvulsant drugs belong to several different chemical groups, but they have similar antiseizure properties. The precise mechanism and site of action are not clear. It is thought, however, that these drugs act in two ways to control seizure activity. First, they may act directly on abnormal neurons to decrease their excitability and responsiveness to stimuli. Consequently, the seizure threshold is raised and seizure activity is decreased. Second, and more commonly, they prevent the spread of impulses to the normal neurons that surround the abnormal ones. This helps to prevent or minimize seizures by confining excessive electrical activity to a small portion of the brain. The ability of the drugs to reduce the responsiveness of normal neurons to stimuli may be related to alterations in the activity of sodium, potassium, calcium, and magnesium ions at the cell membrane. Such ionic activity is necessary for normal conduction of nerve impulses, and changes engendered by the anticonvulsant drugs result in stabilized, less responsive cell membranes.

Most anticonvulsant drugs can be taken orally and are absorbed through the intestinal mucosa. The degree of absorption depends on drug solubility and other chemical or enzymatic conversions in the gastrointestinal tract. After absorption, the drugs pass through the liver and undergo transformation by liver enzymes, during which a portion of the drug is inactivated. All anticonvulsant drugs are metabolized in the liver.

The major clinical indication for anticonvulsant drugs is in prevention or treatment of seizure activity, especially the chronic recurring seizures of epilepsy. *Epilepsy* is a fairly common brain disorder characterized by abnormal and excessive electrical discharges of nerve cells. It is diagnosed by clinical signs and symptoms of seizure activity and by the presence of abnormal brain wave patterns as shown on the electroencephalogram (EEG). The cause of most cases of epilepsy is unknown. When epilepsy begins in infancy, causes include developmental defects, metabolic disease, or birth injury. When it begins in adulthood, it is usually caused by an acquired brain disorder, such as head injury, disease or infection of the brain and spinal cord, cerebrovascular accident (CVA, or stroke), metabolic disorder, primary or metastatic brain tumor, or other recognizable neurologic disease.

Epilepsy is classified in different ways, and different terms are used. Traditionally, it has been described as grand mal, petit mal or absence, psychomotor, and Jacksonian. A more recent and preferred system is the international classification proposed by Gastaut in 1970. In this system, the two major classes are *partial* and *generalized seizures.* Partial or focal seizures begin in a specific area of the brain and produce symptoms ranging from simple motor and sensory manifestations to more complex abnormal movements and bizarre behavior. Movements are usually automatic, repetitive, and inappropriate to the situation, such as chewing, swallowing, or aversive movements. Behavior may be so bizarre that the person is sometimes diagnosed as psychotic or schizophrenic. Generalized seizures are bilateral and symmetric and have no discernible point of origin in the brain. The most common type is the tonic–clonic or major motor seizure, formerly called grand mal epilepsy. The tonic phase involves sustained contraction of skeletal muscles, abnormal postures such as opisthotonos, and absence of respiration, during which the person becomes cyanotic. The clonic phase is characterized by rapid rhythmic and symmetric jerking movements of the body. Tonic–clonic seizures are sometimes preceded by an aura, a brief warning such as a flash of light or a specific sound. Another type of generalized seizure is the absence seizure, also called *petit mal epilepsy,* which is characterized by abrupt alterations in consciousness that last only a few seconds. The person may have a blank, staring expression with or without blinking of the eyelids, twitching of the head or arms, and other motor movements. Other types of generalized seizures include the myoclonic type (contraction of a muscle or group of muscles) and the akinetic type (absence of movement). Some people are subject to mixed seizures.

In addition to maintenance treatment of epilepsy, anticonvulsant drugs are also used to stop acute convulsions and the life-threatening, continuous seizures called *status epilepticus.* The drug of choice for this purpose is diazepam (Valium), given intravenously. Once seizure activity is controlled, long-term drug therapy is begun with other agents to prevent recurrence. Prophylactic use of the drugs is often indicated in people with severe head injuries, following brain surgery, and in children with febrile seizures.

Individual anticonvulsant drugs

BARBITURATES

Phenobarbital is a long-acting barbiturate. It is one of the safest, most effective, and most widely used anticonvulsant drugs. It is most effective in generalized tonic–clonic epilepsy (major motor or grand mal), temporal lobe and other partial seizures, and febrile convulsions in children. It is less effective in absence seizures (petit mal) and in myoclonic and akinetic epilepsy, but it is sometimes helpful because generalized tonic–clonic seizures may complicate other types of seizures. It acts to limit the spread of seizure activity and raise the seizure threshold.

Although phenobarbital is sometimes used alone as initial anticonvulsant drug therapy, especially in children, it is probably more often the second drug added when phenytoin has not controlled seizure activity adequately. Drug dependence and barbiturate intoxication are unlikely to occur with the usual doses of phenobarbital used in epilepsy treatment. Since phenobarbital has a long half-life, it takes about 2 or 3 weeks to reach therapeutic serum levels and about 3 or 4 weeks to reach a steady state concentration. Serum drug levels of about 10 to 25 μg/ml are considered in the therapeutic range; higher concentrations are often accompanied by signs and symptoms of toxicity.

Mephobarbital (Mebaral) and *metharbital* (Gemonil) are two other long-acting barbiturates used clinically in seizure disorders, usually in children who become hyperactive or hyperexcitable with phenobarbital.

For further discussion and anticonvulsant dosages of barbiturates, see Chapter 7.

HYDANTOINS

Phenytoin (Dilantin) is the prototype of a group of anticonvulsant drugs called the hydantoins. It is the most widely used and effective drug for generalized tonic–clonic and some partial seizures such as psychomotor seizures. Phenytoin is usually the initial drug of choice, especially in adults. It is often given with phenobarbital or primidone when a single agent does not control seizures. It is also used to prevent seizures in people who have had brain surgery or brain injury. Phenytoin is not effective in absence, myoclonic, or akinetic seizures. The drug is also used in some cardiac arrhythmias, especially those resulting from digitalis toxicity.

The rate at which phenytoin is metabolized varies, but the average half-life is about 18 to 24 hours. The clinical significance of this relatively long half-life is that phenytoin can be given once or twice daily and that, when it is started at usual maintenance doses, a steady-state concentration in plasma is not reached for about 7 to 21 days. The therapeutic serum level is 10 to 20 μg/ml. Concentrations at or above the upper therapeutic range may be associated with clinical signs of toxicity.

Routes and dosage ranges

Adults: PO 3.5–7 mg/kg/day
IM 8.6 mg/kg/day in multiple sites
IV same as PO dose (should not exceed 50 mg/min)
Children: PO 4–7 mg/kg/day in divided doses

Ethotoin (Peganone) is a hydantoin that may be effective in generalized tonic–clonic and psychomotor seizures. It is both less effective and less toxic than phenytoin. It is usually combined with other anticonvulsant drugs because it is rarely effective alone. Also, it is used as an alternative drug when seizures are not controlled by other agents.

Route and dosage range

Adults: PO 2–3 g daily in 4–6 divided doses
Children: PO 0.5–1 g daily in divided doses

Mephenytoin (Mesantoin) is less effective and more toxic than phenytoin, but it is sometimes used as an alternative drug in treating generalized tonic–clonic and some partial seizures such as psychomotor and Jacksonian.

Route and dosage ranges

Adults: PO 300–600 mg daily
Children: PO 100–400 mg daily

SUCCINIMIDES

Ethosuximide (Zarontin) is the prototype of the succinimide anticonvulsant drugs and is the drug of choice for absence seizures. It may also be effective in myoclonic and akinetic epilepsy but is usually ineffective in psychomotor and generalized tonic–clonic seizures. It is of little value in treating severe organic brain damage. Ethosuximide may be used with other anticonvulsant drugs for treatment of mixed seizures. The therapeutic range of serum drug levels is about 40 to 80 μg/ml, and about 5 days of drug administration are necessary to reach a steady-state serum concentration.

Route and dosage ranges

Adults: PO initially, 500 mg daily, increased by 250 mg at weekly intervals until seizures are controlled or toxicity occurs. Maximal daily dose, approximately 1500 mg
Children: PO initially, 250 mg daily, increased as above. Maximal daily dose, approximately 750–1000 mg

Methsuximide (Celontin) may be used as an alternative drug to ethosuximide in absence, myoclonic and akinetic seizures or in combination with other anticonvulsant drugs for mixed seizures.

Route and dosage range

Adults: PO initially 300 mg daily, usual daily dose 600–1200 mg
Children: same as adults

Phensuximide (Milontin) is the least effective and least toxic of the succinimide drugs. It may be used for absence seizures that do not respond to other drugs. However, because effectiveness is decreased with prolonged use, it is recommended for short-term use.

Route and dosage range

Adults: PO 1–3 g daily in 2–3 divided doses
Children: same as adults

BENZODIAZEPINES (see also Chap. 8)

Clonazepam (Klonopin) is a benzodiazepine drug used as an anticonvulsant. It may be used alone or with other anticonvulsant drugs in myoclonic or akinetic seizures. It is possibly effective in generalized tonic–clonic and psychomotor seizures. Its effectiveness in absence seizures is variable, but it may be helpful in some clients who do not respond to the succinimides. Tolerance to anticonvulsant effects develops with long-term use.

Clonazepam has a long half-life and may require weeks of continued administration to achieve steady-state serum concentrations of 0.013 to 0.072 μg/ml. Clonazepam also produces physical and psychologic dependence as well as withdrawal symptoms. Owing to its long half-life, withdrawal symptoms may appear several days after administration is stopped. Abrupt withdrawal may precipitate seizure activity or status epilepticus.

Route and dosage ranges

Adults: PO 1.5 mg daily, increased by 0.5 mg daily every 3–7 days if necessary, to a maximal daily dose of 20 mg
Children: PO 0.01–0.03 mg/kg/day, increased by 0.25–0.5 mg daily every 3–7 days if necessary, to a maximal daily dose of 0.2 mg/kg

Clorazepate (Tranxene) is a benzodiazepine used for anxiety, acute alcohol withdrawal, and adjunctive therapy in the management of partial seizures.

Route and dosage ranges

Adults: Seizures PO maximal initial dose, 7.5 mg 3 times daily, increased by no more than 7.5 mg/week; maximal dose, 90 mg/day

Children 9–12 years: Seizures PO maximal initial dose, 7.5 mg twice daily, increased by no more than 7.5 mg/week; maximal daily dose, 60 mg

Diazepam (Valium) is a benzodiazepine that is widely used as an antianxiety or sedative agent. In seizure disorders, it is used to terminate acute convulsive seizures. It is the drug of choice for treating the life-threatening seizures of status epilepticus.

Route and dosage ranges

Adults: Acute convulsive seizures, status epilepticus, IV (at a rate not to exceed 5 mg [1 ml]/minute), 5–10 mg. Repeat every 5–10 minutes if needed to a maximum dose of 30 mg. If necessary, repeat regimen in 2–4 hours. Maximal dose in 24 hours, 100 mg

Children: Acute convulsive seizures, status epilepticus, IV (slowly as above), IM 2–5 mg in a single dose. Repeat dose in 2–4 hours if necessary.

OTHER ANTICONVULSANT DRUGS

Acetazolamide (Diamox) is a carbonic anhydrase inhibitor used as an adjunctive drug in many forms of epilepsy, including generalized tonic–clonic (grand mal), absence (petit mal), and partial focal seizures. It is most often used for refractory absence seizures. It is thought to decrease abnormal electrical activity directly by inhibiting carbonic anhydrase or indirectly by producing acidosis. Carbonic anhydrase is an enzyme that catalyzes water and carbon dioxide to form carbonic acid.

Route and dosage range

Adults: PO 8–30 mg/kg/day in 3–4 divided doses
Children: same as adults

Carbamazepine (Tegretol) is related chemically to the tricyclic antidepressants and pharmacologically to the hydantoin anticonvulsants. It is used mainly for psychomotor, generalized tonic–clonic, and mixed seizures. It is not effective for absence, myoclonic, or akinetic seizures.

Since carbamazepine may cause life-threatening blood dyscrasias (*e.g.*, aplastic anemia, agranulocytosis, thrombocytopenia, leukopenia), its use should be reserved for clients whose seizures cannot be controlled with other drugs. Carbamazepine is contraindicated in clients with previous bone marrow depression or hypersensitivity to carbamazepine or tricyclic antidepressants (TCAs) or clients who are receiving monoamine oxidase (MAO) inhibitors. MAO inhibitors should be discontinued at least 14 days before carbamazepine is started. Carbamazepine is also used to treat facial pain associated with trigeminal neuralgia (tic douloureux).

Route and dosage ranges

Adults: Epilepsy, PO 200 mg twice daily initially, increased gradually to 600–1200 mg if needed, in 3–4 divided doses
Trigeminal neuralgia, PO 200 mg daily initially, increased gradually to 1200 mg if necessary

Children: PO 200 mg twice daily initially, gradually increased to 20–30 mg/kg daily if necessary to control seizures

Paramethadione (Paradione) and **trimethadione** (Tridione) are similar drugs used to treat absence seizures that do not respond to other drugs. They cause a high incidence of adverse effects and are alternative drugs rather than primary drugs of choice. The route of administration and dosage are the same for the two drugs.

Route and dosage ranges

Adults: PO 900–2100 mg daily, in single or divided doses
Children: PO 300–900 mg daily (20–60 mg/kg)

Primidone (Mysoline) is converted to two metabolites, phenobarbital and phenylethylmalonamide (PEMA). The parent drug and both metabolites apparently exert anticonvulsant effects. Therefore, measurements of plasma drug levels should include all three chemicals. The therapeutic ranges are phenobarbital, 10 to 20 μg/ml; primidone, 5 to 10 μg/ml; and PEMA, 7 to 15 μg/ml. Primidone can be used in initial drug therapy but is most often used as a substitute for barbiturates in treating clients who do not respond adequately to a barbiturate–hydantoin combination. Because it produces rather marked sedation, primidone is an alternative rather than a primary drug. Excessive sedation is minimized by increasing dosage very gradually. Sedation decreases with continued administration of the drug.

Route and dosage ranges

Adults: PO 500–1500 mg daily in divided doses
Children: PO 5–20 mg/kg/day

Valproic acid (Depakene) is used in treating absence and mixed seizures. It is chemically unrelated to other anticonvulsant drugs and produces a much lower incidence of adverse effects. Its mechanism of action is unknown. Therapeutic plasma levels are approximately 50 to 100 μg/ml.

Route and dosage ranges

Adults: PO 1000–3000 mg daily in divided doses
Children: PO 15–30 mg/kg/day

Principles of therapy: anticonvulsant drugs

ASSESSMENT IN SEIZURE DISORDERS

Assess client status in relation to seizure activity and other factors.

1. If the client has a known seizure disorder and is taking anticonvulsant drugs, helpful assessment data can be obtained by interviewing the client. Some questions and guidelines include the following:
   a. How long has the client had the seizure disorder?
   b. How long has it been since seizure activity occurred, or what is the frequency of seizures?
   c. Does any particular situation or activity seem to cause a seizure?
   d. Does an aura warn of an impending seizure?
   e. How does the seizure affect the client? For example, what parts of the body are involved? Does he lose consciousness? Is he drowsy and tired afterward?
   f. Which anticonvulsant drugs are taken? How do they affect the client? How long has the client taken the drugs? Is the currently ordered dosage the same as that which the client has been taking? Does the client usually take the drugs as prescribed, or does he find it difficult to do so?
   g. What other drugs are taken? This includes both prescription and nonprescription drugs as well as those taken regularly or periodically. This information is necessary because many drugs interact with anticonvulsant drugs to decrease seizure control or increase drug toxicity.
   h. What is the client's attitude toward the seizure disorder? Clues to attitude may include terminology, willingness or reluctance to discuss the seizure disorder, compliance or rejection of drug therapy, and others.
2. Check reports of serum drug levels for abnormal values.
3. People without previous seizure activity may develop seizure disorders with brain surgery, head injury, hypoxia, hypoglycemia, drug overdosage (central nervous system [CNS] stimulants such as amphetamines or local anesthetics such as lidocaine), and withdrawal from CNS depressants such as alcohol and barbiturates.
4. To observe and record seizure activity accurately, note location (localized or generalized), specific characteristics of abnormal movements or behavior, duration, concomitant events such as loss of consciousness and loss of bowel or bladder control, and postseizure behavior.
5. To protect a client experiencing a generalized tonic–clonic seizure
   a. Place a pillow or piece of clothing under the head if injury could be sustained from the ground or floor.
   b. Place a padded tongue depressor, rolled washcloth, or something similar between the teeth to protect the jaws and the tongue. Do not use spoons or similar objects that can be aspirated or increase mouth trauma. If the teeth are clenched tightly, do not try to force them open to insert something. Teeth may be broken off and aspirated.
   c. Do not restrain the client's movements; fractures may result.
   d. Loosen tight clothing, especially around the chest, to promote respiration.
   e. When convulsive movements stop, turn the client to one side so that accumulated secretions can drain from the mouth and the throat. The cyanosis, abnormal movements, and loss of consciousness that characterize a generalized tonic–clonic seizure can be quite alarming to witnesses. Most of these seizures, however, subside within 3 or 4 minutes, and the person starts responding and regaining normal skin color. If the person has one seizure after another (status epilepticus), has trouble breathing or continued cyanosis, or has sustained an injury, further care is needed and a physician should be notified immediately.

NURSING INTERVENTIONS

Use measures to minimize seizure activity. Guidelines include the following:

1. Assist the client to identify conditions under which seizures are likely to occur. These precipitating factors, to be avoided or decreased when possible, may include ingestion of alcoholic beverages or of stimulant drugs such as amphetamines, fever, severe physical or emotional stress, and sensory stimuli such as flashing lights and loud noises.
2. Teach the client such health promotion measures as obtaining sufficient rest and exercise and eating a balanced diet.

3. Assist the client to comply with prescribed drug therapy by
    a. Teaching the client and family members about the seizure disorder and the plan for treatment, including drugs
    b. Involving the client in decision making when possible
    c. Informing the client and family that seizure control is not gained immediately when drug therapy is started. The goal is to avoid unrealistic expectations and excessive frustration while drugs and dosages are being changed in the effort to determine the best combination for the client
    d. Discussing social and economic factors that promote or prevent compliance

DRUG SELECTION AND DOSAGE TO ACHIEVE TREATMENT GOALS

With epilepsy, the only effective treatment modality is long-term drug therapy, and the goal is complete control of seizure activity. To meet this goal, therapy must be individualized.

1. The choice of drug or drugs is determined largely by the type of seizure. Therefore, an accurate diagnosis is essential before drug therapy is started. For generalized convulsive and focal seizures, phenytoin, carbamazepine, and phenobarbital are considered drugs of choice. Valproic acid is also effective. For absence seizures, ethosuximide is the drug of choice; methsuximide, clonazepam, valproic acid, and trimethadione are also effective. For mixed seizures, a combination of drugs is usually necessary. Other factors influencing choice include drug cost, half-life and toxicity, and client characteristics such as willingness to comply with the prescribed regimen.
2. Drug dosage depends on several variables.
    a. Generally, larger doses may be needed for people with a large body mass (assuming normal liver and kidney function) and in cases involving trauma, surgery, and emotional stress.
    b. Smaller doses are usually required when liver disease is present and when multiple drugs are being given.
    c. For most drugs, initial doses are relatively low; doses are gradually increased until seizures are controlled or adverse effects occur.
    d. When phenytoin is used, larger doses may be needed for intramuscular (IM) injection because the drug is deposited in tissues and complete absorption requires about 5 days. The IM route is also very painful. However, phenytoin can be given IM if necessary, preferably for 1 week or less. When substituted for oral phenytoin, the IM dose is 50% larger than the previous oral dose. When oral administration is resumed, the oral dose is about half the dose taken before use of IM phenytoin. This dose can be gradually increased over several days, using the serum drug levels as a guide, until the previous oral maintenance dose is reached. If clients are given full oral doses as soon as IM injections are stopped, toxicity may occur because phenytoin is still being absorbed into the bloodstream from injection sites.
3. The effectiveness of drug therapy is evaluated by client response in terms of therapeutic or adverse effects and by serum drug levels. Each anticonvulsant drug has a therapeutic range of serum levels in which most clients achieve control of seizures. The time required for a drug to reach therapeutic levels may be several days or weeks, depending on drug half-life, rate of metabolism, and other factors.
4. Most anticonvulsant drugs have the potential for causing blood, liver, and kidney disorders. This is especially true of the alternative or "secondary" drugs. For this reason, it is usually recommended that baseline blood studies (complete blood count, platelet count) and liver function tests (*e.g.,* bilirubin, serum protein, serum glutamic oxaloacetic transaminase [SGOT]) be performed before drug therapy and periodically thereafter.
5. When drug therapy fails to control seizures, there are several possible reasons. Probably the most frequent one is client failure to take the anticonvulsant drug as prescribed. Other common causes include inadequate dosage of the prescribed drug(s), failure to use two or more drugs concomitantly when indicated, incorrect diagnosis of the type of seizure, use of the wrong drug for the type of seizure, and too frequent changes or premature withdrawal of drugs (changing or withdrawing a drug before serum concentration has reached therapeutic levels and before the response can be evaluated properly).

DURATION AND DISCONTINUATION OF THERAPY

For most clients, anticonvulsant therapy is life long. For others, drugs may be discontinued, usually after the client remains seizure free for 2 to 5 years. Even if drugs cannot be stopped completely, periodic attempts to decrease number or dosage of drugs are probably desirable to minimize adverse reactions. Discontinuing drugs, changing drugs, or changing dosage must be done gradually over weeks or months. Sudden withdrawal or dosage decreases may cause status epilepticus.

STATUS EPILEPTICUS

Status epilepticus is a life-threatening situation characterized by generalized tonic–clonic convulsions occurring at close intervals. The client does not regain consciousness between seizures, and hypoxia, cardiac arrhythmias, and other problems occur and may result in death. The treatment of choice is intravenous diazepam, injected slowly and stopped when seizure activity ceases. Intravenous phenobarbital or phenytoin may also be used.

USE IN PREGNANCY

Usage of anticonvulsant drugs during pregnancy presents a dilemma. On one hand, infants born to mothers who took the drugs during early pregnancy have a higher-than-usual incidence of birth defects. These teratogenic effects are most clearly associated with phenobarbital, phenytoin, and trimethadione. On the other hand, any seizure activity is potentially harmful to the fetus. Also, if status epilepticus occurs from changes in drug therapy, both mother and fetus are threatened. If anticonvulsant drugs can be avoided or if dosage can be reduced without precipitating seizures, particularly in the first trimester, it is probably safer for the fetus.

PEDIATRIC CONSIDERATIONS

In pediatric anticonvulsant therapy, influencing factors include the following:

1. In newborns, oral drugs are absorbed slowly and inefficiently. If anticonvulsant drugs are necessary during the first 7 to 10 days of life, IM phenobarbital is effective. Metabolism and excretion are also delayed during the first week or two, but rates are more rapid than adult rates by 2 to 3 months of age.
2. In infants and children, oral drugs are absorbed rapidly and have a shorter half-life. Thus, therapeutic serum drug levels are produced earlier than in adults. Drug metabolism and excretion rates are also increased, and children require higher doses per kilogram of body weight than adults. The fast rate of drug elimination from the body persists until approximately 6 years of age, at which time it decreases until it stabilizes around the adult rate by 10 to 14 years of age.
3. A particular concern with children is to avoid excessive sedation and other drug effects that interfere with learning and social development.

GERIATRIC CONSIDERATIONS

In geriatric anticonvulsant therapy, relatively small doses may be necessary because of slowed drug metabolism.

NURSING ACTIONS: ANTICONVULSANT DRUGS

Nursing Actions	*Rationale/Explanation*
1. Administer accurately	
a. Give oral anticonvulsant drugs after meals or with a full glass of water or other fluid.	Most anticonvulsant drugs cause some gastric irritation, nausea, or vomiting. Taking the drugs with food or fluid helps to decrease gastrointestinal side-effects.
b. To give phenytoin	
(1) Shake oral suspensions of the drug vigorously before pouring and always use the same measuring equipment.	When a drug preparation is called a *suspension,* it means that particles of drug are suspended or floating in water or other liquid. On standing, drug particles settle to the bottom of the container. Shaking the container is necessary to achieve a uniform distribution of drug particles in the liquid vehicle. If the contents are not mixed well every time a dose is given, the liquid vehicle will be given initially, and the concentrated drug will be given later. That is, underdosage will occur at first, and little if any therapeutic benefit will result. Overdosage will follow, and the risks of serious toxicity are greatly increased. Using the same measuring container ensures consistent dosage. Calibrated medication cups or measuring tea-

Nursing Actions	Rationale/Explanation
	spoons or tablespoons are acceptable. Regular household teaspoons and tablespoons used for eating and serving are *not* acceptable because sizes vary widely.
(2) Do not mix parenteral phenytoin in the same syringe with any other drug.	Phenytoin solution is highly alkaline (*p*H approximately 12) and physically incompatible with other drugs. A precipitate occurs if mixing is attempted.
(3) Give phenytoin as an undiluted intravenous (IV) bolus injection at a rate not exceeding 50 mg/minute, then flush the IV line with normal saline or dilute in 50 to 100 ml of normal saline (0.9% NaCl) and administer over approximately 30 to 60 minutes. If "piggybacked" into a primary IV line, the primary IV solution must be normal saline or the line must be flushed with normal saline before and after administration of phenytoin.	Phenytoin cannot be diluted or given in IV fluids other than normal saline because it precipitates within minutes. Slow administration and dilution decrease local venous irritation from the highly alkaline drug solution. Rapid administration must be avoided because it may produce myocardial depression, hypotension, cardiac arrhythmias, and even cardiac arrest.
(4) Give IM phenytoin deeply into a large muscle mass and rotate injection sites.	Phenytoin is absorbed slowly when given IM and causes local tissue irritation. Correct administration helps to increase absorption and decrease pain.
2. Observe for therapeutic effects	
a. When drug is given on a long-term basis to prevent seizures, observe for a decrease or absence of seizure activity.	Therapeutic effects begin later with anticonvulsant drugs than with most other drug groups because the anticonvulsant drugs have relatively long half-lives. Optimum therapeutic benefits of phenytoin occur about 7 to 10 days after drug therapy is started. Those of phenobarbital occur in about 2 weeks; those of ethosuximide, in about 5 days.
b. When drug is given to stop an acute convulsive seizure, seizure activity usually slows or stops within a few minutes.	Diazepam is the drug of choice for controlling an acute convulsion because it acts rapidly. Even when given IV, phenytoin and phenobarbital do not act for several minutes.
3. Observe for adverse effects	
a. CNS effects—drowsiness, sedation, ataxia, diplopia, nystagmus	These effects are common, especially during the first week or two of drug therapy.
b. Gastrointestinal effects—anorexia, nausea, vomiting	These common effects of oral drugs can be reduced by taking the drugs with food or a full glass of water.
c. Skin disorders—rash, urticaria, exfoliative dermatitis, Stevens–Johnson syndrome (a severe reaction accompanied by headache, arthralgia, and other symptoms in addition to skin lesions)	These may occur with almost all the anticonvulsant drugs. Some are mild; some are potentially serious but rare. Most skin reactions are apparently caused by hypersensitivity or idiosyncratic reactions and are usually sufficient reason to discontinue the drug.
d. Blood dyscrasias—anemia, leukopenia, thrombocytopenia, agranulocytosis	Most anticonvulsant drugs produce decreases in the levels of folic acid, which may progress to megaloblastic anemia. The other disorders indicate bone marrow depression and are potentially life threatening. They do not usually occur with phenytoin, phenobarbital, or primidone but may infrequently occur with most other anticonvulsant drugs.
e. Respiratory depression	This is not likely to be a significant adverse reaction except when a depressant drug such as diazepam or a barbiturate is given IV to control acute seizures such as status epilepticus. Even then, respiratory depression can be minimized by avoiding overdosage and rapid administration.
f. Liver damage—hepatitis symptoms, jaundice, abnormal liver function tests	Hepatic damage may occur with phenytoin, and fatal hepatotoxicity has been reported with valproic acid.
g. Gingival hyperplasia	Occurs often with phenytoin, especially in children. It may be prevented or delayed by vigorous oral hygiene or treated surgically by gingivectomy.

Nursing Actions	Rationale/Explanation
h. Hypocalcemia	Hypocalcemia may occur when anticonvulsant drugs are taken in high doses and over long periods.
i. Lymphadenopathy resembling malignant lymphoma	This reaction has occurred with several anticonvulsant drugs, most often with phenytoin and other hydantoins.
4. Observe for drug interactions	Most documented drug interactions involve phenytoin, phenobarbital, and valproic acid.
a. Drugs that *increase* effects of anticonvulsants	
(1) CNS depressants	Additive CNS depression
(2) Other anticonvulsants	Additive or synergistic effects
b. Drugs that *decrease* effects of anticonvulsants	
(1) TCAs, antipsychotic drugs, reserpine and other *Rauwolfia* alkaloids	These drugs may lower the seizure threshold and precipitate seizures. Dosage of anticonvulsant drugs may need to be increased.
(2) Barbiturates and other enzyme inducers	These drugs inhibit themselves and other anticonvulsant drugs by activating liver enzymes and accelerating the rate of drug metabolism.
c. Additional drugs that alter effects of phenytoin	
(1) Oral antidiabetic agents, antituberculosis drugs (isoniazid, cycloserine), aspirin and other salicylates, chloramphenicol, oral contraceptives, disulfiram, estrogens, methylphenidate, phenylbutazone, and some sulfonamides increase effects of phenytoin	These drugs generally increase phenytoin toxicity by inhibiting hepatic metabolism of phenytoin or by displacing it from plasma protein binding sites.
(2) Enzyme-inducing drugs (alcohol, sedative–hypnotic drugs) decrease effects of phenytoin.	These agents activate liver enzymes and accelerate phenytoin metabolism with chronic use.
(3) Phenobarbital has variable interactions with phenytoin	Phenytoin and phenobarbital have complex interactions with unpredictable effects. Interactions are considered separately because the two drugs are often used at the same time. Although phenobarbital induces drug metabolism in the liver and may increase the rate of metabolism of other anticonvulsant drugs, its interaction with phenytoin differs. Phenobarbital apparently decreases serum levels of phenytoin and perhaps its half-life. Still, the anticonvulsant effects of the two drugs together are greater than those of either drug given alone. The interaction apparently varies with dosage, route, time of administration, the degree of liver enzyme induction already present, and other factors. Thus, whether a significant interaction will occur in a given client is unpredictable. Probably the most important clinical implication is that close observation of the client is necessary when either drug is being added or withdrawn.
d. Interactions with phenobarbital	
(1) Valproic acid	This anticonvulsant drug may increase plasma levels of phenobarbital as much as 40%, probably by inhibiting liver-metabolizing enzymes.
(2) See Chapter 7.	Many drugs interact with the barbiturates, the drug group of which phenobarbital is a member. These drug interactions are listed in Chapter 7.
e. Interactions with clonazepam, clorazepate, and diazepam	These drugs are benzodiazepines, which are discussed in Chapter 8.
5. Teach clients and parents of children	
a. Take anticonvulsant drugs with food or a full glass of fluid.	To avoid nausea, vomiting and gastric distress, which are adverse reactions to most of these drugs
b. Take these drugs as prescribed.	This is extremely important. These drugs must be taken regularly to maintain blood levels adequate to control seizure activ-

Nursing Actions	Rationale/Explanation
	ity. At the same time, additional doses must not be taken because of increased risks of serious adverse reactions. Also, these drugs must not be stopped abruptly, or seizures are likely to result.
c. Report any difficulties with drug therapy to the prescribing physician or other health-care worker.	These difficulties include seizure activity, excessive drowsiness, or other adverse effects. The physician may be able to adjust dosage or time of administration to relieve the problem.
d. Do not drive a car, operate machinery, or perform other activities requiring physical and mental alertness when drowsy from anticonvulsant drugs.	Drowsiness, sedation, decreased physical coordination, and decreased mental alertness increase the likelihood of injury. Many states do not allow people with seizure disorders to drive automobiles.
e. Do not take other drugs without the physician's knowledge; inform any other physician or dentist about taking anticonvulsant drugs.	There are many potential drug interactions in which the effects of the anticonvulsant drug or other drugs may be altered when drugs are given concomitantly.
f. Carry adequate identification such as a card that contains pertinent medical information.	This is necessary for rapid and appropriate treatment in the event of a seizure, accidental injury, or other emergency situation.
g. A resource for information is the Epilepsy Foundations of America, 1828 L Street, NW, Washington, DC 20036	
h. When taking phenytoin	
(1) Ask for the same brand and form of the drug when renewing prescriptions.	There may be differences in drugs produced by different manufacturers. These differences, such as how fast and how completely the drug is absorbed into the bloodstream, influence both seizure control and likelihood of adverse reactions.
(2) If taking or giving a liquid preparation of phenytoin, always mix thoroughly and use the same size medicine cup or measuring spoon. Do not use household teaspoons or tablespoons.	This is necessary to ensure accurate and consistent dosage. Household spoons vary widely in size, and using them leads to inaccurate dosages.

Selected References

American Academy of Pediatrics (Committee on Drugs): Behavioral and cognitive effects of anticonvulsant therapy. Pediatrics 76:644–647, October 1985

American Medical Association Division of Drugs: AMA Drug Evaluations, 5th ed. New York, John Wiley & Sons, 1983

Anderson PD: Basic Human Anatomy and Physiology: Clinical Implications for the Health Professions. Monterey, CA, Wadsworth, 1984

Clancy PR: Managing epilepsy. II. New developments in evaluation and treatment. Drug Ther 14:121–139, January 1984

Drugs for epilepsy. Med Lett Drug Ther 25:81–84, September 1983

Facts and Comparisons. St Louis, J B Lippincott (Updated monthly)

Groer MW, Shekleton ME: Basic Pathophysiology: A Conceptual Approach, 2d ed. St Louis, C V Mosby, 1983

Guyton AC: Textbook of Medical Physiology, 7th ed. Philadelphia, W B Saunders, 1986

Hansten PD: Drug Interactions: Clinical Significance of Drug–Drug Interactions, 5th ed. Philadelphia, Lea & Febiger, 1985

Hawken M, Ozuna J: Practical aspects of anticonvulsant therapy. Am J Nurs 79:1062–1068, June 1979

Malseed RT: Pharmacology: Drug Therapy and Nursing Considerations, 2d ed. Philadelphia, J B Lippincott, 1985

Parrish MA: A comparison of behavioral side effects related to commonly used anticonvulsants. Pediatr Nurs 10:149–152, March–April 1984

Rodman MJ, Karch AM, Boyd EH, Smith DW: Pharmacology and Drug Therapy in Nursing, 3rd ed. Philadelphia, J B Lippincott, 1985

Rall TW, Schleifer LS: Drugs effective in the therapy of the epilepsies. In Gilman AG, Goodman LS, Rall TW, Murad F (eds): The Pharmacological Basis of Therapeutics, 7th ed, pp 446–472. New York, Macmillan, 1985

12

ANTIPARKINSON DRUGS

Description and uses

Parkinson's disease is a chronic, progressive, degenerative disorder of the central nervous system (CNS) characterized by abnormalities in movement and posture (tremor, bradykinesia, joint and muscular rigidity). The cause of classic parkinsonism is unknown. Signs and symptoms of the disease may also occur with other CNS diseases or trauma and with the use of antipsychotic drugs.

The basal ganglia in the brain normally contain substantial amounts of dopamine, an inhibitory neurotransmitter, and acetylcholine, an excitatory neurotransmitter. The correct balance of dopamine and acetylcholine is important in regulating posture, muscle tone, and voluntary movement. People with Parkinson's disease suffer an imbalance in these neurotransmitters, resulting in a functional and absolute decrease in brain dopamine and a relative increase in acetylcholine.

Drugs used in Parkinson's disease act to increase levels of dopamine (dopaminergic agents) or inhibit the actions of acetylcholine (anticholinergic agents) in the brain. The goal of antiparkinson drug therapy is to control symptoms and improve the client's ability to perform activities of daily living.

DOPAMINERGIC DRUGS

Levodopa, carbidopa, amantadine, and bromocriptine are dopaminergic drugs that exert beneficial effects in Parkinson's disease. Levodopa is the mainstay of drug therapy for classic or idiopathic parkinsonism; carbidopa is used only in conjunction with levodopa; amantadine and bromocriptine are used mainly as adjunctive drugs.

ANTICHOLINERGIC DRUGS

Anticholinergic drugs are discussed in Chapter 21 and listed in Table 12-1. They are described here only in relation to their use in the treatment of Parkinson's disease. Only those anticholinergic drugs that are centrally active (*i.e.,* penetrate the blood–brain barrier) are useful in treating parkinsonism. Trihexyphenidyl (Artane) is the most frequently used drug of this type. Atropine and scopolamine are centrally active but are not used because of a high incidence of adverse reactions. Synthetic anticholinergic–antispasmodic drugs sometimes used in the treatment of gastrointestinal disorders do not penetrate the blood–brain barrier and thus are ineffective in Parkinson's disease.

Anticholinergic drugs may be used in idiopathic parkinsonism to decrease salivation, spasticity, and tremors. Their use has declined with the development of more effective antiparkinson drugs. Currently, they are used primarily for people who have minimal symptoms or who cannot tolerate levodopa or in combination with other antiparkinson drugs. Anticholinergic agents are also used to relieve symptoms of parkinsonism that can occur with the use of antipsychotic drugs.

In addition to the primary anticholinergic drugs, one phenothiazine (ethapropazine [Parsidol]) and three antihistamines (chlorphenoxamine [Phenoxene], diphenhydramine [Benadryl], and orphenadrine [Disi-

TABLE 12-1. ANTICHOLINERGIC ANTIPARKINSON DRUGS

	Generic name	Trade name	Routes and dosage ranges (adults)
Primary agents	Benztropine	Cogentin	PO 0.5–1 mg at bedtime initially, gradually increased to 4–6 mg daily if necessary
	Biperiden	Akincton	Parkinsonism, PO 2 mg 3–4 times daily Drug-induced extrapyramidal reactions, PO 2 mg 1–3 times daily, IM 2 mg repeated q30 minutes if necessary to a maximum of 8 mg in 24 hours
	Procyclidine	Kemadrin	PO 5 mg twice daily initially, gradually increased to 5 mg 3–4 times daily if necessary
	Trihexyphenidyl	Artane	PO 1–2 mg daily initially, gradually increased up to 12–15 mg daily, until therapeutic or adverse effects occur Drug-induced extrapyramidal reactions, PO 1 mg initially, gradually increased to 5–15 mg daily if necessary
Secondary agents	Chlorphenoxamine hydrochloride	Phenoxene	PO 50 mg 3 times daily initially, gradually increased to 100 mg 2–4 times daily if necessary
	Diphenhydramine hydrochloride	Benadryl	PO 25 mg 3 times daily, gradually increased to 50 mg 4 times daily if necessary Drug-induced extrapyramidal reactions, IM, IV 10–50 mg. Maximal single dose, 100 mg; maximal daily dose, 400 mg Children: Drug-induced extrapyramidal reactions, IM 5 mg/kg/day. Maximal daily dose, 300 mg
	Ethopropazine hydrochloride	Parsidol	PO 50 mg once or twice daily initially, gradually increased to a maximal daily dose of 600 mg if necessary
	Orphenadrine hydrochloride	Disipal	PO 50 mg 3 times daily initially, gradually increased up to 250 mg daily if necessary and tolerated

pal]) are also used to treat Parkinson's disease because of their strong anticholinergic effects. (Antihistamines are discussed in Chapter 48.)

Individual antiparkinson drugs

DOPAMINERGIC AGENTS

Levodopa (Larodopa, Dopar) is the most effective drug available for treatment of Parkinson's disease. It relieves all major symptoms of parkinsonism, especially bradykinesia and rigidity. Although levodopa does not alter the underlying disease process, it may improve patients' quality of life.

Levodopa is the immediate precursor to dopamine and acts, at least in part, to replace dopamine in the basal ganglia of the brain. Dopamine cannot be used for replacement therapy because it does not enter the brain in sufficient amounts. Levodopa, in contrast, readily penetrates the CNS and is converted to dopamine by a nonspecific enzyme called L-aromatic amino acid decarboxylase. The concentration of decarboxylase is greater in peripheral tissues than in the brain. Consequently, most levodopa is biotransformed in peripheral tissues, and large amounts are required to obtain therapeutic levels of dopamine in the brain. These large doses contribute to the high incidence of adverse effects experienced during levodopa therapy.

Levodopa is usually rapidly absorbed from the small intestine after oral administration and has a short serum half-life (1 to 3 hours). Absorption is decreased by delayed gastric emptying, hyperacidity of gastric juice, and competition with amino acids (from digestion of protein foods) for sites of absorption in the small intestine. Levodopa is metabolized to 30 or more metabolites, some of which are pharmacologically active and probably contribute to drug toxicity; the metabolites are excreted primarily in the urine, usually within 24 hours.

Because of side-effects and recurrence of parkinsonism symptoms after a few years of levodopa therapy, levodopa is often reserved for clients with significant symptoms and functional disabilities. In addition to treating Parkinson's disease, levodopa may also be useful in other CNS disorders in which symptoms of parkinsonism occur (*e.g.*, juvenile Huntington's chorea, chronic manganese poisoning). Levodopa relieves only parkinsonism symptoms in these conditions.

Levodopa is not effective in drug-induced extrapyramidal reactions and should not be used for this purpose. The drug is also contraindicated in clients with narrow-angle glaucoma, hemolytic anemia, severe angina pectoris, transient ischemic attacks (TIAs), or a history of melanoma or undiagnosed skin disorders and in clients who are taking monoamine oxidase (MAO) inhibitor drugs.

In addition, levodopa must be used with caution in clients with severe cardiovascular, pulmonary, renal, hepatic, or endocrine disorders.

Route and dosage range

Adults: PO 0.5–1 g daily initially in 3–4 divided doses, increased gradually by increments of 100–500 mg daily, every 3–7 days. The rate of dosage increase depends primarily on the client's tolerance of adverse effects, especially nausea and vomiting. Average daily maintenance dose is 3–6 g with a maximum daily dose of 8 g. Therapeutic effects may be increased and adverse effects decreased by frequent administration of small doses.

Carbidopa (Lodosyn) inhibits the enzyme L-aromatic amino acid decarboxylase. As a result, less levodopa is decarboxylated in peripheral tissues, more levodopa reaches the brain, where it is decarboxylated to dopamine, and much smaller doses of levodopa can be given. Carbidopa does not penetrate the blood–brain barrier. A levodopa–carbidopa fixed-dose combination product is marketed under the name *Sinemet.* Sinemet is available in 3 dosages: 10 mg carbidopa/100 mg levodopa, 25 mg carbidopa/100 mg levodopa, and 25 mg carbidopa/250 mg levodopa.

Route and dosage range

Adults: PO initially, levodopa 400 mg and carbidopa 40 mg daily, in divided doses. This dosage can be gradually increased, if necessary, to a daily maximum of 2000 mg of levodopa and 200 mg of carbidopa. When carbidopa is added to a regimen that previously contained levodopa alone, levodopa should be withheld at least 8 hours before Sinemet therapy is begun, and dosage should be about 25% of the previous levodopa dosage.

Amantadine (Symmetrel) is a synthetic antiviral agent initially used to prevent infection from influenza A virus. Amantadine acts to relieve symptoms of Parkinson's disease by causing release of dopamine in the brain. The drug relieves symptoms rapidly, within 1 to 5 days, but it loses efficacy with approximately 6 to 8 weeks of continuous administration. Consequently, it is usually given for 2- to 3-week periods during initiation of drug therapy with longer-acting agents (*e.g.,* levodopa) or when symptoms worsen. Amantadine is often given in conjunction with levodopa. Compared with other antiparkinson drugs, amantadine is considered less effective than levodopa but more effective than anticholinergic agents.

Amantadine is well absorbed from the gastrointestinal tract and has a relatively long duration of action. It is excreted unchanged in the urine. Dosage must be reduced with impaired renal function to avoid drug accumulation.

Route and dosage range

Adults: PO 100 mg twice daily

Bromocriptine (Parlodel) directly stimulates dopamine receptors in the brain. It is used in the treatment of idiopathic or postencephalitic Parkinson's disease. Given concurrently with levodopa or a levodopa–carbidopa combination, bromocriptine may allow reduced dosage of levodopa. Long-term effectiveness of the drug has not been established.

Route and dosage range

Adults: PO 1.25 mg twice daily with meals, increased by 2.5 mg daily every 2–4 weeks if necessary for therapeutic benefit. Reduce dose gradually if severe adverse effects occur.

Principles of therapy: antiparkinson drugs

ASSESSMENT GUIDELINES

Assess for signs and symptoms of Parkinson's disease and drug-induced extrapyramidal reactions. These may include the following, depending on the severity and stage of progression:

1. Slow movements (bradykinesia) and difficulty in changing positions, assuming an upright position, eating, dressing, and other self-care activites
2. Stooped posture
3. Accelerating gait with short steps
4. Tremor at rest (*e.g.,* "pill rolling" movements of fingers)
5. Rigidity of arms, legs, and neck
6. Masklike, immobile facial expression
7. Speech problems (*e.g.,* low volume, monotonous tone, rapid, difficult to understand)
8. Excessive salivation and drooling
9. Dysphagia
10. Excessive sweating
11. Constipation from decreased intestinal motility
12. Mental depression from self-consciousness and embarrassment over physical appearance and activity limitations. The intellect is usually intact until the late stages of the disease process.

NURSING INTERVENTIONS

Use measures to assist the client and family in coping with symptoms and maintaining function. These include the following:

1. Physical therapy for heel-to-toe gait training, widening stance to increase balance and base of support, other exercises

2. Ambulation and frequent changes of position, assisted if necessary
3. Active and passive range-of-motion exercises
4. Encourage self-care as much as possible. Cutting meat, opening cartons, frequent small meals, and allowing privacy during mealtime may be helpful. If the client has difficulty chewing or swallowing, chopped or soft foods may be necessary. Velcro fasteners or zippers are easier to handle than buttons. Slip-on shoes are easier to manage than laced ones.
5. Spend time with client and encourage socialization with other people. Victims of Parkinson's disease tend to become withdrawn, isolated, and depressed.
6. Schedule rest periods. Tremor and rigidity are aggravated by fatigue and emotional stress.
7. Provide facial tissues if drooling is a problem.

DRUG SELECTION AND DOSAGE

Choice of antiparkinson drug depends on the type of parkinsonism (idiopathic or drug induced) and severity of symptoms.

1. Anticholinergic agents may be drugs of choice for early idiopathic parkinsonism, when symptoms are relatively mild, and for drug-induced symptoms. These agents are most effective in decreasing salivation and tremor.
2. Levodopa is the drug of choice in idiopathic parkinsonism, when bradykinesia and rigidity are prominent symptoms.
3. Combination drug therapy may be preferred for many clients. Two advantages of combination therapy are better control of symptoms and reduced dosage of individual drugs. Anticholinergic drugs may be given with levodopa alone or with a levodopa–carbidopa combination. Carbidopa is often used with levodopa so that dosage and adverse effects of levodopa can be reduced. Amantadine and bromocriptine are usually used as adjuncts to other drugs.

Dosage of antiparkinson drugs is highly individualized. The general rule is to start with a low initial dose and gradually increase dosage until therapeutic effects, adverse effects, or maximum drug dosage is achieved. Optimal dosage may not be established for 6 to 8 weeks with levodopa. When combinations of drugs are used, dosage adjustments of individual components are sometimes necessary. When levodopa is added to a regimen of anticholinergic drug therapy, for example, the anticholinergic drug does not need to be discontinued or reduced in dosage. However, when carbidopa is given with levodopa, the dosage of levodopa must be reduced by approximately 75%.

NURSING ACTIONS: ANTIPARKINSON DRUGS

Nursing Actions	*Rationale/Explanation*
1. Administer accurately	
a. Give levodopa and bromocriptine with or just after food intake.	To prevent or reduce anorexia, nausea, and vomiting
2. Observe for therapeutic effects	
a. With anticholinergic agents, observe for decreased tremor, salivation, drooling, and sweating.	Decreased salivation and sweating are therapeutic effects when these drugs are used in Parkinson's disease, but they are adverse effects when the drugs are used in other disorders.
b. With levodopa, observe for improvement in mobility, balance, posture, gait, speech, handwriting, and self-care ability. Drooling and seborrhea may be abolished, and mood may be elevated.	Therapeutic effects are usually evident within 2 to 3 weeks, as dosage approaches 2 to 3 g/day, but may not reach optimum levels for 6 months.
3. Observe for adverse effects	
a. With anticholinergic drugs, observe for atropinelike effects such as	
(1) Tachycardia and palpitations	These effects may occur with usual therapeutic doses but are not likely to be serious except in people with underlying heart disease.

Nursing Actions	***Rationale/Explanation***
(2) Excessive CNS stimulation (tremor, restlessness, confusion, hallucinations, delirium)	This effect is most likely to occur with large doses of trihexyphenidyl (Artane) or benztropine (Cogentin). It may occur with levodopa.
(3) Sedation and drowsiness	These are most likely to occur with benztropine (Cogentin). The drug has antihistaminic as well as anticholinergic properties, and sedation is attributed to the antihistamine effect.
(4) Constipation, impaction, paralytic ileus	These effects result from decreased gastrointesinal motility and muscle tone. They may be severe because decreased intestinal motility and constipation are also characteristics of Parkinson's disease. Thus, additive effects may occur.
(5) Urinary retention	This reaction is caused by loss of muscle tone in the bladder and is most likely to occur in elderly men who have enlarged prostate glands.
(6) Dilated pupils (mydriasis), blurred vision, photophobia	Ocular effects are due to paralysis of accommodation and relaxation of the ciliary muscle and the sphincter muscle of the iris.
b. With levodopa, observe for	
(1) Anorexia, nausea, and vomiting	These symptoms usually disappear after a few months of drug therapy. They may be minimized by giving levodopa with food, gradually increasing dosage, administering smaller doses more frequently, or by adding carbidopa so that dosage of levodopa can be reduced.
(2) Orthostatic hypotension—check blood pressure in both sitting and standing positions, q4h while the client is awake	This effect is common during the first few weeks but usually subsides eventually. It can be minimized by arising slowly from supine or sitting positions and by wearing elastic stockings.
(3) Cardiac arrhythmias (tachycardia, premature ventricular contractions) and increased myocardial contractility	Levodopa and its metabolites stimulate beta-adrenergic receptors in the heart. People with preexisting coronary artery disease may need a beta-adrenergic blocking agent (*e.g.,* propranolol) to counteract these effects.
(4) Dyskinesia—involuntary movements that may involve only the tongue, mouth, and face or the whole body	Dyskinesia eventually develops in most people who take levodopa. It is related to duration of levodopa therapy rather than dosage. Carbidopa may heighten this adverse effect, and there is no way to prevent it except by decreasing levodopa dosage. Many people prefer dyskinesia to lowering drug dosage and subsequent return of parkinsonism symptoms
(5) CNS stimulation—restlessness, agitation, confusion, delirium	This is more likely to occur with levodopa–carbidopa combination drug therapy.
(6) Abrupt swings in motor function (on–off phenomenon)	This fluctuation may indicate progression of the disease process. It often occurs after long-term levodopa use.
c. With amantadine, observe for	
(1) CNS stimulation—insomnia, hyperexcitability, ataxia, dizziness, slurred speech, mental confusion, hallucinations	Compared with other antiparkinson drugs, amantadine produces few adverse effects. The ones that occur are mild, transient, and reversible. However, adverse effects increase if daily dosage exceeds 200 mg.
(2) Livedo reticularis—patchy, bluish discoloration of skin on the legs	This is a benign but cosmetically unappealing condition. It usually occurs with long-term use of amantadine and disappears when the drug is discontinued.
d. With bromocriptine, observe for (1) Nausea (2) Confusion and hallucinations (3) Hypotension	These symptoms are usually mild and can be minimized by starting with low doses and increasing the dose gradually until the desired effect is achieved. If adverse effects do occur, they usually disappear with a decrease in dosage.
4. Observe for drug interactions	
a. Drugs that *increase* effects of anticholinergic drugs	
Antihistamines, disopyramide (Norpace, an antiarrhythmic agent), phenothiazines, thioxanthene agents, and tricyclic antidepressants	These drugs have anticholinergic properties and produce additive anticholinergic effects.

Nursing Actions	Rationale/Explanation
b. Drugs that *decrease* effects of anticholinergic drugs	
Cholinergic agents	These drugs counteract the inhibition of gastrointestinal motility and tone, which is a side-effect of anticholinergic drug therapy.
c. Drugs that *increase* effects of levodopa	
(1) Amantadine, anticholinergic agents, bromocriptine, carbidopa	These drugs are often used in combination for treatment of Parkinson's disease.
(2) Antidepressants, tricyclic	These drugs potentiate levodopa effects and increase the risk of cardiac arrhythmias in people with heart disease.
(3) MAO inhibitors	The combination of a catecholamine precursor (levodopa) and MAO inhibitors that decrease metabolism of catecholamines can result in excessive amounts of dopamine, epinephrine, and norepinephrine. Heart palpitations, headache, hypertensive crisis, and stroke may occur. Levodopa and MAO inhibitors should *not* be given concurrently. Also, levodopa should not be started within 3 weeks after an MAO inhibitor is discontinued. Effects of MAO inhibitors persist for 1 to 3 weeks after their discontinuation.
d. Drugs that *decrease* effects of levodopa	
(1) Anticholinergics	Although anticholinergics are often given with levodopa for increased antiparkinson effects, they may also decrease effects of levodopa by delaying gastric emptying. This causes more levodopa to be metabolized in the stomach and decreases the amount available for absorption from the intestine.
(2) Alcohol, antianxiety agents (*e.g.,* diazepam [Valium] and probably other benzodiazepines), antiemetics, antipsychotic agents (phenothiazines, butyrophenones, and thioxanthenes), and reserpine	The mechanisms by which most of these drugs decrease effects of levodopa are not clear. Phenothiazines block dopamine receptors in the basal ganglia.
(3) Pyridoxine (vitamin B_6)	Pyridoxine stimulates decarboxylase, the enzyme which converts levodopa to dopamine. As a result, more levodopa is metabolized in peripheral tissues and less reaches the CNS, where antiparkinson effects occur. This interaction does not occur when carbidopa is given with levodopa.
5. Teach clients	
a. Do not take other drugs without the physician's knowledge and consent.	To avoid adverse drug interactions. Both prescription and nonprescription drugs may interact with antiparkinson drugs to increase or decrease effects.
b. Excessive mouth dryness can be minimized by maintaining an adequate fluid intake (2000–3000 ml daily if not contraindicated) and using sugarless chewing gum and hard candies.	Both anticholinergics and levodopa may cause mouth dryness. This is usually a therapeutic effect in Parkinson's disease. However, excessive mouth dryness (xerostomia) causes discomfort and dental caries.
c. Avoid driving an automobile or operating other potentially hazardous machinery if vision is blurred or drowsiness occurs with levodopa.	To prevent injury
d. Limit intake of alcohol and high-protein foods (*e.g.,* meat, poultry, fish, milk, eggs, cheese, nuts). Do not take multiple vitamin preparations that contain vitamin B_6 (pyridoxine).	Alcohol, protein, and pyridoxine decrease the therapeutic effects of levodopa alone but not the effects of levodopa–carbidopa in combination. Larobec is a multivitamin preparation available without vitamin B_6.
e. Change positions slowly, especially when assuming an upright position, and wear elastic stockings if needed.	To avoid dizziness
f. Report adverse effects.	Adverse effects can often be reduced by changing drugs or dosages. However, some adverse effects must usually be tolerated for control of disease symptoms.

Selected References

American Medical Association (AMA) Division of Drugs: AMA Drug Evaluations, 5th ed. New York, John Wiley & Sons, 1983

Bianchine JR: Drugs for Parkinson's disease, spasticity, and acute muscle spasms. In Gilman AG, Goodman LS, Rall TW, Murad F (eds): The Pharmacological Basis of Therapeutics, 7th ed, pp 473–490. New York, Macmillan, 1985

Facts and Comparisons. St Louis, J B Lippincott (Updated monthly)

Gresh C: Helpful tips you can give your patients with Parkinson's disease. Nursing 10:26–33, January 1980

Malseed RT: Pharmacology: Drug Therapy and Nursing Considerations, 2d ed. Philadelphia, J B Lippincott, 1985

Rodman MJ, Karch AM, Boyd EH, Smith DW: Pharmacology and Drug Therapy in Nursing, 3rd ed. Philadelphia, J B Lippincott, 1985

Todd B: Drugs and the elderly: Therapy for Parkinson's disease. Geriatr Nurs 6:117–120, March–April 1985

13

SKELETAL MUSCLE RELAXANTS

Description and uses

Skeletal muscle relaxants are used to decrease muscle spasm or spasticity that occurs in certain neurologic and musculoskeletal disorders. (Neuromuscular blocking agents used as adjuncts to general anesthesia for surgery are discussed in Chapter 14.)

Muscle spasm is sudden movement that may involve alternating contraction and relaxation (clonic) or sustained contraction (tonic). Muscle spasm may occur with musculoskeletal trauma or inflammation (*e.g.*, sprains, strains, bursitis, arthritis). It is also encountered with acute or chronic "low back pain," a common condition that is primarily a disorder of posture.

Spasticity involves increased muscle tone or contraction, which produces stiff, awkward movements. Spasticity results from neurologic disorders such as cerebral palsy, stroke, paraplegia, spinal cord injury, and multiple sclerosis.

Almost all skeletal muscle relaxants are centrally active agents. Pharmacologic action is probably caused by general depression of the central nervous system (CNS) but may result from blockage of nerve impulses that cause increased muscle tone and contraction. It is not clear whether relief of pain results from sedative effects, muscular relaxation, or a placebo effect. In addition, although parenteral administration of some drugs (*e.g.*, diazepam [Valium], methocarbamol [Robaxin]) relieves pain associated with acute musculoskeletal trauma or inflammation, it is uncertain whether oral administration of usual doses exerts a beneficial effect in acute or chronic disorders. Dantrolene (Dantrium) is the only skeletal muscle relaxant that acts peripherally, on the muscle itself.

Skeletal muscle relaxants are recommended for use primarily as adjuncts to other treatment measures. Occasionally, parenteral agents are given to facilitate various orthopedic procedures and examinations. In spastic disorders, skeletal muscle relaxants are not generally indicated for use only to relieve spasticity. However, they may be indicated when spasticity causes severe pain or inability to tolerate physical therapy, sit in a wheelchair, or participate in self-care activities of daily living (eating, dressing, and so forth). Drugs should not be given if they cause excessive muscle weakness and impair rather than facilitate mobility and function.

Dantrolene is also indicated for prevention and treatment of malignant hyperthermia. Malignant hyperthermia, a rare but life-threatening complication of anesthesia, is characterized by hypercarbia, metabolic acidosis, skeletal muscle rigidity, fever, and cyanosis. For preoperative prophylaxis in people with previous episodes of malignant hyperthermia, the drug is given orally for 1 to 2 days before surgery. For intraoperative malignant hypertension, the drug is given intravenously. Postoperatively, following occurrences, the drug is given orally for 1 to 3 days to prevent recurrence of symptoms.

Individual skeletal muscle relaxants are listed in Table 13-1.

Principles of therapy: skeletal muscle relaxants

ASSESSMENT GUIDELINES

Assess for muscle spasm and spasticity.

1. With muscle spasm, assess for
   a. Pain. This is a prominent symptom of muscle spasm and is usually aggravated by movement. Try to determine the location as specifically as possible as well as the intensity, duration, and precipitating factors (*i.e.,* traumatic injury, strenuous exercise).
   b. Accompanying signs and symptoms such as bruises (ecchymoses), edema, or signs of inflammation (redness, heat, edema, tenderness to touch).
2. With spasticity, assess for pain and impaired functional ability in self-care (*e.g.,* eating, dressing). In addition, severe spasticity interferes with physical therapy exercises to maintain joint and muscle mobility.

TABLE 13-1. SKELETAL MUSCLE RELAXANTS

Generic name	Trade name	Routes and dosage ranges	
		Adults	*Children*
Baclofen	Lioresal	PO 5 mg 3 times daily initially, increased to 10 mg 3 times daily after 3 days, then gradually increased further if necessary Maximal dose, 20 mg 4 times daily Dosage must be reduced in the presence of impaired renal function.	Under age 12 years, not recommended
Carisoprodol	Rela, Soma	PO 350 mg 4 times daily	Age 5 years and over, PO 25 mg/kg/day in 4 divided doses
Chlorphenesin	Maolate	PO 800 mg 3 times daily until desired effected attained, then 400 mg 4 times daily or less for maintenance, as needed	Dosage not established
Chlorzoxazone	Paraflex	PO 250–750 mg 3–4 times daily	PO 20 mg/kg/day in 3–4 divided doses
Cyclobenzaprine	Flexeril	PO 10 mg 3 times daily. Maximal recommended duration, 3 weeks; maximal recommended dose, 60 mg daily	
Dantrolene	Dantrium	PO 25 mg daily initially, gradually increased weekly (by increments of 50–100 mg/day) to a maximal dose of 400 mg daily in 4 divided doses Preoperative prophylaxis of malignant hyperthermia: PO 4–8 mg/kg/day in 3–4 divided doses for 1 or 2 days before surgery Intraoperative malignant hyperthermia: IV push 1 mg/kg initially, continued until symptoms are relieved or a maximum total dose of 10 mg/kg has been given Postcrisis follow-up treatment: PO 4–8 mg/kg/day in 4 divided doses for 1–3 days	PO 1 mg/kg/day initially, gradually increased to a maximal dose of 3 mg/kg 4 times daily, not to exceed 400 mg daily Same as adult
Diazepam	Valium	PO 2–10 mg 3–4 times daily IM, IV 5–10 mg repeated in 3–4 hours if necessary	PO 0.12–0.8 mg/kg/day in 3–4 divided doses IM, IV 0.04–0.2 mg/kg in a single dose, not to exceed 0.6 mg/kg within an 8-hour period
Metaxalone	Skelaxin	PO 800 mg 3–4 times daily for not more than 10 consecutive days	
Methocarbamol	Robaxin	PO 1.5–2 g 4 times daily for 48–72 hours, reduced to 1.0 g 4 times daily for maintenance IM 500 mg q8h IV 1–3 g daily at a rate not to exceed 300 mg/minute (3 ml of 10% injection). Do not give IV more than 3 days	PO, IM, IV 60–75 mg/kg/day in 4 divided doses
Orphenadrine citrate	Norflex	PO 100 mg twice daily IM, IV 60 mg twice daily	

NURSING INTERVENTIONS

Use adjunctive measures for muscle spasm and spasticity. These include

1. Physical therapy—massage, moist heat, exercises
2. Bed rest for acute muscle spasm
3. Relaxation techniques
4. Correct posture and lifting techniques (*e.g.,* stooping rather than bending to lift objects, holding heavy objects close to the body, and *not* lifting excessive amounts of weight).
5. Regular exercise programs and use of "warm-up" exercises. Strenuous exercise performed on an occasional basis (*e.g.,* weekly or monthly) is more likely to cause acute muscle spasm.

DRUG SELECTION

Choice of skeletal muscle relaxant depends primarily on the disorder being treated.

1. In acute muscle spasm and pain, a drug that can be given parenterally (*e.g.,* diazepam, methocarbamol) is usually the drug of choice.
2. Parenteral agents are preferred for orthopedic procedures because they have greater sedative and pain-relieving effects.
3. Baclofen (Liorcsal) is approved for treatment of spasticity in people with multiple sclerosis. It is variably effective, and its clinical usefulness may be limited by adverse reactions. Baclofen is not recommended for pregnant women or children under 12 years of age.
4. None of the skeletal muscle relaxants has been established as safe for use during pregnancy and lactation.
5. Many of the skeletal muscle relaxants have not been established as safe for use in children. Choice of drug should be limited to those with established pediatric dosages.

NURSING ACTIONS: SKELETAL MUSCLE RELAXANTS

Nursing Actions	*Rationale/Explanation*
1. Administer accurately	
a. Do not mix parenteral diazepam in a syringe with any other drugs.	Diazepam is physically incompatible with other drugs.
b. Inject intravenous (IV) diazepam directly into a vein or the injection site nearest the vein (during continuous IV infusions), at a rate not to exceed 5 mg/minute.	Diazepam may cause a precipitate if diluted. Avoid contact with intravenous solutions as much as possible. A slow rate of injection minimizes risks of respiratory depression and apnea.
c. Avoid extravasation with IV diazepam and inject intramuscular (IM) diazepam deeply into a gluteal muscle.	To prevent or reduce tissue irritation
d. Avoid extravasation with IV methocarbamol and give IM methocarbamol deeply into a gluteal muscle. (Dividing the dose and giving two injections is preferred.)	Parenteral methocarbamol is a hypertonic solution that is very irritating to tissues. Thrombophlebitis may occur at IV injection sites, and sloughing of tissue may occur at sites of extravasation or IM injections.
2. Observe for therapeutic effects	
a. When drug is given for acute muscle spasm, observe for (1) Decreased pain and tenderness (2) Increased mobility (3) Increased ability to participate in activities of daily living	Therapeutic effects usually occur within 30 minutes after IV injection of diazepam or methocarbamol.
b. When drug is given for spasticity in chronic neurologic disorders, observe for (1) Increased ability to maintain posture and balance (2) Increased ability for self care (*e.g.,* eating and dressing) (3) Increased tolerance for physical therapy and exercises	

Nursing Actions	***Rationale/Explanation***
3. Observe for adverse effects	
a. With centrally active agents, observe for	
(1) Drowsiness and dizziness	These are the most common adverse effects.
(2) Blurred vision, lethargy, flushing	These effects occur more often with IV administration of drugs. They are usually transient.
(3) Nausea, vomiting, abdominal distress, constipation or diarrhea, ataxia, areflexia, flaccid paralysis, respiratory depression, tachycardia, hypotension	These effects are most likely to occur with large oral doses.
(4) Hypersensitivity—skin rash, pruritus	The drug should be discontinued if hypersensitivity reactions occur. Serious allergic reactions (*e.g.,* anaphylaxis) are rare.
(5) Psychic or physical dependence with diazepam and other antianxiety agents	Most likely to occur with long-term use of large doses
b. With a peripherally active agent (dantrolene), observe for	Adverse effects are usually transient.
(1) Drowsiness, fatigue, lethargy, weakness, nausea, vomiting	These effects are the most common.
(2) Headache, anorexia, nervousness	Less common effects
(3) Hepatotoxicity	This potentially serious adverse effect is most likely to occur in people more than 35 years of age who have taken the drug 60 days or longer. Women over 35 who take estrogens have the highest risk. Hepatotoxicity can be prevented or minimized by administering the lowest effective dose, monitoring liver enzymes (serum glutamic oxaloacetic transaminase [SGOT], serum glutamic pyruvic transaminase [SGPT]) during therapy, and discontinuing the drug if no beneficial effects occur within 45 days.
4. Observe for drug interactions	
a. Drugs that *increase* effects of skeletal muscle relaxants	
(1) CNS depressants (alcohol, antianxiety agents, antidepressants, antihistamines, antipsychotic drugs, sedative–hypnotics)	Additive CNS depression with increased risks of excessive sedation and respiratory depression or apnea
(2) Monoamine oxidase (MAO) inhibitors	May potentiate effects by inhibiting metabolism of muscle relaxants
5. Teach clients	
a. Do not attempt activities that require mental alertness or physical coordination (*e.g.,* driving an automobile, operating potentially dangerous machinery) if drowsy from medication.	To avoid injury
b. Do not take other drugs without the physician's knowledge, including nonprescription drugs.	The major risk occurs with concurrent use of alcohol, antihistamines, sleeping aids, or other drugs that cause drowsiness.

Selected References

American Medical Association (AMA) Division of Drugs: AMA Drug Evaluations, 5th ed. New York, John Wiley & Sons, 1983

Anderson PD: Basic Human Anatomy and Physiology: Clinical Implications for the Health Professions. Monterey, CA, Wadsworth, 1984

Facts and Comparisons. St. Louis, J B Lippincott (Updated monthly)

Malseed RT: Pharmacology: Drug Therapy and Nursing Considerations, 2d ed. Philadelphia, J B Lippincott, 1985

Rodman MJ, Karch AM, Boyd EH, Smith DW: Pharmacology and Drug Therapy in Nursing, 3rd ed. Philadelphia, J B Lippincott, 1985

14
ANESTHETICS

Description and uses

Anesthesia means loss of sensation with or without loss of consciousness. Anesthetic drugs are given to prevent pain and promote relaxation during surgery, childbirth, and some diagnostic tests and treatment procedures. They interrupt the conduction of painful nerve impulses from a site of injury to the brain. The two basic types of anesthesia are general and regional.

GENERAL ANESTHESIA

General anesthesia is a state of profound central nervous system (CNS) depression during which there is complete loss of sensation, consciousness, pain perception, and memory. It has three components: hypnosis, analgesia, and muscle relaxation. Several different drugs are usually combined to produce desired levels of these components without excessive CNS depression. This so-called balanced anesthesia also allows lower dosage of potent general anesthetics. The four stages of general anesthesia are analgesia (I), excitement and hyperactivity (II), surgical anesthesia (III), and medullary paralysis (IV). General anesthesia is administered so that stage III anesthesia is maintained as long as necessary and stage IV is avoided. Spontaneous breathing stops with stage IV. Death follows unless the anesthetic is discontinued and resuscitative measures are undertaken. These stages were described in relation to ether anesthesia and may not be completely discernible with newer agents. Their importance for the nurse is that people recovering from anesthesia progress through the same stages in reverse. Thus, analgesia or hyperactivity may extend into the postanesthesia recovery period.

General anesthesia is usually induced with an ultra-short-acting barbiturate, given intravenously (IV), and is maintained with a gas mixture of an anesthetic agent and oxygen, given by inhalation. The IV agent produces a rapid loss of consciousness, is not explosive, and provides a pleasant induction and recovery. Its rapid onset of action is attributed to rapid circulation to the brain and accumulation in the neuronal tissue of the cerebral cortex. Duration of action is also very short with a single dose but can be prolonged with continuous IV infusion. These drugs may also be used alone for anesthesia during brief diagnostic tests or surgical procedures.

Inhalation anesthetics vary in the degree of CNS depression produced and thereby vary in rate of induction, anesthetic potency, degree of muscle relaxation, and analgesic potency. CNS depression is determined by the concentration of the drug in the CNS. Drug concentration, in turn, depends on the rate at which the drug is transported from the alveoli to the blood, transported past the blood–brain barrier to reach the CNS, redistributed by the blood to other body tissues, and eliminated by the lungs. Depth of anesthesia can readily be regulated by varying the concentration of the inhaled anesthetic gas. General inhalation anesthetics should be administered only by specially trained persons such as anesthesiologists and nurse anesthetists and only with appropriate equipment.

REGIONAL ANESTHESIA

Regional anesthesia involves loss of sensation and motor activity in localized areas of the body. It is induced by application or injection of local anesthetic drugs. The drugs act to stabilize the cell membrane of nerve cells, thereby preventing the cells from responding to pain impulses and other sensory stimuli.

Regional anesthesia is usually categorized according to the site of application. The area anesthetized may be the site of application or it may be distal to the point of injection. Specific types of anesthesia attained with local anesthetic drugs include the following:

1. Topical or surface anesthesia involves applying local anesthetic agents to skin or mucous membrane. Such application makes sensory receptors unresponsive to pain, itching, and other stimuli. Local anesthetics for topical use are usually ingredients of various ointments, solutions, or lotions designed for use at particular sites. For example, preparations are available for use on eyes, ears, nose, oral mucosa, perineum, hemorrhoids, and skin.
2. Infiltration involves injecting the local anesthetic solution directly into or very close to the area to be anesthetized.
3. Peripheral nerve block involves injecting the anesthetic solution into the area of a larger nerve trunk or a nerve plexus at some access point along the course of a nerve distant from the area to be anesthetized.
4. Field block anesthesia involves injecting the anesthetic solution around the area to be anesthetized.
5. Spinal anesthesia involves injecting the anesthetic agent into the cerebrospinal fluid, usually in the lumbar spine. The anesthetic blocks sensory impulses at the root of peripheral nerves as they enter the spinal cord. Spinal anesthesia is especially useful for surgery involving the lower abdomen and legs.

   The body area anesthetized is determined by the level to which the drug solution rises in the spinal canal. This, in turn, is determined by the site of injection, the position of the client, and the specific gravity, amount, and concentration of the injected solution.

   Solutions of local anesthetic drugs used for spinal anesthesia are either hyperbaric or hypobaric. Hyperbaric or heavy solutions are diluted with dextrose, have a higher specific gravity than cerebrospinal fluid, and gravitate toward the head when the person is tilted in a head-down position. Hypobaric or light solutions are diluted with distilled water, have a lower specific gravity than cerebrospinal fluid, and gravitate toward the lower (caudal) end of the spinal canal when the person is tilted in a head-down position.
6. Epidural or caudal anesthesia involves injecting the anesthetic into the epidural space. In lumbar epidural anesthesia, the injection is usually made between the second lumbar and the first sacral vertebrae to avoid injury to the spinal cord, which ends at the first lumbar vertebra in 95% of clients. In caudal anesthesia, the drug solution is injected into the caudal canal through the sacral area. Epidural or caudal anesthesia is used most often in obstetrics during labor and delivery and occasionally in surgery of the perineal or rectal areas.

   Generally, the area anesthetized is determined by the site of injection (lumbar or caudal), the position of the client, the volume and concentration of the anesthetic solution, the age of the client, whether the client is pregnant, and the extent of arteriosclerosis. A smaller area is anesthetized if the recipient is in a sitting position. A larger area is anesthetized with high volumes and high concentrations of drug solutions, if the client is a child or is elderly, if the client is pregnant and at full term, and if occlusive arterial disease is present.

The extent and duration of anesthesia produced by injection of local anesthetics depend on several factors. Generally, large amounts, high concentrations, or injections into highly vascular areas (*e.g.,* head and neck, intercostal and paracervical sites) produce rapid peak plasma levels. Duration depends on the chemical characteristics of the drug used and the rate at which it leaves nerve tissue. When a vasoconstrictor drug such as epinephrine has been added, both onset and duration of anesthesia are prolonged owing to slowed absorption of the anesthetic agent.

ADJUNCTS TO ANESTHESIA

Several nonanesthetic drugs are used as adjuncts or supplements to anesthetic drugs. Most are discussed elsewhere and are described here only in relation to anesthesia. Drug groups include antianxiety agents (see Chap. 8), sedative–hypnotics (see Chap. 7), anticholinergics (see Chap. 21), and narcotic analgesics (see Chap. 5). The neuromuscular blocking agents are described more fully here because they are not included elsewhere.

Antianxiety agents and sedative–hypnotics are given to decrease anxiety, promote rest, and increase client safety by allowing easier induction of anesthesia and smaller doses of anesthetic agents. These drugs are often given the night before to aid sleep and 1 or 2 hours before the scheduled procedure. Hypnotic doses are usually given for greater sedative effects. Some commonly used drugs are diazepam (Valium), promethazine (Phenergan), hydroxyzine (Vistaril), and pentobarbital (Nembutal).

Anticholinergic drugs are given to prevent excessive activity of the parasympathetic nervous system (vagal stimulation). Vagal stimulation occurs with some inhalation anesthetics such as halothane and cyclopropane; with succinylcholine, a commonly used muscle relaxant; and with surgical procedures in which there is manipulation of the pharynx, trachea, peritoneum, stomach, intestine, or other viscera as well as procedures in which pressure is exerted on the eyeball. If not blocked by anticholinergic drugs, vagal stimulation may cause excessive bradycardia, hypotension, and cardiac arrest. Useful drugs are atropine, scopolamine, and glycopyrrolate (Robinul).

Anticholinergic drugs have also been widely used to decrease secretions in the respiratory tract. Although they are probably still prescribed for this purpose, they are not indicated for routine use. Newer inhalation anesthetics are less irritating to the respiratory tract mucosa and therefore are less likely to produce excessive secretions.

Narcotic analgesics such as morphine and meperidine (Demerol) induce relaxation and pain relief in the preanesthetic period. These drugs potentiate the CNS depression produced by other drugs, and less anesthetic agent is required. Morphine and fentanyl may be given in anesthetic doses in certain circumstances.

Neuromuscular blocking agents cause muscle relaxation, the third component of general anesthesia, and allow usage of smaller amounts of anesthetic agent. Artificial ventilation is necessary because these drugs paralyze muscles of respiration as well as other skeletal muscles. The drugs do not cause sedation. Therefore, unless the client is unconscious, he can see and hear environmental activities.

There are two types of neuromuscular blocking agents: depolarizing and nondepolarizing. The depolarizing drugs such as succinylcholine are similar to acetylcholine, the natural neurotransmitter in the parasympathetic nervous system (see Chap. 17). They combine with cholinergic receptors at the motor endplate to produce depolarization and muscle contraction initially. Repolarization and further muscle contraction is then inhibited as long as an adequate concentration of drug remains at the receptor site.

Muscle paralysis is preceded by muscle spasms, which may damage muscles. Injury to muscle cells may cause postoperative muscle pain and release potassium into the circulation. If hyperkalemia develops, it is usually mild and insignificant but may cause cardiac arrhythmias or even cardiac arrest in some situations. Succinylcholine is normally deactivated by plasma pseudocholinesterase. There is no antidote except reconstituted fresh frozen plasma that contains pseudocholinesterase.

Nondepolarizing neuromuscular blocking agents such as tubocurarine and gallamine are also called competitive blocking agents, curariform drugs, and antidepolarizing agents. They prevent acetylcholine from acting at neuromuscular junctions. Consequently, the nerve cell membrane is not depolarized, the muscle fibers are not stimulated, and skeletal muscle contraction does not occur. Anticholinesterase drugs such as neostigmine (Prostigimin) (see Chap. 20) are antidotes and are often used to reverse muscle paralysis.

Individual anesthetic agents

General anesthetics and neuromuscular blocking agents are listed in Table 14-1. Local anesthetics are listed in Table 14-2.

Principles of therapy: anesthetic drugs

1. The nursing role in relation to anesthetic agents differs from the role associated with other drugs. The nurse provides nursing care before, during, and after anesthetic administration, but the agents are given by anesthesiologists and other physicians (*e.g.*, surgeons and obstetricians), nurse anesthetists, and dentists.
2. Before administration of general anesthesia and some regional anesthesia, most nursing care centers on general preoperative teaching and preparation for surgery. Afterward, nursing care is mainly concerned with general postoperative assessment and actions related to maintenance of respiration, circulation, and other vital functions. (For additional and more specific nursing activities in caring for clients having surgery, the reader is referred to medical–surgical nursing textbooks. In this book, the focus is on the drugs used during this period and the associated nursing role.)
3. Principles for using adjunctive drugs—antianxiety agents, anticholinergics, narcotic analgesics—are the same when these drugs are given preoperatively as at other times. They are usually ordered by an anesthesiologist, sometimes by the surgeon.
4. Many drugs are available for use as anesthetics and adjunctive agents. The anesthesiologist is usually responsible for choosing particular drugs, and his choice depends on a number of factors. Some

(Text continues on p. 129.)

TABLE 14-1. GENERAL ANESTHETICS AND NEUROMUSCULAR BLOCKING AGENTS

	Generic name	Trade name	Characteristics	Remarks
General inhalation anesthetics	Cyclopropane		Explosive, flammable gas; wide margin of safety; good analgesia and muscle relaxation; rapid induction and recovery; minimal myocardial depression; ventricular arrhythmias are uncommon unless ventilation is inadequate or adrenergic drugs are given	Used less often since newer nonexplosive and nonflammable agents have been developed
	Enflurane	Ethrane	Nonexplosive, nonflammable volatile liquid; similar to halothane but may produce better analgesia and muscle relaxation; sensitizes heart to catecholamines—increases risks of cardiac arrhythmias; renal or hepatic toxicity not reported	A frequently used agent
	Ether		Explosive, flammable volatile liquid; slow induction, often with excitement and hyperactivity; slow recovery with excitement and hyperactivity, nausea and vomiting, and increased respiratory tract secretions	Rarely used in the United States; still used in underdeveloped countries
	Fluroxene	Fluoromar	Explosive, flammable volatile liquid derived from ether; nausea and vomiting are common during recovery but excitement is rare	Used mainly for minor surgical procedures that do not require extensive muscle relaxation
	Halothane	Fluothane	Nonexplosive, nonflammable volatile liquid Advantages 1. Produces rapid induction with little or no excitement; rapid recovery with little excitement or nausea and vomiting 2. Does not irritate respiratory tract mucosa; therefore does not increase saliva and tracheobronchial secretions 3. Depresses pharyngeal and laryngeal reflexes, which decreases risk of laryngospasm and bronchospasm Disadvantages 1. Depresses contractility of the heart and vascular smooth muscle, which causes decreased cardiac output, hypotension, and bradycardia 2. Circulatory failure may occur with high doses 3. Causes cardiac arrhythmias. Bradycardia is common; ventricular arrhythmias are uncommon unless ventilation is inadequate 4. Sensitizes heart to catecholamines, increases risk of cardiac arrhythmias 5. Depresses respiration and may produce hypoxemia and respiratory acidosis (hypercarbia) 6. Depresses functions of the kidneys, liver, and immune system 7. May cause jaundice and hepatitis 8. May cause malignant hyperthermia	Halothane is one of the most widely used inhalation anesthetics. It is often used in "balanced" anesthesia with other agents. Although quite potent, it may not produce adequate analgesia and muscle relaxation at a dosage that is not likely to produce significant adverse effects. Therefore, nitrous oxide is given to increase analgesic effects, a neuromuscular blocking agent is given to increase muscle relaxation, and an IV barbiturate is used to produce rapid, smooth induction, after which halothane is given to maintain anesthesia.
	Isoflurane	Forane	Similar to halothane in actions; less likely to cause cardiovascular depression and ventricular arrhythmias than halothane. Isoflurane may cause malignant hyperthermia but apparently does not cause hepatotoxicity.	Used for induction and maintenance of general anesthesia
	Methoxyflurane	Penthrane	Nonexplosive, nonflammable volatile liquid; similar to halothane in most respects but is more analgesic when	Usage as a general anesthetic is limited because of renal toxicity. It is used

TABLE 14-1. GENERAL ANESTHETICS AND NEUROMUSCULAR BLOCKING AGENTS (*Continued*)

	Generic name	Trade name	Characteristics	Remarks
			inhaled at low concentrations, has slower induction and recovery, does not sensitize the heart to catecholamines, and causes renal damage and failure. Renal failure is dose related and increases with drug concentration and length of time administered. It is attributed to metabolites of methoxyflurane.	in dentistry, childbirth, or other procedures in which small amounts can be given for brief periods. This does not allow enough accumulation of the drug or its metabolites to cause renal damage.
	Nitrous oxide		Nonexplosive gas; good analgesic, weak anesthetic; one of oldest and safest anesthetics; causes no appreciable damage to vital organs unless hypoxia is allowed to develop and persist; administered with oxygen to prevent hypoxia; rapid induction and recovery. Note: nitrous oxide is an incomplete anesthetic; that is, by itself, it cannot produce stage III anesthesia.	Often used in "balanced" anesthesia with intravenous barbiturates, neuromuscular blocking agents, narcotic analgesics and more potent inhalation anesthetics such as halothane. It is safer for prolonged surgical procedures (see "Characteristics"). It is used alone for analgesia in dentistry, obstetrics, and brief surgical procedures.
General intravenous anesthetics	Droperidol and fentanyl combination	Innovar	Droperidol (Inapsine) is related to the antipsychotic agent haloperidol. It produces sedative and antiemetic effects. Fentanyl citrate (Sublimaze) is a very potent narcotic analgesic whose actions are similar to those of morphine but of shorter duration. Innovar is a fixed-dose combination of the two drugs. Additional doses of fentanyl are often needed because its analgesic effect lasts about 30 minutes while droperidol effects last 3–6 hours	Either drug may be used alone but they are most often used together for neuroleptanalgesia and combined with nitrous oxide for neuroleptanesthesia. Neuroleptanalgesia is a state of reduced awareness and reduced sensory perception during which a variety of diagnositic tests or minor surgical procedures can be done, such as bronchoscopy and burn dressings. Neuroleptanesthesia can be used for major surgical procedures. Consciousness returns rapidly but respiratory depression may last 3–4 hours into the postoperative recovery period.
	Etomidate	Amidate	A nonanalgesic hypnotic used for induction and maintenance of general anesthesia	May be used with nitrous oxide in oxygen in maintenance of general anesthesia for short operative procedures such as uterine dilation and curettage.
	Ketamine	Ketalar	Rapid-acting, nonbarbiturate anesthetic; produces marked analgesia, sedation, immobility, amnesia and a lack of awareness of surroundings (called dissociative anesthesia); may be given IV or IM; awakening may require several hours; during recovery, unpleasant psychic symptoms may occur, including dreams and hallucinations; vomiting, hypersalivation, and transient skin rashes may also occur during recovery	Used most often for brief surgical, diagnostic or therapeutic procedures. It may also be used to induce anesthesia. If used for major surgery, it must be supplemented by other general anesthetics. It is generally contraindicated in individuals with increased intracranial pressure, severe coronary artery disease, hyperten-

TABLE 14-1. GENERAL ANESTHETICS AND NEUROMUSCULAR BLOCKING AGENTS *(Continued)*

	Generic name	Trade name	Characteristics	Remarks
				sion, or psychiatric disorders. Hyperactivity and unpleasant dreams occur less often with children than adults.
	Sufentanil	Sufenta	A synthetic opioid analgesic–anesthetic related to fentanyl. Compared to fentanyl, it is more potent and faster acting and may allow a more rapid recovery.	May be used as a primary anesthetic or an analgesic adjunct in balanced anesthesia.
	Methohexital sodium Thiamylal sodium Thiopental sodium	Brevital Surital Pentothal	These three drugs are ultra-short-acting barbiturates, used almost exclusively in general anesthesia; excellent hypnotics but do not produce significant analgesia or muscle relaxation; given IV by intermittent injection or by continuous infusion of a dilute solution	Thiopental is commonly used. A single dose produces unconsciousness in less than 30 seconds and lasts 20–30 minutes. Usually given to induce anesthesia. It is used alone only for brief procedures. For major surgery, it is usually supplemented by inhalation anesthetics and muscle relaxants.
Neuromuscular blocking agents	Atracurium	Tracrium	A newer nondepolarizing agent similar to pancuronium, gallamine, and tubocurarine but with a shorter duration of action	Used as an adjunct to general anesthesia
	Gallamine	Flaxedil	A synthetic, nondepolarizing skeletal muscle relaxant. Its effects can be reversed by neostigmine (Prostigmin).	Used only as an adjunct to anesthesia
	Hexafluorenium	Mylaxen	Inhibits plasma cholinesterase and thereby prolongs the effects of succinylcholine	Used only in conjunction with succinylcholine to prolong skeletal muscle relaxation and inhibit muscle twitching
	Metocurine	Metubine	A nondepolarizing skeletal muscle relaxant that is reportedly more potent than tubocurarine	Used as an adjunct to general anesthesia and electroshock therapy. Also used to facilitate mechanical ventilation.
	Pancuronium	Pavulon	A synthetic, nondepolarizing skeletal muscle relaxant. Its effects can be reversed by neostigmine.	Used mainly during surgery after general anesthesia has been induced. Occasionally used to facilitate endotracheal intubation or mechanical ventilation.
	Tubocurarine		A nondepolarizing drug that is the active ingredient of curare, a naturally occurring plant alkaloid that causes skeletal muscle relaxation or paralysis. Its effects can be reversed by neostigmine.	Used mainly as an adjunct to general anesthesia. Also used occasionally to facilitate mechanical ventilation.
	Succinylcholine	Anectine	A depolarizing neuromuscular blocking agent with a short duration of action following a single dose. Duration may be prolonged with intermittent injection or continuous intravenous infusion. Malignant hyperthermia may occur. There is no antidote or antagonist to succinylcholine.	Used for all types of surgery. Its short duration of action makes it useful for endoscopy, endotracheal intubation, and other brief procedures.
	Vercuronium	Norcuron	A newer nondepolarizing agent that is more potent and faster acting and has a shorter duration of action than pancuronium. Vercuronium produced few adverse effects in clinical testing and can be used in all age groups.	Used as an adjunct to general anesthesia. It can be used to facilitate endotracheal intubation and mechanical ventilation.

client-related factors include age; the specific procedure to be done and its anticipated duration; the physical condition of the client, including severity of illness, presence of chronic diseases, and any other drugs being given; and the mental status of the client. Severe anxiety, for example, may be a contraindication for regional anesthesia, and the client may require larger doses of preanesthetic sedative-type medication.

a. General anesthesia can be used for almost any surgical, diagnostic, or therapeutic procedure. If a medical disorder of a vital organ system—cardiovascular, respiratory, renal—is present, it should be corrected before anesthesia is induced when possible. Both general anesthesia and major surgical procedures have profound effects on normal body functioning. When alterations due to other disorders are also involved, the risks of anesthesia and surgery are greatly increased.

b. Regional or local anesthesia is usually safer than general anesthesia because it produces fewer systemic effects. For example, spinal anesthesia is often the anesthesia of choice for surgery involving the lower abdomen and lower extremities, especially in people who are elderly or have chronic lung disease. A major advantage of spinal anesthesia is that it causes less CNS and respiratory depression.

5. Anesthetics should be administered *only* by people with special training in correct usage. This applies especially to general anesthetics and neuromuscular blocking agents, but it is also important with local anesthetics when they are injected. In addition, general and local anesthetics should be given only in locations where personnel, equipment, and drugs are available for emergency use or cardiopulmonary resuscitation.

6. Choice of a local anesthetic drug depends mainly on the reason for use or the type of regional anesthesia desired. Lidocaine is one of the most widely used, and it is available in topical and injectable forms.

GUIDELINES FOR ADMINISTRATION OF A LOCAL ANESTHETIC

1. When local anesthetic solutions are injected, some guidelines for safe use include the following:

   a. Local anesthetic solutions must not be injected into blood vessels because of the high risk of serious adverse reactions involving the cardiovascular and central nervous systems. To prevent accidental injection into a blood vessel, needle placement must be verified by aspirating before injecting the local anesthetic solution. If blood is aspirated into the syringe, another injection site must be selected.

   b. Local anesthetics given during labor cross the placental barrier and may depress muscle strength, muscle tone, and rooting behavior in the newborn. Apgar scores are usually normal. If excessive amounts are used, in paracervical block, for example, local anesthetics may cause fetal bradycardia, increased movement, and expulsion of meconium before birth and marked depression after birth. Dosage used for spinal anesthesia during labor is too small to depress the fetus or the newborn.

   c. For spinal or epidural anesthesia, use only local anesthetic solutions that have been specifically prepared for spinal anesthesia and are in single-dose containers. Multiple-dose containers are not used because of the risk of injecting contaminated solutions.

   d. Use of local anesthetic solutions containing epinephrine requires some special considerations, such as the following:

      (1) This combination of drugs should not be used for nerve blocks in areas supplied by end arteries (fingers, ears, nose, toes, penis) because it may produce ischemia and gangrene.

      (2) This combination should not be given IV or in excessive dosage because both the local anesthetic and epinephrine can cause serious systemic toxicity, including cardiac arrhythmias.

      (3) This combination should not be used with inhalation anesthetic agents that increase myocardial sensitivity to catecholamines. Severe ventricular arrhythmias may result.

      (4) These drugs should probably not be used in people who have severe cardiovascular disease or hyperthyroidism.

      (5) If used in obstetrics, the concentration of epinephrine should be no greater than 1:200,000 because of the danger of producing vasoconstriction in uterine blood vessels. Such vasoconstriction may cause decreased placental circulation, decreased intensity of uterine contractions, and prolonged labor.

2. For topical anesthesia of mucous membranes of the nose, mouth, pharynx, larynx, trachea, bronchi, and urethra, local anesthetics are effective but should be given in reduced dosage. Because drug absorption from these areas is rapid, no more than one fourth to one third of the dose used for infiltration should be given to minimize systemic adverse reactions.

TABLE 14-2. LOCAL ANESTHETICS

Generic name	Trade name	Characteristics	Clinical uses
Benoxinate	Dorsacaine	A short-acting anesthetic that does not alter pupil size or accommodation	Topical anesthesia of the eye for tonometry and removal of sutures and foreign bodies
Benzocaine	Americaine	Poorly water soluble and poorly absorbed; thus anesthetic effects are relatively prolonged and systemic absorption is minimal; available in many prescription and nonprescription preparations, including aerosol sprays, throat lozenges, rectal suppositories, lotions, and ointments	Topical anesthesia of skin and mucous membrane to relieve pain and itching of sunburn, other minor burns and wounds, skin abrasions, earache, hemorrhoids, sore throat, and other conditions. Caution: may cause hypersensitivity reactions.
Bupivacaine	Marcaine	Given by injection; has a relatively long duration of action; may produce systemic toxicity	Regional anesthesia by infiltration, nerve block, and epidural anesthesia during childbirth. It is not used for spinal anesthesia.
Butacaine	Butyn	Too toxic for injection	Topical anesthesia of mucous membranes of nose, mouth, throat, and urethra
Chloroprocaine	Nesacaine	Chemically and pharmacologically related to procaine, but its potency is greater and duration of action is shorter; rapidly metabolized and less likely to cause systemic toxicity than other local anesthetics; given by injection	Regional anesthesia by infiltration, nerve block, and epidural anesthesia
Cocaine		One of the oldest local anesthetics; a naturally occurring plant alkaloid; readily absorbed through mucous membranes; a Schedule II controlled substance with high potential for abuse, largely because of euphoria and other CNS stimulatory effects; produces psychic dependence and tolerance with prolonged use; too toxic for systemic use	Topical anesthesia of ear, nose, and throat
Cyclomethycaine	Surfacaine	Acts on damaged or diseased skin and on mucosa of rectum and urethra to relieve pain and itching; ineffective on mucous membranes of mouth, nose, bronchi and eye	Topical anesthesia for dermatologic, proctologic, and urologic conditions
Dibucaine	Nupercaine, Nupercainal	Potent agent; onset of action slow but duration relatively long; rather high incidence of toxicity	Topical or spinal anesthesia
Dimethisoquin	Quotane	Applied to surface only, not given by injection	Topical anesthesia for various skin conditions such as itching and sunburn
Diperodon	Diothane	As potent as cocaine and has a longer duration of action; may cause local burning, stinging or skin rash	Topical anesthesia for skin and mucous membrane disorders
Dyclonine	Dyclone	Rapid onset of action and duration comparable to procaine; absorbed through skin and mucous membrane	Topical anesthesia in otolaryngology
Etidocaine	Duranest	A derivative of lidocaine that is both more potent and more toxic than lidocaine; long duration of action	Regional nerve blocks and epidural anesthesia
Hexylcaine	Cyclaine	Applied only to intact mucosa; too toxic for injection	Topical anesthesia in endoscopy, intubation, and manipulative procedures involving the respiratory, upper gastrointestinal, and urinary tracts
Lidocaine	Xylocaine	Given topically and by injection; more rapid in onset, intensity, and duration of action than procaine, also more toxic; acts as an antiarrhythmic drug by decreasing myocardial irritability. One of the most widely used local anesthetic drugs.	Topical anesthesia and regional anesthesia by local infiltration, nerve block, spinal, and epidural anesthesia. It is also used intravenously to prevent or treat cardiac arrhythmias (see Chap. 52). (Caution: do

TABLE 14-2. LOCAL ANESTHETICS *(Continued)*

Generic name	Trade name	Characteristics	Clinical uses
			not use preparations containing epinephrine for arrhythmias).
Mepivacaine	Carbocaine	Chemically and pharmacologically related to lidocaine; action slower in onset and longer in duration than lidocaine; effective only in large doses; not used topically	Infiltration, nerve block, and epidural anesthesia
Piperocaine	Metycaine	Pharmacologic effects similar to procaine but is more potent and more toxic; has a faster onset and longer duration of action	Topical anesthesia
Pramoxine	Tronothane	Not injected or applied to nasal mucosa because it irritates tissues	Topical anesthesia for skin wounds, dermatoses, hemorrhoids, endotracheal intubation, sigmoidoscopy
Prilocaine	Citanest	Pharmacologically similar to lidocaine with about the same effectiveness but slower onset, longer duration, and less toxicity because it is more rapidly metabolized and excreted	Regional anesthesia by infiltration, nerve block, and epidural anesthesia
Procaine	Novocain	Most widely used local anesthetic for many years, but it has largely been replaced by lidocaine and other newer drugs. It is rapidly metabolized, which increases safety but shortens duration of action.	Regional anesthesia by infiltration, nerve block, and spinal anesthesia. Not used topically
Proparacaine	Alcaine	Causes minimal irritation of the eye but may cause allergic contact dermatitis of the fingers	Topical anesthesia of the eye for tonometry and for removal of sutures, foreign bodies, and cataracts
Tetracaine	Pontocaine	Applied topically or given by injection	Topical and spinal anesthesia mainly; can be used for local infiltration or nerve block

NURSING ACTIONS: ANESTHETIC DRUGS

Nursing Actions	*Rationale/Explanation*
1. Administer accurately	Drug administration in relation to anesthesia refers primarily to preanesthetic or postanesthetic drugs because physicians, dentists, and nurse anesthetists administer anesthetic drugs.
a. Schedule the administration of preanesthetic medications so that their peak effects are reached at the optimal time, if possible.	Timing is important. It is probably better if these medications are administered so that peak sedative effects occur before administration of anesthetics to avoid excessive CNS depression. If they are given too early, the client may be sedated longer than necessary and the risk of postanesthetic respiratory and circulatory complications is increased. Also, the medication effects may wear off before induction of anesthesia. If they are given too late, the client may suffer needless anxiety and not be relaxed and drowsy when anesthesia is being initiated. Preanesthetic medications are often ordered "on call" rather than for a specific time, and the client may or may not become sedated before being transported to the surgery suite.
b. When a combination of two or three preanesthetic medications is ordered, do *not* mix in the same syringe	A precipitate may develop, or one of the drugs may be inactivated or altered when combined. Although larger amounts

Nursing Actions	Rationale/Explanation
and give as one injection unless the drugs are known to be compatible and the total volume is about 2 ml.	are sometimes given, probably no more than 2 to 3 ml should be given intramuscularly (IM) for both drug absorption and client comfort. About $1\frac{1}{4}$ ml (20 minims) is the upper limit for subcutaneous injections.
(1) Morphine and meperidine (Demerol) mix with promethazine (Phenergan) and hydroxyzine (Vistaril) and may be combined in the same syringe.	These are commonly used drugs.
(2) Atropine and scopolamine mix with all the above drugs. A rather common order is for meperidine, promethazine, and atropine. These can be mixed if the total volume is not excessive.	
(3) Glycopyrrolate (Robinul) is often ordered instead of atropine or scopolamine. It is compatible with morphine, meperidine, Innovar, and hydroxyzine.	
(4) Do *not* mix injectable pentobarbital (Nembutal) or other barbiturates with any other drug.	Parenteral barbiturates are physically incompatible with other parenteral drugs.
(5) If there is any doubt about the compatibility of a drug combination, *do not mix*. Instead, give two or more injections if necessary.	
c. If assisting a physician in injecting a local anesthetic solution, show the drug container to the physician and verbally verify the name of the drug, the percentage concentration, and whether the solution is plain or contains epinephrine.	Although the physician is responsible for drugs he or she administers, the nurse often assists by obtaining and perhaps holding the drug vial while the physician aspirates drug solution into a syringe. Accuracy of administration is essential so that adverse reactions can be avoided or treated appropriately if they do occur. The incidence of adverse reactions increases with the amount and concentration of local anesthetic solution injected. Also, adverse reactions to epinephrine may occur.
d. Have drugs and equipment for resuscitation readily available in any location where local anesthetics are given.	
e. When applying local anesthetics for topical or surface anesthesia, be certain to use the appropriate preparation of the prescribed drug.	Most preparations are used in particular conditions or bodily locations. For example, lidocaine viscous is used only as an oral preparation for anesthesia of the mouth and throat. Other preparations are used only on the skin.
2. Observe for therapeutic effects	Therapeutic effects depend on the type of drug and the reason for use.
a. When adjunctive drugs are given for preanesthetic medication, observe for relaxation, drowsiness, and relief of pain.	Depending on dose and client condition, these effects are usually evident within 20 to 30 minutes after the drugs are given.
b. When local anesthetic drugs are applied for surface anesthesia, observe for relief of the symptom for which the drug was ordered, such as sore mouth or throat, pain in skin or mucous membrane, and itching of hemorrhoids.	Relief is usually obtained within a few minutes. Ask the client if the symptom has been relieved and, if not, assess the situation to determine whether further action is needed.
3. Observe for adverse effects	Serious adverse effects are most likely to occur during and within a few hours after general anesthesia and major surgery. During general anesthesia, the anesthesiologist monitors the client's condition constantly to prevent, detect, or treat hypoxia, hypotension, cardiac arrhythmias, and other problems. The nurse observes for adverse effects in the preanesthetic and postanesthetic periods.

Nursing Actions	Rationale/Explanation
a. With preanesthetic drugs, observe for excessive sedation.	The often-used combination of a narcotic analgesic and a sedative-type drug produces additive CNS depression.
b. After general anesthesia, observe for	
(1) Excessive sedation—delayed awakening, failure to respond to verbal or tactile stimuli	The early recovery period is normally marked by a progressive increase in alertness, responsiveness, and movement.
(2) Respiratory problems—laryngospasm, hypoxia, hypercarbia	Laryngospasm may occur after removal of the endotracheal tube used to administer general anesthesia. Hypoxia and hypercarbia indicate inadequate ventilation and may result from depression of the respiratory center in the medulla oblongata, prolonged paralysis of respiratory muscles with muscle relaxant drugs, or retention of respiratory tract secretions due to a depressed cough reflex.
(3) Cardiovascular problems—hypotension, tachycardia and other cardiac arrhythmias, fluid and electrolyte imbalances	Vital signs are often unstable during the early recovery period and therefore need to be checked frequently. Extreme changes must be reported to the surgeon or the anesthesiologist. These problems are most likely to occur while general anesthesia is being administered and progressively less likely as the patient recovers or awakens.
(4) Other problems—restlessness, nausea, and vomiting. With ketamine, unpleasant dreams or hallucinations may also occur.	Restlessness may be caused by the anesthetic, pain, or hypoxia and should be assessed carefully before action is taken. For example, if caused by hypoxia but interpreted as being caused by pain, administration of analgesics would aggravate hypoxia.
c. After regional anesthesia, observe for	
(1) CNS stimulation at first (hyperactivity, excitement, seizure activity) followed by CNS depression	These symptoms are more likely to occur with large doses, high concentrations, injections into highly vascular areas, or accidental injection into a blood vessel.
(2) Cardiovascular depression–hypotension, arrhythmias	Local anesthetics depress myocardial contractility and the cardiac conduction system. These effects are most likely to occur with high doses. Doses used for spinal or epidural anesthesia usually have little effect on cardiovascular function.
(3) Headache and urinary retention with spinal anesthesia	Headache is more likely to occur if the person does not lie flat for 8 to 12 hours after spinal anesthesia is given. Urinary retention may occur in anyone but is more likely in older men with enlarged prostate glands.
4. Observe for drug interactions	For interactions involving preanesthetic medications, see Antianxiety Drugs (Chap. 8), Anticholinergic Drugs (Chap. 21), Narcotic Analgesics (Chap. 5), and Sedative–Hypnotics (Chap. 7).
a. Drugs that *increase* effects of general anesthetic agents	
(1) Antibiotics—bacitracin, colistimethate, aminoglycosides (gentamicin and related drugs), polymyxin B, viomycin	These antibiotics inhibit neuromuscular transmission. When they are combined with general anesthetics, additive muscle relaxation occurs with increased likelihood of respiratory paralysis and apnea.
(2) Antihypertensives	Additive hypotension, shock, and circulatory failure may occur.
(3) Catecholamines—dopamine, epinephrine, isoproterenol, levarterenol	Increased likelihood of cardiac arrhythmias. Halothane, cyclopropane, and a few rarely used general anesthetics sensitize the myocardium to the effects of catecholamines. If they are combined, ventricular tachycardia or ventricular fibrillation may occur. Such a combination is contraindicated.
(4) CNS depressants—alcohol, antianxiety agents, anticonvulsants, antidepressants, antihistamines,	CNS depressants include many different drug groups and hundreds of individual drugs. Some are used therapeutically

Nursing Actions	Rationale/Explanation
antipsychotics, barbiturates, narcotic analgesics, sedative–hypnotics	for their CNS depressant effects; others are used mainly for other purposes, and CNS depression is a side-effect. Any combination of these drugs with each other or with general anesthetic agents produces additive CNS depression. Extreme caution must be used to prevent excessive CNS depression.
(5) Corticosteroids	Additive hypotension may occur during and after surgery owing to adrenocortical atrophy and reduced ability to respond to stress. For clients who have been receiving corticosteroids, most physicians recommend administration of hydrocortisone before, during, and, in decreasing doses, after surgery.
(6) Monoamine oxidase (MAO) inhibitors—isocarboxazide, isoniazid, procarbazine, tranylcypromine, and others	Additive CNS depression. These drugs should be discontinued at least 10 days to 3 weeks before elective surgery. If emergency surgery is required, clients taking MAO inhibitors should not be given general anesthesia. Although they may be given spinal anesthesia, there is increased risk of hypotension. They should not be given local anesthetic solutions to which epinephrine has been added.
(7) Muscle relaxants—gallamine, pancuronium, succinylcholine, tubocurarine	Additive relaxation of skeletal muscles. These drugs are given for this therapeutic effect so that smaller amounts of general anesthetics may be given.
b. Drugs that *decrease* effects of general anesthetics	Few drugs actually decrease effects of general anesthetics. When clients are excessively depressed and develop hypotension, cardiac arrhythmias, respiratory depression, and other problems, the main treatment is stopping the anesthetic and supporting vital functions rather than giving additional drugs. Effects of general inhalation anesthetics decrease rapidly once administration is discontinued. Effects of IV anesthetics decrease more slowly.
(1) Alcohol	Alcohol is a CNS depressant, and acute ingestion has an additive CNS depressant effect with general anesthetic agents. With chronic ingestion, however, tolerance to the effects of alcohol and general anesthetics develops. That is, larger amounts of general anesthetic agents are required in clients who have developed tolerance to alcohol.
(2) Atropine	Atropine is often given as preanesthetic medication to prevent reflex bradycardia, which may occur with halothane, cyclopropane, and other general anesthetics.
c. Drugs that *increase* effects of local anesthetics	
(1) Cardiovascular depressants—general anesthetics, propranolol (Inderal)	Additive depression and increased risk of hypotension and arrhythmias
(2) CNS depressants	Additive CNS depression with high doses
(3) Epinephrine	Epinephrine is often used in dental anesthesia to prolong anesthetic effects by delaying systemic absorption of the local anesthetic drug. It is contraindicated for this use, however, in clients with hyperthyroidism or severe heart disease or those receiving adrenergic blocking agents such as guanethidine (Ismelin) and reserpine for hypertension.
(4) Succinylcholine (Anectine)	Apnea may be prolonged by the combination of a local anesthetic agent and succinylcholine.
d. Drugs that *decrease* effects of local anesthetics	These are seldom necessary or desirable. If overdosage of local anesthetics occurs, treatment is mainly symptomatic and supportive.

Nursing Actions	***Rationale/Explanation***
Succinylcholine (Anectine)	This drug may be given to treat acute convulsions resulting from toxicity of local anesthetic drugs.
e. Drugs that *increase* effects of neuromuscular blocking agents (muscle relaxants)	
(1) Aminoglycoside antibiotics (*e.g.,* gentamicin), colistin (Coly-Mycin) and related antibiotics	Additive neuromuscular blockade, apnea, and respiratory depression
(2) Diuretics, potassium-losing (*e.g.,* furosemide, hydrochlorothiazide)	Diuretics that produce hypokalemia potentiate skeletal muscle relaxants
(3) General anesthetics	Additive muscle relaxation
(4) Local anesthetics	Prolong apnea from succinylcholine
(5) Monoamine oxidase inhibitors	Additive respiratory depression
(6) Narcotic analgesics	Additive respiratory depression
(7) Procainamide (Pronestyl) and quinidine	Additive neuromuscular blockade with succinylcholine and other peripherally acting muscle relaxants
f. Drugs that *decrease* effects of neuromuscular blocking agents	
Anticholinesterase drugs (*e.g.,* neostigmine)	These drugs are often used to reverse the effects of the nondepolarizing agents gallamine, pancuronium, and tubocurarine. (They do not reverse the effects of succinylcholine and may potentiate them instead).
5. Teach clients	
a. With preanesthetic, sedative-type medications	The medications cause drowsiness and relaxation.
(1) Stay in bed with siderails up. (2) Use call light if help is needed. (3) Do not smoke.	Lying quietly helps the drugs to act. Activities are generally unsafe unless another person is available to provide assistance.
b. With local anesthetics applied topically	
(1) Use the drug preparation only on the part of the body for which it was prescribed.	Most preparations are specifically made to apply on certain areas, and they cannot be used effectively and safely on other body parts.
(2) Use the drug only for the condition for which it was prescribed.	For example, a local anesthetic prescribed to relieve itching may aggravate an open wound.
(3) Apply local anesthetics to clean areas. If needed, wash skin areas or take a sitz bath to cleanse the perineal area.	To enhance drug effectiveness. The drug must have direct contact with the affected area.
(4) Do *not* apply more often than directed.	Local irritation, skin rash, and hives can develop.
(5) With spray preparations, do not inhale vapors, spray near food, or store near any heat source.	
(6) Use local anesthetic preparations for only a short period. If the condition for which it is being used persists, report the condition to the physician.	
(7) Inform dentists or other physicians if allergic to any local anesthetic drug.	To prevent further reactions. Allergic reactions are rare, but if they have occurred, another type of local anesthetic can usually be substituted safely.

Selected References

American Medical Association (AMA) Division of Drugs: AMA Drug Evaluations, 5th ed. New York, John Wiley & Sons, 1983

Atracurium. Med Lett Drugs Ther 26:53–54, May 1984

Condon RE, Nyhus LM (eds): Manual of Surgical Therapeutics, 5th ed. Boston, Little, Brown & Co, 1981

Fraulini KE, Gorski DW: Don't let perioperative medications put you in a spin. Nursing 13:26–30, December 1983
Hahn AB, Oestreich SJK, Barkin RL: Mosby's Pharmacology in Nursing, 16th ed. St Louis, CV Mosby, 1986
Marshall BE, Wollman H: General anesthetics. In Gilman AG, Goodman LS, Rall TW, Murad F (eds): The Pharmacological Basis of Therapeutics, 7th ed, pp 276–301. New York, Macmillan, 1985
Ritchie JM, Greene NM: Local anesthetics, In Gilman AG, Goodman LS, Rall TW, Murad F (eds): The Pharmacological Basis of Therapeutics, 7th ed, pp 302–321. New York, Macmillan, 1985
Rodman MJ, Karch AM, Boyd EH, Smith DW: Pharmacology and Drug Therapy in Nursing, 3rd ed. Philadelphia, J B Lippincott, 1985
Smith BG: Surgery: Drugs used in perioperative care. In Wiener MB, Pepper GA (eds.): Clinical Pharmacology and Therapeutics in Nursing, 2d ed., pp 934–961. New York, McGraw-Hill, 1985
Smith TC, Wollman H: History and principles of anesthesiology. In Gilman AG, Goodman LS, Rall TW, Murad F (eds): The Pharmacological Basis of Therapeutics, 7th ed, pp 260–275. New York, Macmillan, 1985
Sufentanil—a new opioid anesthetic. Med Lett Drugs Ther 26:106, November 1984
Vecuronium. Med Lett Drugs Ther 26:102, November 1984

15 ALCOHOL AND DRUG ABUSE

Abuse of alcohol and drugs is a significant health, social, economic, and legal problem. As used here, the term *drug abuse* refers to self-administration of a drug for prolonged periods or in excessive amounts to the point of producing physical or psychologic dependence and reduced ability to function as a productive member of society. Most drugs of abuse are those that affect the central nervous system (CNS) and alter the state of consciousness. These include prescription and nonprescription, legal and illegal drugs. Alcohol is the primary drug of abuse worldwide. Also commonly abused are other CNS depressants such as narcotic analgesics, antianxiety agents, sedative–hypnotics, CNS stimulants such as amphetamines and cocaine, and other mind-altering drugs such as lysergic acid diethylamide (LSD) and marihuana.

Many terms are used to describe alcohol and drug abuse. In this context, alcohol abuse is synonymous with alcoholism, problem drinking, and other terms that denote excessive use of and preoccupation with alcohol. Similarly, drug abuse is considered synonymous with drug dependence, drug addiction, or other terminology denoting excessive or inappropriate use of a mind-altering drug.

Drug dependence involves compulsive drug-taking behavior. *Psychic dependence* involves feelings of satisfaction and pleasure from taking the drug. These feelings, perceived as extremely desirable by the drug-dependent person, contribute to acute intoxication, development and maintenance of drug abuse patterns, and return to drug-taking behavior after periods of abstinence. *Physical dependence* involves unpleasant and uncomfortable signs and symptoms that occur when the drug is stopped or its action is antagonized by another drug. The withdrawal or abstinence syndrome produces specific manifestations according to the type of drug and does not occur as long as adequate dosage is maintained. Attempts to avoid withdrawal symptoms reinforce psychic dependence and promote continuing drug use and relapses to drug-taking behavior. Tolerance is often an element of drug dependence, and increasing doses are therefore required to obtain psychic effects or avoid physical withdrawal symptoms. A person may be dependent on more than one drug.

Why does drug dependence occur? Various theories have been proposed, but none adequately answers the question. Some influencing factors include a given person's psychologic and physiologic characteristics, environmental or circumstantial characteristics, and characteristics of the drug itself, including amount, frequency, and route of administration. In one study of college students conducted through a self-administered, anonymous questionnaire, the three major reasons given for use of illegal drugs were peer group pressure, pleasure, and curiosity. Some specific factors associated with drug use include the following:

Broken family
Unhappy family relationships
Absence of religious affiliation
Parental use of depressant drugs
Parental use of cigarettes
Excessive alcohol use by parents
Poor academic achievement
Low self-esteem
Lack of ambition for the future
Nonparticipation in extracurricular activities
Involvement in political protest movements
Drug use among friends
Regular cigarette use
Sibling use of illicit drugs

Statistical analysis of these factors indicated that pressure from peer groups outweighed all other factors studied even if all the others were combined. Other important factors were parental use of prescription drugs and tobacco. Children were more likely to use illicit drugs when either parent regularly used tranquilizers or other mood-altering drugs or were heavy cigarette smokers. Keep in mind, however, that statistical correlation does not necessarily imply causation: some underlying factor may have been at the root of both the drug use and the associated factors.

Types of drug dependence

ALCOHOL-TYPE DEPENDENCE

1. It is usually characterized by consumption of alcohol in excess of the limits accepted by the person's culture, at times considered inappropriate by that culture and to the extent that physical health and social relationships are impaired. Psychic dependence, physical dependence, and tolerance are prominent characteristics.
2. It is similar to barbiturate-type dependence. Signs and symptoms of intoxication and withdrawal are similar for alcohol and barbiturates. Cross tolerance develops between these drugs.
3. Signs and symptoms of alcohol withdrawal or abstinence include tremors, sweating, nausea, tachycardia, fever, hyperreflexia, postural hypotension, and, if severe, convulsions and delirium. Delirium tremens (DTs), the most serious form of alcohol withdrawal, is characterized by confusion, disorientation, delusions, visual hallucinations, and other signs of acute psychosis. The intensity of the alcohol withdrawal syndrome probably varies with the duration and amount of alcohol ingestion.
4. Alcohol dependence can cause as much harm to a person as any other type of drug dependence. Alcohol impairs thinking, judgment, and psychomotor coordination. These impairments lead to poor work performance, accidents, and disturbed relationships with other people. Conscious control of behavior is lost, and exhibitionism, aggressiveness, and assaultiveness often result. Alcohol causes severe organic damage as well as mental problems.
5. Alcohol dependence can cause a great deal of damage to other people. Some problems commonly associated with alcohol abuse include automobile accidents, child and spouse abuse, job absenteeism, inability to keep a job, and loss of productivity.

AMPHETAMINE-TYPE DEPENDENCE

1. Amphetamines produce stimulation and euphoria, effects often sought by drug abusers. The user may increase amount and frequency of administration to reach or continue the state of stimulation. Psychologic effects of amphetamines are similar to those produced by cocaine. Effects are largely dose related. Small quantities produce mental alertness, wakefulness, and increased energy. Large quantities, especially if taken intravenously (IV), may produce psychotic behavior (*e.g.*, hallucinations and paranoid delusions). Tolerance develops to amphetamines.
2. Withdrawal from amphetamines or related stimulant drugs whose use has masked underlying problems (such as fatigue or depression) allows these conditions to emerge in an exaggerated form. Exhaustion and depression probably reinforce the compulsion to continue using the drug.
3. Related drugs that produce amphetamine-type drug dependence include methylphenidate (Ritalin) and phenmetrazine (Preludin).
4. Nonmedical use of these drugs is apparently increasing. Users take them alone or to counteract the effects of alcohol or barbiturates. In the latter case, these drugs are part of a pattern of polydrug use in which CNS depressants such as alcohol or barbiturates ("downers") are alternated with CNS stimulants such as amphetamines ("uppers").

BARBITURATE-TYPE DEPENDENCE

1. Drugs that produce dependence of this type include not only the short- and intermediate-acting barbiturates but antianxiety agents and other sedative–hypnotics as well.
2. It resembles alcohol-type dependence in symptoms of intoxication and withdrawal. It is also characterized by strong physical and psychic dependence.

Tolerance and cross tolerance develop with these drugs.

3. Signs and symptoms of withdrawal include anxiety, tremors and muscle twitching, progressive weakness, dizziness, distorted visual perceptions, nausea and vomiting, insomnia, weight loss, postural hypotension, generalized tonic–clonic (grand mal) seizures, and delirium that resembles the DTs of alcoholism or a major psychotic episode. Convulsions are more likely to occur during the first 48 hours of withdrawal and delirium after 48 to 72 hours.

MARIHUANA (CANNABIS)-TYPE DEPENDENCE

1. The amount of psychoactive (mind-altering) substance in a cannabis preparation varies according to specific characteristics of the plant, the place and circumstances of its growth, the age of the harvested material, its preparation, and the storage method used.
2. Cannabis preparations are usually smoked. Hashish, a secretion from the plant's flowers, is also taken orally in candies, cookies, and beverages. Effects appear sooner with smoking; larger amounts are required to produce effects when the drug is taken orally. Specific effects of cannabis preparations depend on the dose to some extent but also on the user's personality, expectations, and physical condition and on the environment in which the drug is used. Low-to-moderate doses usually produce euphoria, sensory and perceptual changes, decreased sense of identity and reality, visual and sometimes auditory hallucinations, increased pulse rate, and decreased muscle strength. These symptoms may be followed by sedation and sleep. Regular smoking for a prolonged period produces inflammatory and other changes in the respiratory tract.
3. Tolerance and psychic dependence do not usually develop with occasional use but may occur with chronic use; physical dependence rarely occurs.

COCAINE-TYPE DEPENDENCE

1. Cocaine is a CNS stimulant that induces euphoria, excitement, hallucinations, and strong psychic dependence.
2. It is usually taken IV or by sniffing drug crystals into the nose, where it is rapidly absorbed. Because cocaine is a strong vasoconstrictor, prolonged use or high doses may lead to damage and necrosis of nasal tissue. "Freebasing" (cooking cocaine, mixing it with ether, and inhaling the fumes) produces the greatest high and is the most addictive and dangerous method of administration.
3. Relatively large quantities are often taken within a short period because the drug is rapidly destroyed in the body and its effects are brief.

HALLUCINOGEN (LSD)-TYPE DEPENDENCE

1. There are many hallucinogenic drugs. Examples are LSD, peyote, phencyclidine (PCP), and psilocybin (obtained from a type of mushroom).
2. Drugs producing this type of dependence cause mood changes, anxiety, distorted visual and other sensory perceptions, hallucinations, delusions, depersonalization, pupil dilation, elevated body temperature, and elevated blood pressure.
3. Tolerance develops, but there is no apparent physical dependence or abstinence syndrome. Psychic dependence probably occurs but is usually not intense. Users may prefer one of these drugs, but they apparently do without or substitute another drug if the one they favor is not available.
4. A major danger with these drugs is their ability to impair judgment and insight, which can lead to panic reactions in which the user is induced to try to injure himself (*e.g.*, by running into traffic).

OPIATE (MORPHINE)-TYPE DEPENDENCE

1. These drugs all produce high degrees of psychic and physical dependence as well as tolerance. Most other drugs that produce dependence do so with prolonged usage of large doses. Morphinelike drugs are somewhat unusual in producing dependence with repeated administration of small doses. This characteristic is especially significant in medical usage of these potent analgesics because it implies that dependence may be induced by usual therapeutic dosages and initiated by the first dose given.
2. Effects of narcotic drugs vary according to dosage, route of administration, and physical and mental characteristics of the user. Usually, though, they produce euphoria, sedation, analgesia, apathy, lethargy, respiratory depression, postural hypotension, vasodilation, pupil constriction (miosis), and decreased gastrointestinal tract motility with constipation.
3. Opiate-type drugs produce a characteristic withdrawal syndrome. With morphine, withdrawal symptoms begin within a few hours of the last dose, reach peak intensity in 24 to 48 hours, and

subside spontaneously. The more severe symptoms usually disappear within 10 days, but some residual symptoms may persist much longer.

4. The abstinence syndrome varies in time of onset, peak intensity, and duration, depending on the specific drug involved. If a narcotic antagonist such as naloxone (Narcan) is given, withdrawal symptoms occur rapidly and are more intense but of shorter duration.
5. Withdrawal produces a wide array of signs and symptoms, including anxiety, restlessness, generalized body aches, insomnia, yawning, lacrimation, rhinorrhea, perspiration, pupil dilation (mydriasis), piloerection (goose flesh), hot flushes, nausea and vomiting, diarrhea, elevation of body temperature, respiratory rate and systolic blood pressure, abdominal and other muscle cramps, dehydration, anorexia, and weight loss.

VOLATILE SOLVENT (INHALANT)-TYPE DEPENDENCE

1. Some general inhalation anesthetics such as nitrous oxide have been used to the point of producing this type of dependence. More recently, however, volatile solvents such as acetone, toluene, and gasoline are being used. These solvents are constituents of various products, including some types of glue, plastic cements, and aerosol sprays.
2. These substances are most often abused by preadolescents and adolescents who squeeze glue into a plastic bag, for example, and sniff the fumes. Suffocation sometimes occurs when the sniffer loses consciousness while the bag covers the face.
3. These substances depress the CNS and produce symptoms somewhat comparable to acute intoxication with alcohol, including initial mild euphoria followed by ataxia, confusion, and disorientation. Some substances in gasoline and toluene may also produce symptoms similar to those produced by the hallucinogens, including euphoria, hallucinations, recklessness, and loss of self-control. Large doses may cause convulsions, coma, and death.

   Substances containing gasoline, benzene, or carbon tetrachloride are especially likely to cause serious damage to the liver, kidneys, and bone marrow.
4. These substances produce psychic dependence, and some produce tolerance. There is some question about whether physical dependence occurs. If it does occur, it is considered less intense than the physical dependence associated with alcohol, barbiturates, and opiates.

Selected individual drugs of abuse

Many drugs are abused for their mind-altering properties. Most of these have clinical usefulness and are discussed individually elsewhere in this text (see Antianxiety Drugs [Chap. 8], Narcotic Analgesics [Chap. 5], Sedative–Hypnotics [Chap. 7], and Central Nervous System Stimulants [Chap. 16]). The individual drugs of abuse included here are those that are commonly abused but have little, if any, clinical usefulness. Except for alcohol, they are illegal.

ALCOHOL (ETHANOL)

Alcohol is a CNS depressant drug and is the most abused drug in the world. It is legal and readily available, and its use is accepted in most societies. There is no clear-cut dividing line between "use" and "abuse" but rather a continuum of progression over several years.

When ingested orally, alcohol is absorbed partly from the stomach but mostly from the upper small intestine. It is rapidly absorbed when the stomach and small intestine are empty. Food delays absorption by diluting the alcohol and by delaying gastric emptying. Once absorbed, alcohol is quickly distributed to all body tissues. The alcohol concentration in the brain rapidly approaches that in the blood, and CNS effects usually occur within a few minutes. These effects depend on the amount ingested, how rapidly it was ingested, whether the stomach was empty, and other factors. Generally, though, effects with acute intoxication progress from a feeling of relaxation to impaired mental and motor functions to stupor and sleep. Excited behavior may occur, due to depression of the cerebral cortex, which normally controls behavior. The person may seem more relaxed, talkative, and outgoing or more impulsive and aggressive because inhibitions have been lessened.

The major factor affecting the duration of the CNS effects of ingested alcohol is the rate at which alcohol is metabolized in the body. Between 90% and 95% of alcohol is oxidized in the liver to acetaldehyde, then to acetate, and finally to carbon dioxide and water. When converted to acetaldehyde, alcohol no longer exerts depressant effects on the CNS. Although the rate of metabolism differs with acute ingestion or chronic intake as well as some other factors, it is generally about 10 ml per hour. This is the amount of alcohol contained in about $\frac{2}{3}$ ounce of whiskey, 3 to 4 ounces of wine, or 8 to 12 ounces of beer. The important point is that alcohol is metabolized at the same rate regardless of the amount present in body tissues. Efforts to find drugs or procedures to increase the rate of metabolism and thereby reverse the effects of alcohol have been unsuccessful thus far.

Chronic alcohol abuse leads to alcoholism, a progressive illness that usually develops over a period of 5 to 20 years. Alcoholism is prevalent in all segments of society. Incidence is highest among people 35 to 55 years old but is increasing in younger people, especially teenagers. Alcohol exerts profound metabolic and physiologic effects on all organ systems of the body. Some of these effects are evident with acute alcohol intake, while others become evident with chronic intake of substantial amounts.

Central and peripheral nervous system effects

1. Sedation ranging from drowsiness to coma
2. Impaired mental processes such as memory and learning
3. Impaired motor coordination—ataxia or staggering gait, altered speech patterns, poor task performance, hypoactivity or hyperactivity
4. Mental depression, anxiety, insomnia
5. Impaired interpersonal relationships
6. Brain damage
7. Polyneuritis and Wernicke–Korsakoff's syndrome, which are attributed to thiamine deficiency

Hepatic effects

1. Chronic alcohol ingestion induces drug-metabolizing enzymes in the liver and thereby increases the rate of metabolism of itself and several other drugs. This mechanism probably accounts for the development of tolerance to alcohol and cross tolerance with other drugs. Once liver damage occurs, however, drug metabolism is slowed and drugs metabolized by the liver may accumulate and produce toxic effects.
2. Decreased use and increased production of lactate by the liver, which leads to accumulation of lactic acid in the blood. This in turn leads to lactic acidosis, decreased renal excretion of uric acid, and secondary hyperuricemia.
3. Decreased use and increased production of lipids, which leads to hyperlipidemia and fatty liver. Fatty liver may be a precursor to hepatic cirrhosis and hepatitis.
4. Hepatomegaly due to accumulation of fat and protein
5. Severe liver injury characterized by necrosis and inflammation (alcoholic hepatitis) or by fibrous bands of scar tissue that alter both structure and function (cirrhosis). Cirrhosis is irreversible.
6. Liver damage from ethanol had been attributed to the malnutrition accompanying alcoholism rather than to direct toxic effects of ethanol on the liver. This view has largely been disproved. The entire progression of liver damage, from early and mild to late and severe, is apparently caused by ethanol itself or to the metabolic changes produced by ethanol. The incidence of liver disease correlates with the amount of alcohol consumed; it does not correlate with dietary deficiencies.

Gastrointestinal effects

1. Slowed gastric emptying time with large concentrations of alcohol
2. Increased intestinal motility, which probably contributes to the diarrhea that often occurs with alcoholism
3. Damage to the epithelial cells of the intestinal mucosa, which alters both structure and function of the cells and may produce inflammatory reactions
4. Multiple nutritional deficiencies, including protein and water-soluble vitamins such as thiamine, folic acid, and vitamin B_{12}
5. Pancreatic disease, which contributes to malabsorption of fat, nitrogen, and vitamin B_{12}
6. All the above factors probably contribute to the malabsorption that often occurs in alcoholism.

Cardiovascular effects

1. Changes in cardiac metabolism and function, apparently due to toxic effects of alcohol on myocardial cells
2. Alcoholic cardiomyopathy, which includes signs and symptoms of cardiomegaly, rales, edema, dyspnea, third and fourth heart sounds, and a cardiac murmur. Electrocardiographic changes include indications of left ventricular hypertrophy, abnormal T waves, and conduction disturbances.
3. Effects of alcohol on coronary blood flow and myocardial contractility are still controversial. Some studies have shown increased coronary blood flow, although others have shown decreased flow or no change. Similarly, some investigators report depressed left ventricular contractility, but others do not. The different results may be at least partly caused by different levels of alcohol in the blood.

Hematologic effects

1. Bone marrow depression due either to alcohol or associated conditions such as malnutrition, infection, and liver disease

2. Several types of anemia result from abnormalities in red blood cells. *Megaloblastic anemia* is caused by folic acid deficiency. Folic acid deficiency is caused, in turn, by alcohol ingestion or inadequate dietary intake in most instances, but gastrointestinal bleeding, hypersplenism, hemolysis, and infection may also contribute. *Sideroblastic anemia* (sideroblasts are precursors of red blood cells) is probably the result of nutritional deficiency. Low-grade *hemolytic anemia* results from abnormalities in the structure of red blood cells and from a shortened life span of red blood cells. *Iron deficiency anemia* is usually caused by gastrointestinal bleeding. Other causes of anemia in people who abuse alcohol include hemodilution, chronic infection, and fatty liver and bone marrow failure associated with cirrhosis.
3. Thrombocytopenia and decreased platelet aggregation due to folic acid deficiency, hypersplenism, and other factors
4. Decreased numbers and impaired function of white blood cells, which leads to decreased resistance to infection. Granulocytopenia sometimes occurs with intoxication in the absence of infection; paradoxical granulocytopenia may occur in alcoholics with severe bacterial infection. The mechanism by which granulocytopenia occurs is unknown. Ethanol may also lower resistance to infection by decreasing the ability of leukocytes to migrate to an area of inflammation or infection. Other factors that probably contribute to lowered resistance include cigarette smoking, depression of cough, and impaired closure of the epiglottis.

Endocrine effects

1. Increased release of cortisol and catecholamines and decreased release of aldosterone from the adrenal glands
2. Hypogonadism, gynecomastia, and feminization in men with cirrhosis due to decreased secretion of male sex hormones
3. Degenerative changes in the anterior pituitary gland and decreased secretion of antidiuretic hormone from the posterior pituitary
4. Hypoglycemia due to impaired glucose synthesis, or hyperglycemia due to glycogenolysis

Skeletal effects

1. Impaired growth and development. This has been most apparent in children born to alcoholic mothers. The so-called fetal alcohol syndrome is usually characterized by low birth weight and length and by birth defects such as cleft palate and cardiac septal defects. Impairment of growth and motor development persists in the postnatal period, and mental retardation becomes apparent.
2. Decreased bone density, osteoporosis, and increased susceptibility to fractures
3. Osteonecrosis due to obstructed blood supply
4. Alcohol affects the skeletal system primarily by altering calcium and phosphorus metabolism. Hypocalcemia often occurs with alcoholism because of poor dietary intake of calcium, impaired absorption, and increased urinary and sometimes fecal losses. Hypocalcemia leads to release of parathyroid hormone, which in turn leads to bone resorption and decreased skeletal mass. Alcohol-induced losses of magnesium often accompany hypocalcemia and may further stimulate parathormone secretion and bone resorption. Hypophosphatemia is often observed in chronic alcoholism and is most likely caused by inadequate dietary intake of phosphorus.

Muscular effects

1. Alcoholic cardiomyopathy produced by chronic damage to the myocardium
2. Myopathy, usually classified as subclinical, acute or chronic. Elevated creatine phosphokinase (CPK) is common with chronic alcoholism and may occur with no other manifestations of myopathy. Acute myopathy may involve acute pain, tenderness, and edema similar to deep vein thrombosis, and it may be accompanied by hyperkalemia. Chronic myopathy may involve muscle weakness, atrophy, and episodes of acute myopathy associated with a drinking spree.

Drug interactions

Many drug interactions of potential clinical significance involve alcohol and other drugs. Alcohol increases or decreases the effects of several other drugs, and other drugs often increase or decrease the effects of alcohol. The interactions are frequently encountered and are complex. In relation to alcohol intake, drug interactions may differ depending on acute or chronic ingestion and, if chronic, how much and for how long. Acute ingestion tends to inhibit drug-metabolizing enzymes. This slows the metabolism rate of some drugs, thereby increasing their effects and the likelihood of toxicity. Chronic ingestion tends to induce metabolizing enzymes. This increases the rate of metabolism and decreases drug effects. Note, however, that long-term ingestion of large amounts of alcohol causes liver damage and impaired ability to metabolize drugs.

Because so many variables influence the incidence and significance of alcohol's interactions with other drugs, it is difficult to predict interactions in particular persons. Generally, though, clinically significant interactions are likely to include the following:

1. Alcohol interacts with other general depressants of the CNS to produce additive CNS depression, sedation, respiratory depression, impaired mental and physical functioning, and other effects. These depressant drug groups include the sedative–hypnotics, narcotic analgesics, antianxiety agents, antipsychotic agents, general anesthetics, and tricyclic antidepressants (TCAs).

   Two additional points must be emphasized regarding these interactions. First, combining alcohol with barbiturates or TCAs is more likely to be lethal and should be avoided. Second, chronic ingestion of large amounts of alcohol produces a cross tolerance with barbiturates and general anesthetics. This means, for example, that the alcoholic client requires larger doses of these drugs when barbiturates are given during alcohol withdrawal syndromes or when a general anesthetic is given for a surgical procedure.
2. Alcohol has a vasodilating effect and thus increases the hypotensive effects of most antihypertensive drugs.
3. Alcohol potentiates hypoglycemic effects of oral antidiabetic drugs.
4. Alcohol's interaction with oral anticoagulants varies. Chronic ingestion of alcohol tends to decrease the effects of anticoagulants by inducing drug metabolizing enzymes in the liver and increasing their rate of metabolism. However, if chronic ingestion has caused liver damage, metabolism of the oral anticoagulants may be slowed. This increases the risk of excessive anticoagulant effect and bleeding.
5. Alcohol interacts with disulfiram (Antabuse) to produce symptoms such as flushing, dyspnea, hypotension, tachycardia, nausea, and vomiting (see Treatment of Alcohol Abuse under Principles of Therapy, below). A disulfiramlike reaction may also occur with other drugs, such as chloramphenicol (Chloromycetin), furazolidone (Furoxone), griseofulvin (Fulvicin), chlorpropamide (Diabinese), tolbutamide (Orinase), and metronidazole (Flagyl).

HEROIN

Heroin is a semisynthetic derivative of morphine and is the opiate most widely used for illicit purposes. It is a potent analgesic and produces rapid, intense euphoria with IV injection. A Schedule I drug in the United States, it is not used therapeutically. It is used medically in other countries. In England, it is an ingredient in Brompton's solution (a combination of drugs used to relieve pain in terminally ill clients). Heroin produces psychic and physical dependence and tolerance within a few weeks of continued abuse. Like other opiates, heroin causes severe respiratory depression with overdose and produces a characteristic abstinence syndrome.

MARIHUANA AND OTHER CANNABIS PREPARATIONS

Marihuana and other cannabis preparations are obtained from *Cannabis sativa,* the hemp plant, which grows in most parts of the world, including the entire United States. Marihuana and hashish are the two cannabis preparations used in the United States. Marihuana is obtained from leaves and stems. Hashish is prepared from plant resin and is five to ten times as potent as commonly available marihuana. These cannabis preparations contain several related compounds called *cannabinoids.* Delta-9-tetrahydrocannabinol (Δ-9-THC) has been thought to be the active ingredient, but metabolites and other constituents may also exert pharmacologic activity.

Cannabis preparations are difficult to classify. Some people call them depressants, some call them stimulants, and others label them as mind altering, hallucinogenic, psychotomimetic, or unique in terms of fitting into drug categories. It is also difficult to predict the effects of these drugs. Many factors apparently influence a person's response. One factor is the amount of active ingredients, which varies with the climate and soil where the plants are grown as well as with the method of preparation. Other factors include dose, route of administration, personality variables, and the environment in which the drug is taken.

Marihuana can be taken orally but is more often smoked and inhaled through the lungs. It is more potent and more rapid in its actions when inhaled. Low doses seem to be mildly intoxicating and similar to small amounts of alcohol. Large doses can produce panic reactions and hallucinations similar to acute psychosis. Many adverse reactions have been reported with marihuana use, including impaired ability to drive an automobile, chronic bronchitis and emphysema with prolonged, heavy use, chromosomal abnormalities, and impairments of cell metabolism, immune responses, and endocrine gland function. The first two reactions seem relatively well documented and accepted; the others are still being evaluated.

Marihuana and other cannabis preparations are illegal and not used therapeutically in the United States except for investigational and research purposes. Some proposed clinical uses are to relieve the nausea, vomiting, and anorexia associated with cancer chemotherapy, to lower intraocular pressure in glaucoma, and to exert a bronchodilating effect in asthma. These uses are still being studied and are not approved by the Food and Drug Administration. The highly refined tetrahydrocannabinol (THC) used in some studies probably bears little resemblance to the cannabis preparations generally available to drug abusers.

HALLUCINOGENS

Lysergic acid diethylamide is a synthetic derivative of lysergic acid, a compound in ergot and some varieties of morning glory seeds. It is very potent, and small doses can alter normal brain functioning. LSD is usually distributed as a soluble powder and ingested in capsule, tablet, or liquid form. The exact mechanism of action is not known, and effects cannot be predicted accurately. Generally, LSD alters sensory perceptions, supposedly enhancing their intensity; alters thought processes; impairs most intellectual functions, such as memory and problem-solving ability; distorts perception of time and space; and produces sympathomimetic reactions including increased blood pressure, heart rate, and body temperature, and pupil dilation. Adverse reactions include self-injury and possibly suicide, violent behavior, psychotic episodes, "flashback" (a phenomenon characterized by psychologic effects and hallucinations that may recur days, weeks, or months after the drug is taken), and possible chromosomal damage resulting in birth defects.

Mescaline is an alkaloid of the peyote cactus. It is the least active of the commonly used psychotomimetic agents, but users are apparently attracted by the vivid visual hallucinations and psychic effects. As with LSD, mescaline produces hallucinations, impairs memory and problem-solving ability, and produces sympathomimetic changes such as increased blood pressure and pulse and pupil dilation. It is usually ingested in the form of a soluble powder and capsule.

Phencyclidine (PCP) emerged as a leading street drug during the late 1970s. Phencyclidine was originally developed for use as an anesthetic. However, it produced excitement, visual disturbances, delirium, and hallucinations and was never approved for use in human beings. It is used as a veterinary anesthetic. It is cheap, widely available, and easily synthesized. It is usually distributed in liquid or crystal form and can be ingested, inhaled, or injected. Usually, though, it is sprayed or sprinkled on marihuana or herbs and smoked.

Phencyclidine produces profound psychologic and physiologic effects, including a state of intoxication similar to that produced by alcohol, altered sensory perceptions, impaired thought processes, impaired motor skills, psychotic reactions, sedation and analgesia, eye disorders such as nystagmus and diplopia, and pressor effects that can cause hypertensive crisis, cerebral hemorrhage, convulsions, coma, and death. Death from overdose has also occurred as a result of respiratory depression. Bizarre murders, suicides, and self-mutilations have been attributed to the schizophrenic reaction induced by PCP, especially in high doses. The drug also produces flashback.

Probably because it is cheap and readily available, phencyclidine is often sold as LSD, mescaline, cocaine, or tetrahydrocannabinol (THC). It is also added to low-potency marihuana without the user's knowledge. Consequently, the drug user may experience severe and unexpected reactions, including death.

Principles of therapy: alcohol and drug abuse

ASSESSMENT GUIDELINES

Assess clients for signs of alcohol and drug abuse, including abuse of prescription drugs such as antianxiety agents, narcotics, and sedative–hypnotics. Helpful information is often included in the physician's medical history of the client, especially regular medications and alcohol use.

1. Interview the client regarding alcohol and drug use to help determine immediate and long-term nursing needs. For example, information may be obtained that would indicate the likelihood of a withdrawal reaction, the risk of increased or decreased effects of a variety of drugs, and the client's susceptibility to drug abuse. People who abuse one drug are likely to abuse others. These and other factors aid effective planning of nursing care.

   Some general, screening-type questions are appropriate for any initial nursing assessment. The overall purpose of these questions is to determine whether a current or potential problem exists and whether additional information is needed. Some clients may refuse to answer or will give answers that contradict other assessment data. Denial of excessive drinking and of problems resulting from alcohol use is a prominent characteristic of alcoholism. It may be an important factor in other types of drug abuse as well. Useful information includes each specific drug, the amount, the frequency of administration and the duration of administration. If answers to general questions reveal problem areas such as long-term use of alcohol or psychotropic drugs, more specific questions can be formulated to assess the scope and depth of the problem.

2. Assess behavior that may indicate drug abuse such as alcohol breath, altered speech patterns, staggering gait, hyperactivity or hypoactivity, and other signs of excessive CNS depression or stimulation. Impairments in work performance and in interpersonal relationships may also be behavioral clues.
3. Assess for disorders that may be caused by alcohol or drug abuse. These disorders may include infections, liver disease, accidental injuries, and psychiatric problems of anxiety or depression. These disorders may be caused by other factors, of course, and are not specific.
4. Check laboratory reports, when available, for abnormal liver function tests, indications of anemia, abnormal white blood cell counts, abnormal electrolytes (hypocalcemia, hypomagnesemia, and acidosis are common in alcoholics), and alcohol and drug levels in the blood.

PREVENTION OF ALCOHOL AND DRUG ABUSE

Use measures to prevent development of alcohol and drug abuse. Although there are difficulties in trying to prevent conditions for which causes are not known, some of the following community-wide and individual measures may be helpful:

1. Decrease supply or availability of commonly abused drugs. Most efforts at prevention have tried to reduce the supply of drugs. For example, various laws designate certain drugs as illegal and provide penalties for possession or use of these drugs. Other laws regulate circumstances in which legal drugs, such as narcotic analgesics and barbiturates, may be used. Also, laws regulate the sale of alcoholic beverages.
2. Decrease demand for drugs. This involves changing attitudes. Consequently, it is likely to be very difficult but more effective in the long run. A number of current attitudes seem to promote drug use, misuse, and abuse. Some of these are as follows:
   a. The widespread belief that a drug is available for every mental and physical discomfort and should be taken in preference to tolerating even minor discomfort. Consequently, society has a permissive attitude toward taking drugs, and this attitude is probably perpetuated by physicians who are quick to prescribe drugs and nurses who are quick to administer them. Of course, there are many appropriate uses of drugs, and clients certainly should not be denied their benefits. The difficulties emerge when there is excessive reliance on drugs as chemical solutions to human problems that are not amenable to chemical solutions.
   b. The widespread acceptance and use of alcohol. In some groups, every social occasion is accompanied by alcoholic beverages of some kind.
   c. The apparently prevalent view that drug abuse refers only to the use of illegal drugs and that using prescription drugs, however inappropriately, does not constitute drug abuse.
   d. The acceptance and use of illegal drugs in certain subgroups of the population. This is especially prevalent in high school and college students.

   Efforts to change attitudes and decrease demand for drugs can be made through education and counseling about such topics as drug effects and nondrug ways to handle the stresses and problems of daily life.
3. Each person must take personal responsibility for drinking alcoholic beverages and taking mind-altering drugs. Initially, conscious, voluntary choices are made to drink or not to drink, to take a drug or not to take it. This period varies somewhat, but drug dependence develops in most instances only after prolonged use. When mind-altering drugs are prescribed for a legitimate reason, the client must use them in prescribed doses and preferably for a short time.
4. Physicians can help prevent drug abuse by prescribing drugs appropriately, prescribing mind-altering drugs in limited amounts and for limited periods, using nondrug measures when they are likely to be effective, educating clients about the drugs prescribed for them, participating in drug

education programs, and recognizing, as early as possible, clients who are abusing or are likely to abuse drugs.
5. Nurses can help prevent drug abuse by administering drugs appropriately, using nondrug measures when possible, teaching clients about drugs prescribed for them, and participating in drug education programs.
6. Parents can help prevent drug abuse in their children by mimimizing their own use of drugs and by avoiding heavy cigarette smoking. Children are more likely to use illegal drugs if their parents have a generally permissive attitude about drug taking, if either parent takes mind-altering drugs regularly, and if either parent is a heavy cigarette smoker.
7. Pregnant women should avoid alcohol in any form, as well as drugs, because of potentially harmful effects on the fetus.

TREATMENT OF ALCOHOL AND DRUG ABUSE

Treatment measures for alcohol and drug abuse have not been especially successful. Even those persons who have been institutionalized and achieved a drug-free state for prolonged periods are apt to resume their drug-taking behavior when released from the institution. Thus far, voluntary groups such as Alcoholics Anonymous and Narcotics Anonymous have been more successful than health professionals in dealing with drug abuse. Health professionals are more likely to be involved in acute situations, such as intoxication or overdose, withdrawal syndromes, or various medical–surgical conditions. As a general rule, treatment depends on the type, extent, and duration of drug-taking behavior plus the particular situation for which treatment is needed. Some general management principles include the following:

1. Psychologic rehabilitation efforts should be part of any treatment program for a drug-dependent person. Several approaches may be useful, including psychotherapy, voluntary groups, and other types of emotional support and counseling.
2. Drug therapy is relatively limited in treating drug dependence for several reasons. First, no specific antagonist drugs offset effects of the abused drug except for the narcotic antagonists such as naloxone (Narcan). Second, there is a high risk of substituting one abused drug for another because it is very likely that a person who has abused one drug will abuse another. Third, there are significant drawbacks to giving CNS stimulants to reverse effects of CNS depressants, and vice versa. Despite these drawbacks, however, there are some clinical indications for drug therapy. These include disulfiram (Antabuse) as deterrent therapy in chronic alcohol abuse, methadone maintenance in treating heroin-type drug dependence, treatment of symptoms during acute drug toxicity or overdose, and treatment of withdrawal syndromes.
3. General care of persons with drug overdose is primarily symptomatic and supportive. The aim of treatment is usually to support vital functions such as respiration and circulation until the drug is metabolized and eliminated from the body. For example, respiratory depression from an overdose of a CNS depressant drug may be treated by insertion of an artificial airway and mechanical ventilation. Removal of some drugs can be hastened by hemodialysis or hemoperfusion.

TREATMENT OF VARIOUS TYPES OF DEPENDENCE

1. Treatment of alcohol abuse can be divided into treatment of chronic alcoholism, acute intoxication, and withdrawal syndromes.
   a. Chronic alcohol abuse is a progressive illness. Therefore, early recognition and treatment are very desirable. They are also quite difficult, at least partly because denial is a prominent characteristic of alcoholism. The alcohol-dependent person is not likely to seek treatment for alcohol abuse until an acute situation forces the issue. He is likely, however, to seek treatment for numerous other disorders such as nervousness, anxiety, depression, insomnia, and gastroenteritis. Thus, health professionals may recognize alcohol abuse in its early stages if they are aware of indicative assessment data.

      If the first step of treatment is recognition or diagnosis of alcohol abuse, the second step is probably confronting the client with evidence of alcohol abuse and trying to elicit cooperation. Unless the client admits that alcohol abuse is a problem and agrees to participate in a treatment program, success is highly unlikely. In fact, the client may fail to make return visits or may seek treatment elsewhere at this point.

      If the client agrees to treatment, the two primary approaches are psychologic counseling and drug therapy. Short-term drug therapy involves use of drugs to control nervousness, insomnia, and other symptoms as well as to prevent withdrawal symptoms. For example, antianxiety drugs such as diazepam (Valium) or chlordiazepoxide (Librium) may be given. The primary purpose of such drug therapy is to help the client participate in rehabilitation programs. Long-term use of these drugs should be avoided because they may also be abused, and the client may simply be trading one type of drug abuse for another. These drugs can be gradually reduced in dosage and discontinued without precipitating withdrawal symptoms.

Long-term drug therapy may involve use of the deterrent drug, disulfiram (Antabuse). Normally, alcohol is metabolized in the liver to acetaldehyde, acetaldehyde is metabolized to acetate by the enzyme aldehyde dehydrogenase, and acetate is metabolized to carbon dioxide and water. When disulfiram is given, it blocks the action of aldehyde dehydrogenase and allows acetaldehyde to accumulate. If alcohol is then ingested, certain signs and symptoms occur. These include flushing of the face, dyspnea, hypotension, tachycardia, nausea and vomiting, syncope, vertigo, blurred vision, headache, and confusion. Severe reactions include respiratory depression, cardiovascular collapse, cardiac arrhythmias, myocardial infarction, congestive heart failure, unconsciousness, convulsions, and death. The severity of the reaction varies but is usually proportional to the amounts of alcohol and disulfiram taken. The duration of the reaction varies from a few minutes to several hours, as long as alcohol is present in the blood. Note that ingestion of prescription and over-the-counter medications that contain alcohol may cause a reaction in the disulfiram-treated alcoholic. Also, such reactions may occur following ingestion of aftershave lotions containing alcohol and of certain foods, such as sauces made with fermented vinegar.

Disulfiram alone may produce adverse reactions of drowsiness, fatigue, impotence, headache, and dermatitis. These are more likely to occur during the first 2 weeks of treatment, after which they usually subside. Disulfiram also interferes with the metabolism of barbiturates, coumarin anticoagulants, and phenytoin as well as alcohol. Concurrent use of disulfiram and these drugs may increase blood levels of the drugs and increase their toxicity. Because of these reactions, disulfiram must be given only with the client's full consent, cooperation, and knowledge.

b. Acute intoxication with alcohol does not usually require treatment. If the client is hyperactive and combative, a sedative-type drug may be given. The client must be closely observed because sedatives potentiate alcohol, and excessive CNS depression may occur. If the client is already sedated and stuporous, he can be allowed to sleep off the alcohol effects. If the client is comatose, supportive measures are indicated. For example, respiratory depression may require insertion of an artificial airway and mechanical ventilation.

c. Abstinence or withdrawal from alcohol is characterized by increased excitability of the nervous system, including both sensory and motor stimulation. Withdrawal of mild-to-moderate severity is characterized by tremors, restlessness, agitation, insomnia, and other signs and symptoms. Withdrawal syndromes of greater severity include the above signs and symptoms plus seizures, hallucinations, and DTs.

   Benzodiazepine antianxiety agents are usually the drugs of choice for treating alcohol withdrawal syndromes. They provide adequate sedation and also have a significant anticonvulsant effect. Seizures require treatment if they are repeated or continuous. Anticonvulsant drugs do not need to be given for more than a few days unless the person has a preexisting seizure disorder. Other treatment measures include vitamins, nutritional therapy, and symptomatic measures.

2. Treatment of barbiturate-type abuse—which also includes abuse of antianxiety agents and nonbarbiturate sedative–hypnotic drugs—can be divided into treatment of overdose and withdrawal syndromes.

   a. Overdose of these drugs produces intoxication similar to that produced by alcohol. There may be a period of excitement and emotional lability followed by progressively increasing signs of CNS depression such as impaired mental function, muscular incoordination, and sedation. Treatment is unnecessary for mild overdose if vital functions are adequate. The client usually sleeps off the effects of the drug. The rate of recovery depends primarily on the amount of drug ingested and its rate of metabolism.

      More severe overdose of these drugs produces impairment of vital functions due to excessive CNS depression. Respiratory depression and coma usually occur. There is no antidote for these drugs. Treatment is symptomatic and supportive. The goals of treatment are to maintain vital functions until the drug is metabolized and eliminated from the body. Insertion of an artificial airway and mechanical ventilation are often necessary. Gastric lavage may help if started within about 3 hours of drug ingestion. If the person is comatose, a cuffed endotracheal tube should be inserted and the cuff inflated before lavage to prevent aspiration. Diuresis helps to eliminate these drugs and can be induced by intravenous fluids or diuretic drugs. Hemodialysis or hemoperfusion is effective in removing most of these drugs. It is most likely to be used in shock, failure to respond to other treatment measures, or the presence of a potentially fatal serum drug level. Hypotension and shock are usually treated with IV fluids rather than vasopressor drugs, but the drugs may be used if necessary.

b. Treatment of withdrawal may involve administration of a dose of the drug to relieve signs and symptoms. Then, the drug is given in gradually reduced doses until it can be discontinued entirely. With dependence on short- or intermediate-acting barbiturates, a long-acting barbiturate such as phenobarbital is often substituted, gradually reduced in dosage, and then discontinued.

Barbiturate withdrawal can be life threatening. The person may experience cardiovascular collapse, generalized tonic–clonic (grand mal) seizures, and acute psychotic episodes. These can be prevented by gradually withdrawing the offending drug. If they do occur, each situation requires specific drug therapy and supportive measures.

3. Treatment of opiate-type dependence can be divided into treatment of overdose and withdrawal or abstinence syndromes.

a. Opiates produce respiratory depression in varying degrees, depending largely on dosage. Overdosage is likely to produce severe respiratory depression and coma. Insertion of an endotracheal tube and mechanical ventilation are often required. Drug therapy consists of a narcotic antagonist such as naloxone (Narcan) to reverse the effects of the opiate. Administration of a narcotic antagonist can precipitate immediate withdrawal symptoms. Also, if there is no apparent response to the narcotic antagonist, the signs and symptoms may be caused by depressant drugs other than opiates. In addition to profound respiratory depression, pulmonary edema, hypoglycemia, pneumonia, cellulitis, and other infections often accompany narcotic overdose and require specific treatment measures.

b. Signs and symptoms of withdrawal from opiates and related drugs can immediately be reversed by giving the drug producing the dependence. Therapeutic withdrawal, which is more comfortable and safer, can be managed by gradually reducing dosage over several days. An alternative method that has been somewhat successful is treating opiate-type drug dependence by methadone maintenance. This method involves daily administration of a single oral dose. Proponents say that methadone blocks euphoria produced by heroin, acts longer, and thereby reduces preoccupation with drug seeking and drug taking. This allows a more nearly normal lifestyle for the client. Also, since methadone is usually furnished free, the heroin addict does not commit crimes to obtain drugs. However, close supervision is required. Opponents of methadone maintenance programs say this method only substitutes one type of drug dependence for another.

A newer treatment modality is naltrexone (Trexan), a narcotic antagonist that prevents opiates from occupying receptor sites and thereby prevents their physiologic effects. Used in the maintenance of opiate-free states in the opiate addict, it is recommended for use in conjunction with psychologic counseling to promote client motivation and compliance.

4. Treatment of amphetamine-type abuse is mainly concerned with overdosage because these drugs supposedly do not produce physical dependence and withdrawal, at least in the sense that alcohol, opiates, and sedative–hypnotic drugs do. Since amphetamines delay gastric emptying, gastric lavage may be helpful even if several hours have passed since drug ingestion. The client is likely to be hyperactive, agitated, and hallucinating (toxic psychosis) and may have tachycardia, fever, and other symptoms. Symptomatic treatment includes sedation, lowering of body temperature, and administration of an antipsychotic drug. Sedative-type drugs must be used with great caution, however, because depression and sleep usually follow amphetamine use, and these after effects can be aggravated by sedative administration.

Selected References

Adverse effects of cocaine abuse. Med Lett Drugs Ther 26:51–52, May 1984

Bernstein JG: Kids and drugs. I. Recreational use. Drug Ther 14:193–208, March 1984

Bluhm J: When you face the alcoholic patient. Nursing 11:71–73, February 1981

Dyke CV, Byck R: Cocaine. Sci Am 246:128–141, March 1983

Geokas MC (ed): Symposium on ethyl alcohol and disease. Med Clin North Am 68:3–246, January 1984

Jaffe JH: Drug addiction and drug abuse. In Gilman AG, Goodman LS, Rall TW, Murad F (eds): The Pharmacological Basis of Therapeutics, 7th ed, pp 532–581. New York, Macmillan, 1985

Kurose K, Anderson TN, Bull W: A standard care plan for alcoholism. Am J Nurs 81:1001–1006, May 1981

Lieber CS (ed): Metabolic Aspects of Alcoholism. Philadelphia, W B Saunders, 1982

Marks VL: Health teaching for recovering alcoholic patients. Am J Nurs 80:2058–2061, November 1980

Mittleman HS, Mittleman RE, Elser B: Cocaine. Am J Nurs 84:1092–1095, September 1984

Ritchie JM: The aliphatic alcohols. In Gilman AG, Goodman LS, Rall TW, Murad F (eds): The Pharmacological Basis of Therapeutics, 7th ed, pp 372–386. New York, Macmillan, 1985

Rodman MJ, Karch AM, Boyd EH, Smith DW: Pharmacology and Drug Therapy in Nursing, 3rd ed. Philadelphia, J B Lippincott, 1985

16

CENTRAL NERVOUS SYSTEM STIMULANTS

Description and uses

Many drugs stimulate the central nervous system (CNS), but only a few are used clinically. These drugs are decreasing in number, and their indications for use are becoming limited. Most CNS stimulants act by facilitating initiation and transmission of nerve impulses that excite other nerve cells. Some act by inhibiting nerve impulses. CNS stimulants are somewhat selective in their actions at lower doses but tend to involve the entire CNS at higher doses. The major groups of CNS stimulants are amphetamines and related drugs, analeptics, and xanthines.

Amphetamines produce mood elevation or euphoria, increase mental alertness and capacity for work, decrease fatigue and drowsiness, and prolong wakefulness. Larger doses, however, tend to produce signs of excessive CNS stimulation such as restlessness, hyperactivity, agitation, nervousness, difficulty in concentrating on a task, and confusion. Overdoses can produce convulsions and psychotic behavior. They also stimulate the sympathetic nervous system, resulting in increases in heart rate and blood pressure, mydriasis, slowed gastrointestinal motility, and other symptoms.

These drugs are commonly abused. They produce tolerance and psychologic dependence. They are Schedule II drugs under the Controlled Substances Act, and prescriptions for them are nonrefillable. Despite efforts to control their distribution, these drugs are widely sold "on the street." In fact, they are used more often for nonmedical purposes than for therapeutic ones. (See Chap. 15 regarding amphetamine-type drug dependence.) For a time, amphetamines were prescribed as anorexiants (appetite suppressants) in treating obesity. The Food and Drug Administration (FDA) withdrew approval for such use in 1979, citing the high incidence of drug abuse. These drugs are clearly indicated only for treating narcolepsy and hyperkinetic behavior in children. Narcolepsy is a rare disorder characterized by periodic "sleep attacks" in which the person has an uncontrollable feeling of drowsiness and goes to sleep any place or any time. Hyperkinetic syndrome (also called minimal brain dysfunction and attention deficit disorder) is characterized by hyperactivity, short attention span, restlessness, and impulsive behavior.

Analeptic drugs stimulate respiration but do not reverse effects of CNS depressant drugs. A major drawback to clinical use is that doses sufficient to stimulate respiration often cause convulsive seizures. Respiratory depression can be more safely and effectively treated with endotracheal intubation and mechanical ventilation than with analeptic drugs.

Xanthine drugs stimulate the cerebral cortex, increasing mental alertness and decreasing drowsiness and fatigue. Other effects include myocardial stimulation with increased cardiac output and heart rate, diuresis, and increased secretion of pepsin and hydrochloric acid. Large doses can impair mental and physical functions by producing restlessness, nervousness, anxiety, agitation, insomnia, and cardiac arrhythmias.

Individual CNS stimulants

AMPHETAMINES AND RELATED DRUGS

Amphetamine, dextroamphetamine (Dexedrine), and **methamphetamine** (Desoxyn) are closely related drugs that share characteristics of the amphetamines as a group. They are more important as drugs of abuse than as therapeutic agents.

Route and dosage ranges

Amphetamine and Dextroamphetamine

Adults: Narcolepsy, PO 5–60 mg daily in divided doses

Children over 6 years: Narcolepsy, PO 5 mg daily to start therapy; raise by 5 mg/week to effective dose
Hyperkinetic syndrome, PO 5 mg 1–2 times daily initially, increased by 5 mg daily at weekly intervals until optimal response is obtained (usually no greater than 40 mg/day). Note: do not initiate dosage with a long-acting preparation.

Children 3–5 years: Hyperkinetic syndrome, PO 2.5 mg daily initially, increased by 2.5 mg daily at weekly intervals until optimal response is obtained. Note: do not initiate dosage with a long-acting preparation.

Methamphetamine

Adults: Narcolepsy, same as amphetamine

Children over 6 years: Narcolepsy, no dosage established
Hyperkinetic syndrome, same as amphetamine

Children under 6 years: no dosage established

Methylphenidate (Ritalin) is chemically related to amphetamines and has similar actions, uses, and adverse reactions. As a CNS stimulant, methylphenidate is considered less potent than amphetamines and more potent than caffeine. It is clearly indicated only in narcolepsy and hyperkinetic syndrome. It has been tested for use in mental depression, in treating overdosage of depressant drugs, and in relieving general lassitude, but its effectiveness in these conditions is doubtful. Methylphenidate is a Schedule II drug because it produces psychic dependence and is a drug of abuse.

Route and dosage ranges

Adults: Narcolepsy, PO 10–60 mg daily in 2–3 divided doses (average daily dose 30 mg)

Children 6 years or older: Hyperkinetic syndrome, PO 5 mg twice daily initially, increased by 5–10 mg at weekly intervals to a maximum daily dose of 60 mg

Pemoline (Cylert) differs chemically from amphetamines and methylphenidate but exerts similar pharmacologic actions. It is used only in treating hyperkinetic syndrome in children. It is a Schedule IV controlled drug.

Route and dosage range

Children over 6 years: PO 37.5 mg daily initially in the morning; increase by 18.75 mg at weekly intervals until desired response is obtained; maximal daily dose, 112.5 mg

ANALEPTIC AGENTS

Doxapram (Dopram) has limited clinical usefulness as a respiratory stimulant. Although it does increase tidal volume and respiratory rate, it also increases oxygen consumption and carbon dioxide production. Limitations include a short duration of action (5 to 10 minutes after a single intravenous dose) and therapeutic dosages near or overlapping those that produce convulsions. Mechanical ventilation is safer and more effective in relieving respiratory depression from depressant drugs or other causes. Doxapram is occasionally used by anesthesiologists and pulmonary specialists. A related drug, nikethamide (Coramine), is still available but is obsolete.

Route and dosage range

Adults: IV 0.5–1.5 mg/kg of body weight in single or divided doses
IV continuous infusion 5 mg/minute initially, decreased to 2.5 mg/minute or more. Dose by infusion should not exceed 3 g.

XANTHINES

Caffeine is commercially prepared from tea leaves. Pharmaceutical preparations include an oral preparation and a solution for injection. Caffeine is usually prescribed as caffeine citrate for oral use and caffeine and sodium benzoate for parenteral use because these forms are more soluble than caffeine itself. Caffeine has limited therapeutic usefulness. It is an ingredient in some nonprescription analgesic preparations (Anacin, A.P.C., Excedrin, Vanquish) and may increase analgesia. It is also an ingredient in some nonprescription stimulant preparations (*e.g.*, No-Doz). It is sometimes combined with an ergot alkaloid to treat migraine headaches (*e.g.,* Cafergot). Caffeine and sodium benzoate is used as a respiratory stimulant in neonatal apnea unresponsive to other therapies. Most caffeine is consumed in beverages such as coffee, tea, cocoa, and cola drinks. One cup of coffee contains about 100 mg to 150 mg of caffeine, analgesic preparations contain 30 mg to 60 mg, and antisleep preparations contain 100 mg to 200 mg. Thus the stimulating effects of caffeine can be obtained as readily with coffee as with a drug preparation. Caffeine produces tolerance to its stimulating effects, and psychologic dependence or habituation occurs.

Theophylline and theophylline salts (aminophylline and others) are xanthine derivatives used therapeutically in the treatment of respiratory disorders such as asthma and bronchitis. In these conditions, the desired effect is bronchodilation and improvement of breathing; CNS stimulation is then an adverse reaction. For additional information, see Chapter 47.

Principles of therapy: central nervous system stimulants

1. Assess the client's behavior carefully. For example, assess behavior of a child with possible hyperkinetic syndrome as specifically and thoroughly as possible. Some authorities believe this condition is diagnosed more often than it actually occurs and that stimulant drugs are prescribed unnecessarily. Also, assess behavior of any client receiving amphetamines or methylphenidate for signs of tolerance and abuse.
2. Counseling and psychotherapy are recommended along with drug therapy for clients with narcolepsy and hyperkinetic syndrome. With narcolepsy, for example, clients must be informed about the risks of driving an automobile and other activities. With hyperkinetic syndrome, parental counseling is indicated. For example, parents may be overmedicating the child in an effort to eliminate hyperactivity completely. If this is the case, they should be advised not to exceed the prescribed dosage. Other parents may fear that the child will become addicted if therapy is continued. They can be reassured that drug dependence does not occur with recommended dosages.
3. Stimulant drugs are often misused and abused by people who want to combat fatigue and delay sleep, such as long-distance drivers, students, and athletes. Use of amphetamines or other stimulants for this purpose is not justified. These drugs are dangerous for drivers and those involved in similar activities, and they have no legitimate use in athletics.
4. When an amphetamine or methylphenidate is prescribed, giving the smallest effective dose and limiting the number of doses obtained with one prescription will decrease the likelihood of drug dependence.
5. Analeptics are not indicated for most clients with depression of the CNS or the respiratory system. Anesthesiologists, if they use analeptic drugs at all, use them only in carefully selected circumstances and with great caution. Doxapram has replaced older analeptics, but it should generally not be used to stimulate ventilation in clients with drug-induced coma or exacerbations of chronic lung disease. Respiration can be more effectively and safely controlled with mechanical ventilation than with drugs.

NURSING ACTIONS: CENTRAL NERVOUS SYSTEM STIMULANTS

Nursing Actions	*Rationale/Explanation*
1. Administer accurately	
a. If possible, give amphetamines and methylphenidate at least 6 hours before bedtime.	To avoid interference with sleep
2. Observe for therapeutic effects	Therapeutic effects depend on the reason for use.
a. Fewer "sleep attacks" with narcolepsy	
b. Improved task performance with hyperkinetic syndrome	
c. Increased mental alertness and decreased fatigue	

Nursing Actions	***Rationale/Explanation***
3. Observe for adverse effects	Adverse effects may occur with acute or chronic ingestion of excessive amounts of coffee as well as with other forms of CNS stimulant drugs.
a. Excessive CNS stimulation—hyperactivity, nervousness, insomnia, anxiety, tremors, convulsions, psychotic behavior	These reactions are more likely to occur with large doses.
b. Cardiovascular effects—tachycardia, other arrhythmias, hypertension	These reactions are caused by the sympathomimetic effects of the drugs.
c. Gastrointestinal effects—anorexia, weight loss, nausea, diarrhea, constipation	
4. Observe for drug interactions	
a. Drugs that *increase* effects of amphetamines	
(1) Alkalinizing agents (sodium bicarbonate, antacids, some diuretics)	Drugs that increase the alkalinity of the gastrointestinal tract increase intestinal absorption of amphetamines, and urinary alkalinizers decrease urinary excretion. Increased absorption and decreased excretion both serve to potentiate drug effects.
(2) Monoamine oxidase (MAO) inhibitors	Potentiate amphetamines by slowing drug metabolism. These drugs thereby increase the risks of headache, subarachnoid hemorrhage, and other signs of a hypertensive crisis. A variety of neurologic toxic effects and malignant hyperpyrexia may occur. The combination may cause death.
b. Drugs that *decrease* effects of amphetamines	
(1) Acidifying agents	Urinary acidifying agents (*e.g.,* ammonium chloride) increase urinary excretion and lower blood levels of amphetamines. Both decreased absorption and increased excretion serve to decrease drug effects.
(2) Antipsychotic agents	Decrease or antagonize the excessive CNS stimulation produced by amphetamines. Chlorpromazine (Thorazine) or haloperidol (Haldol) is sometimes used in treating amphetamine overdose.
c. Drugs that *increase* effects of doxapram	
MAO inhibitors; sympathomimetic or adrenergic drugs (*e.g.,* epinephrine, norepinephrine)	Synergistic vasopressor effects may occur.
d. Drugs that *decrease* effects of doxapram	
Barbiturates	These CNS depressant drugs (sedative–hypnotics) may be used to manage excessive CNS stimulation caused by doxapram overdosage.
5. Teach clients	
a. Take amphetamines and methylphenidate only as prescribed by a physician.	These drugs have a high potential for abuse. The risks of drug dependence are lessened if the drugs are taken correctly.
b. Do not take stimulant drugs to delay fatigue and sleep.	Fatigue and sleep are normal "resting" mechanisms for the body.
c. Get adequate rest and sleep.	This is a much safer and more effective way to function than preventing rest and sleep by taking drugs or drinking large amounts of coffee or other caffeine-containing beverages.
d. Prevent nervousness, anxiety, tremors, and insomnia from excessive caffeine intake by decreasing consumption of coffee and other caffeine-containing beverages or by drinking decaffeinated coffee, tea, and cola.	Brewed coffee generally has a larger amount of caffeine than instant coffee, tea, and other beverages.

Selected References

American Medical Association (AMA) Division of Drugs: AMA Drug Evaluations, 5th ed. New York, John Wiley & Sons, 1983

Curatolo PW, Robertson D: The health consequences of caffeine. Ann Intern Med 98:641–653, May 1983

Facts and Comparisons. St. Louis, J B Lippincott (Updated monthly)

Franz DN: Central nervous system stimulants. In Gilman AG, Goodman LS, Rall TW, Murad F (eds): The Pharmacological Basis of Therapeutics, 7th ed, pp 582–588. New York, Macmillan, 1985

Laska EM, Sunshine A, Mueller F, et al: Caffeine as an analgesic adjunct. JAMA 251:1711–1718, April 1984

Rall TW: Central nervous system stimulants: The methylxanthines. In Gilman AG, Goodman LS, Rall TW, Murad F (eds): The Pharmacological Basis of Therapeutics, 7th ed, pp 589–603. New York, Macmillan, 1985

Rodman MJ, Karch AM, Boyd EH, Smith DW: Pharmacology and Drug Therapy in Nursing, 3rd ed. Philadelphia, J B Lippincott, 1985

III

DRUGS AFFECTING THE AUTONOMIC NERVOUS SYSTEM

17

PHYSIOLOGY OF THE AUTONOMIC NERVOUS SYSTEM

The autonomic nervous system (ANS) is a branch of the nervous system regulated mainly by centers in the spinal cord, brain stem, and hypothalamus. These centers serve to alter and integrate activities of the ANS. The ANS automatically, without conscious thought or effort, regulates many body functions. These functions can broadly be described as mechanisms designed to maintain a constant internal environment (homeostasis), to respond to stress or emergencies, and to repair body tissues.

Autonomic nerve impulses are transmitted to body tissues through two major subdivisions of the ANS, called the *sympathetic nervous system* and the *parasympathetic nervous system.* More specifically, nerve impulses are carried through *preganglionic fibers, ganglia,* and *postganglionic fibers.* Preganglionic impulses travel from the central nervous system (CNS) to ganglia (cell bodies of postganglionic fibers located outside the brain and spinal cord); postganglionic impulses travel from ganglia to effector tissues of the heart, blood vessels, glands, other visceral organs, and smooth muscle. Motor nerves of the ANS innervate all body structures except skeletal muscle, which is innervated by the somatic nerves.

Neurotransmitter substances, primarily norepinephrine and acetylcholine, are necessary for transmission of nerve impulses through the ANS. Preganglionic fibers of both the sympathetic and the parasympathetic systems secrete acetylcholine. Postganglionic fibers of the parasympathetic system also secrete acetylcholine, and those of the sympathetic system secrete norepinephrine. The nerve fibers that secrete acetylcholine are called *cholinergic fibers;* those secreting norepinephrine are called *adrenergic fibers.*

Acetylcholine and norepinephrine act on body organs and tissues to cause parasympathetic or sympathetic effects, respectively. Stimulation of both systems causes excitatory effects in some organs but inhibitory effects in others. However, most organs are predominantly controlled by one system. Also, when the sympathetic system excites a particular organ, the parasympathetic system often inhibits it. For example, sympathetic stimulation of the heart causes an increased rate and force of myocardial contraction. Parasympathetic stimulation decreases rate and force of contraction, thereby resting the heart.

Characteristics and functions of the sympathetic nervous system

The sympathetic nervous system is stimulated by physical or emotional stress such as strenuous exercise or work, pain, hemorrhage, intense emotions, and temperature extremes. Increased capacity for vigorous muscle activity in response to a perceived threat, whether real or imaginary, is often called the "fight or flight" reaction. Specific body responses include the following:

1. Increased arterial blood pressure and cardiac output
2. Increased blood flow to the brain, heart, and skeletal muscles; decreased blood flow to viscera and organs not needed for "fight or flight"
3. Increased rate of cellular metabolism—increased oxygen consumption and carbon dioxide production
4. Increased breakdown of muscle glycogen for energy
5. Increased blood sugar
6. Increased mental activity and ability to think clearly
7. Increased muscle strength
8. Increased rate of blood coagulation
9. Increased rate and depth of respiration
10. Pupil dilation to aid vision

These responses are protective mechanisms designed to help the person cope with the stress or get away from it. Intensity and duration of responses depend on the amounts of norepinephrine and epinephrine present. Norepinephrine and epinephrine are naturally occurring substances called catecholamines that function as neurotransmitters and hormones. As a neurotransmitter, norepinephrine is secreted when adrenergic nerve endings are stimulated. It exerts intense but brief effects. Then it is taken up again by the nerve endings and reused as a neurotransmitter, or it diffuses into surrounding body fluids and subsequently into the bloodstream. As a hormone, norepinephrine is secreted by the adrenal medulla, along with epinephrine, in response to sympathetic nerve stimulation. These hormones are secreted into the bloodstream and transported to all body tissues. They are continually present in arterial blood in amounts that vary according to the degree of stress present and the ability of the adrenal medulla to respond to stimuli. The circulating hormones exert the same effects as those caused by direct stimulation of the sympathetic nervous system. However, these effects last longer because the hormones are removed from the blood more slowly. These hormones are metabolized mainly in the liver by the enzymes monoamine oxidase (MAO) and catecholomethyl transferase (COMT).

When norepinephrine and epinephrine act on body cells that respond to adrenergic or sympathetic nerve stimulation, they interact with two distinct adrenergic receptors, alpha and beta. Norepinephrine acts mainly on alpha receptors to cause vasoconstriction and increased blood pressure, pupil dilation, and gastrointestinal relaxation. Epinephrine acts on both alpha and beta receptors. Beta-adrenergic activity includes increased heart rate and force of contraction, vasodilation of arterioles supplying skeletal muscles, relaxation of bronchial smooth muscle, and glycogenolysis and lipolysis. Large arteries and veins contain both alpha and beta receptors; the heart contains only beta receptors. Beta receptors have been further subdivided into $beta_1$ receptors, which predominate in the heart, and $beta_2$ receptors, which are present mainly in the smooth muscle of the bronchioles and in gland cells. The existence of different kinds of alpha receptors (called $alpha_1$ and $alpha_2$ receptors) is also being postulated.

Characteristics and functions of the parasympathetic nervous system

Functions stimulated by the parasympathetic nervous system are often described as resting, reparative, or vegetative functions. They include digestion, excretion, cardiac deceleration, anabolism, and near vision.

About 75% of all parasympathetic nerve fibers are in the vagus nerves. These nerves supply the thoracic and abdominal organs; their branches go to the heart, lungs, esophagus, stomach, and small intestine, the proximal half of the colon, the liver, gallbladder, and pancreas, and the upper portions of the ureters. Other parasympathetic fibers supply pupillary sphincters and ciliary muscles; lacrimal, nasal, submaxillary and parotid glands; descending colon and rectum; lower portions of the ureters and bladder; and genitalia.

Specific body responses to parasympathetic stimulation include the following:

1. Dilation of blood vessels in the skin; no particular effect on systemic blood vessels
2. Decreased heart rate and force of myocardial contraction
3. Increased secretion of digestive enzymes and motility of the gastrointestinal tract
4. Constriction of bronchi
5. Increased glandular secretions generally
6. Constricted pupils
7. No apparent effects on blood coagulation, blood sugar, mental activity, or muscle strength

These responses are very brief (milliseconds) because acetylcholine is rapidly split into acetate ion and choline by acetylcholinesterase, an enzyme present in the nerve ending and on the surface of the receptor organ.

Characteristics of autonomic drugs

The terminology used to describe autonomic drugs is often confusing because different terms are used to refer to the same phenomenon. Thus *sympathomimetic* and *adrenergic* are used to describe a drug that has the same effects on the human body as stimulation of the sympathetic nervous system. *Parasympathomimetic* and *cholinergic* are used to describe a drug that has the same effects on the body as stimulation of the parasympathetic nervous system. There are also drugs that oppose or block stimulation of these systems. *Sympatholytic, antiadrenergic,* and, more recently, *alpha-* and *beta-blocking* drugs inhibit sympathetic stimulation. *Parasympatholytic, anticholinergic,* and *cholinergic blocking* drugs inhibit parasympathetic stimulation. In this book, the terms *adrenergic, antiadrenergic, cholinergic,* and *anticholinergic* are used.

Drugs that act on the ANS generally affect the entire body rather than certain organs and tissues. Drug effects depend on which branch of the ANS is involved and whether it is stimulated or inhibited by drug therapy. Thus, knowledge of the physiology of the ANS is required if drug effects are to be understood and predicted. Also note that when the effects of one division are blocked by drugs, the other division may become dominant.

Selected References

Anderson PD: Basic Human Anatomy and Physiology: Clinical Implications for the Health Professions. Monterey, CA, Wadsworth, 1984

Boyd EH, Karch AM: Anatomy and physiology of the autonomic nervous system. In Wiener MB, Pepper GA (eds): Clinical Pharmacology and Therapeutics in Nursing, 2d ed., pp 153–167. New York, McGraw-Hill, 1985

Guyton AC: Textbook of Medical Physiology, 7th ed. Philadelphia, W B Saunders, 1986

Weiner N, Taylor P: Neurohumoral transmission: The autonomic and somatic motor nervous systems. In Gilman AG, Goodman LS, Rall TW, Murad F (eds): The Pharmacological Basis of Therapeutics, 7th ed, pp 66–99. New York, Macmillan, 1985

18

ADRENERGIC DRUGS

Description and uses

Adrenergic (sympathomimetic) drugs are those that produce effects similar to those produced by stimulation of the sympathetic nervous system. As discussed in Chapter 17, stimulation of alpha-adrenergic receptors produces vasoconstriction, and stimulation of beta-adrenergic receptors produces cardiac stimulation ($beta_1$ receptors) and bronchodilation ($beta_2$ receptors).

The drugs discussed in this chapter are epinephrine, ephedrine, isoproterenol, and phenylephrine. Epinephrine and ephedrine stimulate both alpha- and beta-adrenergic receptors. As a result, these drugs have widespread effects on body tissues and multiple clinical uses. Isoproterenol stimulates beta-adrenergic receptors (both $beta_1$ and $beta_2$) and is used in the treatment of several clinical conditions. Phenylephrine stimulates alpha-adrenergic receptors and is used to induce vasoconstriction in several conditions.

Other adrenergic drugs act mainly on specific adrenergic receptors or are given topically to produce more selective effects. These drugs have relatively restricted clinical indications and are discussed more extensively elsewhere (agents used in hypotension and shock, Chap. 54; bronchodilators, Chap. 47; nasal decongestants, Chap. 49; mydriatics, Chap. 65). Table 18-1 provides an overview of commonly used adrenergic drugs in relation to adrenergic receptor activity and clinical use.

Epinephrine is the prototype of adrenergic drugs. When epinephrine is given systemically, the effects may be therapeutic or adverse, depending on the reason for use and route of administration. Specific effects include the following:

1. Increased systolic blood pressure due primarily to increased force of myocardial contraction and vasoconstriction in skin, mucous membranes, and kidneys
2. Vasodilation and increased blood flow to skeletal muscles, heart, and brain
3. Increased heart rate and possibly arrhythmias due to stimulation of conducting tissues in the heart. A reflex bradycardia may occur when blood pressure is raised.
4. Relaxation of gastrointestinal smooth muscle
5. Relaxation or dilation of bronchial smooth muscle
6. Increased glucose, lactate, and fatty acids in the blood due to metabolic effects
7. Inhibition of insulin secretion
8. Miscellaneous effects, including increased total leukocyte count, increased rate of blood coagulation, and decreased intraocular pressure in wide-angle glaucoma. When given locally, the main effect is vasoconstriction.

CLINICAL INDICATIONS

Clinical indications for the use of adrenergic drugs stem mainly from their effects on the heart, blood vessels, and bronchi. They are often used as emergency

TABLE 18-1. ADRENERGIC DRUGS

	Generic name	Trade name	Major clinical uses
Alpha and beta activity	Dopamine	Intropin	Hypotension and shock
	Epinephrine	Adrenalin	Allergic reactions, hypotension and shock, local vasoconstriction, bronchodilation, cardiac stimulation, ophthalmic conditions
	Ephedrine		Bronchodilation, cardiac stimulation, nasal decongestion
Alpha activity	Levarterenol	Levophed	Hypotension and shock
	Metaraminol	Aramine	Hypotension and shock
	Methoxamine	Vasoxyl	Hypotension and shock
	Naphazoline hydrochloride	Privine	Nasal decongestion
	Oxymetazoline hydrochloride	Afrin	Nasal decongestion
	Phenylephrine	Neo-Synephrine	Hypotension and shock, nasal decongestion, ophthalmic conditions
	Phenylpropanolamine hydrochloride	Propadrine	Nasal decongestion
	Propylhexedrine	Benzedrex	Nasal decongestion
	Tetrahydrozoline hydrochloride	Tyzine, Visine	Nasal decongestion, local vasoconstriction in the eye
	Tuaminoheptane	Tuamine	Nasal decongestion
	Xylometazoline hydrochloride	Otrivin	Nasal decongestion
Beta activity	Albuterol	Salbutamol, Proventil	Bronchodilation
	Bitolterol	Tornalate	Bronchodilation
	Dobutamine	Dobutrex	Cardiac stimulation
	Isoproterenol	Isuprel	Bronchodilation, cardiac stimulation
	Isoetharine	Bronkosol	Bronchodilation
	Metaproterenol	Alupent	Bronchodilation
	Methoxyphenamine	Orthoxine	Bronchodilation
	Terbutaline	Brethine	Bronchodilation

drugs in the treatment of acute cardiovascular, respiratory, and allergic disorders. In hypotension and shock, they may be given as cardiac stimulants and vasopressor agents. (Vasopressors cause the muscles of capillaries and arteries to contract; contraction increases the resistance of vessels to the flow of blood, resulting in an increase in blood pressure.) In bronchial asthma and other obstructive pulmonary diseases, the drugs are given as bronchodilators to relieve bronchoconstriction and bronchospasm. In allergic disorders, the drugs are given for vasoconstricting or decongestant effects to relieve edema in the respiratory tract, skin, and other tissues. Other clinical uses include topical application to skin and mucous membrane for vasoconstriction and hemostatic effects, to the eyes for vasoconstriction (decongestant) and mydriatic effects, and to nasal mucosa for decongestant effects in upper respiratory infections or allergic disorders.

CONTRAINDICATIONS

Contraindications to using adrenergic drugs include cardiac arrhythmias, angina pectoris, hypertension, hyperthyroidism, and narrow-angle glaucoma. They should be used with caution in hemorrhagic or hypovolemic shock.

Individual adrenergic drugs

Epinephrine (Adrenalin) stimulates both alpha and beta receptors. As the prototype of adrenergic drugs, effects and clinical indications for epinephrine are the same as for adrenergic drugs. In addition, epinephrine is the adrenergic drug of choice for relieving the acute bronchospasm and laryngeal edema of anaphylactic shock, the most life-threatening allergic reaction. Epinephrine is used in cardiac arrest for its cardiac stimulant effects. It is also added to local anesthetics for vasoconstrictive effects to slow absorption and prolong action of the local anesthetic drug.

Epinephrine is not given orally because it is destroyed by enzymes in the gastrointestinal tract and liver. It may be given by inhalation, injection, or topical application. Numerous epinephrine solutions are available for various uses and routes of administration. Solutions vary widely in the amount of drug contained. These must be used correctly to avoid potentially serious hazards to recipients. Epinephrine is the active ingredient in several over-the-counter inhalation products for asthma (Asthma Nefrin, Asthma-Meter Mist, Micro Nefrin, Primatene Mist, Bronkaid Mist, and others). These products are very hazardous if used incorrectly.

Sus-phrine is an aqueous suspension of epinephrine that is given subcutaneously only. Some of the epinephrine is in solution and acts rapidly; some is suspended in crystalline form for slower absorption and relatively prolonged activity.

Routes and dosage ranges

Epinephrine Injection, 1:1000 (1 mg/ml) Aqueous Solution

Adults: IM, SC 0.1–0.5 ml q2h if necessary
IV 1 ml diluted to 10 ml with sodium chloride injection. Final concentration, 1:10,000
Intracardiac, 0.1–0.2 ml

Children: SC 0.01 ml/kg q4h if necessary

Epinephrine Inhalation, 1:100 (1%) Aqueous Solution

Adults: Oral inhalation by aerosol, nebulizer, or intermittent positive pressure breathing (IPPB) machine. This is not a preferred route of administration for epinephrine.

Epinephrine Nasal Solution, 1:1000 Solution

Adults: Topical application to nasal mucosa by drops (1–2 drops/nostril q4–6h)
Topical application to skin and mucous membranes for hemostasis, nasal solution diluted to 1:50,000–1:2000

Sus-Phrine Injection, 1:200 Suspension

Adults: SC *only,* 0.1 ml initially, maximal dose 0.3 ml. Do not repeat for at least 6 hours.

Children: SC 0.005 ml/kg (maximal dose, 0.15 ml)

Ephedrine is an adrenergic drug that acts by stimulating alpha and beta receptors and causing release of norepinephrine. Ephedrine can be given orally, and its actions are less potent but longer lasting than those of epinephrine. Ephedrine produces more central nervous system (CNS) stimulation than other adrenergic drugs. It is often used in treatment of bronchial asthma to prevent bronchospasm, but it is less effective than epinephrine for acute bronchospasm and respiratory distress. Ephedrine is a common ingredient in over-the-counter asthma tablets (Bronkaid, Primatene, and others). The tablets contain about 24 mg of ephedrine and 100 mg to 130 mg of theophylline, a xanthine bronchodilator.

Other clinical uses include shock associated with spinal or epidural anesthesia, Stokes–Adams syndrome (sudden attacks of unconsciousness caused by heart block), allergic disorders, nasal congestion, and eye disorders. *Pseudoephedrine* (Sudafed) is a related drug with similar actions. It is used for bronchodilating and nasal decongestant effects. Formerly a prescription drug, pseudoephedrine is now available over the counter.

Routes and dosage ranges

Ephedrine

Adults: Asthma, PO 25–50 mg q4h
Hypotension, SC, IM 25–50 mg; IV 20 mg. Maximal dose should not exceed 150 mg/24 hours
Mydriasis, eyedrops of 0.1%
Nasal congestion, nose drops of 0.5%, 1%, and 3% solutions; PO 25–50 mg q4h

Children 6–12 years: PO 6.25–12.5 mg q4–6h

Children 2–6 years: PO 0.3–0.5 mg/kg q4–6h

Pseudoephedrine

Adults: PO 60 mg 3–4 times daily

Children 6–12 years: PO 30 mg q6h

Children 2–6 years: PO 15 mg q6h

Isoproterenol (Isuprel) is a synthetic catecholamine that acts on beta-adrenergic receptors. Its main actions are to stimulate the heart, dilate blood vessels in skeletal muscle, and relax bronchial smooth muscle. It is well absorbed when given by injection or as an aerosol. However, absorption is unreliable with sublingual and oral preparations, and their use is not recommended. Isoproterenol is used clinically as a bronchodilator in respiratory conditions characterized by bronchospasm and as a cardiac stimulant in heart block and cardiogenic shock. Too frequent use may lead to tachyphylaxis and a reversal of bronchodilating effects.

Routes and dosage ranges

Adults: Bradycardia and heart block, IV 1–2 mg (5–10 ml of 1:5000 solution), diluted in 5% dextrose injection, infused at 0.5–5 μg/minute initially, then changed according to heart rate as indicated by continuous monitoring of the electrocardiogram

Hypotension and shock, IV 1–2 mg (5–10 ml of 1:5000 solution) diluted in 5% dextrose injection, infused at 1–10 μg/minute

Bronchospasm during anesthesia, IV 0.01–0.02 mg or 0.5–1 ml of diluted solution initially (1 ml of 1:5000 solution, diluted to 10 ml with sodium chloride or 5% dextrose injection for a final concentration of 1:50,000), repeated as necessary

Bronchodilation, *inhalation* by nebulizer, 5–15 deep inhalations of a mist of 1:200 solution, repeated in 10–30 minutes if necessary; by oxygen aerosol, up to 0.5 ml of 1:200 solution or 0.3 ml of 1:100 solution with oxygen flow at 4 liters/minute for 15–20 minutes; by measured-dose inhalers (Mistometer, Medihaler), 1–2 inhalations (second inhalation is given 2–5 minutes after first). These treatments should generally be given no more often than q4h; *sublingual tablets,* 10–15 mg 3–4 times daily, maximum of 60 mg daily. This route is not recommended because absorption is unpredictable.

Children: Bronchodilation, *inhalation,* generally the same as above, with adult supervision; *sublingual,* 5–10 mg 3–4 times daily, maximum of 30 mg daily. Not a preferred route because of erratic absorption.

Phenylephrine (Neo-Synephrine and others) is a synthetic drug that acts on alpha-adrenergic receptors to produce vasoconstriction with little cardiac stimulation. It is given to raise blood pressure in hypotension and shock. Compared with epinephrine, phenylephrine produces longer lasting elevation of blood pressure (20 to 50 minutes with injection). When given systemically, phenylephrine produces a reflex bradycardia. This effect may be used therapeutically to relieve paroxysmal atrial tachycardia. Other uses include local application for nasal decongestant and mydriatic effects. Various preparations are available for different uses. Phenylephrine is often an ingredient in mixtures used for symptoms of the common cold and allergic rhinitis, both prescription and nonprescription.

Routes and dosage ranges

Adults: Hypotension and shock, IM, SC 5–10 mg; IV 0.25–0.5 mg diluted in sodium chloride injection and given slowly, or 10 mg diluted in 500 ml 5% dextrose injection and infused slowly, according to blood pressure readings

Orthostatic hypotension, PO 20 mg 3 times daily

Nasal congestion, nasal solutions of 0.125%, 0.25%, 0.5%, and 1.0%

Mydriasis, ophthalmic solutions of 2.5% and 10%

Principles of therapy: adrenergic drugs

ASSESSMENT GUIDELINES

Assess the client's condition in relation to allergic disorders, asthma and other obstructive lung diseases, and cardiovascular status.

1. It is standard procedure to question a client about allergies on initial contact or admission to a health care agency. If the client reports a previous allergic reaction, try to determine what caused it and what specific symptoms occurred. It may be helpful to ask if swelling, breathing difficulty, or hives occurred.
2. If the client is a known asthmatic, assess the frequency of the attacks, the specific signs and symptoms experienced, the precipitating factors, the actions taken to obtain relief, and the use of bronchodilators or other medications on a long-term basis. Acute asthma attacks or bronchoconstriction may be precipitated by exposure to allergens. Clients with asthma are also susceptible to respiratory infections.
3. Emphysema and bronchitis are characterized by respiratory difficulty and bronchospasm. Acute or chronic respiratory acidosis is a common feature as well. Acidosis decreases effectiveness of adrenergic drugs in relieving bronchoconstriction. Acidosis can be accurately assessed by arterial blood gas analysis. Check reports for decreased oxygen (hypoxemia), increased carbon dioxide (hypercarbia) and *p*H under 7.35.
4. In emergencies, rapid action is necessary because signs and symptoms are acute, dramatic, and life threatening. With acute bronchospasm, respiratory distress is clearly evidenced by loud, rapid, gasping respirations. With anaphylactic shock, severe respiratory distress (from bronchospasm and laryngeal edema) and profound hypotension commonly occur. In other types of shock, which involves inadequate tissue perfusion, low blood pressure is only one assessment factor.

NURSING INTERVENTIONS

Use measures to prevent or minimize conditions for which adrenergic drugs are required.

1. Decrease exposure to allergens. Allergens include cigarette smoke, foods, drugs, air pollutants, plant pollens, insect venoms, and animal dander. Specific allergens must be determined for each person.
2. For people with chronic lung disease, use measures to prevent respiratory infections. These include measures to aid removal of respiratory secretions such as adequate hydration, ambulation, deep breathing and coughing exercises, and chest physiotherapy (percussion and postural drainage). Annual influenza vaccination is also recommended.
3. When administering substances that are known to produce hypersensitivity reactions—penicillin and other antibiotics, allergy extracts, vaccines, local anesthetics—observe the recipient carefully for at least 30 minutes after administration. Have adrenergic and other emergency drugs and equipment readily available in case a reaction occurs.

DRUG SELECTION AND ADMINISTRATION

Choice of drug, dosage, and route of administration depends largely on the reason for use. Epinephrine, injected intravenously (IV) or subcutaneously, is the drug of choice in anaphylactic shock. Isoproterenol by oral inhalation is often effective for producing bronchodilation. Adrenergic drugs are given IV only for emergencies such as cardiac arrest, severe arterial hypotension, circulatory shock, and anaphylactic shock. No standard doses of individual adrenergic drugs are always effective; dosage must be individualized according to the client's response. This is especially necessary in emergencies, but it also applies to long-term usage.

USE IN SPECIFIC SITUATIONS

Adrenergic drugs are often used in crises. Therefore, they must be readily available in health care areas such as hospitals, nursing homes, clinics, and physicians' offices. All health care personnel should know where emergency drugs are stored.

Hypotension and shock

In hypotension and shock, initial efforts involve identifying and treating the cause when possible. Such treatments include blood transfusions, fluid and electrolyte replacement, treatment of infection, and administration of corticosteroids. If these measures are ineffective in raising blood pressure enough to maintain tissue perfusion, vasopressor drugs may be used. The usual goal of vasopressor drug therapy is to maintain tissue perfusion and a systolic blood pressure of 80 to 100 mm Hg.

Cardiac arrest

In treating cardiac arrest, adrenergic drugs are less effective in the presence of metabolic acidosis. Metabolic acidosis develops rapidly in the presence of hypoxia and depresses cardiac function. It must be corrected by parenteral administration of sodium bicarbonate, a systemic alkalinizing agent. Epinephrine, the most commonly used adrenergic drug, is physically incompatible with sodium bicarbonate, and the two drugs must not come in contact with each other. However, the sodium bicarbonate may be given by injection into an established IV line and followed by enough fluid to thoroughly rinse the tubing. Then, epinephrine may be injected.

Bronchial asthma

In bronchial asthma, adrenergic drugs are usually given by inhalation or orally for chronic prophylactic and maintenance therapy. IPPB machines are sometimes used to administer adrenergic bronchodilators by inhalation. There is little evidence that IPPB delivers bronchodilators to the tracheobronchial tree more effectively than other methods of aerosolization. Only about 10% of an aerosolized drug dose reaches the tracheobronchial tree. The remainder is deposited in the upper respiratory tract and swallowed or exhaled.

NURSING ACTIONS: ADRENERGIC DRUGS

Nursing Actions	*Rationale/Explanation*
1. Administer accurately	
a. Check package inserts or other references if not absolutely sure about the preparation/concentration and method of administration for an adrenergic drug.	The many different preparations and concentrations available for various routes of administration increase the risk of medication error unless extreme caution is used. Preparations for intravenous, subcutaneous, inhalation, ophthalmic, or nasal routes must be used by the designated route only.
b. To give epinephrine subcutaneously, use a tuberculin syringe, aspirate, and massage the injection site.	The tuberculin syringe is necessary for accurate measurement of the small doses usually given (often less than 0.5 ml).

Nursing Actions	***Rationale/Explanation***
	Aspiration is necessary to avoid inadvertent IV administration of the larger, undiluted amount of drug intended for subcutaneous use. Massaging the injection site accelerates drug absorption and thus relief of symptoms.
c. Give Sus-Phrine subcutaneously only, and shake well before using (both vial and syringe).	Sus-Phrine is a suspension preparation of epinephrine, and suspensions must not be given IV. Rotating or shaking the container ensures that the medication is evenly distributed throughout the suspension.
d. For inhalation, be sure to use the correct drug concentration, and use the nebulizing device properly.	Inhalation medications are often administered by clients themselves or by respiratory therapists if IPPB is used. The nurse may need to demonstrate and supervise self-administration initially.
e. Do *not* give epinephrine and isoproterenol at the same time or within 4 hours of each other.	Both these drugs are potent cardiac stimulants, and the combination could cause serious cardiac arrhythmias. However, they have synergistic bronchodilating effects, and doses can be alternated and given safely if the drugs are given no more closely together than 4 hours.
f. For IV administration of epinephrine, dilute 1 ml of 1:1000 solution to a total volume of 10 ml with sodium chloride injection, or use a commercial preparation of 1:10,000 concentration. Use parenteral solutions of epinephrine only if clear.	Dilution increases safety of administration. A solution that is brown or contains a precipitate should not be used. Discoloration indicates chemical deterioration of epinephrine.
g. For IV infusion of isoproterenol and phenylephrine:	
(1) Administer in an intensive care unit when possible.	These drugs are given IV in emergencies, during which the client's condition must be carefully monitored. Frequent recording of blood pressure and pulse as well as continuous electrocardiographic monitoring are needed.
(2) Use only clear drug solutions.	A brownish color or precipitate indicates deterioration, and such solutions should not be used.
(3) Dilute the drugs in 500 ml of 5% dextrose injection. Do not add the drug until ready to use.	A 5% dextrose solution is compatible with the drugs. Mixing solutions when ready for use helps to ensure drug stability. Note that drug concentration varies with the amount of drug and the amount of dextrose solution to which it is added.
(4) Use an infusion device to regulate flow rate accurately.	Flow rate usually requires frequent adjustment according to blood pressure measurements. An infusion device helps to regulate drug administration, so that wide fluctuations in blood pressure are avoided.
(5) Use a "piggyback" IV apparatus.	Only one bottle contains an adrenergic drug, and it can be regulated or discontinued without disruption of the primary IV line.
(6) Start the adrenergic drug solution slowly and increase flow rate according to the client's response (*e.g.,* blood pressure, color, mental status). Slow or discontinue gradually as well.	To avoid abrupt changes in circulation and blood pressure
h. When giving adrenergic drugs as eye drops or nose drops, do not touch the dropper to the eye or nose.	Contaminated droppers can be a source of bacterial infection.
2. Observe for therapeutic effects	These depend on the reason for use.
a. When the drug is used as a bronchodilator, observe for absence or reduction of wheezing, less labored breathing, and decreased rate of respirations.	Indicates prevention or relief of bronchospasm. Acute bronchospasm is usually relieved within 5 minutes by injected or inhaled epinephrine or inhaled isoproterenol.
b. When epinephrine is given in anaphylactic shock, observe for decreased tissue edema and improved breathing and circulation.	Epinephrine injection usually relieves laryngeal edema and bronchospasm within 5 minutes and lasts for about 20 minutes.

Nursing Actions	Rationale/Explanation
c. When isoproterenol or phenylephrine is given in hypotension and shock, observe for increased blood pressure, stronger pulse, and improved urine output, level of consciousness, and color.	These are indicators of improved circulation.
d. When a drug is given nasally for decongestant effects, observe for decreased nasal congestion and ability to breathe through the nose.	The drugs act as vasoconstrictors to reduce engorgement of nasal mucosa.
e. When given as eye drops for vasoconstrictor effects, observe for decreased redness. When given for mydriatic effects, observe for pupil dilation.	
3. Observe for adverse effects	Adverse effects depend to some extent on the reason for use. For example, cardiovascular effects are considered adverse reactions when the drugs are given for bronchodilation. Adverse effects occur with usual therapeutic doses and are more likely to occur with higher doses.
a. Cardiovascular effects—cardiac arrhythmias, hypertension	Tachycardia and hypertension are common; if severe or prolonged, myocardial ischemia or heart failure may occur. Premature ventricular contractions and other serious arrhythmias may occur. Propranolol (Inderal) or another beta blocker may be given to decrease heart rate and hypertension resulting from overdosage of adrenergic drugs. Phentolamine (Regitine) may be used to decrease severe hypertension.
b. Excessive CNS stimulation—nervousness, anxiety, tremor, insomnia	These effects are more likely to occur with ephedrine or high doses of other adrenergic drugs. Sometimes, a sedative-type drug is given concomitantly to offset these effects.
c. Rebound nasal congestion, rhinitis, possible ulceration of nasal mucosa	These effects occur with excessive use of nasal decongestant drugs.
4. Observe for drug interactions	
a. Drugs that *increase* effects of adrenergic drugs	Most of these drugs increase incidence or severity of adverse reactions.
(1) Anesthetics, general (halothane, cyclopropane)	Increased risk of cardiac arrhythmias. Potentially hazardous.
(2) Anticholinergics (*e.g.,* atropine)	Increased bronchial relaxation. Also increased mydriasis and therefore contraindicated with narrow angle glaucoma.
(3) Antidepressants, tricyclic (*e.g.,* amitriptyline [Elavil])	Increased pressor response with intravenous epinephrine.
(4) Antihistamines	May increase pressor effects
(5) Cocaine	Increases pressor and mydriatic effects by inhibiting uptake of norepinephrine by nerve endings. Cardiac arrhythmias, convulsions, and acute glaucoma may occur.
(6) Digitalis	Sympathomimetics, especially beta adrenergics like epinephrine and isoproterenol, increase the likelihood of cardiac arrhythmias due to ectopic pacemaker activity.
(7) Doxapram (Dopram)	Increased pressor effect
(8) Ergot alkaloids (*e.g.,* Gynergen)	Increased vasoconstriction. Extremely high blood pressure may occur. There may also be decreased perfusion of fingers and toes.
(9) Monoamine oxidase (MAO) inhibitors (*e.g.,* isocarboxazid [Marplan])	Contraindicated. The combination may cause death. When these drugs are given concurrently with adrenergic drugs, there is danger of cardiac arrhythmias, respiratory depression, and acute hypertensive crisis with possible intracranial hemorrhage, convulsions, coma, and death. Effects of MAO inhibitors may not occur for several weeks after treatment is started and may last up to 3 weeks after the drug is stopped. Every client taking MAO inhibitors should be warned against

Nursing Actions	Rationale/Explanation
	taking any other medication without the advice of a physician or pharmacist.
(10) Methylphenidate (Ritalin)	Increased pressor and mydriatic effects. The combination may be hazardous in glaucoma.
(11) Thyroid preparations (*e.g.,* Synthroid)	Increased adrenergic effects, resulting in increased likelihood of arrhythmias
(12) Xanthines (in caffeine-containing substances such as coffee, tea, cola drinks; theophylline)	Synergistic bronchodilating effect. Sympathomimetics with CNS-stimulating properties (*e.g.,* ephedrine, isoproterenol) may produce excessive CNS stimulation with cardiac arrhythmias, emotional disturbances, and insomnia.
(13) Beta-adrenergic blocking agents (*e.g.,* propranolol [Inderal])	May augment hypertensive response to epinephrine (see also b[4] below)
b. Drugs that *decrease* effects of adrenergics	
(1) Anticholinesterases (*e.g.,* neostigmine [Prostigmin], pyridostigmine [Mestinon]) and other cholinergic drugs	Decrease mydriatic effects of adrenergics; thus the two groups should not be given concurrently in ophthalmic conditions
(2) Antihypertensives (*e.g.,* methyldopa [Aldomet])	Generally antagonize pressor effects of adrenergics, which act to increase blood pressure while antihypertensives act to lower it.
(3) Antipsychotic drugs (*e.g.,* haloperidol [Haldol], chlorpromazine [Thorazine])	Block the vasopressor action of epinephrine. Therefore, epinephrine should not be used to treat hypotension induced by these drugs.
(4) Beta-adrenergic blocking agents (*e.g.,* propranolol [Inderal])	Decrease bronchodilating effects of adrenergics and may exacerbate asthma. Contraindicated with asthma.
(5) Phentolamine (Regitine)	Antagonizes vasopressor effects of adrenergics
5. Teach clients	
a. Use these drugs only as directed.	The potential for abuse of these drugs is high, especially for the client with asthma or other chronic lung disease who is seeking relief from labored breathing. Also, some of these drugs are often prescribed for long-term use. However, excessive use does not increase therapeutic effects. Instead, it increases the incidence and severity of adverse reactions and causes tolerance and decreased benefit from usual doses.
b. Take no other medications without the physician's knowledge and approval.	Many cold remedies available on an over-the-counter or nonprescription basis contain adrenergic drugs. Use of these along with prescribed adrenergic drugs can result in overdose and serious cardiovascular or CNS problems. In addition, adrenergic drugs interact with numerous other drugs to increase or decrease effects. Some of these interactions may be life threatening.
c. Inhaled solutions of isoproterenol may turn saliva and sputum pink.	This harmless discoloration is caused by the medication, not by bleeding.
d. Report adverse reactions such as fast pulse, palpitations, chest pain.	So that drug dosage can be reevaluated and therapy changed if needed.
e. Report if previously effective dose becomes ineffective.	This may indicate that drug tolerance has developed. This is more likely to occur with long-term use of ephedrine and isoproterenol for bronchodilation. Tolerance can be prevented or treated by discontinuing the individual drug for a few days or by substituting another adrenergic drug.
f. For clients receiving intravenous adrenergic drugs for cadiac stimulation or vasopressor effects, explain the necessity for cardiac monitoring, frequent checks of flow rate, blood pressure, urine output, and so on.	An explanation may help decrease anxiety in a seriously ill patient. He or she should know that these measures increase the safety and benefits of drug therapy rather than indicate the presence of a critical condition.

Selected References

American Medical Association (AMA) Division of Drugs: AMA Drug Evaluations, 5th ed. New York, John Wiley & Sons, 1983

Anderson PD: Basic Human Anatomy and Physiology: Clinical Implications for the Health Professions. Monterey, CA, Wadsworth, 1984

Dalgas P: Understanding drugs that affect the autonomic nervous system. Nursing 15:58–63, October 1985

Facts and Comparisons. St. Louis, J B Lippincott (updated monthly)

Groer MW, Shekleton ME: Basic Pathophysiology: A Conceptual Approach, 2d ed. St. Louis, C V Mosby 1983

Guidelines for nursing care of the pulmonary patient. Los Angeles, CA, Thoracic Society, 1984

Guyton AC: Textbook of Medical Physiology, 7th ed. Philadelphia, W B Saunders, 1986

Hansten PD: Drug Interactions: Clinical Significance of Drug–Drug Interactions, 5th ed. Philadelphia, Lea & Febiger, 1985

Kirilloff LH, Tibbals SC: Drugs for asthma: A complete guide. Am J Nurs 83:55–61, January 1983

Malseed RT: Pharmacology: Drug Therapy and Nursing Considerations, 2d ed. Philadelphia, J B Lippincott, 1985

Phenylpropanolamine for weight reduction. Med Lett Drugs Ther 26:55–56, June 1984

Rodman MJ, Karch AM, Boyd EH, Smith DW: Pharmacology and Drug Therapy in Nursing, 3rd ed. Philadelphia, J B Lippincott, 1985

Wang VA, Dworetzky M: How to manage your asthmatic patient: Recent advances. Drug Ther 13:79–102, September 1983

Webber-Jones JE, Bryant MK: Over-the-counter bronchodilators: What are the risks of "relief in seconds"? Nursing 10:34–39, January 1980.

Weiner N: Norepinephrine, epinephrine, and the sympathomimetic amines. In Gilman AG, Goodman LS, Rall TW, Murad F (eds): The Pharmacological Basis of Therapeutics, 7th ed, pp 145–180. New York, MacMillan, 1985

19

ANTIADRENERGIC DRUGS

Description and uses

Antiadrenergic drugs (also called adrenergic blocking or sympatholytic agents) block the effects of sympathetic nerve stimulation and adrenergic drugs. Centrally active antiadrenergic drugs (*e.g.*, clonidine, methyldopa) and ganglionic blocking agents (*e.g.*, guanethidine, reserpine) are used almost exclusively in the treatment of hypertension. These drugs are discussed in Chapter 55. Peripherally active antiadrenergic agents (alpha- and beta-adrenergic blocking agents) are used for various clinical purposes. These drugs act by occupying alpha and beta receptor sites in tissues and organs innervated by the sympathetic nervous system. By doing so, they prevent catecholamines and other sympathomimetic amines from occupying these sites and exerting their stimulating action. Thus, blocking agents can prevent the action of naturally occurring (endogenous) or externally administered (exogenous) catecholamines such as epinephrine, norepinephrine, isoproterenol, and other adrenergic agents. A basal level of sympathetic tone is necessary to maintain normal body functioning, including regulation of blood pressure, blood glucose, and stress response. Therefore, the goal of antiadrenergic drug therapy is to suppress pathologic stimulation, not the normal, physiologic response to activity, stress, and other stimuli.

ALPHA-ADRENERGIC BLOCKING DRUGS

Alpha-adrenergic blocking agents occupy alpha-adrenergic receptor sites in smooth muscles and glands innervated by sympathetic nerve fibers. These drugs act primarily in arterioles of the skin, mucosa, intestines, and kidneys to prevent alpha-mediated vasoconstriction. Specific effects include dilation of arterioles, increased local blood flow, decreased blood pressure, constriction of pupils, and increased motility of the gastrointestinal tract. Clinically, the effects on arteriolar smooth muscle are most important.

Clinical indications for use of these drugs are limited. Prazosin is used only in the management of hypertension; it is discussed in Chapter 55. Phenoxybenzamine and phentolamine are not used as antihypertensive drugs except in hypertension caused by excessive catecholamines. Excessive catecholamines may result from overdosage of adrenergic drugs or from pheochromocytoma, a rare tumor of the adrenal medulla that secretes epinephrine and norepinephrine and causes hypertension, tachycardia, and cardiac arrhythmias. Although the treatment of choice for pheochromocytoma is surgical excision, alpha-adrenergic blocking drugs are useful adjuncts. They are given before and during surgery, usually in conjunction with beta blockers. Alpha blockers are also used in vascular diseases characterized by vasospasm such as Raynaud's disease and frostbite.

BETA-ADRENERGIC BLOCKING DRUGS

Beta-adrenergic blocking agents occupy beta-adrenergic receptor sites and prevent the receptors from responding to sympathetic nerve impulses, circulating catecholamines, and beta-adrenergic drugs (Fig. 19-1). Specific effects include the following:

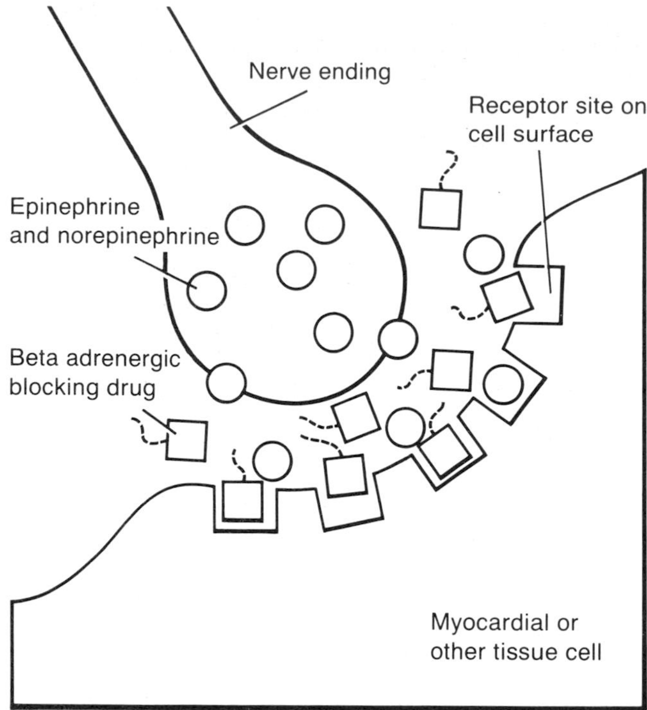

Figure 19-1. *Beta adrenergic blocking agents prevent epinephrine and norepinephrine from occupying receptor sites on cell membranes. This action alters cell functions normally stimulated by epinephrine and norepinephrine, according to the number of receptor sites occupied by the beta blocking drugs. (Adapted by J. Harley from Encyclopedia Brittanica Medical and Health Annual. Chicago, Encyclopedia Brittanica, 1983)*

1. Decreased heart rate (negative chronotropy)
2. Decreased force of myocardial contraction (negative inotropy)
3. Decreased cardiac output at rest and with exercise
4. Slowed conduction through the atrioventricular (AV) node
5. Decreased automaticity of ectopic pacemakers
6. Decreased blood pressure in supine and standing positions
7. Bronchoconstriction from blockade of $beta_2$ receptors in bronchial smooth muscle. This effect occurs primarily in people with asthma or other chronic lung diseases with a bronchospastic component.
8. Less effective metabolism of glucose (decreased glycogenolysis) when needed by the body, especially in people who are taking beta-blocking agents along with antidiabetic drugs. These people may experience more severe and prolonged hypoglycemia. In addition, early symptoms of hypoglycemia (*e.g.,* tachycardia) may be blocked, delaying recognition of the hypoglycemia.

Clinical indications for use of beta-blocking agents include cardiac arrhythmias, hypertension, angina pectoris, and myocardial infarction. In arrhythmias, drug effects depend on the sympathetic tone of the heart; that is, the degree of adrenergic stimulation of the heart that the drug must block or overcome. The drugs slow the sinus rate and prolong conduction through the AV node. In hypertension their major mechanism is related to the inhibition of renin and central sympathetic outflow. (Renin, an enzyme found mainly in the cortex of the kidneys, leads to the formation of angiotensin II, a powerful vasoconstrictor.) Beta-blocking drugs are often combined with vasodilator antihypertensive drugs (*e.g.,* hydralazine, minoxidil). When blood pressure is lowered by the vasodilator drugs, the sympathetic nervous system is stimulated and produces tachycardia, increased cardiac output, and increased renin release. These effects tend to cancel antihypertensive actions unless a beta-adrenergic blocking drug is given. In angina pectoris, beta blockers decrease the oxygen requirement of the heart by decreasing heart rate, blood pressure, and myocardial contractility during activity or exercise. In myocardial infarction, the drugs help to protect the heart from reinfarction, possibly by preventing or decreasing the incidence of catecholamine-induced dysrhythmias.

Propranolol (Inderal) is the prototype of beta-adrenergic blocking agents. It is also the oldest, most widely used, and most extensively studied beta blocker. In addition to its use in the treatment of hypertension, arrhythmias, angina pectoris, and myocardial infarction, propranolol is also used in hypertrophic obstructive cardiomyopathies, in which it improves exercise tolerance; pheochromocytoma, in which it decreases tachycardia and arrhythmias but must be used along with an alpha-adrenergic blocking agent; hyperthyroidism, in which it decreases heart rate, cardiac output, and tremor; and prevention of migraine headaches by an unknown mechanism (it is not helpful in acute attacks of migraine). The drug also relieves palpitation and tremor associated with anxiety, but it is not approved for clinical use as an antianxiety drug.

Contraindications to the use of beta-blocking agents include bradycardia, heart block, congestive heart failure, and asthma and other allergic or pulmonary conditions characterized by bronchoconstriction.

Individual antiadrenergic drugs

ALPHA-ADRENERGIC BLOCKING DRUGS

Phenoxybenzamine (Dibenzyline) blocks $alpha_1$-adrenergic receptor sites to decrease blood pressure and increase blood flow to the skin, mucosa, and viscera. Thus, it may be used to aid arterial blood flow in peripheral vasospastic disorders such as Raynaud's disorder and frostbite. It may also be given in hypertension resulting from pheochromocytoma, either during the perioperative period or during long-term treatment of clients who are not candidates for surgical excision. Phenoxybenzamine is long acting; effects of a single dose persist for 3 to 4 days.

Route and dosage range

Adults: PO 10 mg daily initially, gradually increased by 10 mg every 4 days until therapeutic effects are obtained or adverse effects become intolerable. Two weeks are usually required to reach the optimal dosage level. Usual maintenance dose, 20–60 mg daily

Phentolamine (Regitine) blocks $alpha_1$ and $alpha_2$ receptor sites. It dilates both arteries and veins to decrease peripheral vascular resistance and decrease venous return to the heart. It generally has the same action, uses, and adverse effects as phenoxybenzamine. In addition, certain unique characteristics make it more useful clinically than phenoxybenzamine. Phentolamine is short acting. Effects last only a few hours and can be reversed by an alpha-adrenergic stimulant drug such as levarterenol (Levophed). It is recommended for intravenous administration before and during surgical excision of pheochromocytoma. Phentolamine can also be used to prevent tissue necrosis from extravasation of potent vasoconstrictors (*e.g.*, levarterenol, dopamine) into subcutaneous tissues.

Routes and dosage ranges

Before and during surgery, IV, IM 5–20 mg as needed to control blood pressure

Prevention of tissue necrosis, IV 10 mg in each liter of IV solution containing a potent vasoconstrictor

Treatment of extravasation, SC 5–10 mg in 10 ml saline, infiltrated into the area within 12 hours

BETA-ADRENERGIC BLOCKING DRUGS

Eleven beta-blocking agents are currently approved for clinical use in the United States. Although they produce similar effects, they differ in several characteristics, including clinical indications for use, receptor selectivity, intrinsic sympathomimetic activity, membrane-stabilizing effects, lipid solubility, routes of excretion, routes of administration, and duration of action. Characteristics of subgroups and individual drugs are described in the following paragraphs and Table 19-1.

Clinical indications

Nine of the currently approved beta blockers are approved for the treatment of hypertension. A beta blocker may be used alone or with another antihypertensive drug, such as a diuretic. Labetalol (Trandate) is the only beta-blocking agent approved for treatment of hypertensive emergencies. Only propranolol (Inderal), nadolol (Corgard), and atenolol (Tenormin) are approved as antianginal agents; only propranolol and acebutolol (Sectral) are approved as antidysrhythmic agents. Propranolol, metoprolol (Lopressor), and timolol (Blocadren) are used to prevent myocardial infarction or reinfarction. Timolol (Timoptic), betaxolol (Betoptic), and levobunolol (Betagan) are approved for use in glaucoma. The drugs apparently reduce intraocular pressure by binding to beta adrenergic receptors in the ciliary body of the eye and decreasing formation of aqueous humor.

Receptor selectivity

Propranolol, nadolol, pindolol (Visken), timolol, and levobunolol are nonselective beta blockers. A sixth drug, oxprenolol, is approved for treatment of hypertension but is not yet marketed. The term *nonselective* indicates that the drugs block both $beta_1$ (cardiac) and $beta_2$ (mainly smooth muscle in the bronchi and blood vessels) receptors. Blockade of $beta_2$ receptors is associated with adverse effects such as bronchoconstriction and interference with glycogenolysis.

Acebutolol, metoprolol, atenolol, and betaxolol are "cardioselective" agents. This means that they have more effect on $beta_1$ receptors than on $beta_2$ receptors. As a result, they may cause less bronchospasm, less impairment of glucose metabolism, and less peripheral vascular insufficiency. These drugs are preferred when beta blockers are needed by clients with asthma or other bronchospastic pulmonary disorders, with diabetes mellitus, and with peripheral vascular disorders. Note, however, that cardioselectivity is lost at higher doses, probably because most organs have both $beta_1$ and $beta_2$ receptors rather than one or the other exclusively.

Labetalol is a unique drug that blocks $alpha_1$ receptors to cause vasodilation and $beta_1$ and $beta_2$ receptors to cause all the effects of the nonselective agents. Both alpha- and beta-adrenergic blocking actions contribute to its antihypertensive effects, but it is not clear whether labetalol has any definite advantage over other beta blockers. It may cause less bradycardia but more postural hypotension than other beta-blocking agents, and it may cause less reflex tachycardia than other vasodilators.

Intrinsic sympathomimetic activity

Pindolol, acebutolol, and oxprenolol exert a stimulating effect as well as beta blockade. Consequently, they

TABLE 19-1. BETA-ADRENERGIC BLOCKING AGENTS

Receptor activity	Generic name	Brand name	Clinical indications	Routes and dosage ranges
Nonselective	Levobunolol	Betagan	Glaucoma	Topically to each eye, 1 drop once or twice daily
	Propranolol	Inderal	Hypertension Angina pectoris Cardiac arrhythmias Myocardial infarction Hypertrophic obstructive cardiomyopathy Migraine prophylaxis Thyrotoxicosis Pheochromocytoma	Hypertension, PO 40 mg twice daily, gradually increased to 160–480 mg daily in divided doses; maximal daily dose, 960 mg Angina pectoris, dysrhythmias, PO 10–30 mg in divided doses, q4–6h Migraine prophylaxis, PO 40 mg daily in divided doses Life-threatening arrhythmias, IV 1–3 mg at a rate not to exceed 1 mg/minute, with electrocardiographic and blood pressure monitoring
	Nadolol	Corgard	Hypertension Angina pectoris	Hypertension, PO 40 mg once daily initially, gradually increased. Usual daily maintenance dose, 80–320 mg Angina, PO 40 mg once daily initially, increased by 40–80 mg at 3- to 7-day intervals. Usual daily maintenance dose, 80–240 mg
	Pindolol	Visken	Hypertension	PO 5 mg twice daily initially, increased by 10 mg every 3–4 weeks, to a maximal daily dose of 60 mg
	Timolol	Blocadren, Timoptic	Hypertension Myocardial infarction Glaucoma	Hypertension, PO 10 mg twice daily initially, increased at 7-day intervals to a maximum of 60 mg/day in 2 divided doses; usual maintenance dose, 20–40 mg daily Myocardial infarction, PO 10 mg twice daily Glaucoma, topically to eye, 1 drop of 0.25% or 0.5% solution (Timoptic) in each eye twice daily
Cardioselective	Acebutolol	Sectral	Hypertension Ventricular arrhythmia	Hypertension, PO 400 mg daily in 1 or 2 doses; usual maintenance dose, 400–800 mg daily Arrhythmia, PO 400 mg daily in 2 divided doses; usual maintenance dose, 600–1200 mg daily
	Atenolol	Tenormin	Hypertension	PO 50–100 mg daily
	Betaxolol	Betoptic	Glaucoma	Topically to each eye, 1 drop twice daily
	Metoprolol	Lopressor	Hypertension Myocardial infarction	Hypertension, PO 100 mg daily in single or divided doses, increased at 7-day or longer intervals; usual maintenance dose, 100–450 mg daily Myocardial infarction, early treatment, IV 5 mg every 2 minutes for total of 3 doses (15 mg), then 50 mg PO q6h for 48 hours, then 100 mg PO twice daily. MI, late treatment, PO 100 mg twice daily, at least 3 months, up to 1–3 years
Alpha–Beta	Labetalol	Trandate, Normodyne	Hypertension, including hypertensive emergencies	PO 100 mg twice daily IV 20 mg over 2 minutes then 40–80 mg every 10 minutes until desired blood pressure achieved or 300 mg given IV infusion 2 mg/minute (*e.g.,* add 200 mg of drug to 250 ml 5% dextrose solution for a 2 mg/3 ml concentration)

are less likely to cause bradycardia and may be useful for clients experiencing bradycardia with other beta blockers.

Membrane stabilizing ability

Propranolol, labetalol, pindolol, and possibly metoprolol have a membrane-stabilizing effect that has been described as quinidinelike, namely, direct myocardial depressant activity. The clinical significance of this property is not clear. Some sources indicate a contribution to antiarrhythmic activity; others say that the doses required to produce this effect are substantially higher than those used clinically and thus that the effect is not significant.

Lipid solubility

Propranolol has high lipid solubility; labetalol, metoprolol, and pindolol have moderate lipid solubility. These drugs penetrate the central nervous system (CNS) more readily than other beta blockers and are more likely to cause CNS adverse effects such as mental depression, insomnia, nightmares, hallucinations, and short-term memory loss. Paranoia, disorientation, and combativeness have been reported in elderly clients.

Routes of excretion

Most beta-blocking agents are metabolized in the liver. Nadolol, atenolol, and an active metabolite of acebutolol, are excreted by the kidneys, and dosage must be reduced in the presence of renal failure.

Routes of administration

Most beta blockers can be given orally. Propranolol, metoprolol, and labetalol can also be given intravenously, and ophthalmic solutions are applied topically to the eye.

Duration of action

Acebutolol, atenolol, and nadolol have long serum half-lives and can usually be given once daily. Labetalol, metoprolol, pindolol, and timolol are usually given twice daily. Propranolol required administration several times daily until development of a sustained-release capsule allowed once-daily dosing.

Principles of therapy: antiadrenergic drugs

ASSESSMENT GUIDELINES

Assess the client's condition in relation to disorders in which antiadrenergic drugs are used. That is, check blood pressure for elevation, pulse for tachycardia or arrhythmia, and determine the presence or absence of chest pain, migraine headache, or hyperthyroidism. If the client reports or medical records indicate one or more of these disorders, assess for specific signs and symptoms.

NURSING INTERVENTIONS

Use measures to prevent or decrease need for antiadrenergic drugs. Because the sympathetic nervous system is stimulated by physical and emotional stress, efforts to decrease stress may indirectly decrease the need for drugs to antagonize sympathetic effects. Such efforts may include the following:

1. Assisting the client to stop or decrease cigarette smoking. Nicotine stimulates both the CNS and the sympathetic nervous system to cause tremors, tachycardia, and elevated blood pressure.
2. Measures to relieve pain, anxiety, and other stresses
3. Counseling regarding relaxation techniques
4. Assisting in avoiding temperature extremes
5. Assisting in avoiding excessive caffeine in coffee or other beverages
6. Assisting to develop a reasonable balance between rest and exercise, work and recreation

PRINCIPLES OF USING ALPHA-ADRENERGIC BLOCKING DRUGS

1. When phenoxybenzamine is given on a long-term basis, dosage must be carefully individualized. Because the drug is long acting and accumulates in the body, dosage is small initially and gradually increased at intervals of about 4 days. Several weeks may be required for full therapeutic benefit, and drug effects persist for several days after the drug is discontinued.
2. If circulatory shock develops from overdosage or hypersensitivity, levarterenol can be given to overcome the blockade of alpha-adrenergic receptors in arterioles and to raise blood pressure. Epinephrine is contraindicated because it stimulates both alpha- and beta-adrenergic receptors, with a net result of increased vasodilation and hypotension.

PRINCIPLES OF USING BETA-ADRENERGIC BLOCKING AGENTS

1. For most people, a nonselective beta blocker that can be taken on a convenient schedule, once or twice daily, is acceptable. For others, the choice of a beta-blocking agent depends largely on the client's condition and response to the drugs. For example, cardioselective drugs are preferred for clients with pulmonary disorders and diabetes mellitus; water-soluble agents may be preferred for those who experience CNS adverse effects with lipid-soluble beta blockers; a drug with intrinsic sympathomimetic activity may be preferred for those who experience significant bradycardia with beta blockers lacking this property.
2. Dosage of beta-blocking agents must be individualized because of wide variations in plasma levels from comparable doses. Variations are attributed

to initial metabolism in the liver, the high level of binding to plasma proteins, and the degree of beta-adrenergic stimulation that the drugs must overcome. Generally, low doses should be used initially and increased gradually until therapeutic or adverse effects occur.

3. When a beta blocker is used to prevent myocardial infarction, it should be started as soon as the client is hemodynamically stable after a definite or suspected acute myocardial infarction. The drug should be continued at least 3 months and possibly 1 to 3 years.
4. Beta-blocking agents should not be discontinued abruptly because of increased sensitivity to catecholamines and possible exacerbation of angina and ventricular dysrhythmias or occurrence of myocardial infarction. Instead, dosage should be reduced gradually over 1 to 2 weeks.
5. Opinions differ regarding use of beta blockers before anesthesia and major surgery. On one hand, the drugs block arrhythmogenic properties of some general inhalation anesthetics. On the other hand, there is a risk of excessive myocardial depression. If feasible, the drug may be tapered gradually and discontinued before the scheduled surgery. If the drug is continued, the lowest effective dosage should be given. If emergency surgery is necessary, the effects of beta blockers can be reversed by administration of beta-receptor stimulants such as isoproterenol, dopamine, dobutamine, or norepinephrine.
6. If bradycardia occurs, atropine can be given to increase heart rate. Digitalis and diuretics can be given for congestive heart failure. Vasopressor agents can be given to raise the blood pressure, and bronchodilator drugs can be given to relieve bronchospasm.
7. *Use in pregnancy.* Effects of beta blockers during pregnancy are not clear. Animal studies with high doses have indicated embryotoxicity with atenolol, nadolol, propranolol, and timolol but not with acebutolol, metoprolol, and pindolol. Most clinical experience has been with propranolol, and it has been used successfully in the management of hypertension, thyrotoxicosis, hypertrophic cardiomyopathy, paroxysmal atrial tachycardia, dysfunctional uterine activity, and fetal tachycardia. Some reports indicate adverse effects on the fetus (*e.g.,* impaired placental blood supply, apnea at birth, prolonged labor, bradycardia, hypoglycemia, polycythemia, and hyperbilirubinemia), but it is not clear whether the effects were caused by the drug or by the high-risk pathologic conditions that required use of the drug. Although data are limited, some studies indicate that metoprolol, atenolol, and labetalol are associated with few maternal or neonatal adverse effects.
8. *Use in lactation.* During lactation, some beta blockers are excreted in breast milk. Although only small amounts of drug are involved, it is recommended that nursing mothers do not take beta blockers.
9. *Pediatric considerations.* In pediatric drug therapy, little reliable information is available, and safety and effectiveness of beta-blocking agents have not been established.
10. *Geriatric considerations.* In geriatric drug therapy, beta blockers may produce higher plasma levels. This effect is related to slower drug distribution to the tissues and impaired hepatic metabolism. Low initial doses and gradual increases are recommended.
11. In the presence of hepatic disease (*e.g.,* cirrhosis) or impaired blood flow to the liver (*e.g.,* reduced cardiac output from any cause), dosage of propranolol, metoprolol, and timolol should be substantially reduced because these drugs are extensively metabolized in the liver. Atenolol or nadolol is preferred in liver disease because they are eliminated primarily by the kidneys.
12. In renal failure, dosage of acebutolol, atenolol, and nadolol must be reduced because they are eliminated mainly through the kidneys. Dosage of acebutolol and nadolol should be reduced if creatinine clearance is <50 ml/minute; dosage of atenolol should be decreased if creatinine clearance is <35 ml/minute.

GUIDELINES IN TREATMENT OF PHEOCHROMOCYTOMA

For pheochromocytoma, both alpha- and beta-adrenergic blocking drugs may be used because the tumor secretes epinephrine, which acts to stimulate both alpha- and beta-adrenergic receptors. When propranolol is given to decrease the tachycardia and hypertension associated with pheochromocytoma, it must not be given until alpha-adrenergic blocking agents have been given. If propranolol alone were given, the peripheral vasodilating (beta) effect of epinephrine would be blocked, and its vasoconstrictor (alpha) effect would be unopposed. Vasoconstriction could lead to a life-threatening rise in blood pressure.

Both types of drugs are indicated during surgical excision of a pheochromocytoma. Otherwise, excessive hypertension or hypertensive crisis could occur because manipulation of the tumor during surgery causes catecholamines to be released.

NURSING ACTIONS: ANTIADRENERGIC DRUGS

Nursing Actions	*Rationale/Explanation*
1. Administer accurately	
a. With alpha-adrenergic blocking agents	
(1) Reconstitute parenteral phentolamine (5 mg/1 ml sterile water for injection) at the time it is to be used.	The reconstituted solution should not be stored.
(2) To treat extravasation of levarterenol or dopamine, phentolamine, 5–10 mg, may be diluted in 10 ml of sodium chloride injection and injected subcutaneously around the area of extravasation.	This should be done as soon as extravasation is detected. It may prevent tissue necrosis if done within 12 hours.
b. With beta-adrenergic blocking agents	
(1) Check blood pressure and pulse frequently, especially when dosage is being increased. It is probably best to omit the drug and report to the physician if systolic pressure is below 100 mm Hg and resting pulse rate is below 60.	To monitor both therapeutic effects and the occurrence of adverse reactions
(2) See Table 19-1 and manufacturers' literature regarding intravenous administration.	Specific instructions vary with individual drugs.
2. Observe for therapeutic effects	
a. With alpha-adrenergic blocking agents	
(1) In pheochromocytoma, observe for decreased pulse rate, blood pressure, sweating, palpitations, and blood sugar.	Because symptoms of pheochromocytoma are caused by excessive sympathetic nervous system stimulation, blocking stimulation with these drugs produces a decrease or absence of symptoms.
(2) In Raynaud's disease or frostbite, observe affected areas for improvement in skin color and skin temperature and in the quality of peripheral pulses.	These conditions are characterized by vasospasm, which diminishes blood flow to the affected part. The drugs improve blood flow by vasodilation.
b. With beta-adrenergic blocking drugs	
(1) When given in hypertension, observe for lowering of blood pressure toward normal ranges.	
(2) When given in tachyarrhythmias, observe for slowing of heart rate.	
(3) When given in angina pectoris, observe for decreased chest pain and increased exercise tolerance.	
3. Observe for adverse effects	Adverse effects are usually extensions of therapeutic effects.
a. With alpha-blocking agents	
(1) Hypotension	Hypotension may range from transient postural hypotension to a more severe hypotensive state resembling shock.
(2) Tachycardia	Tachycardia occurs as a reflex mechanism to increase blood supply to body tissues in hypotensive states.
b. With beta-blocking agents	
(1) Bradycardia and heart block	These are extensions of the therapeutic effects, which slow conduction of electrical impulses through the AV node, particularly in clients with compromised cardiac function.
(2) Congestive heart failure—edema, dyspnea, fatigue	Caused by reduced force of myocardial contraction
(3) Bronchospasm—dyspnea, wheezing	Caused by drug-induced constriction of bronchi and bronchioles. It is much more likely to occur in people with bronchial asthma or other obstructive lung disease.

Nursing Actions	*Rationale/Explanation*
(4) Fatigue and dizziness, especially with activity or exercise	These symptoms occur because the usual sympathetic nervous system stimulation in response to activity or stress is blocked by drug action.
(5) CNS effects—depression, insomnia, vivid dreams and hallucinations	The mechanism by which these effects is produced is unknown. Depression is particularly likely to occur in clients with a history of mood alterations.
4. Observe for drug interactions	
a. Drugs that alter effects of alpha-adrenergic blocking agents	
(1) Epinephrine	Epinephrine *increases* the hypotensive effects of alpha-adrenergic blocking agents and should not be given to treat shock caused by phenoxybenzamine or phentolamine. Because epinephrine stimulates both alpha- and beta-adrenergic receptors, the net effect is vasodilation and a further drop in blood pressure.
(2) Levarterenol	Levarterenol *decreases* effects of alpha adrenergic blocking agents and is the drug of choice for treating shock caused by overdosage of or hypersensitivity to phenoxybenzamine or phentolamine.
b. Drugs that *increase* effects of beta-adrenergic blocking agents (*e.g.,* propranolol, nadolol)	
(1) Alpha-adrenergic blocking drugs	Synergistic effects to prevent excessive hypertension before and during surgical excision of pheochromocytoma.
(2) Chlorpromazine, cimetidine, furosemide	Increase plasma levels by slowing hepatic metabolism
(3) Digitalis	Additive bradycardia, heart block
(4) Hydralazine, prazosin	Synergistic antihypertensive effects. Clients who do not respond to beta blockers or vasodilators alone may respond well to the combination. Also, beta blockers prevent reflex tachycardia, which usually occurs with vasodilator antihypertensive drugs. Note: prazosin produces relatively little tachycardia compared to hydralazine.
(5) Phenytoin	Potentiates cardiac depressant effects of propranolol
(6) Quinidine	The combination may be synergistic in treating cardiac arrhythmias. However, additive cardiac depressant effects may also occur (bradycardia, negative inotropy, decreased cardiac output).
(7) Verapamil, intravenous	The combination of intravenous verapamil and intravenous propranolol causes additive bradycardia and hypotension.
c. Drugs that *decrease* effects of beta-adrenergic blocking agents	
(1) Atropine	Increases heart rate and may be used to counteract excessive bradycardia caused by propranolol and other beta-blocking agents.
(2) Isoproterenol	Stimulates beta-adrenergic receptors and therefore antagonizes effects of beta-blocking agents. Isoproterenol can also be used to counteract excessive bradycardia.
5. Teach clients	
a. With alpha-adrenergic blocking agents	
(1) The adverse reactions of palpitations, weakness, and dizziness usually disappear with continued use. However, they may recur with conditions promoting vasodilation (exercise, dosage increase, ingesting alcohol or a large meal).	These are symptoms of postural hypotension and reflex tachycardia.

Nursing Actions	***Rationale/Explanation***
(2) If the above reactions occur, sit down or lie down immediately and flex arms and legs. Change positions slowly, especially from supine to standing.	To prevent falls and injuries due to postural hypotension
b. With beta-adrenergic blocking agents	
(1) Report weight gain (more than 2 pounds within a week), ankle edema, shortness of breath, or excessive fatigue.	These are signs of congestive heart failure. If they occur, the drug will be stopped.
(2) Report fainting spells, excessive weakness, or difficulty in breathing.	Beta-blocking drugs decrease the usual adaptive responses to exercise or stress. Syncope may result from hypotension or bradycardia and heart block. Occurrence will probably indicate stopping or decreasing the dose of the drug.
(3) Adverse effects may occur if beta-blocking drugs are suddenly discontinued. Therefore, the drugs should not be discontinued without medical advice. Also, dosage should be gradually decreased over several days.	Tapering of drug dosage is especially indicated when these drugs are used for angina pectoris or in elderly clients. If the drugs are stopped suddenly, "rebound" chest pain from myocardial ischemia and myocardial infarction may occur.

Selected References

American Medical Association (AMA) Division of Drugs: AMA Drug Evaluations, 5th ed. New York, John Wiley & Sons, 1983

Dalgas P: Understanding drugs that affect the autonomic nervous system. Nursing 15:58–63, October 1985

Ewy GA, Bressler R (eds): Cardiovascular Drugs and the Management of Heart Disease. New York, Raven Press, 1982

Facts and Comparisons. St. Louis, J B Lippincott (Updated monthly)

Fenster PE, Bressler R: Treating cardiovascular disease in the elderly. I. Digitalis glycosides and beta blockers. Drug Ther 14:125–132, February 1984

Groer MW, Shekleton ME: Basic Pathophysiology: A Conceptual Approach, 2d ed. St. Louis, C V Mosby, 1983

Guyton AC: Textbook of Medical Physiology, 7th ed. Philadelphia, W B Saunders, 1986

Hansten PD: Drug Interactions: Clinical Significance of Drug–Drug Interactions, 5th ed. Philadelphia, Lea & Febiger, 1985

Johnson GP, Johanson BC: Beta blockers. Am J Nurs 83:1034–1043, July 1983

Labetalol for hypertension. Med Lett Drugs Ther 26:83–85, September 1984

Malseed RT: Pharmacology: Drug Therapy and Nursing Considerations, 2d ed. Philadelphia, J B Lippincott, 1985

Needleman P, Corr PB, Johnson EM Jr: Drugs used for the treatment of angina; organic nitrates, calcium channel blockers, and beta-adrenergic antagonists. In Gilman AG, Goodman LS, Rall TW, Murad F (eds): The Pharmacological Basis of Therapeutics, 7th ed, pp 806–826. New York, Macmillan, 1985

Rodman MJ, Karch AM, Boyd EH, Smith DW: Pharmacology and Drug Therapy in Nursing, 3rd ed. Philadelphia, J B Lippincott, 1985

Weiner N: Drugs that inhibit adrenergic nerves and block adrenergic receptors. In Gilman AG, Goodman LS, Rall TW, Murad F (eds): The Pharmacological Basis of Therapeutics, 7th ed, pp 181–214. New York, Macmillan, 1985

20
CHOLINERGIC DRUGS

Description and uses

Cholinergic drugs, also called parasympathomimetics and cholinomimetics, stimulate the parasympathetic nervous system (PNS) in the same manner as acetylcholine. Some drugs act directly to stimulate cholinergic receptors; others act indirectly by slowing acetylcholine metabolism at autonomic nerve synapses and terminals.

Acetylcholine is formed from choline, an aminoalcohol involved in carbohydrate, fat, and protein metabolism. The enzyme necessary for formation of acetylcholine is choline acetylase; the enzyme necessary for its metabolism is acetylcholinesterase. Acetylcholinesterase rapidly splits acetylcholine into inactive acetate and choline, which are then released into the systemic circulation.

DIRECT-ACTING CHOLINERGIC DRUGS

Direct-acting cholinergic drugs are synthetic derivatives of choline. These drugs are able to exert their therapeutic effects because they are highly resistant to metabolism or breakdown by acetylcholinesterase. Their action is longer than the action of acetylcholine. They have widespread, systemic effects when they combine with receptors in cardiac muscle, smooth muscle, and glands. Specific effects include the following:

1. Decreased heart rate, vasodilation, and unpredictable changes in blood pressure
2. Increased tone and contractility in gastrointestinal smooth muscle, relaxation of sphincters, increased salivary gland and gastrointestinal secretions
3. Increased tone and contractility of smooth muscle (detrusor) in the urinary bladder and relaxation of the sphincter
4. Increased tone and contractility of bronchial smooth muscle
5. Increased respiratory secretions
6. Constriction of pupils and contraction of ciliary muscle

These drugs are used primarily to treat conditions of the gastrointestinal and genitourinary systems that are characterized by decreased smooth muscle tone and to treat glaucoma. Thus, they are used in urinary retention and postoperative hypoperistalsis or paralytic ileus. Paralytic ileus is a complication of abdominal surgery that may occur after surgery on the gastrointestinal tract or any surgery in which the bowels are extensively manipulated. These drugs are rarely used therapeutically for other effects. Drug effects on the cardiovascular and respiratory systems and on the eye are generally undesirable effects. An exception is decreased intraocular pressure, an effect sought in treatment of glaucoma (see Chap. 65).

Contraindications to use include urinary or gastrointestinal tract obstruction, asthma, peptic ulcer disease, coronary artery disease, hyperthyroidism, pregnancy, and inflammatory abdominal conditions.

INDIRECT-ACTING CHOLINERGIC AGENTS (ANTICHOLINESTERASES)

Indirect-acting cholinergic or anticholinesterase drugs act at the neuromuscular junction by decreasing metabolism of acetylcholine. These agents compete with acetylcholine for attachment sites on the enzyme acetylcholinesterase. This prolongs the effect of acetylcholine by preventing inactivation of acetylcholine in the synaptic cleft. Acetylcholine is then able to accumulate and stimulate receptors. The longer period of acetylcholine activity decreases skeletal muscle weakness, improves contractility of skeletal and smooth muscle, and restores other physiologic responses. Anticholinesterase drugs have parasympathetic, sympathetic, and somatic effects. They stimulate skeletal muscle and increase the strength of muscle contraction. This effect is used therapeutically to treat myasthenia gravis, a neuromuscular disorder characterized by skeletal muscle weakness. Clinical indications for use of these drugs include urinary retention, paralytic ileus, and glaucoma (see Chap. 65) as well as myasthenia gravis.

Individual cholinergic drugs

DIRECT-ACTING CHOLINERGICS

Bethanechol (Urecholine) is a synthetic derivative of choline with relatively specific effects on smooth muscle of the urinary and gastrointestinal tracts. It is used to relieve urinary retention, gastric atony, paralytic ileus, and gastroesophageal reflux, which occurs with hiatal hernia or incompetent cardioesophageal sphincter. Because the drug produces smooth-muscle contractions, it should not be used in obstructive conditions. Oral bethanechol is not well absorbed from the gastrointestinal tract. Consequently, oral doses are much larger than subcutaneous doses. Because severe adverse effects may occur with intramuscular or intravenous administration, the drug is not given by these routes.

Routes and dosage ranges

Adults: PO 10–30 mg 2–4 times daily; maximal daily dose, 120 mg
SC 2.5–5 mg 3–4 times daily
Children: PO 0.2 mg/kg of body weight 3 times daily
SC 0.05 mg/kg of body weight 3 times daily

INDIRECT-ACTING CHOLINERGICS (ANTICHOLINESTERASES)

Neostigmine (Prostigmin) is the prototype and the most widely used anticholinesterase agent. It is used for urinary retention, paralytic ileus, and myasthenia gravis and as an antidote for tubocurarine and other nondepolarizing skeletal muscle relaxants used in surgery. Neostigmine is poorly absorbed from the gastrointestinal tract. Consequently, oral doses are much larger than parenteral doses. When it is used for long-term treatment of myasthenia gravis, resistance to its action may occur and larger doses may be required.

Routes and dosage ranges

Adults: Myasthenia gravis, PO 15–30 mg q4h while awake
Exacerbation of myasthenia gravis, IM, SC 0.25–2 mg q2–3h
Prevention and treatment of urinary retention, IM, SC 0.25–0.5 mg q4–6h (up to 2–3 days)
Children: Myasthenia gravis, PO 0.3–0.6 mg/kg q3–4h while awake
Exacerbation of myasthenia gravis, IM, SC 0.01–0.04 mg/kg q2–3h

Edrophonium (Tensilon) is a very short-acting cholinergic drug. It is used only to diagnose myasthenia gravis, to differentiate between myasthenic crisis and cholinergic crisis, and to reverse the neuromuscular blockade produced by nondepolarizing skeletal muscle relaxants. It is not effective in the neuromuscular blockade produced by depolarizing agents such as succinylcholine (Anectine). It is given intramuscularly or intravenously by a physician who remains in attendance. Atropine, an antidote, and life-support equipment such as respirators and endotracheal tubes must be available when the drug is given.

Routes and dosage ranges

Adults: Diagnosis of myasthenia gravis, IV 2–4 mg initially, may be repeated and increased up to a total dose of 10 mg if no response is elicited by smaller amounts after 45 seconds. Or, IM 10 mg as a single dose
Differential diagnosis of myasthenic crisis or cholinergic crisis, IV 1–2 mg
Children: Diagnosis of myasthenia gravis, IV 0.2 mg/kg
Diagnosis in infants, IM 0.1 mg/kg

Ambenonium (Mytelase) is used therapeutically only for treatment of myasthenia gravis. It has the longest duration of action of indirect-acting agents. It is used less frequently than neostigmine and pyridostigmine. It may be useful in clients who are allergic to bromides, however, because the other drugs are both bromide salts. Ambenonium may increase respiratory secretions to a lesser degree than other anticholinesterase drugs and therefore may be useful for myasthenic clients on respirators.

Route and dosage range

Adults: PO 5 mg initially, increased to 10–30 mg q3–4h while awake
Dosage varies considerably, depending on client; dosage range, 5–75 mg/day
Children: PO 0.1 mg/kg of body weight initially, increased if necessary to 0.4 mg/kg q4h while awake

Physostigmine salicylate (Antilirium) is used clinically as an antidote for overdosage of anticholinergic drugs ("atropine poisoning"), including tricyclic antidepressants. Some other preparations of physostigmine are used in glaucoma.

Routes and dosage ranges

Adults: IV, IM 0.5–2 mg. Give slowly IV, no faster than 1 mg/minute

Pyridostigmine (Mestinon) is similar to neostigmine in actions, uses, and adverse effects. It may have a longer duration of action than neostigmine. Pyridostigmine is the maintenance drug of choice for clients with myasthenia gravis. An added advantage is the availability of a slow-release form, which is effective for 8 to 12 hours. When this form is taken at bedtime, the client does not have to take other medication during the night and does not awaken too weak to swallow.

Routes and dosage ranges

Adults: PO 60–120 mg q3–4h when awake; maximal single dose, 180 mg; or 1 timespan tablet (180 mg) at bedtime. Up to 1500 mg daily may be necessary
IM (exacerbations of myasthenia gravis or when oral administration is contraindicated) 2 mg
Children: PO 1–2 mg/kg of body weight q3–4h when awake
Newborns whose mothers have myasthenia gravis, IM 0.05–0.15 mg/kg

Principles of therapy: cholinergic drugs

ASSESSMENT GUIDELINES

Assess the client's condition. In clients known to have myasthenia gravis, assess for muscle weakness. This may be manifested by ptosis (drooping of the upper eyelid) and diplopia (double vision) caused by weakness of the eye muscles. More severe disease may be indicated by difficulty in chewing, swallowing, and speaking; accumulation of oral secretions, which the person may not be able to expectorate or swallow; decreased skeletal muscle activity, including impaired chest expansion; and eventual respiratory failure. In clients with possible urinary retention, check for bladder distention and time and amount of previous urination and assess fluid intake. For clients with decreased tone and motility of the gastrointestinal tract, assess for abdominal distention, cramping, and pain.

NURSING INTERVENTIONS

1. Use measures to prevent or decrease need for cholinergic drugs. Ambulation, adequate fluid intake, and judicious use of narcotic analgesics or other sedative-type drugs help to prevent postoperative urinary retention and paralytic ileus. For paralytic ileus, nasogastric intubation and suction, along with no food or fluids by mouth, are used more often than cholinergic drugs. In myasthenia gravis, muscle weakness is aggravated by exercise and improved by rest. Therefore, scheduling activities to avoid excessive fatigue and to allow adequate rest periods may be beneficial.
2. Before giving cholinergic drugs for bladder atony and urinary retention or gastrointestinal atony, abdominal distention, and "gas pains," be sure there is no obstruction in the urinary or gastrointestinal tract.

USE IN MYASTHENIA GRAVIS

Guidelines for use of anticholinesterase drugs in myasthenia gravis include the following:

1. Drug dosage should be gradually increased until maximal benefit is obtained. Larger doses are often required with increased physical activity, emotional stress, infections, and sometimes premenstrually.
2. Some clients with myasthenia gravis cannot tolerate optimal doses of anticholinesterase drugs unless atropine is given to decrease the severity of adverse reactions. However, atropine should be given only if necessary because it may mask the sudden increase of side-effects. This increase is the first sign of overdose.
3. Drug dosage in excess of the amount needed to maintain muscle strength and function can produce a cholinergic crisis. A cholinergic crisis is characterized by excessive stimulation of the PNS.

If early symptoms are not treated, hypotension and respiratory failure may occur. At high doses, anticholinesterase drugs weaken rather than strengthen skeletal muscle contraction because excessive amounts of acetylcholine accumulate at motor end-plates and reduce nerve impulse transmission to muscle tissue.

a. Treatment for cholinergic crisis includes withdrawal of anticholinesterase drugs, administration of atropine, and measures to maintain respiration. Endotracheal intubation and mechanical ventilation may be necessary owing to profound skeletal muscle weakness, including muscles of respiration, which is not counteracted by atropine.

b. Differentiating myasthenic crisis from cholinergic crisis may be difficult because both are characterized by respiratory difficulty or failure. It is necessary to differentiate between them, however, because they require opposite treatment measures. Myasthenic crisis requires more anticholinesterase drug, whereas cholinergic crisis requires discontinuing any anticholinesterase drug the person has been receiving. The physician may be able to make an accurate diagnosis from signs and symptoms and when they occur in relation to medication. That is, signs and symptoms having their onset within about 1 hour after a dose of anticholinesterase drug are more likely to be caused by cholinergic crisis (too much drug). Signs and symptoms beginning 3 hours or more after a drug dose are more likely to be caused by myasthenic crisis (too little drug).

c. If the differential diagnosis cannot be made on the basis of signs and symptoms, the client can be intubated, mechanically ventilated, and observed closely until a diagnosis is possible. Still another way to differentiate between the two conditions is for the physician to inject a small dose of edrophonium intravenously. If the edrophonium causes a dramatic improvement in breathing, the diagnosis is myasthenic crisis; if it makes the patient even weaker, the diagnosis is cholinergic crisis. Note, however, that edrophonium or any other pharmacologic agent should be administered only after endotracheal intubation and controlled ventilation have been instituted.

4. Some people develop partial or total resistance to anticholinesterase drugs after taking them for months or years. Therefore, do not assume that drug therapy that is effective initially will continue to be effective over the long-term course of the disease.

ANTIDOTE TO CHOLINERGIC AGENTS

Atropine, an anticholinergic drug, is a specific antidote to cholinergic agents. The drug and equipment for injection should be readily available whenever cholinergic drugs are given.

NURSING ACTIONS: CHOLINERGIC DRUGS

Nursing Actions	*Rationale/Explanation*
1. Administer accurately	
a. Give parenteral bethanechol by the subcutaneous route *only*.	Intramuscular and intravenous injections may cause acute, severe hypotension and circulatory failure. Cardiac arrest may occur.
b. With pyridostigmine and other drugs for myasthenia gravis, give at regularly scheduled intervals.	For consistent control of symptoms
2. Observe for therapeutic effects	
a. When the drug is given for postoperative hypoperistalsis, observe for bowel sounds, passage of flatus through the rectum, or a bowel movement.	These are indicators of increased gastrointestinal muscle tone and motility.
b. When bethanechol or neostigmine is given for urinary retention, micturition usually occurs within about 60 minutes. If it does not, urinary catheterization may be necessary.	

Nursing Actions	**Rationale/Explanation**
c. When the drug is given in myasthenia gravis, observe for increased muscle strength as shown by (1) Decreased or absent ptosis of eyelids (2) Decreased difficulty with chewing, swallowing, and speech (3) Increased skeletal muscle strength, increased tolerance of activity, less fatigue	With neostigmine, onset of action is 2–4 hours after oral administration and 10–30 minutes after injection. Duration is about 3–4 hours. With pyridostigmine, onset of action is about 30–45 minutes after oral use, 15 minutes after intramuscular (IM) injection, and 2–5 minutes after intravenous (IV) injection. Duration is about 4–6 hours. The long-acting form of pyridostigmine lasts 8–12 hours.
3. Observe for adverse effects	Adverse effects occur with usual therapeutic doses but are more likely with large doses. They are caused by stimulation of the PNS.
a. Respiratory effects—increased secretions, bronchospasm, respiratory failure	
b. Gastrointestinal effects—nausea and vomiting, diarrhea, increased peristalsis, abdominal cramping, hypersalivation	
c. Cardiovascular effects—arrhythmias, bradycardia, hypotension	These may be detected early by regular assessment of blood pressure and heart rate.
d. Other effects—increased frequency and urgency of urination, increased sweating, miosis, skin rash	Skin rashes are most likely to occur from formulations of neostigmine or pyridostigmine that contain bromide.
4. Observe for drug interactions **a.** Drugs that *decrease* effects of cholinergic agents	
(1) Anticholinergic drugs (*e.g.,* atropine)	Antagonize effects of cholinergic drugs (miosis, increased tone and motility in smooth muscle of the gastrointestinal tract, bronchi and urinary bladder, bradycardia). Atropine is the specific antidote for overdosage with cholinergic drugs.
(2) Antihistamines	Most antihistamines have anticholinergic properties that antagonize effects of cholinergic drugs.
5. Teach persons with myasthenia gravis and at least one responsible family member	Cholinergic drugs are not prescribed for long-term therapeutic use except for clients with myasthenia gravis, certain types of hypotonic bladder disorders, and glaucoma.
a. Take drugs as directed.	Underdosage will not relieve muscle weakness enough for adequate function; overdosage can cause severe, even life-threatening reactions.
b. Record symptoms of myasthenia and effects of drug therapy, especially when drug therapy is initiated and medication doses are being titrated.	Clients vary widely in the amounts of medication required. The physician usually aims for the lowest effective dose to minimize adverse drug reactions. Information provided by the client can allow the physician to prescribe more effectively.
c. Rest between activities; do not carry on activities to the point of extreme fatigue or exhaustion.	Although the dose of medication may be increased during periods of increased activity, spacing activities is probably more desirable to obtain optimal benefit from the drug while avoiding adverse reactions.
d. Have atropine readily available.	Atropine (0.6 mg IM or IV) is a specific antidote for overdosage with cholinergic drugs.
e. Report increased muscle weakness or recurrence of myasthenic symptoms to the physician.	Drug dosage may need to be increased or other alterations made in treatment.
f. Report adverse reactions, including abdominal cramps, diarrhea, excessive oropharyngeal secretions, difficulty in breathing, and muscle weakness.	These are signs of drug overdosage (cholinergic crisis) and require immediate discontinuation of drugs and treatment by the physician. Respiratory failure can result if this condition is not recognized and treated appropriately.

Selected References

American Medical Association (AMA) Division of Drugs: AMA Drug Evaluations, 5th ed. New York, John Wiley & Sons, 1983

Dalgas P: Understanding drugs that affect the autonomic nervous system. Nursing 15:58–63, October 1985

Facts and Comparisons. St. Louis, J B Lippincott (Updated monthly)

Groer MW, Shekleton ME: Basic Pathophysiology: A Conceptual Approach, 2d ed. St. Louis, Mosby, 1983

Ress R: Suddenly in crisis—unpredictable myasthenia gravis. Am J Nurs 84:994–998, August 1984

Rodman MJ, Karch AM, Boyd EH, Smith DW: Pharmacology and Drug Therapy in Nursing, 3rd ed. Philadelphia, J B Lippincott, 1985

Taylor P: Cholinergic agonists. In Gilman AG, Goodman LS, Rall TW, Murad F (eds): The Pharmacological Basis of Therapeutics, 7th ed, pp 100–109. New York, Macmillan, 1985

21

ANTICHOLINERGIC DRUGS

Description and uses

Anticholinergic drugs, also called cholinergic blocking and parasympatholytic agents, are those which block the action of acetylcholine on the parasympathetic nervous system (PNS). This drug class includes belladonna alkaloids, their derivatives, and many synthetic substitutes. The prototype drug is atropine, an alkaloid of the potato plant family.

These drugs act by occupying receptor sites at parasympathetic nerve endings, thereby leaving fewer receptor sites free to respond to acetylcholine. Parasympathetic response is absent or decreased, depending on the number of receptors blocked by anticholinergic drugs and the underlying degree of parasympathetic activity.

Anticholinergic drugs have widespread effects on the body, including smooth muscle relaxation, decreased glandular secretions, and mydriasis. Specific effects on body tissues and organs include the following:

1. Central nervous system (CNS) stimulation followed by depression, which may result in coma and death. This is most likely to occur with large doses of anticholinergic drugs that cross the blood–brain barrier (atropine, scopolamine, and antiparkinson agents).
2. Decreased cardiovascular response to parasympathetic (vagal) stimulation that slows heart rate. Atropine is the anticholinergic drug most used for its cardiovascular effects. Usual clinical doses may produce a slight and temporary decrease in heart rate; moderate-to-large doses (0.5 to 1 mg) increase heart rate. This effect may be therapeutic in bradycardia or an adverse effect in other types of heart disease. Atropine usually has little or no effect on blood pressure. Large doses cause facial flushing due to dilation of blood vessels in the neck.
3. Bronchodilation and decreased respiratory tract secretions.
4. Antispasmodic effects in the gastrointestinal tract due to decreased muscle tone and motility. Little inhibitory effect on acidity and amount of gastric secretions, at least in usual doses. Insignificant effects on pancreatic and intestinal secretions.
5. Mydriasis and cycloplegia in the eye. Normally, anticholinergics do not change intraocular pressure. With glaucoma, however, they may increase intraocular pressure. When the pupil is fully dilated, photophobia may be bothersome, and reflexes to light and accommodation may disappear.
6. Miscellaneous effects include decreased secretions from salivary and sweat glands; relaxation of ureters, urinary bladder, and the detrusor muscle; and relaxation of smooth muscle in the gallbladder and bile ducts.

Clinical usefulness of anticholinergic drugs has been limited by their far-reaching actions. Consequently, numerous synthetic drugs have been developed in an effort to increase selectivity of action on particular body tissues, especially to retain antispasmodic and antisecretory effects of atropine while eliminating adverse effects. This effort has been less than successful. All the synthetic drugs produce atropinelike adverse effects when given in sufficient dosage.

One group of synthetic drugs is used for antispasmodic effects in gastrointestinal disorders. These drugs are listed in Table 21-1. They are quaternary ammonium compounds, which do not readily cross the blood–brain barrier. They are therefore less likely to cause CNS effects than the natural alkaloids, which readily enter the CNS.

Another group of synthetic drugs includes centrally active anticholinergics used in the treatment of Parkinson's disease (see Chap. 12). They balance the relative cholinergic dominance that causes the movement disorders associated with parkinsonism.

Clinical indications for use of anticholinergic drugs include gastrointestinal and ophthalmic conditions, bradycardia, Parkinson's disease, genitourinary disorders, and preoperative use.

Gastrointestinal disorders in which anticholinergics have been used include peptic ulcer disease, gastritis, pylorospasm, diverticulitis, ileitis, and ulcerative colitis. These conditions are often characterized by excessive gastric acid and abdominal pain due to increased motility and spasm of gastrointestinal smooth muscle. In peptic ulcer disease, use of anticholinergic drugs has been based more on tradition than scientific rationale. The drugs are weak inhibitors of gastric acid secretion even in maximal doses (which usually produce intolerable adverse effects). There is no evidence that they aid healing or prevent ulcer recurrence and complications. They may, however, relieve abdominal pain by relaxing gastrointestinal smooth muscle.

Anticholinergics may be helpful in treating irritable colon or colitis, but they may be contraindicated in chronic inflammatory disorders (*e.g.*, diverticulitis, ul-

TABLE 21-1. SYNTHETIC ANTICHOLINERGIC–ANTISPASMODICS USED IN GASTROINTESTINAL DISORDERS

Generic name	Trade name	Routes and dosage ranges	
		Adults	*Children*
Anisotropine methylbromide	Valpin	PO 50 mg 3 times daily	Dosage not established
Clidinium bromide	Quarzan	PO 2.5–5 mg 3–4 times daily Geriatric: PO 2.5 mg TID before meals	Dosage not established
Dicyclomine hydrochloride	Bentyl	PO, IM 10–20 mg 3–4 times daily	PO, IM 10 mg 3–4 times daily Infants: 5 mg 3–4 times daily
Glycopyrrolate	Robinul	PO 1–2 mg 3 times daily initially, 1 mg 2 times daily for maintenance IM, IV, SC 0.1–0.2 mg 3–4 times daily at 4-hour intervals	Dosage not established
Hexocyclium methylsulfate	Tral	PO 25 mg 3–4 times daily before meals and at bedtime	Not for use in children
Isopropamide chloride	Darbid	PO 5–10 mg q12h	Not recommended for children under 12 years
Mepenzolate bromide	Cantil	PO 25 mg 4 times daily with meals and at bedtime, increased gradually to 50 mg if necessary	Dosage not established
Methantheline bromide	Banthine	PO 50–100 mg q6h initially, reduced to 25–50 mg q6h for maintenance IM 50 mg q6h	PO, IM 6 mg/kg/day in 4 divided doses
Oxyphencyclimine bromide	Daricon	PO 10 mg 2 times daily (morning and at bedtime), gradually increased to 50 mg if no adverse effects	Dosage not established
Oxyphenonium bromide	Antrenyl	PO 10 mg 4 times daily	PO 0.8 mg/kg of body weight daily in 4 divided doses
Propantheline bromide	Pro-Banthine	PO 15 mg 3 times daily before meals and 30 mg at bedtime IM, IV 30 mg q6h	PO 1.5 mg/kg/day in 4 divided doses

cerative colitis) or acute intestinal infections (*e.g.*, bacterial, viral, amebic). Other drugs are used to decrease diarrhea and intestinal motility in these conditions.

In ophthalmology, anticholinergic drugs are applied topically for mydriatic and cycloplegic effects to aid examination or surgery. They are also used to treat some inflammatory disorders. Anticholinergic preparations used in ophthalmology are discussed further in Chapter 65.

In cardiology, atropine may be given to increase heart rate in bradycardia and heart block characterized by hypotension and shock.

In respiratory disorders characterized by bronchoconstriction (*i.e.*, asthma, chronic bronchitis), atropine may be given by inhalation for bronchodilating effects.

In Parkinson's disease, anticholinergic drugs are given for their central effects in decreasing salivation, spasticity, and tremors. Their use is declining because more effective antiparkinson drugs have been developed. They are used mainly in clients who have minimal symptoms, who do not respond to levodopa, or who cannot tolerate levodopa because of adverse reactions or contraindications. An additional use of these drugs is to relieve parkinsonlike symptoms that sometimes occur with antipsychotic drugs.

In genitourinary disorders, anticholinergic drugs may be given for antispasmodic effects on smooth muscle. In infections such as cystitis, urethritis, and prostatitis, the drugs decrease the frequency and pain of urination. The drugs are also given to increase bladder capacity in enuresis, paraplegia, or neurogenic bladder.

Anticholinergics are often given preoperatively. The traditional reason is to reduce respiratory tract secretions. This is no longer valid because newer general inhalation anesthetics are less irritating and do not increase secretions significantly. However, the drugs are rationally used to prevent vagal stimulation, which may in turn cause excessive bradycardia, hypotension, and even cardiac arrest. Vagal stimulation occurs with halothane and related anesthetics; with succinylcholine (Anectine), a skeletal muscle relaxant; and with surgical procedures requiring manipulation of the pharynx, trachea, peritoneum, stomach, or intestines as well as procedures in which pressure is applied to the eye.

Contraindications to the use of anticholinergic drugs include any condition characterized by symptoms that would be aggravated by the drugs. Some of these are prostatic hypertrophy, glaucoma, and tachyarrhythmias as well as myocardial infarction and congestive heart failure unless bradycardia is present. They should not be given in hiatal hernia or other conditions contributing to reflux esophagitis because the drugs delay gastric emptying, relax the cardioesophageal sphincter, and increase esophageal reflux.

Individual anticholinergic drugs

BELLADONNA ALKALOIDS AND DERIVATIVES

Atropine is the prototype of anticholinergic drugs. It produces the same effects and has the same clinical indications for use and the same contraindications as those described above. It is a naturally occurring belladonna alkaloid that can be extracted from the belladonna plant or prepared synthetically. It is usually prepared as atropine sulfate. This salt is very soluble in water. It is well absorbed from the gastrointestinal tract and distributed throughout the body. It crosses the blood–brain barrier to enter the CNS, where large doses produce stimulant effects and toxic doses produce depressant effects. Atropine is also absorbed systemically when applied locally to mucous membranes. The drug is rapidly excreted in the urine. Pharmacologic effects are of short duration except for ocular effects, which may last for several days.

Routes and dosage ranges

Adults: Gastrointestinal disorders, PO, SC 0.3–1.2 mg q4–6h
Preoperatively, IM 0.4–0.6 mg in a single dose 45–60 minutes before anesthesia
Bradyarrhythmias, IV 0.4–1 mg q1–2h as necessary.
Bronchoconstriction, 0.025 mg/kg diluted with 3–5 ml saline and given by nebulizer 3–4 times daily
Topically to eye, one drop of 1% or 2% ophthalmic solution

Children: Gastrointestinal disorders, SC 0.01 mg/kg of body weight q4–6h
Preoperatively, IM 0.4 mg for children 3–14 years, less for younger children and infants
Bradyarrhythmias, IV 0.01–0.03 mg/kg of body weight
Bronchoconstriction, 0.05 mg/kg diluted with 3–5 ml saline and given by nebulizer 3–4 times daily
Topically to eye, one drop of 0.5% or 1% ophthalmic solution

Belladonna tincture is a mixture of alkaloids in an aqueous-alcohol solution. It is most often used in gastrointestinal disorders for antispasmodic effect. It is an ingredient in several drug mixtures.

Route and dosage range

Adults: PO 0.6–1 ml 3–4 times daily
Children: PO 0.03 ml/kg/day in 3–4 divided doses

Homatropine methylbromide (Homapin) is a semisynthetic derivative of atropine. It is administered topically as eye drops to produce mydriasis and cycloplegia. Homatropine is sometimes preferable to atropine because ocular effects do not last as long.

Routes and dosage ranges

Adults: Topically to eye, one drop of 5% ophthalmic solution every 5 minutes for 2–3 doses for refraction; one drop of 2% to 5% solution 2–3 times daily for uveitis

Hyoscyamine (Anaspaz) is a belladonna alkaloid used in gastrointestinal disorders characterized by spasm, increased secretion, and increased motility. It has the same effects as other atropinelike drugs.

Routes and dosage ranges

Adults: PO 0.125–0.25 mg q4–6h
IM, SC, IV 0.25–0.5 mg q4–6h until symptoms are controlled
Children: PO 0.062–0.125 mg q4–6h for children 2–10 years; half this dosage for children under 2 years

Methscopolamine (Pamine) is a belladonna derivative used almost exclusively in treating peptic ulcer disease. It lacks the central action of scopolamine and is less potent and longer acting than atropine.

Routes and dosage ranges

Adults: PO 2.5–5 mg 4 times daily
Children: PO 0.2 mg/kg/day in 4 divided doses

Scopolamine is very similar to atropine and has the same uses and adverse reactions for the most part. More specifically, scopolamine has similar peripheral effects but different central effects. When given parenterally, scopolamine depresses the CNS and usually causes drowsiness, euphoria, relaxation, amnesia, and sleep. Some over-the-counter sleeping pills contain small amounts of scopolamine. Effects of scopolamine appear more quickly and disappear more readily than those of atropine. Scopolamine may be preferred over atropine in obstetrics owing to its amnesic effects and preoperatively to increase the pain relief of narcotic analgesics without a proportionate increase in respiratory depression. Scopolamine is also used in motion sickness. It is available as oral tablets and as a transdermal adhesive disc that is placed behind the ear. The disc (Transderm-V) protects against motion sickness for 72 hours.

Routes and dosage ranges

Adults: Preoperatively, IM 0.4 mg
Motion sickness, PO 0.25–0.8 mg 1 hour before travel; transdermally 1 disc q72h
Mydriasis, topically to the eye, 1 drop of 0.2% to 0.25% ophthalmic solution, repeated as necessary
Children: Preoperatively, 6 months–3 years, IM 0.1–0.15 mg; 3–6 years, IM 0.15–0.2 mg; 6–12 years, 0.2–0.3 mg
Mydriasis, same as for adults

SYNTHETIC ANTICHOLINERGICS USED IN PARKINSON'S DISEASE

Trihexyphenidyl (Artane) is usually the anticholinergic drug of choice for initiating treatment of moderate or severe parkinsonism. It is also effective in treating extrapyramidal reactions caused by phenothiazines and some other antipsychotic drugs. Trihexyphenidyl relieves smooth muscle spasm by a direct action on the muscle and by inhibiting the PNS. Trihexyphenidyl supposedly has fewer side-effects than atropine, but about half the recipients report mouth dryness, blurring of vision, and other side-effects common to anticholinergic drugs. Trihexyphenidyl requires the same precautions as other anticholinergic drugs. It is contraindicated in glaucoma. Biperiden (Akineton) and procyclidine (Kemadrin) are chemical derivatives of trihexyphenidyl and have similar actions, uses, and adverse effects.

Routes and dosage ranges

Biperiden

Adults: Parkinsonism, PO 2 mg 3–4 times daily
Drug-induced extrapyramidal reactions, IM 2 mg, repeated q30 minutes if necessary. Maximum of 4 consecutive doses in 24 hours
Children: Drug-induced extrapyramidal reactions, IM, 0.04 mg/kg, repeated as above if necessary

Procyclidine

Adults: Parkinsonism, PO 5 mg 2 times daily initially, gradually increased to 5 mg 3–4 times daily if necessary
Drug-induced extrapyramidal reactions, PO 2–2.5 mg 3 times daily, gradually increased to 10–20 mg daily if necessary

Trihexyphenidyl

Adults: Parkinsonism, PO 2 mg 2–3 times daily initially, gradually increased until therapeutic effects or severe adverse effects occur
Drug-induced extrapyramidal reactions, PO 1 mg initially, gradually increased to 5–15 mg daily in divided doses

Benztropine (Cogentin) is a synthetic drug with both anticholinergic and antihistaminic effects. Its anticholinergic activity approximates that of atropine. A major clinical use is to treat acute dystonic reactions caused by antipsychotic drugs and to prevent their recurrence in clients receiving long-term antipsychotic drug therapy. It may also be given in small doses to supplement other antiparkinson drugs. In full dosage, adverse reactions are common.

Routes and dosage ranges

Adults: PO 0.5–1 mg at bedtime, initially, gradually increased to 4–6 mg daily if required and tolerated
Drug-induced extrapyramidal reactions, PO, IM, IV 1–4 mg once or twice daily

Principles of therapy: anticholinergic drugs

ASSESSMENT GUIDELINES

Assess the client's condition in relation to disorders for which anticholinergic drugs are used. That is, check for bradycardia or heart block, diarrhea, dysuria, abdominal pain, and other disorders. If the client reports or medical records indicate a specific disorder, assess for signs and symptoms of that disorder (*e.g.*, Parkinson's disease).

NURSING INTERVENTIONS

Use measures to decrease need for anticholinergic drugs. For example, with peptic ulcer disease, teach the client to avoid factors known to increase gastric secretion and gastrointestinal motility (alcohol, cigarette smoking, caffeine-containing beverages such as coffee, tea, and cola drinks, ulcerogenic drugs such as aspirin). Late evening snacks should also be avoided because increased gastric acid secretion occurs about 90 minutes after eating and may cause pain and awakening from sleep. Although milk is traditionally an "ulcer" food, it contains protein and calcium, which promote acid secretion, and is a poor buffer of gastric acid. Thus, drinking large amounts of milk should be avoided.

USE IN SPECIFIC CONDITIONS

Renal or biliary colic

Atropine is sometimes given with morphine or meperidine to relieve the severe pain of renal or biliary colic. It acts mainly to decrease the spasm-producing effects of the narcotic analgesics. It has little antispasmodic effect on the involved muscles and is not used alone for this purpose.

Preoperative use in clients with glaucoma

Glaucoma is usually listed as a contraindication for anticholinergic drugs because the drugs impair outflow of aqueous humor and may cause an acute attack of glaucoma (increased intraocular pressure). However, anticholinergic drugs can safely be given preoperatively to clients with open-angle glaucoma (80% of clients with primary glaucoma) if they are receiving miotic drugs such as pilocarpine. If anticholinergic preoperative medication is needed in clients predisposed to angle closure, the hazard of causing acute glaucoma can be minimized by also giving pilocarpine eye drops and acetazolamide (Diamox).

Gastrointestinal disorders

When anticholinergic drugs are given for gastrointestinal disorders, larger doses may be given at bedtime to prevent pain and awakening during sleeping hours.

Parkinsonism

When these drugs are used in parkinsonism, small doses are given initially and gradually increased. This regimen decreases adverse reactions.

Extrapyramidal reactions

When used in drug-induced extrapyramidal reactions (parkinsonlike symptoms), these drugs should be prescribed only if symptoms occur. That is, anticholinergic drugs are used to treat extrapyramidal reactions. They are not used routinely to prevent extrapyramidal reactions because fewer than half the persons taking antipsychotic drugs experience such reactions. Most drug-induced reactions last about 3 months and do not recur if anticholinergic drugs are discontinued at that time. An exception is tardive dyskinesia, which does not respond to anticholinergic drugs and may, in fact, be aggravated by them.

TREATMENT OF ATROPINE OVERDOSAGE

Atropine overdosage produces the usual pharmacologic effects in a severe and exaggerated form. Physostigmine salicylate (Antilirium) is a specific antidote. It is given intravenously at a slow rate of injection in dosages of 1 to 4 mg for adults and 0.5 mg to 1 mg for children. Diazepam (Valium) or a similar drug may be given for excessive stimulation of the CNS (delirium, excitement). Cardiopulmonary resuscitation measures are used if excessive depression of the CNS causes coma and respiratory failure.

NURSING ACTIONS: ANTICHOLINERGIC DRUGS

Nursing Actions	*Rationale/Explanation*
1. Administer accurately	
a. For gastrointestinal disorders, give most oral anticholinergic drugs about 30 minutes before meals and at bedtime.	To allow the drugs to reach peak antisecretory effects by the time ingested food is stimulating gastric acid secretion. Bedtime administration helps prevent awakening with abdominal pain.
b. When given preoperatively, parenteral preparations of atropine can be mixed in the same syringe with several other common preoperative medications such as meperidine (Demerol), morphine, oxymorphone (Numorphan), and promethazine (Phenergan).	The primary reason for mixing medications in the same syringe is to decrease the number of injections and thus decrease client discomfort. Note, however, that extra caution is required when mixing drugs to be sure that the dosage of each drug is accurate. Also, if any question exists regarding compatibility with another drug, it is safer not to mix the drugs, even if two or three injections are required.
c. When applying topical atropine solutions or ointment to the eye, be sure to use the correct concentration and blot any excess from the inner canthus.	Atropine ophthalmic preparations are available in several concentrations (usually 1%, 2%, and 3%). Excess medication should be removed so that the drug will not enter the nasolacrimal (tear) ducts and be absorbed systemically through the mucous membrane of the nasopharynx or be carried to the throat and swallowed.
d. If propantheline is to be given intravenously, dissolve the 30-mg dose of powder in no less than 10 ml of sterile water for injection.	Parenteral administration is reserved for clients who cannot take the drug orally.
e. Instruct clients to swallow oral propantheline tablets, not to chew them.	The tablets have a hard sugar coating to mask the bitter taste of the drug.
f. Parenteral glycopyrrolate can be given through the tubing of a running intravenous infusion of physiologic saline or lactated Ringer's solution.	
2. Observe for therapeutic effects	Therapeutic effects depend primarily on the reason for use. Thus, a therapeutic effect in one condition may be a side-effect or an adverse reaction in another condition.
a. When a drug is given for peptic ulcer disease or other gastrointestinal disorders, observe for decreased abdominal pain.	Relief of abdominal pain is due to the smooth muscle relaxant or antispasmodic effect of the drug.
b. When the drug is given for diagnosing or treating eye disorders, observe for pupil dilation (mydriasis) and blurring of vision (cycloplegia).	Note that these ocular effects are side-effects when the drugs are given for problems not related to the eyes.
c. When the drug is given for symptomatic bradycardia, observe for increased pulse rate.	These drugs increase heart rate by blocking action of the vagus nerve.
d. When the drug is given for urinary tract disorders such as cystitis or enuresis, observe for decreased fre-	Anticholinergic drugs decrease muscle tone and spasm in the smooth muscle of the ureters and urinary bladder.

Nursing Actions	Rationale/Explanation
quency of urination. When the drug is given for renal colic due to stones, observe for decreased pain.	
e. When the centrally acting anticholinergics are given for Parkinson's disease, observe for decrease in tremor, salivation, and drooling.	Decreased salivation is a therapeutic effect with parkinsonism but an adverse reaction in most other conditions.
3. Observe for adverse effects	These depend on reasons for use and are dose related.
a. Tachycardia	Tachycardia may occur with usual therapeutic doses because anticholinergic drugs block vagal action, which normally slows heart rate. Tachycardia is not likely to be serious except in clients with underlying heart disease. For example, in clients with angina pectoris, prolonged or severe tachycardia may increase myocardial ischemia to the point of causing an acute attack of angina (chest pain) or even myocardial infarction. In clients with congestive heart failure, severe or prolonged tachycardia can increase the work load of the heart to the point of causing acute heart failure or pulmonary edema.
b. Excessive CNS stimulation (tremor, restlessness, confusion, hallucinations, delirium) followed by excessive CNS depression (coma, respiratory depression)	These effects are more likely to occur with large doses of atropine because atropine crosses the blood–brain barrier. Large doses of trihexyphenidyl (Artane) may also cause CNS stimulation.
c. Sedation and amnesia with scopolamine or benztropine (Cogentin)	This may be a therapeutic effect but becomes an adverse reaction if severe or if the drug is given for another purpose. Benzotropine has both anticholinergic and antihistaminic properties. Apparently, drowsiness and sedation are caused by the antihistaminic component.
d. Constipation or paralytic ileus	These effects are the result of decreased gastrointestinal motility and muscle tone. Constipation is more likely with large doses or parenteral administration. Paralytic ileus is not likely unless the drugs are given to clients who already have decreased gastrointestinal motility.
e. Decreased oral and respiratory tract secretions, which cause mouth dryness and thick respiratory secretions	Mouth dryness is more annoying than serious in most cases and is caused by decreased salivation. However, clients with chronic lung diseases, who usually have excessive secretions, tend to retain them with the consequence of frequent respiratory tract infections.
f. Urinary retention	This reaction is caused by loss of bladder tone and is most likely to occur in elderly men with enlarged prostate glands. Thus, the drugs are generally contraindicated with prostatic hypertrophy.
g. Hot, dry skin, fever, heat stroke	These effects are due to decreased sweating and impairment of the normal heat loss mechanism. Fever may occur with any age group. Heat stroke is more likely to occur with cardiovascular disease, strenuous physical activity and high environmental temperatures, especially in elderly people.
h. Ocular effects—mydriasis, blurred vision, photophobia	These are adverse effects when anticholinergic drugs are given for conditions not related to the eyes.
4. Observe for drug interactions	
a. Drugs that *increase* effects of anticholinergic drugs	
(1) Antihistamines, disopyramide, phenothiazines, thioxanthene agents, and tricyclic antidepressants	These drugs have anticholinergic properties and produce additive anticholinergic effects.

Nursing Actions	***Rationale/Explanation***
b. Drugs that *decrease* effects of anticholinergic drugs (1) Cholinergic drugs	These drugs counteract the inhibition of gastrointestinal motility and tone induced by atropine. They are sometimes used in atropine overdose.
5. Teach clients	
a. Mouth dryness commonly occurs. Use sugarless chewing gum and hard candy if not contraindicated.	To relieve mouth dryness
b. The importance of dental hygiene (*e.g.,* regular brushing of teeth)	Dental caries and loss of teeth may result from drug-induced xerostomia (dry mouth from decreased saliva production). This is more likely to occur with long-term use of these drugs.
c. Blurring of vision is also common. Avoid potentially hazardous activities (*e.g.,* driving a car or operating machinery) when this occurs.	To prevent injury
d. Dark glasses can be worn outdoors in strong light.	To reduce sensitivity to light (photophobia)
e. Do not take other drugs without the physician's knowledge.	Several drugs have anticholinergic properties, and combining them may cause overdosage or excessive anticholinergic effects. Also, some over-the-counter sleeping pills (*e.g.,* Sleep-Eze) contain small amounts of scopolamine, and over-the-counter antihistamines have anticholinergic properties. Taking any of these concurrently could cause additive anticholinergic effects.
f. Prevent heat stroke by (1) Maintaining fluid and salt intake if not contraindicated (2) Limiting exposure to direct sunlight (3) Limiting physical exertion (4) Taking frequent sponge baths (5) Ensuring adequate ventilation, with fans or air conditioners if necessary	This is most important in elderly people.

Selected References

American Medical Association (AMA) Division of Drugs: AMA Drug Evaluations, 5th ed. New York, John Wiley & Sons, 1983

Dalgas P: Understanding drugs that affect the autonomic nervous system. Nursing 15:58–63, October 1985

Facts and Comparisons. St. Louis, J B Lippincott (Updated monthly)

Hansten PD: Drug Interactions: Clinical Significance of Drug–Drug Interactions, 5th ed. Philadelphia, Lea & Febiger, 1985

Middleton E, Reed CE, Ellis EF (eds): Allergy Principles and Practice. St. Louis, C V Mosby, 1984

Rodman MJ, Karch AM, Boyd EH, Smith DW: Pharmacology and Drug Therapy in Nursing, 3rd ed. Philadelphia, J B Lippincott, 1985

Tetrault GA, Weintraub M: How to handle drug-related dry mouth. Drug Ther 14:159–166, February 1984

Weiner N: Atropine, scopolamine, and related antimuscarinic drugs. In Gilman AG, Goodman LS, Rall TW, Murad F (eds): The Pharmacological Basis of Therapeutics, 7th ed, pp 130–144. New York, Macmillan, 1985

IV

DRUGS AFFECTING THE ENDOCRINE SYSTEM

22

PHYSIOLOGY OF THE ENDOCRINE SYSTEM

The endocrine system is composed of the hypothalamus, pituitary, thyroid, parathyroids, pancreas, adrenals, ovaries, and testes. The system works in harmony with the nervous system to regulate body functions. Generally, the nervous system regulates rapid muscular and sensory activities, and the endocrine system regulates slow metabolic activities. Specific endocrine organs are discussed in the following chapters. Some general characteristics of the endocrine system include the following:

1. Endocrine glands produce hormones, chemical substances that are manufactured by specialized cells, released into the bloodstream, and circulated to other cells, where they act. Growth hormone (produced by the anterior pituitary) and thyroid hormone affect almost all body cells. Other hormones affect specific or "target" tissues. For example, corticotropin from the anterior pituitary stimulates the adrenal cortex, and ovarian hormones affect the endometrial lining of the uterus.
2. There are many interrelationships between the nervous system and the endocrine system. For example, secretion of almost all pituitary hormones (by the pituitary gland) is controlled by the hypothalamus. Special nerve fibers originating in the hypothalamus and ending in the posterior pituitary gland control secretions of the posterior pituitary. The hypothalamus secretes hormones called *releasing* and *inhibitory factors,* which regulate functions of the anterior pituitary. The anterior pituitary, in turn, secretes corticotropin (ACTH), a hormone that stimulates functions of the adrenal cortex. This complex interrelationship is often referred to as the *hypothalamic–pituitary–adrenocortical* (HPA) axis. It functions by a negative feedback system, in which hormone secretion is stimulated when hormones are needed and inhibited when they are not needed. The hypothalamic–pituitary–thyroid axis also functions by a negative feedback mechanism.
3. Major hormones and their general functions are listed as follows:
   a. Anterior pituitary hormones are growth hormone (also called somatotropin), corticotropin, thyroid-stimulating hormone (TSH), follicle-stimulating hormone (FSH), luteinizing hormone (LH), and prolactin. Most of these hormones function by stimulating secretion of other hormones.
   b. Posterior pituitary hormones are antidiuretic hormone (ADH or vasopressin) and oxytocin. ADH helps maintain fluid balance; oxytocin stimulates uterine contractions during childbirth.
   c. Adrenal cortex hormones, commonly called corticosteroids, include the glucocorticoids such as cortisol and the mineralocorticoids

such as aldosterone. Glucocorticoids influence carbohydrate storage, exert anti-inflammatory effects, suppress corticotropin secretion, and increase protein catabolism. Mineralocorticoids help regulate electrolyte balance, mainly by promoting sodium retention and potassium loss. The adrenal cortex also produces sex hormones. Adrenal medulla hormones are epinephrine and norepinephrine (see Chap. 18).

d. Thyroid hormones include triiodothyronine (T_3 or liothyronine) and tetraiodothyronine (T_4 or thyroxine). These hormones regulate the metabolic rate of the body and greatly influence growth and development.
e. Parathyroid hormone, also called parathormone and PTH, regulates calcium and phosphate metabolism.
f. Pancreatic hormones are insulin and glucagon, which regulate the metabolism of glucose, lipids, and proteins.
g. Ovarian hormones (female sex hormones) are estrogens and progesterone. Estrogens promote growth of specific body cells and development of most secondary sexual characteristics in females. Progesterone helps prepare the uterus for pregnancy and the mammary glands for lactation.
h. Testicular hormone (male sex hormone) is testosterone, which regulates development of masculine characteristics.
i. Placental hormones are chorionic gonadotropin, estrogen, progesterone, and human placental lactogen, all of which are concerned with reproductive functions.

4. Although all body cells are exposed to all hormones, only certain cells respond to a particular hormone. It is believed that the hormone combines with a specific receptor at the membrane of the target cell. The receptor determines which hormone will affect the target cell. In addition to their actions on cell membranes, hormones may alter enzyme activity and protein synthesis within the cell.
5. Hormones are extremely important in regulating body activities. Their normal secretion and function help to maintain the internal environment and determine response and adaptation to the external environment. Hormones participate in complex interactions with other hormones and nonhormone chemical substances in the body to influence every aspect of life. Abnormal secretion and function of hormones, even minor alterations, can affect physical well being and, in some cases, thought processes and emotional stability. Malfunction of an endocrine organ is usually associated with hyposecretion, hypersecretion, or inappropriate secretion of its hormones. Any malfunction can produce serious disease or death.
6. Physiologic effects of hormones vary in onset and duration. Some occur immediately; others occur in minutes or hours. Some disappear as soon as the hormone leaves the bloodstream, although others persist for hours.
7. Not all hormones are secreted by the major endocrine organs. For example, the gastrointestinal mucosa produces several hormones that are important in the digestive process. These hormones include gastrin, enterogastrone, secretin, and cholecystokinin. In addition, the kidneys produce erythropoietin, a hormone that stimulates the bone marrow to produce red blood cells, and renin, which regulates angiotensin II levels. These tissues are not traditionally described as endocrine glands but are usually said to have an endocrine function that is secondary to their main functions.
8. Hormones or hormonelike substances may be produced by some neoplasms. In endocrine tissues, neoplasms may be an added source of the hormone normally produced by the organ. In nonendocrine tissues, various hormones may be produced. For example, lung tumors may produce corticotropin, antidiuretic hormone, or parathyroid hormone; kidney tumors may produce parathyroid hormone. The usual effects are those of excess hormone secretion.

General characteristics of hormonal drugs

1. Hormone preparations given for therapeutic purposes include natural hormones from human or animal sources and synthetic hormones. Many of the most important hormones have been synthesized, and these preparations may have more potent and prolonged effects than the naturally occurring hormones.
2. Hormones are given for physiologic or pharmacologic effects. Physiologic use involves giving rather small doses as a replacement or substitute for the amount ordinarily secreted by a normally functioning endocrine gland. Such usage is indicated only when a gland is unable to secrete an adequate amount of hormone. Examples of physiologic use include insulin administration in diabetes mellitus and adrenal corticosteroid administration in Addison's disease. Pharmacologic use involves relatively large doses for greater-than-physiologic effects. For example, adrenal corticosteroids are

widely used for anti-inflammatory effects in both endocrine and nonendocrine disorders.
3. Hormones are powerful drugs that produce widespread therapeutic and adverse effects.
4. Administration of one hormone may alter effects of other hormones. These alterations result from the complex interactions among hormones.
5. Hormonal drugs are more often given for disorders resulting from endocrine gland hypofunction than for those related to hyperfunction.

Selected References

Anderson PD: Basic Human Anatomy and Physiology: Clinical Implications for the Health Professions. Monterey, CA, Wadsworth, 1984

Guyton AC: Textbook of Medical Physiology, 7th ed. Philadelphia, W B Saunders, 1986

Rodman MJ, Karch AM, Boyd EH, Smith DW: Pharmacology and Drug Therapy in Nursing, 3rd ed. Philadelphia, J B Lippincott, 1985

23
HYPOTHALAMIC AND PITUITARY HORMONES

Description and uses

The hypothalamus and pituitary gland (hypophysis) interact to control most metabolic functions of the body and to maintain homeostasis. They are anatomically connected by the hypophyseal stalk. The hypothalamus controls secretions of the pituitary gland. The pituitary gland, in turn, regulates secretions or functions of other body tissues called "target" issues. The pituitary gland is actually two glands, each with different structures and functions. The anterior pituitary (adenohypophysis) is composed of different types of glandular cells that synthesize and secrete different hormones. The posterior pituitary (neurohypophysis) is anatomically an extension of the hypothalamus and is composed largely of nerve fibers. It does not manufacture any hormones itself but stores and releases hormones synthesized in the hypothalamus.

HYPOTHALAMIC HORMONES

The hypothalamus produces a releasing hormone (also called factor) or an inhibiting hormone that corresponds to each of the six major hormones of the anterior pituitary gland. Specifically, they are as follows:

1. *Corticotropin-releasing hormone* (CRH), which causes release of corticotropin in response to stress and threatening stimuli
2. *Growth hormone–releasing factor* (GRF), which causes release of growth hormone in response to low blood levels of the hormone. A growth hormone–inhibiting hormone, *somatostatin,* is also secreted, which inhibits release of growth hormone.
3. *Thyrotropin-releasing hormone* (TRH), which causes release of thyroid-stimulating hormone (TSH or thyrotropin) in response to stress such as exposure to cold
4. *Follicle-stimulating hormone-releasing factor* (FRF), which causes release of follicle-stimulating hormone (FSH)
5. *Luteinizing hormone-releasing factor* (LRF), which causes release of luteinizing hormone
6. *Prolactin-inhibitory factor* (PIF), which prevents secretion of prolactin. There is also a *prolactin-releasing factor* (PRF). Usually the inhibitory factor is more important. During lactation after childbirth, the releasing factor is active.

PITUITARY HORMONES

The anterior pituitary gland produces six major hormones. Two of these, growth hormone and prolactin, act directly on their target tissues. The other four act indirectly by stimulating target tissues to produce other hormones.

1. *Corticotropin,* also called adrenocorticotropic hormone, stimulates the adrenal cortex to produce

adrenocorticosteroids. Secretion is controlled by the hypothalamus and by plasma levels of cortisol, the major adrenocorticosteroid. When plasma levels are adequate for body needs, the anterior pituitary does not release corticotropin (negative feedback mechanism).

2. *Growth hormone,* also called somatotropin, stimulates growth of all body tissues that are capable of responding. It promotes an increase in cell size and number, largely by affecting metabolism of carbohydrate, protein, fat, and bone tissue.

   Deficient growth hormone in children produces dwarfism, a condition marked by severely decreased linear growth and, frequently, severely delayed mental, emotional, dental, and sexual growth as well. Excessive growth hormone in preadolescent children produces gigantism, marked by heights of 8 or 9 feet if untreated. Excessive growth hormone in adults produces acromegaly.
3. *Thyrotropin,* also called thyroid-stimulating hormone or TSH, regulates secretion of thyroid hormones. Thyrotropin secretion is controlled by a negative feedback mechanism in proportion to metabolic needs. Thus, increased thyroid hormones in body fluids inhibit secretion of thyrotropin by the anterior pituitary and of TRH by the hypothalamus.
4. *Follicle-stimulating hormone* (FSH), one of the gonadotropins, stimulates functions of sex glands. It is produced by the anterior pituitary gland of both males and females, beginning at puberty. FSH acts on the ovaries in a cyclical fashion during reproductive years, stimulating growth of ovarian follicles. These follicles then produce estrogen, which prepares the endometrium for implantation of a fertilized ovum. FSH acts on the testes to stimulate the production and growth of sperm (spermatogenesis), but it does not stimulate secretion of male sex hormones.
5. *Luteinizing hormone* (LH), also called *interstitial cell-stimulating hormone* (ICSH), is another gonadotropin that stimulates hormone production by the gonads of both sexes. LH is important in the maturation and rupture of the ovarian follicle (ovulation). After ovulation, LH acts on the cells of the collapsed sac to produce the corpus luteum, which then produces progesterone during the last half of the menstrual cycle. When blood progesterone levels rise, a negative feedback effect is exerted on hypothalamic and anterior pituitary secretion of gonadotropins. Decreased pituitary secretion of LH causes the corpus luteum to die and stop producing progesterone. Lack of progesterone causes slough and discharge of the endometrial lining as menstrual flow. Of course, if the ovum has been fertilized and attached to the endometrium, menstruation does not occur.

   In males, LH stimulates the Leydig cells in the spaces between the seminiferous tubules. These cells then secrete androgens, mainly testosterone.
6. *Prolactin* plays a part in milk production by nursing mothers. It is not usually secreted in nonpregnant women because of the hypothalamic hormone PIF. During late pregnancy and lactation various stimuli, including suckling, inhibit the production of PIF, and thus prolactin is synthesized and released.

The posterior pituitary gland stores and releases two hormones that are actually synthesized by nerve cells in the hypothalamus. These two hormones and their functions are as follows:

1. *Antidiuretic hormone* (ADH), which is also called vasopressin. It functions in regulation of water balance. When ADH is secreted, it makes renal tubules more permeable to water. This allows water in renal tubules to be reabsorbed into the plasma and so conserves body water. In the absence of ADH, little water is reabsorbed and large amounts are lost in the urine.

   ADH is secreted when body fluids become concentrated (high amounts of electrolytes in proportion to the amount of water) and when blood volume is low. In the first instance, ADH causes reabsorption of water, dilution of extracellular fluids, and restoration of normal osmotic pressure. In the second instance, ADH raises blood volume and arterial blood pressure toward homeostatic levels.
2. *Oxytocin,* which functions in childbirth and lactation. It initiates uterine contractions at the end of gestation to induce childbirth, and it causes milk to move from breast glands to nipples so the infant can obtain the milk by suckling.

THERAPEUTIC LIMITATIONS

There are no approved clinical uses for hypothalamic hormones and few for pituitary hormones. There are several reasons why pituitary hormones are not used extensively. First, other effective agents are available for some potential uses. When there is a deficiency of target gland hormones (*e.g.,* adrenocorticosteroids, thyroid hormones, male or female sex hormones), it is usually more convenient and effective to administer those hormones than the anterior pituitary hormones that stimulate their secretion. Second, some pituitary hormones must be obtained from natural sources, which tends to be inconvenient and relatively expensive. For example, corticotropin, thyrotropin, and ADH are obtained from the pituitary glands of domestic animals slaughtered for food; gonadotropins are obtained from the urine of pregnant or menopausal women. A third reason for the infrequent use of pituitary hormones is that most conditions in which pituitary hormones are indicated are fortunately uncommon.

Despite their limitations, pituitary hormones carry out important functions when indicated for clinical use. These hormones and the clinical disorders for which they are used are discussed in the following section.

Individual hormonal agents

ANTERIOR PITUITARY HORMONES

Corticotropin (ACTH, Acthar) is obtained from pituitary glands of cattle and hogs. It is purified and standardized. Corticotropin is composed of 39 amino acids, 24 of which exert the characteristic physiologic effects. Because it is a protein substance, corticotropin is destroyed by proteolytic enzymes in the digestive tract and must therefore be given parenterally. Corticotropin has a short duration of action and must be administered frequently. There are, however, repository preparations (Cortrophin gel, Cortrophin-zinc) that are slowly absorbed, have a longer duration of action, and can be given once daily.

Corticotropin is given to stimulate synthesis of hormones by the adrenal cortex (glucocorticoids, mineralocorticoids, sex hormones). It is not effective unless the adrenal cortex is able to respond. Adrenocortical response is variable, and dosage of corticotropin must be individualized. When corticotropin therapy is being discontinued, dosage is gradually reduced to avoid the steroid withdrawal syndrome characterized by muscle weakness, fatigue, and hypotension. Corticotropin is also used in laboratory tests of adrenal function.

Cosyntropin (Cortrosyn) is a synthetic drug with biologic activity similar to that of corticotropin. It is used as a diagnostic test in suspected adrenal insufficiency.

Routes and dosage ranges

Corticotropin

Adults: Therapeutic use, IM, SC 20 units 4 times daily
Diagnostic use, IM 40–80 units daily for 1–3 days; IV 10–25 units in 500 ml of 5% dextrose or 0.9% sodium chloride solution, infused over 8 hours once daily. A continuous infusion with 40 units q12h for 48 hours may also be used

Cortrophin Gel

Adults: Therapeutic use, IM 40–80 units q24–72h
Diagnostic use, IM 40–80 units daily for 1–3 days

Cosyntropin

Adults: Diagnostic use, IM, IV 0.25 mg (equivalent to 25 units ACTH)

Growth hormone (Asellacrin) is obtained from the pituitary gland of human cadavers. This source provides limited amounts of very expensive growth hormone. Experiments using mutant bacteria may lead to eventual mass production. The only clinical use of growth hormone is for treatment of children with dwarfism caused by inadequate pituitary function. It is not effective when dwarfism results from other causes or after puberty when epiphyses of the long bones have closed. Excessive administration can cause excessive growth (gigantism). This preparation is available only for children with documented deficiency (impaired growth, low plasma levels of hormone) and for scientists doing research studies of pituitary disorders.

Route and dosage range

Children: IM 2 IU 3 times/week, 48 hours apart initially. If growth rate does not exceed 2.5 cm in a 6-month period, the dose is doubled for the next 6 months.

Human chorionic gonadotropin (HCG [Follutein]) is a placental hormone obtained from the urine of pregnant women. In men, HCG produces physiologic effects similar to those of the naturally occurring LH. HCG is used clinically to evaluate the ability of the Leydig cells to produce testosterone and to treat cryptorchidism (undescended testicle) in preadolescent boys. Excessive doses or prolonged administration can lead to sexual precocity, edema, and breast enlargement caused by oversecretion of testosterone and, possibly, of estrogen. In women, HCG is used in combination with menotropins to induce ovulation in treatment of infertility.

Route and dosage ranges

Cryptorchidism and hypogonadism in males, IM 500–4000 units 2–3 times weekly for several weeks
To induce ovulation, IM 5,000–10,000 units in 1 dose, 1 day after treatment with menotropins

Menotropins (Pergonal), a gonadotropin preparation obtained from the urine of postmenopausal women, contains both FSH and LH. It is usually combined with HCG to induce ovulation in treatment of infertility caused by lack of pituitary gonadotropins.

Route and dosage range

IM 1 ampule (75 units FSH and 75 units LH) daily for 9–12 days, followed by HCG to induce ovulation

Thyrotropin (Thytropar) is obtained from the anterior pituitary glands of cattle. It is used as a diagnostic agent to distinguish between primary hypothyroidism (hypothyroidism caused by a thyroid disorder) and secondary hypothyroidism (hypothyroidism caused by pituitary malfunction). If thyroid hormones in serum are elevated after the administration of thyrotropin, then the hypothyroidism is secondary to inadequate pituitary function. Thyrotropin must be used cautiously in clients with coronary artery disease, congestive heart failure, or adrenocortical insufficiency.

Route and dosage ranges

Adults: IM, SC 10 units daily for 1–3 days, followed by ^{131}I in 18–24 hours. Twenty-four hours after iodine administration, thyroid uptake of iodine is measured. Accumulation is greater in hypopituitarism than in primary hypothyroidism.

POSTERIOR PITUITARY HORMONES

Desmopressin acetate (DDAVP, Stimate) is a synthetic analog of ADH. A major clinical use is the treatment of neurogenic diabetes insipidus, a disorder characterized by a deficiency of ADH and the excretion of large amounts of dilute urine. Diabetes insipidus may be idiopathic, hereditary, or acquired as a result of trauma, surgery, tumor, infection, or other conditions that impair the function of the hypothalamus or posterior pituitary. Parenteral desmopressin is also used as a hemostatic in clients with hemophilia A or mild-to-moderate von Willebrand's disease (type 1). The drug is effective in controlling spontaneous or trauma-induced bleeding as well as intraoperative and postoperative bleeding when given 30 minutes before the procedure.

Routes and dosage ranges

Adults: Diabetes insipidus, intranasally, 0.1–0.4 ml daily, usually in 2 divided doses
Hemophilia A, von Willebrand's disease, IV 0.3 μg/kg in 50 ml sterile saline, infused over 15–30 minutes

Children 3 months–2 years: Diabetes insipidus, intranasally, 0.05–0.3 ml daily in 1–2 doses

Children weighing over 10 kg: Hemophilia A, von Willebrand's disease, same as adult dosage

Children weighing 10 kg or less: Hemophilia A, von Willebrand's disease, IV 0.3 μg/kg in 10 ml of sterile saline

Lypressin is a synthetic vasopressin that has several advantages over the natural product. It is free of oxytocin impurity and foreign proteins. Consequently, it is less likely to produce allergic reactions and other side-effects than vasopressin, which is derived from animal sources. Lypressin is also advantageous in that it is given intranasally rather than by injection. It is used only for controlling the excessive water loss of diabetes insipidus caused by inadequate function of the posterior pituitary gland.

Route and dosage ranges

Adults: Intranasal spray, 1 or 2 sprays, to one or both nostrils, 3–4 times daily

Vasopressin (Pitressin) is available as an extract derived from animal pituitary glands and as a synthetic preparation. The synthetic preparation is preferred because it contains no oxytocin. Until lypressin was developed, vasopressin was the most widely used drug for diabetes insipidus caused by hypofunction of the posterior pituitary gland. Vasopressin has a short duration of action (a few hours). This short action is sometimes an advantage, for example, when acutely ill patients require precise control of fluid balance after brain surgery or trauma. It is a disadvantage when long-term treatment of diabetes insipidus is necessary. Vasopressin tannate is a long-acting oil suspension that must also be injected; its effects last 1 to 3 days. Vasopressin has a vasoconstrictor effect and is also used in treatment of bleeding esophageal varices.

Routes and dosage ranges

Vasopressin

Adults: IM, SC, intranasally on cotton pledgets, 0.25–0.5 ml (5–10 units) 2–3 times daily

Children: IM, SC, intranasally on cotton pledgets, 0.125–0.5 ml (2.5–10 units) 3–4 times daily

Vasopressin Tannate

Adults: IM 0.3–1.0 ml (1.5–5 units) every 1–3 days

Children: IM 0.25–0.5 ml (1.25–2.5 units) every 1–3 days

Oxytocin (Pitocin) is a synthetic drug that exerts the same physiologic effects as the posterior pituitary hormone. Thus, it promotes uterine contractility and is used clinically to induce labor and in the postpartum period to control bleeding. Oxytocin must be used only when clearly indicated and when the recipient can be supervised by well-trained personnel. It is usually given in a hospital setting.

Routes and dosage ranges

Induction of labor, IV 1-ml ampule (10 units) in 1000 ml of 5% dextrose injection (10 units/1000 ml = 10 mU/ml), infused at 0.2–2 mU/min initially, then regulated according to frequency and strength of uterine contractions

Prevention or treatment of postpartum bleeding, IV 10–40 units in 1000 ml of 5% dextrose injection, infused at 125 ml/hr (40 mU/min) *or* 0.6–1.8 units (0.06–0.18 ml) diluted in 3–5 ml sodium chloride injection and injected slowly

IM 0.3–1.0 ml (3–10 units)

Principles of therapy: pituitary hormones

1. Most drug therapy with pituitary hormones is given to replace or supplement naturally occurring hormones in situations involving inadequate function of the pituitary gland (hypopituitarism). Conditions resulting from excessive amounts of pituitary hormones (hyperpituitarism) are more often treated with surgery or irradiation.
2. Diagnosis of suspected pituitary disorders should be as complete and as specific as possible. This promotes more specific and more effective treatment measures, including drug therapy.
3. Even though manufacturers recommend corticotropin for treatment of diseases that respond to glucocorticoids, corticotropin is less predictable and less convenient than glucocorticoids and has no apparent advantages over them.
4. Dosage of any pituitary hormone must be individualized because responsiveness of affected tissues varies.

NURSING ACTIONS: PITUITARY HORMONES

Nursing Actions	*Rationale/Explanation*
1. Administer accurately	
a. Read the manufacturer's instructions and drug labels carefully before drug preparation and administration.	These hormone preparations are given infrequently and often require special techniques of administration.
2. Observe for therapeutic effects	Therapeutic effects vary widely, depending on the particular pituitary hormone given and the reason for use.
a. With corticotropin, therapeutic effects stem largely from increased secretion of adrenal cortex hormones, especially the glucocorticoids, and include anti-inflammatory effects (see Chap. 24).	Corticotropin is usually not recommended for the numerous nonendocrine inflammatory disorders that respond to glucocorticoids. Administration of glucocorticoids is more convenient and effective than administration of corticotropin.
b. With chorionic gonadotropin and menotropins given in cases of female infertility, ovulation and conception are therapeutic effects.	
c. With chorionic gonadotropins given in cryptorchidism, the therapeutic effect is descent of the testicles from the abdomen to the scrotum.	
d. With antidiuretics (desmopressin, lypressin, and vasopressin), observe for decreased urine output, increased urine specific gravity, decreased signs of dehydration, decreased thirst.	These effects indicate control of diabetes insipidus.
e. With oxytocin given to induce labor, observe for the beginning or the intensifying of uterine contractions.	
f. With oxytocin given to control postpartum bleeding, observe for a firm uterine fundus and decreased vaginal bleeding.	

Nursing Actions	***Rationale/Explanation***
3. Observe for adverse effects	
a. With corticotropin, observe for sodium and fluid retention; edema; hypokalemia; hyperglycemia; osteoporosis; increased susceptibility to infection; myopathy; behavioral changes.	These adverse reactions are generally the same as those produced by adrenal cortex hormones. Severity of adverse reactions tends to increase with dosage and duration of corticotropin administration.
b. With human chorionic gonadotropin given to preadolescent boys, observe for sexual precocity, breast enlargement, and edema.	Sexual precocity results from stimulation of excessive testosterone secretion at an early age.
c. With menotropins, observe for symptoms of ovarian hyperstimulation such as abdominal discomfort, weight gain, ascites, pleural effusion, oliguria, and hypotension.	Adverse effects can be minimized by frequent pelvic examinations to check for ovarian enlargement and by laboratory measurement of estrogen levels. Multiple gestation (mostly twins) is a possibility and is related to ovarian overstimulation.
d. With desmopressin, observe for headache, nasal congestion, nausea, and occasionally a slight increase in blood pressure. A more serious adverse reaction is water retention and hyponatremia.	Adverse reactions usually occur only with high dosages and tend to be relatively mild. Water intoxication (headache, nausea, vomiting, confusion, lethargy, coma, convulsions) may occur with any antidiuretic therapy if excessive fluids are ingested.
e. With lypressin, observe for headache and congestion of nasal passages, dyspnea and coughing (if the drug is inhaled), and water intoxication if excessive amounts of lypressin or fluid are taken.	Adverse effects are usually mild and occur infrequently with usual doses.
f. With vasopressin, observe for water intoxication (headache, nausea, vomiting, confusion, lethargy, coma, convulsions); allergic reactions; chest pain, myocardial infarction, increased blood pressure; abdominal cramps, nausea, and diarrhea.	Adverse reactions to vasopressin are likely to be more widespread and to occur more often than reactions to the synthetic agents, desmopressin and lypressin. With high doses, vasopressin constricts blood vessels, especially coronary arteries, and stimulates smooth muscle of the gastrointestinal tract. Special caution is necessary in clients with heart disease, asthma, or epilepsy.
g. With oxytocin, observe for excessive stimulation or contractility of the uterus, uterine rupture, and cervical and perineal lacerations.	Severe adverse reactions are most likely to occur when oxytocin is given to induce labor and delivery.
4. Observe for drug interactions	
a. Drugs that *increase* effects of vasopressin	
(1) General anesthetics, chlorpropamide (Diabinese)	Potentiate vasopressin
(2) Ganglionic blocking agents (*e.g.,* trimethaphan [Arfonad])	Markedly increase the pressor effects of vasopressin
b. Drugs that *decrease* effects of vasopressin	
(1) Lithium	Inhibits the renal tubular reabsorption of water normally stimulated by vasopressin
c. Drugs that *increase* effects of oxytocin	
(1) Estrogens	With adequate estrogen levels, oxytocin increases uterine contractility. When estrogen levels are low, the effect of oxytocin is reduced.
(2) Vasoconstrictors or vasopressors (*e.g.,* ephedrine, epinephrine, norepinephrine)	Severe, persistent hypertension with rupture of cerebral blood vessels may occur because of additive vasoconstrictor effects. This is a potentially lethal interaction and should be avoided.
5. Teach clients	
a. Take the drug as directed.	To increase therapeutic effects and decrease potentially serious adverse reactions

Nursing Actions	Rationale/Explanation
b. Report adverse effects.	The drug may need to be discontinued or reduced in dosage.
c. With corticotropin,	
(1) Follow a low-sodium, high-potassium diet.	To decrease sodium retention and potassium loss
(2) Weigh regularly.	Weight gain may indicate fluid retention. Edema may occur.
(3) Avoid exposure to infections, when possible.	Corticotropin increases susceptibility to infections.
(4) Follow instructions when the drug is being discontinued.	Corticotropin is gradually reduced in dosage to avoid symptoms such as fatigue, muscle weakness, and hypotension, which may occur with abrupt withdrawal.
(5) Test urine for glycosuria.	This is probably not indicated for all clients but may be helpful in those who have family histories of diabetes mellitus or who are obese. Corticotropin may cause hyperglycemia, activate latent diabetes mellitus, or aggravate existing diabetes mellitus.
d. With antidiuretics	
(1) Reduce fluid intake when starting an antidiuretic drug.	To avoid water intoxication
(2) Regulate dosage in accordance with physician's instructions and with occurrence of excessive urination and thirst.	The purpose of the drugs is to control symptoms of diabetes insipidus. The amount of drug necessary to achieve this purpose varies among clients.

Selected References

American Medical Association (AMA) Division of Drugs: AMA Drug Evaluations, 5th ed. New York, John Wiley & Sons, 1983

Anderson PD: Basic Human Anatomy and Physiology: Clinical Implications for the Health Professions. Monterey, CA, Wadsworth, 1984

Malseed RT: Pharmacology: Drug Therapy and Nursing Considerations, 2d ed. Philadelphia, J B Lippincott, 1985

Murad F, Haynes RC Jr: Adenohypophyseal hormones and related substances. In Gilman AG, Goodman LS, Rall TW, Murad F (eds): The Pharmacological Basis of Therapeutics, 7th ed, pp 1362–1388. New York, Macmillan, 1985

Stewarts ML: When the patient has the "other" diabetes. RN 48:54–58, May 1985

24
CORTICOSTEROIDS

Description and uses

Corticosteroids, also called adrenocorticosteroids and steroids, are hormones produced by the adrenal cortex. These hormones are extremely important in maintaining homeostasis when secreted in normal amounts. Disease results from inadequate or excessive secretion. Exogenous corticosteroids are used as drugs in a variety of endocrine and nonendocrine disorders. Few other drug groups produce such profound therapeutic benefits or adverse reactions as the corticosteroids. Consequently, their use must be carefully regulated and their effects closely monitored. To understand the effects of corticosteroids used as drugs, it is necessary to understand the physiologic effects and other characteristics of the endogenous hormones.

ENDOGENOUS CORTICOSTEROIDS

The adrenal cortex produces about 30 steroid hormones. These hormones are divided into glucocorticoids, mineralocorticoids, and adrenal sex hormones. Glucocorticoids have important roles in the metabolism of carbohydrates, proteins, and fats. Mineralocorticoids are important in maintaining fluid and electrolyte balance. The adrenal sex hormones are secreted in small amounts and are considered relatively unimportant in the normal functioning of the body.

Chemically, all corticosteroids are derived from cholesterol and all have similar chemical formulas. Despite their similarities, however, very slight differences in structure cause them to have different functions.

Corticosteroids are unique in the endocrine system because they are necessary for life. The rate of corticosteroid secretion is normally maintained within relatively narrow limits but changes according to need. For example, rate of secretion accelerates rapidly in response to stress, then decreases when the need has passed.

Secretion of corticosteroids

Corticosteroid secretion is controlled by the hypothalamus, anterior pituitary, and adrenal cortex (the hypothalamic–pituitary–adrenal, or HPA, axis). Various stimuli (*e.g.*, low plasma levels of corticosteroids, pain, anxiety, trauma, illness, anesthesia) activate the system. These stimuli cause the hypothalamus to secrete corticotropin-releasing hormone (CRH). CRH stimulates the anterior pituitary to secrete corticotropin, and corticotropin stimulates the adrenal cortex to secrete corticosteroids.

When plasma corticosteroid levels rise to an adequate level, secretion of corticosteroids slows or stops. The mechanism by which the hypothalamus and anterior pituitary are informed that no more corticosteroids are currently needed is called a *negative feedback mechanism.*

This negative feedback mechanism is normally very important, but it does not work during stressful situations; that is, during stress, it does not prevent further production of corticosteroids when blood levels are already adequate or high. Secretion of corticosteroids, especially cortisol, may be as much as ten times the normal amount during periods of stress. Apparently, stress stimuli causing increased production of corticosteroids are much stronger than the negative feedback stimuli to decrease production. Usually, this is a protective mechanism that helps the person to cope with stress. When corticosteroid secretion is excessive and prolonged, however, body tissues are damaged.

Corticosteroids are secreted directly into the bloodstream. They have a half-life in the circulation of about $1\frac{1}{2}$ hours. They are metabolized primarily in the liver to water-soluble products, which are then rapidly excreted in the urine. Major secretory products can be measured in the urine. For example, measurement of 17-hydroxycorticosteroids in urine gives an estimate of cortisol production, and measurement of 17-ketosteroids gives an estimate of androgen (male sex hormone) secretion.

Glucocorticoids

The term *corticosteroids* refers to all secretions of the adrenal cortex but is often used to designate the glucocorticoids. Glucocorticoids include cortisol, corticosterone, and cortisone. Cortisol accounts for at least 95% of glucocorticoid activity, and approximately 15 to 25 mg is secreted daily. Corticosterone has a small amount of activity, and about 1.5 to 4 mg is secreted daily. Cortisone has little activity and is secreted in minute quantities. Glucocorticoids are secreted cyclically, with the largest amount being produced during early morning and the smallest amount during the evening hours (in people with a normal day–night schedule). Glucocorticoids account for many of the effects ascribed to the corticosteroids as a group, including the following:

1. Effects on carbohydrate metabolism
   a. Glucocorticoids stimulate formation of glucose (gluconeogenesis) by causing the breakdown of protein into amino acids. The amino acids are then transported to the liver, where they are acted on by enzymes that convert them to glucose. The glucose is then returned to the circulation for utilization by body tissues or storage in the liver as glycogen.
   b. Glucocorticoids also cause a moderate decrease in cell utilization of glucose (anti-insulin effect) by an unknown mechanism.
   c. Both increased production and decreased use of glucose promote higher levels of glucose in the blood (hyperglycemia) and may lead to diabetes mellitus. These actions also increase the amount of glucose stored as glycogen in the liver, skeletal muscles, and other tissues.
2. Effects on protein metabolism
   a. Glucocorticoids increase breakdown of protein into amino acids (catabolic effect). They further increase the rate at which amino acids are transported to the liver and converted into glucose.
   b. Glucocorticoids decrease the rate at which new proteins are formed from dietary and other amino acids (antianabolic effect).
   c. Both the increased breakdown of cell protein and decreased protein synthesis produce protein depletion in virtually all body cells except those of the liver. Thus, glycogen stores in the body are increased, while protein stores are decreased.
3. Effects on lipid metabolism
   a. Glucocorticoids increase breakdown of adipose tissue into fatty acids in much the same way as they increase catabolism of protein into amino acids. These fatty acids are transported in the plasma and used as a source of energy by body cells.
   b. Glucocorticoids also stimulate oxidation of fatty acids within body cells.
4. Other effects
   a. Glucocorticoids suppress inflammation. The inflammatory process is the normal bodily response to tissue damage and involves three stages. First, a large amount of plasmalike fluid leaks out of capillaries into the damaged area and becomes clotted. Second, leukocytes migrate into the area. Third, tissue healing occurs, largely by growth of fibrous scar tissue. Normal or physiologic amounts of glucocorticoids probably do not significantly affect inflammation and healing. However, large amounts of glucocorticoids apparently inhibit all three stages of the inflammatory process. Despite extensive study, the precise mechanisms by which glucocorticoids exert their anti-inflammatory effects are still not clear.
   b. Glucocorticoids suppress secretion of CRH by the hypothalamus and secretion of corticotropin by the anterior pituitary gland. This results in suppression of further glucocorticoid secretion by the adrenal cortex.
   c. Glucocorticoids decrease the number of circulating lymphocytes and eosinophils, decrease the rate of conversion of lymphocytes into antibodies, and decrease the amount of lymphoid tissue. These effects influence immune and allergic responses and help to account for the

immunosuppressive and antiallergic actions of the glucocorticoids.

d. Glucocorticoids help to maintain muscle strength when present in physiologic amounts, but they cause muscle atrophy (from protein breakdown) when present in excessive amounts.
e. Glucocorticoids inhibit bone formation and growth. They also decrease intestinal absorption and increase renal excretion of calcium. These effects contribute to bone demineralization (osteoporosis) in adults and to decreased linear growth in children.
f. Glucocorticoids decrease the viscosity of gastric mucus. This effect may decrease protective properties of the mucus and contribute to the development of peptic ulcer disease.
g. Glucocorticoids act synergistically with epinephrine and norepinephrine during stressful situations.
h. Endogenous glucocorticoids also have mineralocorticoid effects that promote retention of sodium and water. Edema, hypertension, and hypokalemia may result.

Mineralocorticoids

Mineralocorticoids play a vital role in maintaining fluid and electrolyte balance. Aldosterone is the main mineralocorticoid and is responsible for 95% of mineralocorticoid activity. Characteristics and physiologic effects of mineralocorticoids, especially aldosterone, include the following:

1. The overall physiologic effects are to conserve sodium and water and eliminate potassium. Aldosterone increases sodium reabsorption from kidney tubules, and water is reabsorbed along with the sodium. When sodium is conserved, another cation must be excreted to maintain electrical neutrality of body fluids; potassium, not sodium, is the cation excreted. This is the only potent mechanism for controlling the concentration of potassium ions in extracellular fluids.
2. Secretion of aldosterone is controlled by several factors, most of which are related to kidney function. Generally, secretion is increased when the potassium level of extracellular fluid is high, the sodium level of extracellular fluid is low, the renin–angiotensin system of the kidneys is activated, or the anterior pituitary gland secretes corticotropin.
3. Inadequate secretion of aldosterone causes hyperkalemia, hyponatremia, and extracellular fluid volume deficit (dehydration). Hypotension and shock may result from decreased cardiac output. Absence of mineralocorticoids causes death.
4. Excessive secretion of aldosterone produces hypokalemia, hypernatremia, and extracellular fluid volume excess (water intoxication). Edema and hypertension may result.

Adrenal sex hormones

The adrenal cortex secretes both male (androgens) and female (estrogens and progesterone) sex hormones. The adrenal sex hormones are relatively insignificant compared with those produced by the testes and ovaries. Adrenal androgens, secreted continuously in small quantities by both men and women, are responsible for most of the physiologic effects exerted by the adrenal sex hormones. They increase protein synthesis (anabolism), which increases mass and strength of muscle and bone tissue; they affect development of male secondary sex characteristics; and they increase hair growth and libido in women. Excessive secretion of adrenal androgens in women causes masculinizing effects (*e.g.*, hirsutism, acne, breast atrophy, deepening of the voice, and amenorrhea). Female sex hormones are secreted in small amounts and normally exert few physiologic effects. Excessive secretion may produce feminizing effects in men (*e.g.*, breast enlargement, decreased hair growth, voice changes).

Disorders of the adrenal cortex

Disorders of the adrenal cortex involve increased or decreased production of corticosteroids, especially cortisol as the primary glucocorticoid and aldosterone as the primary mineralocorticoid. These disorders include the following:

1. Primary adrenocortical insufficiency (Addison's disease) is associated with destruction of the adrenal cortex by disorders such as tuberculosis, cancer, or hemorrhage, with atrophy of the adrenal cortex caused by autoimmune disease or excessive and prolonged administration of exogenous corticosteroids, and with surgical excision of the adrenal glands. In this condition, there is inadequate production of both cortisol and aldosterone.
2. Secondary adrenocortical insufficiency, produced by inadequate secretion of corticotropin, is most often caused by prolonged administration of corticosteroids. This condition is largely a glucocorticoid deficiency. Mineralocorticoid secretion is not significantly impaired.

3. Congenital adrenogenital syndromes and adrenal hyperplasia result from deficiencies in one or more enzymes required for cortisol production. Low plasma levels of cortisol lead to excessive corticotropin secretion, which leads in turn to excessive adrenal secretion of androgens and hyperplasia.
4. Androgen-producing tumors of the adrenal cortex are usually benign. They produce masculinizing effects.
5. Adrenocortical hyperfunction (Cushing's disease) may result from excessive corticotropin or a primary adrenal tumor. Adrenal tumors may be benign or malignant. Benign tumors often produce one corticosteroid normally secreted by the adrenal cortex, but malignant tumors often secrete several corticosteroids.
6. Hyperaldosteronism is a rare disorder caused by adenoma or hyperplasia of the adrenal cortex cells that produce aldosterone. It is characterized by hypokalemia, hypernatremia, hypertension, thirst, and polyuria.

EXOGENOUS CORTICOSTEROIDS

When corticosteroids are administered from sources outside the body, they are given for replacement, therapeutic, or diagnostic purposes. When given to replace or substitute for the endogenous hormones, they are given in relatively small doses to correct a deficiency state, and their purpose is to restore normal function. When given for therapeutic purposes, they are given in relatively large doses to exert pharmacologic effects. Drug effects involve extension of the physiologic effects of endogenous corticosteroids as well as new effects that do not occur with small, physiologic doses. The most frequently desired effects are anti-inflammatory, immunosuppressive, and antiallergic. These are glucocorticoid effects. Mineralocorticoid and androgenic effects are usually considered adverse reactions.

All adrenal corticosteroids are commercially available for use as drugs, as are many synthetic derivatives. The newer corticosteroids have been developed by chemically altering the basic steroid molecule in efforts to increase therapeutic effects while minimizing adverse effects. These efforts have been most successful in decreasing mineralocorticoid activity. Despite considerable progress, however, synthetic corticosteroids can produce all the adverse reactions associated with the natural corticosteroids.

Exogenous corticosteroids are palliative. They control many symptoms but do not cure the underlying disease process. In chronic disorders, for example, they may enable a client to continue the usual activities of daily living and delay disability. However, the disease may continue to progress. Long-term use of corticosteroids inevitably produces adverse effects.

Exogenous corticosteroids have widely different actions on body tissues and fluids, so a specific effect may be considered therapeutic in one client but adverse in another. For example, an increased blood suger level is therapeutic for the client with adrenocortical insufficiency or an islet cell adenoma of the pancreas, but this is an adverse reaction for the client with diabetes mellitus. In addition, some clients respond more favorably or develop adverse reactions more readily than others taking equivalent doses. This is partially caused by individual differences in the rate at which corticosteroids are metabolized.

Administration of exogenous corticosteroids suppresses the HPA axis. This decreases secretion of corticotropin, which in turn causes atrophy of the adrenal cortex and decreased production of endogenous adrenal corticosteroids. Daily administration of physiologic doses (approximately 20 mg of hydrocortisone or its equivalent) or administration of pharmacologic doses (more than 20 mg of hydrocortisone or its equivalent) for a few days suppresses the HPA axis. Recovery may take 1 to 2 years after corticosteroids are discontinued. During that time, the client's ability to respond to stress is impaired unless additional corticosteroids are given.

Hydrocortisone, the exogenous equivalent of endogenous cortisol, is the prototype of corticosteroid drugs. When a new corticosteroid is developed, it is compared with hydrocortisone to determine its potency in producing anti-inflammatory and antiallergic responses, increasing deposition of liver glycogen, and suppressing secretion of corticotropin.

Exogenous mineralocorticoid drugs are infrequently used for therapeutic purposes. Even with adrenocortical insufficiency in Addison's disease or adrenalectomy, many physicians prefer to use a glucocorticoid with high mineralocorticoid activity rather than separate drugs.

Characteristics of Glucocorticoid Drugs

Glucocorticoids compose the largest subgroup of corticosteroids by far, and they account for almost all clinical usage of corticosteroid drugs. Specific characteristics of the glucocorticoids include the following:

1. Pharmacologic effects sought from glucocorticoid drugs are largely antistress, anti-inflammatory, antiallergic, and immunosuppressive. The mechanisms by which glucocorticoids produce these effects are not clearly understood but may include the following:

a. Strengthening or stabilizing biologic membranes. This inhibits capillary permeability and thus prevents leakage of fluid into the injured area and development of edema. It further inhibits release of bradykinin, histamine, lysosomal enzymes, and perhaps other substances that normally cause vasodilation and tissue irritation.
b. Impaired ability of phagocytic cells to migrate into the injured area from the blood
c. Interference with lymphocyte function and antibody production
d. Shrinkage of lymphoid tissues
e. Decreased growth of new capillaries, fibroblasts, and collagen

2. Important differences among glucocorticoid drugs are duration of action, relative glucocorticoid potency, and relative mineralocorticoid potency. Anti-inflammatory potency of the various glucocorticoids is approximately equal when the drugs are given in equivalent doses. Mineralocorticoid activity is intermediate to high in the older drugs, cortisone and hydrocortisone, and low in newer agents.
3. There are many glucocorticoid preparations available for use in different clinical problems, and routes of administration vary. Several of these drugs can be given by more than one route; others can be given only orally or topically. For intramuscular (IM) or intravenous (IV) injections, sodium phosphate or sodium succinate salts are used because they are most soluble in water. For intra-articular or intralesional injections, acetate salts are used because they have low solubility in water and provide prolonged local action.

CLINICAL INDICATIONS

Corticosteroids are used to treat many different disorders that have few characteristics in common and produce a vast array of clinical signs and symptoms. Corticosteroid preparations applied topically in ophthalmic and dermatologic disorders are discussed in Chapters 65 and 66, respectively. The corticosteroids discussed in this chapter are primarily those given systemically or by local injection in potentially serious or disabling disorders. Individual corticosteroids are listed in Table 24-1. These disorders are as follows:

1. Endocrine disorders such as adrenocortical insufficiency and congenital adrenal hyperplasia. Corticosteroids are given to replace or substitute for the natural hormones (both glucocorticoids and mineralocorticoids) in cases of insufficiency and to suppress corticotropin when excess secretion causes adrenal hyperplasia. These conditions are rare and account for only a small amount of corticosteroid usage.
2. Collagen disorders such as rheumatoid arthritis, systemic lupus erythematosus, scleroderma, and periarteritis nodosa. Collagen is the basic structural protein of connective tissue, tendons, cartilage, and bone, and it is therefore present in almost all body tissues and organ systems. The collagen disorders are characterized by inflammation of various body tissues. Signs and symptoms depend on which body tissues or organs are affected and the severity of the inflammatory process. Rheumatoid arthritis is a frequently encountered collagen disorder.
3. Allergic disorders such as bronchial asthma, status asthmaticus, allergic reactions to drugs, serum and blood transfusions, and dermatoses with an allergic component.
4. Dermatologic disorders such as pemphigus, exfoliative dermatitis, and severe psoriasis
5. Neurologic conditions such as cerebral edema, brain tumor, and myasthenia gravis
6. Hematologic disorders such as idiopathic thrombocytopenic purpura or acquired hemolytic anemia
7. Neoplastic disease such as acute and chronic leukemias, Hodgkin's disease, other lymphomas, and multiple myeloma. The effectiveness of corticosteroids in these conditions probably stems from their ability to suppress lymphocytes and other lymphoid tissue.
8. Gastrointestinal disorders such as ulcerative colitis and regional enteritis (Crohn's disease)
9. Renal disorders characterized by edema, such as the nephrotic syndrome
10. Liver disorders characterized by edema, such as cirrhosis and ascites
11. Some eye disorders, such as optic neuritis, sympathetic ophthalmia, and chorioretinitis
12. Other conditions such as organ or tissue transplants and grafts. Corticosteroids are used as immunosuppressants to prevent rejection of the transplanted tissue. Corticosteroids have also been used to treat shock of various types. However, they are clearly indicated only for shock resulting from adrenocortical insufficiency (Addisonian crisis). Maximal levels of corticosteroids are already being produced in hemorrhagic or cardiogenic shock as well as other forms of severe stress, and administration of exogenous corticosteroids has no apparent therapeutic benefit. There is some evidence of effectiveness when corticosteroids are used to treat septic or gram-negative shock.

(Text continues on p. 213.)

TABLE 24-1. CORTICOSTEROIDS*

Generic name	Trade name	Routes and dosage ranges	Anti-inflammatory dose equivalent to 20 mg of hydrocortisone (mg)	Mineralo-corticoid activity	Duration of action (hr)
Glucocorticoids					
Beclomethasone	Vanceril	Adults: Oral inhalation, 2 inhalations (84 μg) 3–4 times daily (maximal daily dose is 20 inhalations or 840 μg) Children 6–12 years: Oral inhalation, 1–3 inhalations (42–84 μg) 3–4 times daily (maximal daily dose is 10 inhalations or 420 μg)			
Betamethasone	Celestone	Adults: PO 0.6–7.2 mg daily initially, depending on the disease being treated, gradually reduced to lowest effective maintenance dose.	0.6	Low	48
Betamethasone acetate and sodium phosphate	Celestone Soluspan	Adults: IM 1–2 ml (3–6 mg each of betamethasone acetate and betamethasone sodium phosphate) Intra-articular injection 0.25–2 ml Soft-tissue injection 0.25–1.0 ml			
Cortisone	Cortone	Chronic adrenocortical insufficiency, PO 15–30 mg daily Congenital adrenal hyperplasia, PO 15–50 mg daily Anti-inflammatory effects, PO 25–50 mg daily for mild, chronic disorders; 125–300 mg daily in 4 or more doses for acute, life-threatening disease Anti-inflammatory effects, IM 75–300 mg daily for serious disease	25	High	12
Dexamethasone	Decadron	PO 0.75–9 mg daily in 2–4 doses. Dosages in higher ranges are used for serious diseases (leukemia, pemphigus)	0.75	Low	48
Dexamethasone acetate		IM 8–16 mg (1–2 ml) in single dose, repeated every 1–3 weeks if necessary Intralesional 0.8–1.6 mg (0.1–0.2 ml) Intra-articular or soft-tissue injection, 4–16 mg (0.5–2 ml), repeated every 1–3 weeks if necessary			
Dexamethasone sodium phosphate		IM, IV 0.5–9 mg, depending on severity of the disease Intra-articular, soft-tissue injection 0.2–6 mg, depending on size of affected area or joint			
	Decadron Turbinaire	Intranasal, 2 sprays in each nostril 2–3 times daily			
	Decadron Respihaler	2–3 inhalations 3–4 times daily			

TABLE 24-1. CORTICOSTEROIDS* (*Continued*)

Generic name	Trade name	Routes and dosage ranges	Anti-inflammatory dose equivalent to 20 mg of hydrocortisone (mg)	Mineralo-corticoid activity	Duration of action (hr)
Dexamethasone/ lidocaine	Decadron with Xylocaine	Soft-tissue injection, 0.5–0.75 ml			
Fluprednisolone	Alphadrol	PO 1.5–30 mg daily, initially, reduced to lowest effective amount for maintenance	1.5	Low	?
Flunisolide	AeroBid	Adults: Oral inhalation, 2 inhalations (500 μg) twice daily Children 6–15 years: Same as adults			
Hydrocortisone	Hydrocortone, Cortef	Chronic adrenocortical insufficiency, PO 10–20 mg daily in 3–4 doses Chronic nonfatal diseases, PO 20–40 mg daily in 3–4 doses Congenital adrenal hyperplasia, PO 10–30 mg daily in 3–4 doses Chronic, potentially fatal diseases, PO 60–120 mg daily in 3–4 doses Acute, nonfatal diseases, PO 60–120 mg daily in 3–4 doses Acute life-threatening diseases, PO 100–240 mg daily in at least 4 divided doses Disorders other than shock, IV 100–500 mg initially, repeated if necessary Intra-articular injections, 5–50 mg depending on size of joint Soft-tissue injection, 25–75 mg Rectally, one enema (100 mg) nightly for 21 days or until an optimal response is obtained	20	Intermediate	18
Methylprednisolone	Medrol	PO 4–48 mg daily initially, gradually reduced to lowest effective level	4	Low	18–36
Methylprednisolone sodium succinate	Solu-Medrol	IM 40–120 mg as needed IV 100–250 mg q4–6h for shock; 10–40 mg as needed for other conditions Intra-articular and soft-tissue injection, 4–80 mg as needed, depending on size of the affected area Intralesional injection, 20–60 mg Rectally, 40 mg as retention enema 3–7 times weekly for two or more weeks			
Paramethasone	Haldrone	PO 2–24 mg daily until response obtained, then gradually reduced to lowest effective level	2	Low	48
Prednisolone	Sterane, Delta-Cortef	PO 5–60 mg daily initially, adjusted for maintenance	5	Intermediate	18–36

TABLE 24-1. CORTICOSTEROIDS* (*Continued*)

Generic name	Trade name	Routes and dosage ranges	Anti-inflammatory dose equivalent to 20 mg of hydrocortisone (mg)	Mineralo-corticoid activity	Duration of action (hr)
Prednisolone acetate	Fernisolone, others	IM 4–60 mg daily initially, adjusted for maintenance Intra-articular or soft-tissue injection, 4–60 mg daily, depending on the disease			
Prednisolone sodium phosphate	Hydeltrasol	IM 4–60 mg daily initially, adjusted for maintenance Emergencies, IV 20–100 mg, repeated if necessary, to a maximal daily dose of 400 mg. When the client's condition improves, 10–20 mg in single doses may be given Intra-articular or soft-tissue injection, 2–30 mg from once every 3–5 days to once every 2–3 weeks			
Prednisolone sodium succinate	Meticortelone soluble	IM 4–60 mg daily initially, adjusted for maintenance Emergencies, IV 20–100 mg, repeated if necessary to a maximal daily dose of 480 mg. When the client's condition improves, 10–20 mg in single doses may be given			
Prednisolone tebutate	Hydeltra-TBA	Intra-articular or soft-tissue injection, 4–60 mg daily, depending on the disease			
Prednisone	Deltasone	PO 5–60 mg daily initially, reduced for maintenance	5	Intermediate	18–30
Triamcinolone	Aristocort, Kenacort	PO 4–48 mg daily initially; dosage reduced for maintenance	4	Low	18–36
Triamcinolone acetonide	Kenalog-40	IM (deep) 2.5–60 mg daily, depending on the disease. When the client's condition improves, dosage should be reduced and oral therapy instituted when feasible Intra-articular or intrabursal injection, 2.5–15 mg every 1–8 weeks depending on the size of the joint and the disease being treated Soft-tissue injection, 5–48 mg			
	Azmacort	Adults: Oral inhalation, 2 inhalations (200 μg) 3 times daily Children 6–12 years: Oral inhalation, 1 or 2 inhalations (100 or 200 μg) 3 times daily			
Triamcinolone diacetate	Aristocort diacetate, Kenacort diacetate	PO 4–48 mg daily initially; dosage reduced for maintenance IM (deep) 20–80 mg initially Intra-articular injection, 2.5–80 mg every 1–8 weeks, depending on size of joint or affected area			

TABLE 24-1. CORTICOSTEROIDS* (*Continued*)

Generic name	Trade name	Routes and dosage ranges	Anti-inflammatory dose equivalent to 20 mg of hydrocortisone (mg)	Mineralocorticoid activity	Duration of action (hr)
		Soft-tissue injection, 5–48 mg			
Triamcinolone hexacetonide	Aristospan	Intra-articular injection, 2.5–80 mg every 1–8 weeks, depending on size of joint or affected area			
Mineralocorticoids					
Desoxycorticosterone	Percorten, Doca	Addison's disease, IM 1–5 mg daily (solution in oil) Salt-losing adrenogenital syndromes, IM 5–6 mg for 3–4 days, then adjusted according to clinical response and serum electrolyte levels Subcutaneous pellet implantation every 8–12 months, depending on maintenance dosage established with solution in oil IM (pivalate preparation) every 4 weeks, depending on daily maintenance dose established with solution in oil			
Fludrocortisone	Florinef	Chronic adrenocortical insufficiency, PO 0.05–0.1 mg daily Salt-losing adrenogenital syndromes PO 0.1–0.2 mg daily			

* Ophthalmic and dermatologic preparations are discussed in Chapters 65 and 66, respectively.

Principles of therapy: corticosteroid drugs

RISK/BENEFIT FACTORS

1. Because corticosteroid drugs can cause serious adverse reactions, indications for their clinical use should be as clear-cut as possible. They are relatively safe for short-term treatment of self-limiting conditions, such as allergic reactions or acute exacerbations of chronic conditions. Long-term use of pharmacologic doses (more than 20 mg of hydrocortisone daily or its equivalent) is almost always accompanied by adverse reactions of variable severity. For this reason, long-term corticosteroid therapy should be reserved for life-threatening conditions or severe, disabling symptoms that do not respond to treatment with more benign drugs or other measures. Both physician and client should be convinced that the anticipated benefits of long-term therapy are worth the risks.
2. The goal of corticosteroid therapy is usually to reduce symptoms to a tolerable level. Total suppression of symptoms is likely to require excessively large doses and produce excessive adverse effects.

ASSESSMENT RELATED TO INITIATION OF CORTICOSTEROID THERAPY

1. Each client should be thoroughly assessed before long-term corticosteroid therapy is initiated. Assessment may include diagnostic tests for diabetes mellitus, tuberculosis, and peptic ulcer disease because these conditions may develop from or be exacerbated by administration of corticosteroid drugs. If one of these conditions is present, corticosteroid therapy must be altered and other drugs given concomitantly.
2. If acute infection is found on initial assessment, it should be treated with appropriate antibiotics either before corticosteroid drugs are started or concomitantly with corticosteroid therapy. This is

necessary because corticosteroids may mask symptoms of infection and impair healing. Thus, even relatively minor infections can become serious if left untreated during corticosteroid therapy. If infection occurs during long-term corticosteroid therapy, appropriate antibiotic therapy (as determined by culture of the causative microorganism and antibiotic sensitivity studies) is again indicated. Also, increased doses of corticosteroids are usually indicated to cope with the added stress of the infection.

ASSESSMENT RELATED TO PREVIOUS OR CURRENT CORTICOSTEROID THERAPY

Initial assessment of every client should include information about previous or current corticosteroid therapy. This can usually be determined by questioning the client or reviewing medical records.

1. If the nurse determines that the client has taken corticosteroids in the past, additional information is needed regarding the specific drug and dosage taken, the purpose and length of therapy, and when therapy was stopped. Such information is necessary for planning nursing care. If the client had an acute illness and received an oral corticosteroid for 1 to 2 weeks or received corticosteroids by local injection or application to skin lesions, no special nursing care is likely to be required. If, however, the client took systemic corticosteroids for more than a week or two during the past year, approximately, nursing observations must be especially vigilant. Such a client is at high risk for developing acute adrenocortical insufficiency during stressful situations. If the client is having surgery, corticosteroid therapy is restarted either before or on the day of surgery and continued, in decreasing dosage, for a few days after surgery. In addition to anesthesia and surgery, potentially significant sources of stress include hospitalization, various diagnostic tests, concurrent infection or other illnesses, and family problems.
2. If the client is currently taking a systemic corticosteroid drug, again the nurse must identify the drug, the dosage and schedule of administration, the purpose for which the drug is being taken, and the length of time involved. Once this basic information is obtained, the nurse can further assess client status and plan nursing care. Some specific factors include the following:
   a. If the person will undergo anesthesia and surgery, expect that higher doses of corticosteroids will be given for several days. This may be done by changing the drug and the route of administration as well as the dosage. Specific regimens vary according to type of anesthesia, surgical procedure, client condition, physician preference, and other variables. A client having major abdominal surgery may be given 300 to 400 mg of hydrocortisone (or its equivalent dosage of other agents) on the day of surgery and then be tapered back to maintenance dosage within a few days.
   b. Note that additional corticosteroids may be given in other situations as well. One extra dose may be adequate for a short-term stress situation such as an angiogram or other invasive diagnostic test.
   c. Using all available data, assess the likelihood of the client's having acute adrenal insufficiency (sometimes called adrenal crisis).
   d. Assess for signs and symptoms of adrenocortical excess (hypercorticism, Cushing's disease).
   e. Assess for signs and symptoms of the disease for which long-term corticosteroid therapy is being given.

NURSING INTERVENTIONS

Use supplementary drugs as ordered and nondrug measures to decrease dosage and side-effects of corticosteroid drugs. Some specific measures include the following:

1. In clients with bronchial asthma, bronchodilating drugs and other treatment measures should be continued during corticosteroid therapy.
2. In clients with rheumatoid arthritis, rest, physical therapy, salicylates or other nonsteroid antiinflammatory drugs, and local injections of corticosteroid drugs into joints when only one or two are involved are continued during systemic corticosteroid therapy.
3. Assist the client to identify stressors and to find ways to modify or avoid stressful situations when possible. For example, most clients probably do not think of extreme heat or cold or minor infections as significant stressors. They can be, however, for people taking corticosteroid drugs. This assessment of potential stressors must be individualized because a situation viewed as stressful by one client may not be stressful to another.
4. Encourage activity, if not contraindicated, to slow demineralization of bone (osteoporosis). This is especially important in postmenopausal women, who are very susceptible to osteoporosis. Walking is preferred if the client is able. Range-of-motion

exercises are indicated in immobilized or bedfast persons. Also, bedfast clients taking corticosteroid drugs should have their positions changed frequently because these drugs thin the skin and increase the risk of pressure sores. This risk is further increased if edema is also present.

5. Dietary changes may be beneficial in some clients. Salt restriction may help prevent hypernatremia, fluid retention, and edema. Foods high in potassium may help prevent hypokalemia. A diet high in protein, calcium, and vitamin D may help to prevent osteoporosis. Increased intake of vitamin C may help to decrease bleeding in the skin and soft tissues.
6. Avoid exposing the client to potential sources of infection by washing hands frequently, using aseptic technique when changing dressings, keeping health care personnel and visitors with colds or other infections away from the client, and following other appropriate measures. Reverse or protective isolation of the client is sometimes indicated, commonly for those who have had organ transplants and are receiving corticosteroids to help prevent rejection of the transplanted organ.

DRUG SELECTION

Choice of corticosteroid drug is influenced by many factors, including the purpose for use, characteristics of specific drugs, desired route of administration, characteristics of individual clients, and expected side-effects. Some guidelines for rational drug choice include the following:

1. Treatment for adrenocortical insufficiency, whether caused by Addison's disease, adrenalectomy or inadequate corticotropin, requires replacement of both glucocorticoids and mineralocorticoids. Hydrocortisone and cortisone are usually the drugs of choice because they have greater mineralocorticoid activity compared with other corticosteroids. If additional mineralocorticoid activity is required, fludrocortisone is most convenient because it can be given orally.
2. Nonendocrine disorders, in which anti-inflammatory, antiallergic, antistress, and immunosuppressive effects are desired, can be treated by a corticosteroid drug with primarily glucocorticoid activity. Prednisone is often the glucocorticoid of choice. It has less mineralocorticoid activity than hydrocortisone and is less expensive than newer synthetic glucocorticoids.
3. Treatment of acute, life-threatening situations with corticosteroids requires a drug that can be given parenterally, usually IV. This limits the choice of drugs because not all are available in injectable preparations. Hydrocortisone, dexamethasone, and methylprednisolone are among those that may be given parenterally.
4. Dexamethasone is usually considered the corticosteroid of choice in cerebral edema. It is most effective in cerebral edema caused by brain tumors such as metastatic lesions and glioblastomas; it is less effective in those caused by astrocytomas and meningiomas.

DOSAGE FACTORS

Dosage of corticosteroid drugs is influenced by many factors, such as the specific drug to be given, the desired route of administration, the reason for use, expected adverse effects, and client characteristics. Generally, the smallest effective dose should be given for the shortest effective time. Dosage guidelines include the following:

1. Dosage must be individualized according to the severity of the disorder being treated, whether the disease is acute or chronic, and the client's response to drug therapy. If life-threatening disease is present, high doses are usually given until acute symptoms are brought under control. Then, dosage is gradually reduced until a maintenance dose is determined or the drug is discontinued. If the disease is not life threatening, the physician may still choose to prescribe relatively high doses initially and reduce to maintenance doses, or he may choose to start with low doses and increase to a maintenance level.
2. Physiologic doses (approximately 20 mg of hydrocortisone or its equivalent daily) are given to replace or substitute for endogenous adrenocortical hormone. Pharmacologic doses (multiples of physiologic doses) are usually required for anti-inflammatory, antiallergic, and immunosuppressive effects.
3. New drugs are compared to hydrocortisone. They are more potent than hydrocortisone on a weight basis but are equipotent in anti-inflammatory effects when given in equivalent doses (see Table 24-1). Statements of equivalency with hydrocortisone are helpful in evaluating new drugs, comparing different drugs, and changing drugs or dosages. However, dosage equivalents generally apply only to those drugs given orally or IV. When the drugs are given by other routes, equivalency relationships are likely to be changed.

4. Dosage for children is calculated according to severity of disease rather than weight.
5. Dosage must be reduced if hypoalbuminemia is present. Normally, corticosteroids are highly bound to serum proteins, especially albumin. With hypoalbuminemia, more drug is unbound and pharmacologically active. This increases incidence and severity of adverse effects if dosage is not reduced.
6. For people receiving chronic corticosteroid therapy, dosage must be increased during periods of stress. Although an event that is stressful for one client may not be stressful for another, some common sources of stress for most people include surgery and anesthesia, infections, anxiety, and even extremes of temperature. Some guidelines for corticosteroid dosage during stress include the following:
   a. During minor stress or relatively mild illness (viral upper respiratory infection, any febrile illness, strenuous exercise, gastroenteritis with vomiting and diarrhea, minor surgery), doubling the daily maintenance dose is usually adequate. Once the stress period is over, dosage may be reduced abruptly to the usual maintenance dose.
   b. During major stress or severe illness, even larger doses are necessary. For example, a client undergoing abdominal surgery may require 300 to 400 mg of hydrocortisone on the day of surgery. This dose can gradually be reduced to usual maintenance doses within about 5 days if postoperative recovery is uncomplicated. As a general rule, it is better to administer excessive doses temporarily than to risk inadequate doses and adrenal insufficiency. The client may also require sodium chloride and fluid replacement, antibiotic therapy if infection is present, and supportive measures if shock occurs.

      An acute stress situation of short duration, such as traumatic injury of invasive diagnostic tests (angiograms, pneumoencephalograms), can usually be treated with a single dose of about 100 mg of hydrocortisone immediately after the injury or before the diagnostic test.
   c. Many chronic diseases that require long-term corticosteroid therapy are characterized by exacerbations and remissions. Dosage of corticosteroids must usually be increased during acute flare-ups of disease symptoms but can then be gradually decreased to maintenance levels.

SELECTION OF ROUTE OF ADMINISTRATION

Corticosteroid drugs can be given by several different routes to achieve local or systemic effects. When feasible, corticosteroids should be given locally rather than systemically to prevent or decrease systemic toxicity. When it is necessary to give corticosteroids systemically, the oral route is preferred. Parenteral administration is indicated only for clients who are seriously ill or unable to take oral medications.

SCHEDULING GUIDELINES

Scheduling of drug administration is more important with corticosteroids than with most other drug classes. Most adverse effects occur with long-term administration of high doses. A major adverse reaction is suppression of the HPA axis and subsequent loss of adrenocortical function. Although opinions differ, the following schedules are often recommended to prevent or minimize HPA suppression:

1. For short-term use (10 days or less) in acute situations, corticosteroids can be given in relatively large, divided doses for about 48 to 72 hours until the acute situation is brought under control. At times, also, continuous IV infusions may be given. After acute symptoms subside or 48 to 72 hours have passed, the dosage is tapered so that a slightly smaller dose is given each day until the drug can be discontinued completely. Such a regimen may be useful in allergic reactions, contact dermatitis, exacerbations of chronic conditions (*e.g.*, rheumatoid arthritis, bronchial asthma) and stressful situations such as surgery.
2. For replacement therapy in cases of chronic adrenocortical insufficiency, daily administration is preferred. The entire daily dose can be taken each morning, between 6 AM and 9 AM. This schedule simulates normal endogenous corticosteroid secretion.
3. In other chronic conditions, alternate day therapy (ADT) is usually preferred. ADT involves giving a double dose every other morning. This schedule allows rest periods so that adverse effects are decreased while anti-inflammatory effects continue. Other characteristics include the following:
   a. ADT seems to be as effective as more frequent administration in most clients with bronchial asthma, ulcerative colitis, and other conditions for which long-term corticosteroid therapy is prescribed.
   b. ADT is used only for maintenance therapy; that is, clinical signs and symptoms are con-

trolled initially with more frequent drug administration. ADT can be started once symptoms have subsided and stabilized.

c. ADT does not retard growth in children as do other schedules.

d. ADT probably decreases susceptibility to infection.

e. Intermediate-acting glucocorticoids such as prednisone, prednisolone, and methylprednisolone are the drugs of choice for ADT.

f. ADT is not usually indicated in clients who have received long-term corticosteroid therapy. First, these clients already have maximal HPA suppression, so a major advantage of ADT is lost. Second, if they are transferred to ADT, recurrence of symptoms and considerable discomfort may occur on days when drugs are omitted. Clients with severe disease and very painful or disabling symptoms may also experience severe discomfort with ADT.

NURSING ACTIONS: CORTICOSTEROID DRUGS

Nursing Actions	*Rationale/Explanation*
1. Administer accurately	
a. Read the drug label carefully to be certain of having the correct preparation for the intended route of administration.	Many corticosteroid drugs are available in several different preparations. For example, hydrocortisone is available in formulations for IV or IM administration, for intra-articular injection, and for topical application in creams and ointments of several different strengths. These preparations cannot be used interchangeably without causing potentially serious adverse reactions as well as decreasing therapeutic effects. Some drugs are available for only one use. For example, several preparations are for topical use only; beclomethasone is prepared only for oral inhalation.
b. With oral corticosteroid drugs, give with or after meals.	Opinion seems divided regarding the effectiveness of this scheduling in relation to meals. The rationale is to decrease gastric irritation and prevent development or aggravation of peptic ulcer disease. Corticosteroid drugs have long been considered ulcerogenic, but there is no valid evidence to substantiate this claim. Many physicians prescribe antacids to be given at the same time as the corticosteroid drug.
c. For IV or IM administration	
(1) Follow the manufacturer's directions on the drug vial for the type and amount of diluent to add.	Instructions vary with specific preparations.
(2) Give direct IV injection over at least 1 minute.	To increase safety of administration
(3) Follow the manufacturer's directions for diluting and administering by continuous IV infusions.	Instructions vary with specific preparations.
d. For oral inhalation of a corticosteroid, check the instruction leaflet that accompanies the inhaler. If the client is also receiving a bronchodilator, administer it first, then wait a few minutes before giving the corticosteroid inhalation.	Giving a bronchodilating drug by inhalation before giving the beclomethasone increases penetration of the beclomethasone into the tracheobronchial tree and increases its therapeutic effectiveness. Waiting a few minutes between the drugs decreases the likelihood of toxicity from the inhaled fluorocarbon propellants of the aerosol drugs.
2. Observe for therapeutic effects	The primary objective of corticosteroid therapy is to relieve signs and symptoms, since the drugs are not curative. Therefore, therapeutic effects depend largely on the reason for use.
a. With adrenocortical insufficiency, observe for absence or decrease of weakness, weight loss, anorexia, nausea, vomiting, hyperpigmentation, hypotension, hypoglycemia, hyponatremia, and hyperkalemia.	These signs and symptoms of impaired metabolism do not occur with adequate replacement of corticosteroids.

Nursing Actions	Rationale/Explanation
b. With rheumatoid arthritis, observe for decreased pain and edema in joints, greater capacity for movement, and increased ability to perform usual activities of daily living.	
c. With bronchial asthma, observe for decrease in respiratory distress and increased tolerance of activity.	
d. With skin lesions, observe for decreasing inflammation.	
e. When the drug is given to suppress the immune response to organ transplants, therapeutic effect is the absence of signs and symptoms indicating rejection of the transplanted tissue.	
3. Observe for adverse effects	These are uncommon with replacement therapy but common with long-term administration of the pharmacologic doses used for many disease processes. Adverse reactions may affect every body tissue and organ.
a. Adrenocortical insufficiency—fainting, weakness, anorexia, nausea, vomiting, hypotension, shock, and, if untreated, death	This reaction is likely to occur in clients receiving daily corticosteroid drugs who encounter stressful situations. It is caused by drug-induced suppression of the HPA axis, which makes the client unable to respond to stress by increasing adrenocortical hormone secretion.
b. Adrenocortical excess (hypercorticism or Cushing's disease)	Most adverse effects result from excessive corticosteroids.
(1) "Moon face," "buffalo hump" contour of shoulders, obese trunk, thin extremities	This appearance is caused by abnormal fat deposits in cheeks, shoulders, breasts, abdomen, and buttocks. These changes are more cosmetic than physiologically significant. However, the alterations in self-image can lead to psychologic problems. These changes cannot be prevented, but they may be partially reversed if corticosteroid therapy is discontinued or reduced in dosage.
(2) Diabetes mellitus—glycosuria, hyperglycemia, polyuria, polydipsia, polyphagia, impaired healing, and other signs and symptoms	Corticosteroid drugs can cause hyperglycemia and diabetes mellitus or aggravate preexisting diabetes mellitus by their effects on carbohydrate metabolism.
(3) Central nervous system effects—euphoria, psychologic dependence, nervousness, insomnia, depression, personality and behavioral changes, aggravation of preexisting psychiatric disorders	Some clients enjoy the drug-induced euphoria so much that they resist attempts to withdraw the drug or decrease its dosage.
(4) Musculoskeletal effects—osteoporosis, pathologic fractures, muscle weakness and atrophy, decreased linear growth in children	Demineralization of bone produces thin, weak bones that fracture easily. Fractures of vertebrae, long bones, and ribs are relatively common, especially in postmenopausal women and immobilized persons. Myopathy results from abnormal protein metabolism. Decreased growth in children results from impaired bone formation and protein metabolism.
(5) Cardiovascular, fluid, and electrolyte effects—fluid retention, edema, hypertension, congestive heart failure, hypernatremia, hypokalemia, metabolic alkalosis	These effects result largely from mineralocorticoid activity, which causes retention of sodium and water. They are more likely to occur with older corticosteroids such as hydrocortisone and prednisone.
(6) Gastrointestinal effects—nausea, vomiting, possible peptic ulcer disease, increased appetite, obesity	
(7) Increased susceptibility to infection and delayed wound healing	Caused by suppression of normal inflammatory and immune processes and impaired protein metabolism
(8) Menstrual irregularities, acne, excessive facial hair	Caused by excessive sex hormones, primarily androgens

Nursing Actions	**Rationale/Explanation**
(9) Ocular effects—increased intraocular pressure, glaucoma, cataracts	
(10) Integumentary effects—skin becomes reddened, thinner, has stretch marks, and is easily injured	
4. Observe for drug interactions	
a. Drugs that *increase* effects of corticosteroids	
(1) Adrenergics (*e.g.,* epinephrine), anticholinergics (*e.g.,* atropine), tricyclic antidepressants (*e.g.,* amitriptyline [Elavil]), antihistamines, and meperidine	Potentiation of increased intraocular pressure. The combinations are hazardous in glaucoma and should be avoided if possible.
(2) Diuretics	Excessive potassium depletion may occur because both diuretics and corticosteroids can cause hypokalemia.
(3) Estrogens	Potentiate glycosuria and anti-inflammatory effects of hydrocortisone but not those of dexamethasone, methylprednisolone, prednisolone, or prednisone
(4) Indomethacin	Increase ulcerogenic effects
(5) Phenylbutazone	Increase amounts of free, pharmacologically active corticosteroids owing to displacement from plasma protein binding sites. All effects of corticosteroids may be potentiated.
(6) Salicylates	See Indomethacin and Phenylbutazone.
b. Drugs that *decrease* effects of corticosteroids	
(1) Antihistamines, barbiturates, chloral hydrate, glutethimide, phenytoin, rifampin	These drugs induce microsomal enzymes in the liver and increase the rate at which corticosteroids are metabolized or deactivated.
5. Teach clients	
a. With long-term systemic corticosteroid therapy	
(1) Take as directed.	This is extremely important with these drugs. Missing a dose or two, stopping the drug, changing the amount or time of administration, or taking extra drug (except as specifically directed during stress situations) or any other alterations may result in complications. Some complications are relatively minor; several are serious, even life threatening. When these drugs are being discontinued, the dosage is gradually reduced over a period of several weeks. They should not be abruptly stopped.
(2) Recognize stress situations that necessitate increases in drug dosage. Clarify with the physician predictable sources of stress and the amount of drug to be taken if the stress cannot be avoided.	This requires commitment and cooperation between the client and health care personnel. Close supervision is necessary, especially during the first few months of corticosteroid therapy. Common stresses include infections such as the common cold, extremes of heat or cold, surgical procedures, illness, or death of a family member. However, many stress situations are acute and unpredictable and elicit different responses from different clients.
(3) Wear a special alert bracelet or tag or carry an identification card stating the drug being taken, the dosage, the physician's name, address, and telephone number, and instructions for emergency treatment.	If an accident or emergency situation occurs, the physician providing treatment must know about corticosteroid drug therapy to give additional amounts during the stress of the emergency.
(4) Take no other drugs, prescription or nonprescription, without notifying the physician who is supervising corticosteroid therapy.	Corticosteroid drugs influence reactions to many other drugs, and many other drugs interact with corticosteroids to either increase or decrease their effects. Thus, taking other drugs can either cancel or decrease the expected therapeutic benefits or increase the incidence or severity of adverse reactions.
(5) Report to all physicians consulted that corticosteroid drugs are being taken or have been taken within the past year.	Either current or previous corticosteroid therapy can influence treatment measures. Such knowledge on the physician's part greatly increases his ability to provide appropriate treatment.

Nursing Actions	Rationale/Explanation
(6) Avoid exposure to infection when possible. That is, avoid crowds and persons known to have an infection. Also, wash hands frequently and thoroughly.	These drugs increase the likelihood of infection, so preventive measures are necessary. Also, if infection does occur, healing is likely to be slow.
(7) Practice safety measures to avoid accidents	To avoid falls and possible fractures due to osteoporosis; to avoid cuts or other injuries because of delayed wound healing; to avoid soft tissue trauma because of increased tendency to bruise easily.
(8) Weigh frequently when starting corticosteroid therapy and at least weekly during long-term maintenance.	An initial weight gain is likely to occur and is usually attributed to increased appetite. Later weight gains may be caused by fluid retention.
(9) Follow instructions for other measures used in treatment of the particular condition. For example, other drugs and physical therapy may be prescribed for rheumatoid arthritis.	Such measures may allow smaller doses of corticosteroids. Smaller doses are greatly to the client's advantage in decreasing adverse reactions.
(10) Ask the physician about the amount and kind of activity or exercise needed.	As a general rule, being as active as possible helps to prevent or delay osteoporosis, a rather common adverse reaction. However, increased activity may not be desirable for everyone. A client with rheumatoid arthritis, for example, may become too active when drug therapy relieves joint pain and increases mobility.
(11) Muscle weakness and fatigue or disease symptoms may occur when drug dosage is reduced, withdrawn, or omitted (*e.g.,* the nondrug day of ADH).	Although these symptoms may cause some discomfort, they should be tolerated if possible rather than increasing corticosteroid dose. If severe, of course, dosage or time of administration may have to be changed.
(12) Dietary changes, if indicated. Possible changes include decreasing salt and increasing potassium, calcium, protein, and vitamins D and C.	These changes may not be necessary in all clients. Limiting salt intake may be important if fluid retention or edema is a problem. The simplest way to do this is to avoid adding table salt to foods and avoid obviously salty foods, such as many snack foods and prepared sandwich meats. If more stringent restrictions seem indicated, consult a dietitian or diet manual. When sodium is retained, potassium is lost. It may be desirable for the client to increase intake of high-potassium foods such as citrus fruits and juices or bananas. Protein, calcium, and vitamin D may help to prevent or delay osteoporosis, and vitamin C may help to prevent excessive bruising. Meat and dairy products are good sources of protein, calcium and vitamin D; citrus fruits are good sources of vitamin C. Any diet teaching should be specific to the needs of the individual client and should consider food preferences and usual eating habits.
(13) Maintain regular medical supervision	This is extremely important so that the physician can detect adverse reactions, evaluate disease status, and evaluate drug response and indications for dosage change as well as other responsibilities that can be carried out only with personal contact between the physician and the client. Periodic blood tests, x-ray studies, and other tests may be done during long-term corticosteroid therapy.
(14) Report to the physician (a) Stress situations (b) Sore throat, fever, or other signs of infection (c) Weight gain of 5 pounds or more in a week (d) Swelling in ankles or elsewhere in the body (e) Persistent backache or chest pain (f) Mental depression or other mood changes (g) Changes in sleeping patterns	As previously indicated, clients experiencing stress situations require larger doses of corticosteroids. It would be helpful if the physician would instruct the client on what kinds of stress situations the client can handle and for which the physician should be notified. All the other symptoms to be reported indicate adverse reactions such as infection, sodium and fluid retention, fractures of vertebrae or ribs, and psychologic problems. If these occur, they must be assessed by the physician to see if any changes in corticosteroid therapy are indicated.

Nursing Actions	***Rationale/Explanation***
(15) Also, report to the physician if unable to take a dose orally because of vomiting or some other problem.	In some circumstances, the physician may prescribe one or more injections to prevent potentially serious problems.
(16) If diabetes mellitus results from corticosteroid therapy, teach the client as you would any other diabetic. That is, teach about drug therapy, diet, and urine testing and provide other necessary information.	
b. With local applications of corticosteroids	
(1) Use the drug preparation only as directed and for the purpose intended.	To increase therapeutic effects and decrease adverse reactions. As a general rule, not enough drug is absorbed to cause systemic toxicity. However, systemic toxicity can occur if excess beclomethasone is inhaled or if occlusive dressings are used over skin lesions. Local reactions may occur, especially with large doses. Most of the time, different drug preparations are used for specific purposes, such as eye drops or ear drops or application to skin lesions. These preparations must not be used interchangeably.

Selected References

American Medical Association (AMA) Division of Drugs: AMA Drug Evaluations, 5th ed. New York, John Wiley & Sons, 1983

Anderson PD: Basic Human Anatomy and Physiology: Clinical Implications for the Health Professions. Monterey, CA, Wadsworth, 1984

Baylink DJ: Glucocorticoid-induced osteoporosis. N Engl J Med 309:306–309, August 1984

Corticosteroid aerosols for asthma. Med Lett Drugs Ther 27:5–6, January 1985

Facts and Comparisons. St. Louis, J B Lippincott (Updated monthly)

Gotch PM: Teaching patients about adrenal corticosteroids. Am J Nurs 81:78–81, January 1981

Groer MW, Shekleton ME: Basic Pathophysiology: A Conceptual Approach, 2d ed. St. Louis, C V Mosby, 1983

Guyton AC: Textbook of Medical Physiology, 7th ed. Philadelphia, W B Saunders, 1986

Hansten PD: Drug Interactions: Clinical Significance of Drug–Drug Interactions, 5th ed. Philadelphia, Lea & Febiger, 1985

Haynes RC Jr, Murad F: Adrenocorticotropic hormone; adrenocortical steroids and their synthetic analogs; inhibitors of adrenocortical steroid biosynthesis. In Gilman AG, Goodman LS, Rall TW, Murad F (eds): The Pharmacological Basis of Therapeutics, 7th ed., pp 1459–1489. New York, Macmillan, 1985

Larson CA: The critical path of adrenocortical insufficiency. Nursing 14:66–69, October 1984

Malseed RT: Pharmacology: Drug Therapy and Nursing Considerations, 2d ed. Philadelphia, J B Lippincott, 1985

Messer J, Reitman D, Sacks HS, et al: Association of adrenocorticosteroid therapy and peptic ulcer disease. N Engl J Med 309:21–24, July 1983

Middleton E, Reed CE, Ellis EF (eds): Allergy Principles and Practice. St. Louis, C V Mosby, 1983

Rodman MJ, Karch AM, Boyd EH, Smith DW: Pharmacology and Drug Therapy in Nursing, 3rd ed. Philadelphia, J B Lippincott, 1985

25

THYROID AND ANTITHYROID DRUGS

Description and uses

The thyroid gland produces three hormones: thyroxine, triiodothyronine, and calcitonin. Thyroxine contains four atoms of iodine and is also called T_4. Triiodothyronine contains three atoms of iodine and is called T_3. Compared to thyroxine, triiodothyronine is more potent and has a more rapid but shorter duration of action. Despite these minor differences, the two hormones produce the same physiologic effects and have the same actions and uses. They are often considered collectively as thyroid hormone. Calcitonin functions in calcium metabolism and is discussed in Chapter 26.

Production of thyroxine and triiodothyronine depends on the presence of iodine and tyrosine in the thyroid gland. Plasma iodide is derived from dietary sources and from the metabolic breakdown of thyroid hormone, which allows some iodine to be reused. The thyroid gland extracts iodide from the circulating blood, concentrates it, and secretes enzymes that change the chemically inactive iodide to free iodine atoms. Tyrosine is an amino acid derived from dietary protein. It forms the basic structure of thyroglobulin. In a series of chemical reactions, iodine atoms become attached to tyrosine to form the thyroid hormones T_3 and T_4. Once formed, the hormones are stored within the chemically inactive thyroglobulin molecule.

Thyroid hormones are released into the circulation when the thyroid gland is stimulated by thyrotropin from the anterior pituitary gland. Because the thyroglobulin molecule is too large to cross cell membranes, proteolytic enzymes break down the molecule so that the active hormones can be released. After their release from thyroglobulin, the hormones become largely bound to plasma proteins. Only the small amounts left unbound are biologically active. The bound thyroid hormones are released to tissue cells very slowly. Once in the cells, the hormones combine with intracellular proteins so that they are again stored. They are released slowly within the cell and used over a period of days or weeks. Once used by the cells, the thyroid hormones release the iodine atoms. Most of the iodine is reabsorbed and used to produce new thyroid hormones; the remainder is excreted in the urine.

Thyroid hormones control the rate of cell metabolism and thereby influence the functioning of virtually every body tissue, organ, and system. Specific physiologic effects include the following:

1. Increased rate of bone growth and epiphyseal closure
2. Stimulation of carbohydrate and fat metabolism
3. Increased rate of tissue metabolism
4. Increased rate and depth of respiration
5. Increased absorption of foodstuffs, secretion of di-

gestive juices, and motility in the gastrointestinal tract
6. Stimulation of the central nervous system (CNS)

THYROID DISORDERS

Thyroid disorders requiring drug therapy are goiter, hypothyroidism, and hyperthyroidism. Hypothyroidism and hyperthyroidism produce opposing effects on body tissues, depending on the levels of circulating thyroid hormone. Specific effects and clinical manifestations are listed in Table 25-1.

Simple goiter

Simple goiter is an enlargement of the thyroid gland resulting from iodine deficiency. Inadequate iodine decreases thyroid hormone production. To compensate, the anterior pituitary gland secretes more thyrotropin, which causes the thyroid to enlarge and produce more hormone. If the enlarged gland secretes enough hormone, disfigurement, psychologic distress, dyspnea, and dysphagia are the main problems. If the gland is unable to secrete enough hormone despite enlargement, hypothyroidism results. Simple or endemic goiter is a common condition in some geo-

TABLE 25-1. THYROID DISORDERS

Effects on body systems	Hypothyroidism	Hyperthyroidism
Cardiovascular effects	Increased capillary fragility Decreased cardiac output Decreased blood pressure Decreased heart rate Cardiac enlargement Congestive heart failure Anemia More rapid development of arteriosclerosis and its complications (*e.g.*, coronary artery and peripheral vascular disease)	Tachycardia Increased cardiac output Increased blood volume Increased systolic blood pressure Cardiac arrhythmias Congestive heart failure
Central nervous system effects	Apathy and lethargy Emotional dullness Slow speech, perhaps slurring and hoarseness as well Hypoactive reflexes Forgetfulness and mental sluggishness Excessive drowsiness and sleeping	Nervousness Emotional instability Restlessness Anxiety Insomnia Hyperactive reflexes
Metabolic effects	Intolerance of cold Subnormal temperature Increased serum cholesterol Weight gain	Intolerance of heat Low-grade fever Weight loss despite increased appetite
Gastrointestinal effects	Decreased appetite Constipation	Increased appetite Abdominal cramps Diarrhea Nausea and vomiting
Muscular effects	Weakness Fatigue Vague aches and pains	Weakness Fatigue Muscle atrophy Tremors
Integumentary effects	Skin dry, coarse, and thickened Puffy appearance of face and eyelids Hair dry and thinned Nails thick and hard	Skin moist, warm, flushed owing to vasodilation and increased sweating Hair and nails soft
Reproductive effects	Prolonged menstrual periods Infertility or sterility Decreased libido	Amenorrhea or oligomenorrhea
Miscellaneous effects	Increased susceptibility to infection Increased sensitivity to narcotics, barbiturates, and anesthetics owing to slowed metabolism of these drugs	Dyspnea Polyuria Hoarse, rapid speech Increased susceptibility to infection Excessive perspiration Localized edema around the eyeballs, which produces characteristic eye changes, including exophthalmos

graphic areas. It is not common in the United States, largely because of the widespread use of iodized table salt.

Treatment of simple goiter involves administration of iodine preparations and thyroid hormones to prevent further enlargement and promote regression in gland size. Large goiters may require surgical excision.

Hypothyroidism

Primary hypothyroidism occurs when disease or destruction of thyroid gland tissue causes inadequate production of thyroid hormones. Some causes of primary hypothyroidism include acute viral thyroiditis, chronic (Hashimoto's) thyroiditis, an autoimmune disorder, and overtreatment of hyperthyroidism with antithyroid drugs, radiation therapy, or surgery. Secondary hypothyroidism occurs when there is decreased thyrotropin from the anterior pituitary gland.

Congenital hypothyroidism (cretinism) occurs when a child is born without a thyroid gland or with a poorly functioning gland. Cretinism is uncommon in the United States but may occur with a lack of iodine in the mother's diet. Symptoms are rarely present at birth. They develop gradually during infancy and early childhood and include poor growth and development, lethargy and inactivity, feeding problems, slow pulse, subnormal temperature, and constipation. If the disorder is untreated until the child is several months old, permanent mental retardation is likely to result.

Adult hypothyroidism (myxedema) produces variable signs and symptoms, depending on the amount of functioning thyroid tissue and hormone production. Initially, manifestations are mild and vague. They usually increase in incidence and severity over time as the thyroid gland gradually atrophies and functioning glandular tissue is replaced by nonfunctioning fibrous connective tissue (see Table 25-1.)

Regardless of the cause of hypothyroidism and the age at which it occurs, the specific treatment is replacement of thyroid hormone from an exogenous source. Desiccated thyroid obtained from the thyroid glands of domestic animals has long been used for hypothyroidism and is the prototype thyroid drug. However, it has largely been replaced by synthetic preparations of the thyroid hormones. One of the difficulties with using thyroid is that potency is largely unpredictable. Thyroid is standardized only by its content of organic iodide. Preparations containing similar amounts of iodide may contain markedly different amounts of T_4 and T_3 and thus vary widely in biologic activity. Synthetic preparations are consistent in potency and clinical effects; they differ primarily in onset and duration of action.

The most clear-cut clinical indication for use of thyroid drugs is hypothyroidism manifested by signs and symptoms and confirmed by diagnostic tests of thyroid function. They may also be used to suppress secretion of thyrotropin by the anterior pituitary gland. In addition to these rational uses of thyroid drugs, they have often been used irrationally to treat obesity, menstrual disorders, male and female infertility, and fatigue. There is no evidence that thyroid drugs are beneficial in any of these situations unless hypothyroidism is present. Thyroid drugs should not be used in euthyroid clients (*i.e.*, those having a normally functioning thyroid gland).

Hyperthyroidism

Hyperthyroidism is characterized by excessive secretion of thyroid hormones. It may be associated with Graves' disease, nodular goiter, thyroiditis, overtreatment with thyroid drugs, functioning thyroid carcinoma, and pituitary adenoma that secretes excessive thyrotropin. Hyperthyroidism usually involves an enlarged thyroid gland that has an increased number of cells and an increased rate of secretion. The hyperplastic thyroid gland may secrete five to fifteen times the normal amount of thyroid hormone. As a result, body metabolism is greatly increased. Specific physiologic effects and clinical manifestations of hyperthyroidism are listed in Table 25-1. These effects vary, depending on the amount of circulating thyroid hormone, and they usually increase in incidence and severity over time if hyperthyroidism is not treated. Thyroid storm or thyrotoxic crisis is a rare but severe complication characterized by extreme symptoms of hyperthyroidism such as severe tachycardia, fever, dehydration, heart failure, and coma. It is most likely to occur in clients with hyperthyroidism that has been inadequately treated, especially when stressful situations occur (*e.g.*, trauma, infection, surgery, emotional upsets).

Hyperthyroidism is treated by antithyroid drugs, radioactive iodine, surgery, or a combination of these therapeutic methods. The drugs act by decreasing production or release of thyroid hormones. Radioactive iodine acts by emitting rays that destroy thyroid gland tissue. Subtotal thyroidectomy involves surgical excision of thyroid tissue. All these methods reduce the amount of thyroid hormones circulating in the bloodstream. No one method is clearly superior, and each has advantages and disadvantages.

Drug therapy is probably the treatment of choice, at least initially, for most clients. The antithyroid drugs include the thioamide derivatives (propylthiouracil and methimazole) and iodine preparations. The thioamide drugs are preferred by many physicians for clients up to age 30 years and possibly up to age 40. These drugs are inexpensive and relatively safe, and they do not damage the thyroid gland.

Although iodine preparations are the oldest antithyroid drugs, they are no longer used in long-term treatment of hyperthyroidism. They are indicated when a rapid clinical response is needed. For example, they can be used to treat thyroid storm and acute hyperthyroidism. They are also used in the preparation of a hyperthyroid person for thyroidectomy. A thioamide drug is given to produce a euthyroid state, and an iodine preparation is given to reduce the size and vascularity of the thyroid gland so that risk of excessive bleeding is reduced.

Iodine preparations inhibit release of thyroid hormones and cause them to be stored within the gland. They reduce blood levels of thyroid hormones more quickly than thioamide drugs or radioactive iodine. Maximal effects are reached in about 10 or 15 days of continuous therapy, and this is probably the primary advantage. Several disadvantages, however, include the following:

1. They may produce goiter, hypothyroidism, or both.
2. They cannot be used alone. Therapeutic benefits are temporary, and symptoms of hyperthyroidism may reappear and even be intensified if other treatment methods are not also used.
3. Radioactive iodine cannot be used effectively for a prolonged period in a client who has received iodine preparations. Even if the iodine preparation is discontinued, the thyroid gland is saturated with iodine and will not attract enough radioactive iodine for treatment to be effective. Also, if radioactive iodine is given later, acute hyperthyroidism is likely to result because the radioactive iodine causes the stored hormones to be released into the circulation.
4. Although giving a thioamide drug followed by an iodine preparation is standard preparation for thyroidectomy, the opposite sequence of administration is unsafe. That is, if the iodine preparation is given first and followed by propylthiouracil or methimazole, the client is likely to experience acute hyperthyroidism because the thioamide drug causes release of the stored thyroid hormones.

Propranolol is used as an adjunctive drug in the treatment of hyperthyroidism. It does not decrease blood levels of thyroid hormones but relieves tachycardia, cardiac palpitations, excessive sweating, and other symptoms. Propranolol is especially helpful during the several weeks required for therapeutic results from antithyroid drugs or from radioactive iodine administration.

Radioactive iodine is effective, inexpensive, and convenient. Probably its main disadvantage is eventual hypothyroidism. A second disadvantage is the delay in therapeutic benefits. Results may not be apparent for 3 months or longer, during which time severe hyperthyroidism must be brought under control with one of the thioamide antithyroid drugs.

Subtotal thyroidectomy is also effective in relieving hyperthyroidism, but this treatment method also has several disadvantages. First, preparation for surgery requires several weeks of drug therapy. Second, there are risks involved in anesthesia and surgery as well as potential postoperative complications. Third, there is a high risk of eventual hypothyroidism.

Individual drugs

THYROID AGENTS (DRUGS USED IN HYPOTHYROIDISM)

Desiccated thyroid tablets available for clinical use are produced from the thyroid glands of animals used for food. The preparation contains iodine, levothyroxine (T_4), thyroglobulin and triiodothyronine (T_3), which are normally present in the human thyroid gland. Thyroid is the prototype of thyroid drugs and the least expensive preparation. Despite some advantages, however, thyroid is becoming obsolete because it contains varying amounts of thyroid hormones. This preparation is standardized by organic iodine content, not the amount of T_4 or T_3 or metabolic potency. As a result, preparations may have similar amounts of iodine but very different amounts of the metabolically active T_4 and T_3. Therapeutic benefits may be lacking or unpredictable. **Thyroglobulin** (Proloid) is a purified extract of animal thyroid gland standardized according to iodine content. It is given in the same dosages as thyroid.

Route and dosage ranges

Adults: PO 16–32 mg daily initially, increased by 16–32 mg every 2 weeks until desired response is obtained; maintenance dose is usually 65–195 mg daily in a single dose

Older adults: PO 8–16 mg daily initially, doubled every 6–8 weeks until desired response is obtained

Children: PO 32–65 mg daily for infants up to 1 year of age; 65–195 mg daily for older children, depending on clinical response

Levothyroxine (Synthroid, Levothroid) is a synthetic preparation of T_4. It is more potent than thyroid, contains a uniform amount of hormone, and can be given parenterally. Compared with liothyronine, levothyroxine has a slower onset and longer duration of action. Levothyroxine is usually considered the drug of choice for long-term treatment of hypothyroidism.

Routes and dosage ranges

Adults: PO 0.05–0.1 mg daily initially, increased every 1–3 weeks until the desired response is obtained
Usual maintenance dose is 0.1–0.2 mg daily
Myxedema coma, IV 0.2–0.5 mg (0.1 mg/ml) in a single dose; 0.1–0.3 mg may be repeated on the second day if necessary

Older adults, clients with cardiac disorders, and clients with hypothyroidism of long duration: PO 0.0125–0.025 mg daily for 6 weeks, then dose is doubled every 6–8 weeks until the desired response is obtained
Myxedema coma, same as adult dosage

Children: PO no more than 0.05 mg daily initially, then increased by 0.05–0.1 mg every 2 weeks until the desired response is obtained; usual daily dosage range, 0.3–0.4 mg
Myxedema coma, same as adult dosage

Liothyronine (Cytomel) is a synthetic preparation of T_3. It is more potent than thyroid on a weight basis and contains a uniform amount of thyroid hormone. Compared with levothyroxine, liothyronine has a more rapid onset and shorter duration of action. Consequently, it may be more likely to produce high concentrations in blood and tissues and cause adverse reactions. Also, it requires more frequent administration if used for long-term treatment of hypothyroidism.

Route and dosage ranges

Adults: PO 25 μg daily initially, increased by 12.5–25 μg q1–2 weeks until desired response is obtained

Older adults: 2.5–5 μg daily for 3–6 weeks, then doubled q6 weeks until the desired response is obtained

Children: PO 5 μg daily initially, increased by 5 μg daily q3–4 days until the desired response is obtained. Doses as high as 20–80 μg may be required in cretinism.

Liotrix (Euthroid, Thyrolar) contains levothyroxine and liothyronine in a 4:1 ratio, resembling the makeup of natural thyroid hormone. The mixture has the same indications for use and the same adverse effects as desiccated thyroid tablets. Euthroid and Thyrolar are available in several different strengths ranging from 15 to 180 mg in thyroid equivalency. Euthroid-1 and Thyrolar-1 are equivalent to 60 mg (1 gr) of desiccated thyroid.

Route and dosage ranges

Adults: 15–30 mg daily initially, increased gradually every 1–2 weeks until response is obtained

Older adults, clients with cardiac disorders, and clients with hypothyroidism of long duration: one fourth to one half the usual adult dose initially, doubled every 8 weeks if necessary

Children: Same as adult dosage, increased every 2 weeks if necessary

ANTITHYROID AGENTS (DRUGS USED IN HYPERTHYROIDISM)

Propylthiouracil is the prototype of the thioamide antithyroid drugs. It can be used alone to treat hyperthyroidism, as part of the preoperative preparation for a thyroidectomy, before or after radioactive iodine therapy, and in the treatment of thyroid storm or thyrotoxic crisis. Propylthiouracil acts by inhibiting production of thyroid hormones and peripheral conversion of T_4 to the more active T_3. It does not interfere with release of thyroid hormones previously produced and stored. Thus, therapeutic effects do not occur for several days or weeks until the stored hormones have been used. **Methimazole** (Tapazole) is similar to propylthiouracil in actions, uses, and adverse reactions, except that it lacks peripheral activity.

Route and dosage ranges

Propylthiouracil

Adults: PO 300–400 mg daily, in divided doses q8h, until the client is euthyroid. Then 100–150 mg daily, in three divided doses, given for maintenance

Children over 10 years: PO 150–300 mg daily, in divided doses q8h; usual maintenance dose, 100–300 mg daily, in two divided doses, q12h

Children 6–10 years: 50–150 mg daily in divided doses q8h
Neonatal thyrotoxicosis, 10 mg/kg/day, in divided doses

Methimazole

Adults: PO 15–60 mg daily initially, in divided doses q8h until the client is euthyroid. For maintenance, 5–15 mg daily in 2–3 doses

Children: PO 0.4 mg/kg/day initially, in divided doses every 8 hours; maintenance dose, $\frac{1}{2}$ initial dose

Strong iodine solution (Lugol's solution) and **saturated solution of potassium iodide** (SSKI) are iodine preparations that are sometimes used in short-term treatment of hyperthyroidism. The drugs inhibit release of thyroid hormones, causing them to accumulate in the thyroid gland. Lugol's solution is generally used to treat thyrotoxic crisis and to decrease the size and vascularity of the thyroid gland before thyroidectomy. SSKI is more often used as an expectorant but may be given as preparation for thyroidectomy. Iodine preparations should not be followed by propylthiouracil, methimazole, or radioactive iodine because the latter drugs cause release of stored thyroid hormone and may precipitate acute hyperthyroidism. **Sodium iodide** may be given intravenously (IV) for thyrotoxic crisis.

Routes and dosage ranges

Strong iodine solution

Adults: PO 2–6 drops 3 times daily for 10 days before thyroidectomy
Children: Same as adult dosage

Potassium iodide solution

Adults: PO 5 drops 3 times daily for 10 days before thyroidectomy
Children: Same as adult dosage

Sodium iodide

Adults: Thyrotoxic crisis, IV 0.5–2 g every 2–6 days, if necessary

Sodium iodide ^{131}I (Iodotope) is a radioactive isotope of iodine. The thyroid gland cannot differentiate between regular iodide and radioactive iodide so it picks up the radioactive iodide from the circulating blood. As a result, small amounts of radioactive iodide can be used as a diagnostic test of thyroid function, and larger doses are used therapeutically to treat hyperthyroidism. Therapeutic doses act by emitting beta and gamma rays, which destroy thyroid tissue and thereby decrease production of thyroid hormones. It is also used to treat thyroid cancer.

Radioactive iodide is usually given in a single dose on an outpatient basis. For most clients, no special radiation precautions are necessary. If a very large dose is given, the client may be isolated for 8 days, which is the half-life of radioactive iodide. Therapeutic effects are delayed for several weeks or up to 6 months. During this time, symptoms may be controlled with thioamide drugs or propranolol. Radioactive iodide is usually given to middle-aged and elderly people; it should not be given during pregnancy and lactation.

Routes and dosage ranges

Adults and Children: PO, IV, dosage as calculated by a radiologist trained in nuclear medicine

Propranolol (Inderal) is an antiadrenergic, not an antithyroid, drug. It does not affect thyroid function, hormone secretion, or hormone metabolism. It is most often used to treat cardiovascular conditions such as arrhythmias, angina pectoris, and hypertension. When given to clients with hyperthyroidism, propranolol blocks beta-adrenergic receptors in various organs and thereby controls symptoms of hyperthyroidism resulting from excessive stimulation of the sympathetic nervous system. These symptoms include tachycardia, palpitations, excessive sweating (hyperhidrosis), tremors, and nervousness. Propranolol is useful for controlling symptoms during the delayed response to thioamide drugs and radioactive iodine, before thyroidectomy, and in treating thyrotoxic crisis. When the client becomes euthyroid and hyperthyroid symptoms are controlled by definitive treatment measures, propranolol should be discontinued.

Routes and dosage ranges

Adults: PO 40–160 mg daily in divided doses

Principles of therapy: thyroid and antithyroid drugs

THYROID DRUGS

Assessment guidelines for hypothyroidism

When thyroid drugs are given in the treatment of hypothyroidism, some guidelines include the following: Initially, assess for signs and symptoms of hypothyroidism (see Table 25-1). Also check diagnostic test reports when available. After drug therapy has been instituted, assess for therapeutic effects (euthyroidism) and adverse effects (hyperthyroidism).

Nursing interventions in hypothyroidism

Use nondrug measures to control symptoms of hypothyroidism, increase effectiveness of thyroid drug therapy, and decrease adverse reactions. Some helpful measures may include the following:

1. Provide warmth by regulating room temperature, adding blankets, or furnishing suitable clothes such as socks, robes, and sweaters. Clients with hypothyroidism are very intolerant of cold owing to their slow metabolism rate. Chilling and shivering should be prevented because of added strain on the heart.
2. Assist in implementing a low-calorie diet and weight reduction program. Most people with hy-

pothyroidism are overweight despite a poor appetite.

3. Use soap sparingly and lotions or other lubricants liberally when the client's skin is dry.
4. When edema is present, inspect pressure points, turn often, and avoid trauma when possible. Edema increases the likelihood of skin breakdown and decubitus ulcer formation. Also, increased capillary fragility increases the likelihood of bruising from seemingly minor trauma.
5. Encourage the client to force fluids and eat fruits, vegetables, and other foods that increase bulk and roughage in the gastrointestinal tract. These measures help to prevent constipation and fecal impactions, which are common in hypothyroidism and are related to decreased gastrointestinal secretion and motility.

Selection of thyroid drug

Choice of drug for thyroid hormone replacement is largely based on the physician's preference. All the drugs have similar pharmacologic characteristics and produce the same physiologic effects as the naturally occurring endogenous thyroid hormones.

For a client starting to receive thyroid replacement therapy, a synthetic preparation such as levothyroxine is probably preferable because of uniform potency. For a client who has been taking thyroid or thyroglobulin and has achieved adequate therapeutic effects, there would probably be no advantage in changing to a synthetic product. The drugs are inexpensive, so cost is rarely a significant factor.

Dosage factors

Dosage is influenced by the choice of drug, the client's age, general condition, severity and duration of hypothyroidism, and clinical response to drug therapy. Specific factors include the following:

1. Dosage must be individualized to approximate the amount of thyroid hormone needed to make up the deficit in endogenous hormone production.
2. As a general rule, initial dosage is relatively small. Dosage is gradually increased at about 2-week intervals in most clients until an optimum response is obtained and symptoms are relieved. Maintenance dosage for long-term therapy is based on the client's clinical status and periodic laboratory tests, such as measurement of serum T_3 and T_4.
3. Thyroid 60 mg, thyroglobulin 60 mg, levothyroxine 0.1 mg or less, and liothyronine 0.025 mg produce approximately the same clinical response.
4. Infants requiring thyroid hormone replacement need relatively large doses. After thyroid drugs are started, maintenance dosage is determined by periodic radioimmunoassay of serum T_4 and by periodic x-ray studies to follow bone development.
5. Clients who are elderly or have cardiovascular disease are given small initial doses. Also, increments are smaller and made at longer intervals, usually about 8 weeks. The primary reason for very cautious thyroid replacement in such clients is the high risk of adverse effects on the cardiovascular system.

Hypothyroidism and the metabolism of other drugs

Changes in the rate of body metabolism affect the metabolism of various drugs. Most drugs given to a client with hypothyroidism have a prolonged effect because drug metabolism in the liver is delayed and the glomerular filtration rate of the kidneys is decreased. Also, drug absorption from the gastrointestinal system or a parenteral injection site may be slowed. As a result, dosage of most other drugs should be reduced. For example, people with hypothyroidism are especially sensitive to narcotics, barbiturates and other sedative-type drugs, and anesthetics. If these drugs are necessary, they are given very cautiously and in dosages of about one third to one half the usual dose. Even then, clients must be observed very closely for respiratory depression.

Once thyroid replacement therapy is started and stabilized, the client becomes euthyroid, has a normal rate of metabolism, and can tolerate usual doses of most drugs if other influencing factors are not present. On the other hand, excessive doses of thyroid drugs may produce hyperthyroidism and a greatly increased rate of metabolism. In this instance, larger doses of most other drugs are necessary to produce the same effects. Rather than increasing dosage of other drugs, though, dosage of thyroid drugs should be reduced so that the client is euthyroid again.

Duration of replacement therapy

Thyroid replacement therapy in the client with hypothyroidism is lifelong. Medical supervision is needed frequently during early treatment and at least annually after the client's condition has stabilized and maintenance dosage has been determined.

Adrenal insufficiency

If adrenal insufficiency is present in a client who needs thyroid drugs, that insufficiency must be corrected by giving corticosteroid drugs before starting thyroid replacement, since thyroid hormones increase tissue metabolism and tissue demands for adrenocortical hormones. If adrenal insufficiency is not treated first, administration of thyroid hormone may cause acute adrenocortical insufficiency.

ANTITHYROID DRUGS

Assessment guidelines for hyperthyroidism

When antithyroid drugs and iodine preparations are given in the treatment of hyperthyroidism, some guidelines include the following. Initially, assess for signs and symptoms of hyperthyroidism (see Table 25-1). Also check diagnostic test reports when available. After drug therapy has been started, assess for therapeutic effects (euthyroidism) and adverse effects (hypothyroidism).

Nursing interventions in hyperthyroidism

Use nondrug measures to control symptoms of hyperthyroidism, increase effectiveness of antithyroid drug therapy, and decrease adverse reactions. Some helpful measures include the following:

1. Provide a cool environment and lightweight clothing. Clients with hyperthyroidism are very intolerant of heat and perspire excessively owing to their rapid metabolic rate. Cooling baths may also be helpful.
2. Assist in implementing a well-balanced diet containing extra calories and nutrients. Clients may need extra meals and between-meal snacks to satisfy hunger and prevent tissue breakdown. Usually, clients are hungry because of hyperactive metabolism, but they may still lose weight. Other dietary changes that may be helpful include avoiding highly seasoned and high-fiber foods because they may increase diarrhea and avoiding caffeine-containing beverages because they may aggravate the already overexcited state. Weigh every other day and report any weight loss.
3. Force fluids to 3000 to 4000 ml/day unless contraindicated by cardiac or renal disease. Large amounts of fluids are needed to eliminate heat and waste products produced by the hypermetabolic state. Much of the client's fluid loss is visible as excessive perspiration and urine output.
4. Assist in planning and implementing periods of rest and quiet, nonstrenuous activity. Since persons differ in what they find restful, this must be assessed with each client. A quiet room, reading, and soft music may be helpful. Mild sedative-type drugs are often given. The client with hyperthyroidism is caught in the dilemma of needing rest because of the high metabolic rate but being unable to rest because of nervousness and excitement.
5. In mild exophthalmos, use measures to protect the eyes. For example, dark glasses, local lubricants, and patching of the eyes at night may be needed. Diuretic drugs and elevating the head of the bed may help reduce periorbital edema and eyeball protrusion. If the client cannot close his eyelids, they are sometimes taped shut to avoid corneal ulceration. In severe exophthalmos, the above measures are taken, and large doses of corticosteroids are usually given.

Dosage factors

Dosage of the thioamide antithyroid drugs is relatively large until a euthyroid state is reached, in approximately 6 to 8 weeks. Then a maintenance dose, in the smallest amount that prevents recurrent symptoms of hyperthyroidism, is given for 1 year or longer. Dosage should be decreased if the thyroid gland enlarges or signs and symptoms of hypothyroidism occur.

Duration of antithyroid therapy

No clear-cut guidelines exist regarding duration of antithyroid drug therapy because exacerbations and remissions occur. It is usually continued until the client is euthyroid for 6 to 12 months. Then diagnostic tests to evaluate thyroid function or a trial withdrawal may be implemented to determine whether the client is likely to remain euthyroid without further drug therapy. If the drug is to be discontinued, this is usually done gradually over weeks or months.

Use in pregnancy

When iodine preparations and thioamide antithyroid drugs are used during pregnancy, they can cause goiter and hypothyroidism in the fetus or newborn.

Hyperthyroidism and the metabolism of other drugs

Treatment of hyperthyroidism changes the rate of body metabolism, including the rate of metabolism of many drugs. During the hyperthyroid state, drug metabolism may be very rapid, and higher doses of most drugs may be necessary to achieve therapeutic results. When the client becomes euthyroid, the rate of drug metabolism is decreased. Consequently, doses of all medications should be evaluated and probably reduced to avoid severe adverse reactions.

Iodine ingestion and hyperthyroidism

Iodine is present in foods, especially seafoods, in many medications used to treat pulmonary and other diseases (*e.g.*, Calcidrine, Organidin, Quadrinal), and in many contrast dyes used for gallbladder and other radiologic procedures. Ingestion of large amounts of iodine from these sources may result in goiter and hyperthyroidism. These conditions can develop in clients with no history of thyroid disease, but they are probably more likely in those with underlying thyroid problems.

NURSING ACTIONS: THYROID AND ANTITHYROID DRUGS

Nursing Actions	*Rationale/Explanation*
1. Administer accurately	
a. With thyroid drugs	
(1) Administer in a single daily dose, usually before breakfast.	This allows peak drug activity during daytime hours and is less likely to interfere with sleep.
(2) Check the pulse rate before giving the drug. If the rate is over 100 per minute or if any changes in cardiac rhythm are noted, consult the physician before giving the dose.	Tachycardia or other cardiac arrhythmias may indicate adverse cardiac effects. Dosage may need to be reduced or the drug stopped temporarily.
b. With antithyroid and iodine drugs	
(1) Administer q8h	All these drugs have rather short half-lives and must be given frequently and regularly to maintain therapeutic blood levels. In addition, if iodine preparations are not given every 8 hours, symptoms of hyperthyroidism may recur.
(2) Dilute iodine solutions in a full glass of fruit juice or milk, if possible, and have the client drink the medication through a straw.	Dilution of the drug reduces gastric irritation and masks the unpleasant taste. Using a straw prevents staining the teeth.
2. Observe for therapeutic effects	
a. With thyroid drugs, observe for	
(1) Increased energy and activity level, less lethargy and fatigue (2) Increased alertness and interest in surroundings (3) Increased appetite (4) Increased pulse rate and temperature (5) Decreased constipation (6) Reversal of coarseness and other changes in skin and hair (7) With cretinism, increased growth rate (record height periodically) (8) With myxedema, diuresis, weight loss, and decreased edema (9) Increased serum T_4	Therapeutic effects result from a return to normal metabolic activities and relief of the symptoms of hypothyroidism. Therapeutic effects may be evident as early as 2 or 3 days after drug therapy is started or delayed up to about 2 weeks. All signs and symptoms of myxedema should disappear in about 3 to 12 weeks.
(10) Decreased serum cholesterol and possibly decreased creatine phosphokinase, lactic dehydrogenase, and serum glutamic-oxaloacetic transaminase	These tests are often elevated with myxedema and may return to normal when thyroid replacement therapy is begun.
b. With antithyroid and iodine drugs, observe for	
(1) Slower pulse rate (2) Slower speech (3) More normal activity level (slowing of hyperactivity) (4) Decreased nervousness	With propylthiouracil and methimazole, some therapeutic effects are apparent in 1 or 2 weeks, but euthyroidism may not occur for 6 or 8 weeks. With iodine solutions, therapeutic effects may be apparent within 24 hours. Maximal effects occur in about 10 to 15

Nursing Actions	***Rationale/Explanation***
(5) Decreased tremors (6) Improved ability to sleep and rest (7) Weight gain	days. However, therapeutic effects may not be sustained. Symptoms may reappear if the drug is given longer than a few weeks, and they may be more severe than initially.
3. Observe for adverse effects	
a. With thyroid drugs, observe for tachycardia and other cardiac arrhythmias, angina pectoris, myocardial infarction, congestive heart failure, nervousness, hyperactivity, insomnia, diarrhea, abdominal cramps, nausea and vomiting, weight loss, fever, intolerance to heat.	Most adverse reactions stem from excessive doses, and signs and symptoms produced are the same as those occurring with hyperthyroidism. Excessive thyroid hormones make the heart work very hard and fast in attempting to meet tissue demands for oxygenated blood and nutrients. Symptoms of myocardial ischemia occur when the myocardium does not get an adequate supply of oxygenated blood. Symptoms of congestive heart failure occur when the increased cardiac workload is prolonged. Cardiovascular problems are more likely to occur in clients who are elderly or who already have heart disease.
b. With propylthiouracil and methimazole, observe for (1) Hypothyroidism—bradycardia, congestive heart failure, anemia, coronary artery and peripheral vascular disease, slow speech and movements, emotional and mental dullness, excessive sleeping, weight gain, constipation, skin changes, and others	
(2) Blood disorders—leukopenia, agranulocytosis, hypoprothrombinemia	Leukopenia may be difficult to evaluate because it may occur with hyperthyroidism as well as with antithyroid drugs. Agranulocytosis occurs rarely but is the most severe adverse reaction; the earliest symptoms are likely to be sore throat and fever. If these occur, report them to the physician immediately.
(3) Integumentary system—skin rash, pruritus, alopecia (4) CNS—headache, dizziness, loss of sense of taste, drowsiness, paresthesias (5) Gastrointestinal system—nausea, vomiting, abdominal discomfort, gastric irritation, cholestatic hepatitis (6) Other—lymphadenopathy, edema, joint pain, drug fever	
c. With iodine preparations, observe for (1) Iodism—metallic taste, burning in mouth, soreness of gums, excessive salivation, gastric or respiratory irritation, rhinitis, headache, redness of conjunctiva, edema of eyelids	Adverse effects are uncommon with short-term use.
(2) Hypersensitivity—acneiform skin rash, pruritus, fever, jaundice, angioedema, serum sickness	Allergic reactions rarely occur.
(3) Goiter with hypothyroidism	Uncommon but may occur in adults and newborns whose mothers have taken iodides for long periods
4. Observe for drug interactions	
a. Drugs that *increase* effects of thyroid hormones (1) Antidepressants (tricyclic), epinephrine, levarterenol	These drugs primarily increase catecholamines. When combined with thyroid hormones, excessive cardiovascular stimulation may occur and cause myocardial ischemia, cardiac arrhythmias, hypertension, and other adverse cardiovascular effects.
(2) Clofibrate, phenobarbital, and phenytoin	Potentiate thyroid drugs by displacement from plasma protein binding sites or by slowing liver metabolism

Nursing Actions	Rationale/Explanation
b. Drugs that *decrease* effects of thyroid hormones	
(1) Antihypertensives	These agents decrease the cardiovascular effects of catecholamines (epinephrine and norepinephrine) and thyroid hormone so that angina pectoris is less likely to occur.
(2) Cholestyramine resin (Questran)	This drug decreases gastrointestinal absorption of thyroid hormones. Cholestyramine binds both T_4 and T_3 almost irreversibly. If it is necessary to give these drugs concurrently, give the resin at least 4 or 5 hours before or after giving the thyroid drug.
(3) Estrogens, including oral contraceptives containing estrogens	Estrogens inhibit thyroid hormones by increasing thyroxine-binding globulin. This serves to increase the amount of bound, inactive thyroid hormone in clients with hypothyroidism. This decreased effect does not occur in clients with adequate thyroid hormone secretion because the increased binding is offset by increased T_4 production. Women taking oral contraceptives may need larger doses of thyroid hormone replacement than would otherwise be needed.
(4) Propranolol (Inderal)	This drug decreases cardiac effects of thyroid hormones. It is used in hyperthyroidism to reduce tachycardia and other symptoms of excessive cardiovascular stimulation.
c. Drugs that *increase* effects of antithyroid drugs	
(1) Chlorpromazine, phenylbutazone, sulfonamides, oral antidiabetic drugs, xanthines	Increased risk of goiter
(2) Lithium	Acts synergistically to produce hypothyroidism
5. Teach clients	
a. Take thyroid and antithyroid drugs as directed.	Thyroid replacement hormones must be continued throughout life. Thioamide antithyroid drugs must be taken 1 year or longer.
b. Report adverse effects (hyperthyroidism, hypothyroidism, iodism, and others).	Drug dosage may need to be reduced or the drug discontinued.
c. Avoid over-the-counter drugs or consult with physician before taking them.	Many preparations contain iodide, which can increase the likelihood of goiter with thioamides and the risk of adverse reactions from excessive doses of iodide. For example, cough syrups, some asthma medications, and some multivitamins contain iodide.
d. Ask the physician if it is necessary to avoid or restrict amounts of seafoods or iodized salt.	These sources of iodide may need to be reduced or omitted during antithyroid drug therapy.

Selected References

American Medical Association (AMA) Division of Drugs: AMA Drug Evaluations, 5th ed. New York, John Wiley & Sons, 1983

Cooper DS: Antithyroid drugs. N Engl J Med 311:1353–1362, 1984

Facts and Comparisons. St. Louis, J B Lippincott (Updated monthly)

Guyton AC: Textbook of Medical Physiology, 7th ed. Philadelphia, W B Saunders, 1986

Haynes RC Jr, Murad F: Thyroid and antithyroid drugs. In Gilman AG, Goodman LS, Rall TW, Murad F (eds): The Pharmacological Basis of Therapeutics, 7th ed., pp 1389–1411. New York, Macmillan, 1985.

Potency of oral thyroxine preparations. Med Lett Drugs Ther 26:41, 1984

Rodman MJ, Karch AM, Boyd EH, Smith DW: Pharmacology and Drug Therapy in Nursing, 3rd ed. Philadelphia, J B Lippincott, 1985

26

HORMONES THAT REGULATE CALCIUM AND PHOSPHORUS METABOLISM

Description and uses

Calcium and phosphorus metabolism is regulated primarily by three hormones: parathyroid hormone, calcitonin, and vitamin D. These hormones are interrelated in a complex homeostatic mechanism whose main goal is to maintain normal serum levels of calcium.

PARATHYROID HORMONE

Parathyroid hormone, also called parathormone, is secreted by the parathyroid glands, located immediately behind the thyroid gland. The primary function of parathyroid hormone is to maintain normal calcium levels in the serum or extracellular fluid. Parathyroid hormone secretion is stimulated by low serum calcium levels and inhibited by normal or high levels. Thus, secretion is controlled by a negative feedback system, as are most other hormonal secretions. Because phosphate is closely related to calcium in body functions, parathyroid hormone also regulates phosphate metabolism. As a general rule, when serum calcium levels go up, serum phosphate levels go down, and vice versa. Thus, an inverse relationship between calcium and phosphate is maintained.

When the serum calcium level falls below the normal range, parathyroid hormone raises the level by acting on bone, intestines, and kidneys. The effect of parathyroid hormone on bone is to increase bone breakdown or resorption, thereby causing calcium to move from bone into the serum. The effect on intestines is to increase absorption of calcium ingested in food, and the effect on the kidneys is to increase reabsorption of calcium in the renal tubules. The net result of these mechanisms is increased serum calcium and decreased urinary calcium. The opposite effects occur with phosphate; that is, parathyroid hormone decreases serum phosphate and increases urinary phosphate levels.

Disorders of parathyroid function are related to deficient production of parathyroid hormone (hypoparathyroidism) or excessive production (hyperparathyroidism). Hypoparathyroidism is most often caused by removal of or damage to the parathyroid glands during thyroidectomy or other neck surgery. There are normally four parathyroid glands. Removal of two causes little, if any, change in normal function. If even a small amount of parathyroid tissue remains, a transient hypoparathyroidism may occur, but the tissue usually enlarges and secretes sufficient parathyroid hormone to meet body requirements. Hyperparathyroidism is most often caused by a tumor or hyperplasia of one of the glands. It may also result from ectopic secretion of parathyroid hormone by malignant tumors (*e.g.*, carcinomas of the lung, pancreas, kidney, ovary, prostate gland, or bladder).

Clinical manifestations and treatment of hypoparathyroidism are the same as those of hypocalcemia, which is discussed later in this chapter. Treatment of hypocalcemia includes a calcium preparation and perhaps vitamin D. Clinical manifestations of hyperparathyroidism are those of hypercalcemia, discussed in the second half of this chapter. When hypercalcemia is caused by a tumor of parathyroid tissue, the usual treatment of choice is surgical excision. When it is caused by malignant tumor, treatment of the tumor with surgery, irradiation, or chemotherapy may reduce production of parathyroid hormone.

CALCITONIN

Calcitonin is a hormone secreted by the thyroid gland. Its secretion is controlled by the concentration of ionized calcium in the blood flowing through the thyroid gland. When the serum level of ionized calcium is increased, secretion of calcitonin is increased. Calcitonin lowers serum calcium levels primarily by decreasing movement of calcium from bone to serum. Calcitonin also increases renal excretion of calcium, phosphate, sodium, and chloride, but its primary function is to lower serum calcium in the presence of hypercalcemia. Its action is rapid but of short duration. Thus, it has little effect on long-term calcium metabolism. A synthetic preparation of calcitonin (Calcimar) is available for clinical use in the treatment of hypercalcemia and Paget's disease.

VITAMIN D

Vitamin D is a fat-soluble vitamin obtained from foods and exposure of skin to sunlight. It has many characteristics of a hormone as well. Whether considered a vitamin or hormone, vitamin D plays an important role in calcium metabolism. The main action of vitamin D is to raise serum calcium levels by increasing intestinal absorption of dietary calcium and probably by mobilizing calcium from bone. Vitamin D is not physiologically active in the body. It must be converted to an active metabolite (1,25-dihydroxycholecalciferol) by a series of reactions in the liver and kidneys. Parathyroid hormone and adequate renal function are required to produce the active metabolite.

The recommended daily intake of vitamin D for all age groups is 400 units. Milk that has been fortified with vitamin D is the best food source. Exposure of skin to sunlight is also needed to supply adequate amounts of vitamin D.

Deficiency of vitamin D causes inadequate absorption of calcium and phosphorus. This, in turn, leads to low levels of serum calcium and stimulation of parathyroid hormone secretion, which raises serum calcium levels by moving calcium from bone into serum. In children, this sequence of events produces inadequate mineralization of bone (rickets), a condition now rare in the United States. In adults, vitamin D deficiency causes osteomalacia, a condition characterized by decreased bone density and strength. Osteomalacia is more likely to occur during times of increased need for calcium, such as pregnancy and lactation.

Clinical indications for use of vitamin D supplements include prevention and treatment of rickets and osteomalacia, treatment of hypoparathyroidism, and treatment of chronic hypocalcemia when calcium supplements fail to maintain normal serum calcium levels. The major adverse reaction resulting from high dosage or prolonged administration is hypervitaminosis D. This condition of excessive accumulation of vitamin D produces signs and symptoms of hypercalcemia. The first step in treatment is to stop the administration of vitamin D. Other treatment measures are the same as for hypercalcemia from other causes and are described later in this chapter.

CALCIUM AND PHOSPHORUS

Calcium and phosphorus are discussed together because they are closely related in terms of body function. They are both required, as calcium phosphate, in formation and maintenance of bones and teeth. They are also found in many of the same foods, are absorbed together, and are both regulated by parathyroid hormone.

Calcium

1. Calcium is the most abundant cation in the body. Approximately 98% of calcium is located in the bones and teeth. The remainder is located in the extracellular fluid and soft tissues. About half the total serum calcium is ionized and physiologically active. This seemingly small amount of calcium performs vital functions. Small fluctuations in the amount of ionized calcium have profound effects on body organs. The other half of serum calcium is bound, mostly to serum proteins, and is physiologically inactive. There is constant shifting of calcium

among the different forms. This is part of the homeostatic mechanism that acts to maintain serum calcium levels at about 8.5 mg to 10 mg/100 ml.

2. Calcium performs vital functions in the body, among which are the following:
   a. Building and maintaining bones and teeth. Bone calcium is mainly composed of calcium phosphate and calcium carbonate. In addition to these bound forms, a small amount of calcium is available for exchange with serum. This acts as a reserve supply of calcium. Calcium is constantly shifting between bone and serum as bone is formed and broken down. Calcium is taken from the serum and used in the formation of new bone by osteoblast cells; it is transferred from bone to the serum when bone is broken down by osteoclast cells. The latter process is called *bone resorption.* When serum calcium levels become low, calcium moves into serum at the expense of bone calcium.
   b. Participating in many metabolic processes. Calcium regulates cell membrane permeability, excitability of nerve fibers, transmission of nerve impulses, muscle contraction, blood coagulation, and hormone and enzyme activities.
3. The calcium requirement of normal adults is approximately 1000 mg daily. Increased amounts, about 1200 mg daily, are required by growing children and pregnant or lactating women, and 1500 mg daily is recommended for postmenopausal women who do not take replacement estrogens, to prevent osteoporosis.

   The best source of calcium is milk or milk products. Three 8-ounce glasses of milk daily contain approximately the amount needed by healthy adults. Calcium in milk is readily used by the body because milk also contains lactose and vitamin D, both of which are involved in calcium absorption. Other sources of calcium include vegetables (*e.g.,* broccoli, spinach, kale, mustard greens) and seafoods (*e.g.,* clams, oysters).

   Only about 30% of dietary calcium is absorbed. Some factors that aid calcium absorption include the presence of vitamin D, increased acidity of gastric secretions, the presence of lactose, moderate amounts of fat, high protein intake, and a physiologic need. Factors that inhibit calcium absorption include the following: vitamin D deficiency; high-fat diet, which leads to formation of insoluble calcium salts in the intestine; the presence of oxalic acid (from beet greens, chard), which combines with calcium to form insoluble calcium oxalate in the intestine; alkalinity of intestinal secretions, which leads to formation of insoluble calcium phosphate; diarrhea or other conditions of rapid intestinal motility, which do not allow sufficient time for absorption; immobilization; and mental or emotional stress.

   Calcium is lost from the body in feces, urine, and sweat. In lactating women, relatively large amounts are lost in breast milk.

Phosphorus

1. Phosphorus is the second most abundant cation in the body and one of the most essential elements in normal body function. Most phosphorus is combined with calcium in bones and teeth as calcium phosphate (about 80%). The remainder is distributed in every body cell and in extracellular fluid. It is combined with carbohydrates, lipids, proteins, and a variety of other compounds.
2. Most phosphorus is located intracellularly (as the phosphate ion), where it performs many metabolic functions:
   a. It is an essential component of deoxyribonucleic acid (DNA), ribonucleic acid (RNA), and other nucleic acids in body cells. Thus, it makes replication of cells and body growth possible.
   b. It combines with fatty acids to form phospholipids, which are required in the structure of all cell membranes in the body. This reaction also prevents excessive amounts of free fatty acids.
   c. It forms a phosphate buffer system, which helps to maintain acid-base balance. When excess hydrogen ions are present in kidney tubules, phosphate combines with them and allows their excretion in urine. At the same time, bicarbonate is retained by the kidneys and contributes to alkalinity of body fluids. Although there are other buffering systems in the body, failure of the phosphate system leads to metabolic acidosis (retained hydrogen ions or acid and lost bicarbonate ions or base).
   d. It is necessary for cell utilization of glucose and production of energy.
   e. It is necessary for proper function of several B vitamins; that is, the vitamins function as coenzymes in various chemical reactions only when combined with phosphate.
3. Daily requirements for phosphorus are about 800 mg for normal adults and about 1200 mg for growing children and pregnant or lactating women. Phosphorus is widely available in foods. Good sources are milk and dairy products, meat,

poultry, fish, eggs, and nuts. There is little risk of phosphorus deficiency with an adequate intake of calcium and protein.

About 70% of dietary phosphorus is absorbed from the gastrointestinal tract. The most efficient absorption occurs when calcium and phosphorus are ingested in approximately equal amounts. Because this equal ratio is present in milk, milk is probably the best source of phosphorus. Generally, factors that increase or decrease calcium absorption act the same way on phosphorus absorption. Vitamin D enhances, but is not essential for, phosphorus absorption. Large amounts of calcium or aluminum in the gastrointestinal tract may combine with phosphate to form insoluble compounds and thereby decrease absorption of phosphorus.

Phosphorus is lost from the body primarily in urine. In clients with chronic renal failure, phosphorus intake is restricted because excretion is impaired.

HYPOCALCEMIA

Hypocalcemia may result from several causes, including inadequate dietary intake of calcium and vitamin D, inadequate absorption of calcium and vitamin D with diarrhea or malabsorption syndromes, hypoparathyroidism, impaired renal function, and transfusions of large amounts of citrated blood. Hypocalcemia associated with renal failure is caused by two mechanisms. First, inability to excrete phosphate in urine leads to accumulation of phosphate in the blood (hyperphosphatemia). Because phosphate levels are inversely related to calcium levels, hyperphosphatemia induces hypocalcemia. Second, when kidney function is impaired, vitamin D conversion to its active metabolite is impaired. This results in decreased intestinal absorption of calcium.

Clinical manifestations of hypocalcemia are characterized by increased neuromuscular irritability, which may progress to tetany. Tetany is characterized by numbness and tingling of the lips, fingers, and toes; twitching of facial muscles; spasms of skeletal muscle; carpopedal spasm; laryngospasm; and convulsions. In young children, hypocalcemia may be manifested by convulsions rather than tetany and erroneously diagnosed as epilepsy. This may be a serious error because anticonvulsant drugs used for epilepsy may further decrease serum calcium levels.

Individual drugs used in hypocalcemia

The drugs used to treat hypocalcemia are calcium and vitamin D preparations (Table 26-1). Several calcium salts may be used, intravenously for acute hypocalcemia and orally for less severe or chronic hypocalcemia. These preparations differ mainly in the amounts of calcium they contain and the routes by which they may be given. Vitamin D is used in chronic hypocalcemia if calcium preparations alone are unable to maintain serum calcium levels within normal range.

Principles of therapy: drugs used in hypocalcemia

ASSESSMENT GUIDELINES

Assess for current or potential hypocalcemia.

1. Observe for the previously described clinical manifestations.
2. Check serum calcium reports for decreased values. Although laboratories differ slightly in normal values, normal serum calcium level is approximately 8.5–10 mg/100 ml.
3. Check once daily for Chvostek's sign: tap the facial nerve just below the temple, in front of the ear. If facial muscles twitch, hyperirritability of the nerve and potential tetany are indicated.
4. Check for Trousseau's sign: constrict blood circulation in an arm (usually done with a blood pressure cuff) for 3 to 5 minutes. This produces ischemia and increased irritability of peripheral nerves, which causes spasms of the lower arm and hand muscles (carpal spasm) if tetany is present.

DIETARY PREVENTIVE MEASURES

Prevent hypocalcemia when possible by assisting the client to maintain an adequate dietary intake of calcium. The best dietary source is milk and other dairy products. Unless contraindicated by the client's condition, teach the client to drink at least two 8-ounce glasses of milk daily. This will furnish about half the daily calcium requirement; the remainder will probably be obtained from other foods. During the rapid growth period in children and during pregnancy or

TABLE 26-1. DRUGS USED IN HYPOCALCEMIA

	Generic name	Trade name	Routes and dosage ranges: Adults	Routes and dosage ranges: Children
Calcium preparations	Calcium carbonate, precipitated (40% calcium)	Os-Cal 500	PO 1–1.5 g 3 times daily with meals (maximal daily dose, 8 g)	
	Calcium chloride (27% calcium)		PO 6–8 g daily in 4 divided doses IV 500 mg–1 g (5–10 ml of 10% solution) by slow injection	PO 300 mg/kg/day of a 2% solution in 4 divided doses
	Calcium glubionate (6% calcium)	Neo-Calglucon	PO 15 ml 3 times daily Pregnancy or lactation, PO 15 ml 4 times daily	PO 10 ml 3 times daily
	Calcium gluceptate (8% calcium)		IV 5–20 ml IM 2–5 ml	IM 2–5 ml
	Calcium gluconate (9% calcium)	Kalcinate	PO 1–2 g 3–4 times daily IV 5–20 ml of 10% solution	PO, IV 500 mg/kg/day in divided doses
	Calcium lactate (13% calcium)		PO 1–3 g 3 times daily with meals	PO 500 mg/kg/day in divided doses
	Calcium phosphate dibasic (30% calcium)	Dical-D	PO 0.5–1.5 g 2–3 times daily with meals	Dosage not established
Vitamin D preparations	Calcifediol	Calderol	PO 50–100 μg daily	Dosage not established
	Calcitriol	Rocaltrol	PO 0.25 μg daily initially, then adjusted according to serum calcium levels (usual daily maintenance dose, 0.5–1 μg)	
	Dihydrotachysterol	Hytakerol	PO 0.8–2.4 mg daily, then decreased for maintenance according to serum calcium levels (usual daily maintenance dose, 0.2–1.0 mg)	
	Ergocalciferol (vitamin D)	Drisdol	PO 50,000–200,000 units daily initially (average daily maintenance dose, 25,000–100,000 units)	

lactation, about four glasses of milk or milk plus other calcium-containing foods are needed to meet increased needs. Some dietary supplements of vitamins and minerals contain only 250 mg of a calcium salt. This does not go very far in meeting a requirement of about 1200 mg. With an adequate protein and calcium intake, a sufficient amount of phosphorus will also be obtained.

TREATMENT OF HYPOCALCEMIA

1. If hypocalcemia is caused by diarrhea or malabsorption, treatment of the underlying condition will decrease loss of calcium from the body and increase absorption.
2. In severe, acute hypocalcemia, intravenous calcium gluconate is usually the drug of choice. For less acute situations or for long-term treatment of chronic hypocalcemia, oral calcium supplements are preferred. Vitamin D is given also if a calcium preparation alone is unable to maintain serum calcium levels within a normal range.
3. When vitamin D is given to treat hypocalcemia, dosage is determined by frequent measurement of serum calcium levels. Usually, higher doses are given initially, then decreased to smaller doses for maintenance therapy.

CALCIUM/VITAMIN D COMBINATIONS

Calcium salts and vitamin D are combined in a number of commercial preparations. These are promoted as dietary supplements for children and for women during pregnancy and lactation. There is no evidence that these fixed amounts of calcium and vitamin D meet the dietary needs of most people. Therefore, calcium and vitamin D should be prescribed individually. Also, these mixtures are not indicated for maintenance therapy in chronic hypocalcemia.

DRUG INTERACTIONS

1. Calcium preparations and digitalis preparations have similar effects on the myocardium. Therefore, if calcium is given to a digitalized client the risks of digitalis toxicity and cardiac arrhythmias are increased. Such usage must be done very cautiously.
2. Oral calcium preparations decrease effects of oral tetracycline drugs by combining with the antibiotic and preventing its absorption. They should not be given at the same time or within 2 to 3 hours of each other.

NURSING ACTIONS: DRUGS USED IN HYPOCALCEMIA

Nursing Actions	*Rationale/Explanation*
1. Administer accurately	
a. Give oral calcium preparations 30 minutes before meals or at bedtime.	To increase absorption
b. With intravenous (IV) calcium preparations, inject slowly, over at least 2 minutes, check pulse and blood pressure closely, and preferably monitor the electrocardiogram (ECG).	Arrhythmias and hypotension may occur. Hypercalcemia is indicated on the ECG by a prolonged QT interval associated with an inverted T wave.
c. Do not mix IV calcium preparations with any other drug in the same syringe.	Calcium reacts with some other drugs and forms a precipitate.
2. Observe for therapeutic effects	
a. Relief of symptoms of neuromuscular irritability and tetany, such as decreased muscle spasms and decreased paresthesias	
b. Serum calcium levels within normal range (8.5 to 10 mg/100 ml)	
c. Absence of Chvostek's and Trousseau's signs	
3. Observe for adverse effects	
a. Hypercalcemia (1) Gastrointestinal effects—anorexia, nausea, vomiting, abdominal pain, constipation (2) Central nervous system (CNS) effects—apathy, poor memory, depression, drowsiness, disorientation, coma (3) Other effects—weakness and decreased tone in skeletal and smooth muscles, dysphagia, polyuria, polydipsia, cardiac arrhythmias (4) Increased serum calcium	
b. Hypervitaminosis D—produces hypercalcemia and the clinical manifestations listed above	This is most likely to occur with chronic ingestion of 50,000 or more units of vitamin D daily. In children, accidental ingestion may lead to acute toxicity.
4. Observe for drug interactions	
a. Drugs that *increase* effects of calcium	
(1) Vitamin D	Increases intestinal absorption of calcium from both dietary and supplemental drug sources

Nursing Actions	***Rationale/Explanation***
b. Drugs that *decrease* effects of calcium	
(1) Adrenocorticosteroids (prednisone, others), calcitonin, mithramycin, and phosphates	These drugs lower serum calcium levels by various mechanisms. They are used in the treatment of hypercalcemia and are discussed further in the next section of this chapter.
(2) Antacids	Oral calcium preparations are more soluble and better absorbed in an acid medium. Antacids decrease acidity of gastric secretions and therefore may decrease absorption of calcium.
(3) Laxatives	These drugs decrease absorption of calcium from the intestinal tract by increasing motility. This allows less time for calcium absorption.
c. Drugs that *increase* effects of vitamin D	
(1) Thiazide diuretics	Thiazide diuretics administered to hypoparathyroid clients may cause hypercalcemia (potentiate vitamin D effects).
d. Drugs that *decrease* effects of vitamin D	
(1) Anticonvulsants (*e.g.,* phenytoin [Dilantin], primidone [Mysoline], phenobarbital)	These drugs accelerate and change the metabolism of vitamin D in the liver. As a result, vitamin D deficiency, hypocalcemia, and rickets or osteomalacia are likely to develop in clients receiving anticonvulsant drugs for seizure disorders. These problems can be prevented by increasing intake of vitamin D.
(2) Cholestyramine resin (Questran)	May decrease intestinal absorption of calcitriol (Rocaltrol).
(3) Mineral oil	Mineral oil is a fat and therefore combines with fat-soluble vitamins, such as vitamin D, and prevents its absorption from the gastrointestinal tract.
5. Teach clients	
a. Do not take calcium or vitamin D unless prescribed by a physician.	These substances are not usually needed if dietary intake is adequate. Taking more than needed to maintain normal body function serves no beneficial purpose and may lead to serious problems.
b. If calcium or vitamin D is prescribed, take as directed.	To obtain the greatest therapeutic effect with the least likelihood of adverse effects from overdosage.
c. With chronic hypocalcemia, increase dietary intake of calcium and vitamin D with milk and other dairy products. Note that foods that contain oxalic acid (*e.g.,* spinach, rhubarb) and phytic acid (*e.g.,* bran) may decrease absorption of calcium.	
d. Report signs and symptoms of hypercalcemia.	See 3(a) above.

HYPERCALCEMIA

Hypercalcemia occurs with hyperparathyroidism, excessive ingestion of vitamin D, multiple myeloma and several other malignant neoplasms, prolonged immobilization, and adrenocortical insufficiency.

Clinical manifestations are caused by decreased ability of nerves to respond to stimuli and decreased ability of muscles to contract and relax. Hypercalcemia has a depressant effect on nerve and muscle function.

Gastrointestinal problems with hypercalcemia include anorexia, nausea, vomiting, constipation, and abdominal pain. CNS problems include apathy, depression, poor memory, headache, and drowsiness. Severe hypercalcemia may produce lethargy, syncope, disorientation, hallucinations, coma, and death. Other signs and symptoms include weakness and decreased tone in skeletal and smooth muscle, dysphagia, polyuria, polyphagia, and cardiac arrhythmias. In addition, calcium may be deposited in various tissues, such as the conjunctiva, cornea, and kidneys. Calcium deposits in the kidneys (renal calculi) may lead to irreversible damage and impairment of function.

Individual drugs used in hypercalcemia

The agents used in hypercalcemia belong to several therapeutic classes and act by different mechanisms to lower serum calcium levels.

Calcitonin-salmon (Calcimar) is a drug used in the treatment of hypercalcemia, Paget's disease, and postmenopausal osteoporosis. In hypercalcemia, calcitonin lowers serum calcium levels by inhibiting bone resorption, (*i.e.*, movement of calcium from bone to serum). It is most likely to be effective in hypercalcemia caused by hyperparathyroidism, prolonged immobilization, or certain malignant neoplasms. In acute hypercalcemia, calcitonin may be used along with other measures to rapidly lower serum calcium levels. In chronic hypercalcemia, it may lose its effectiveness after several weeks.

Paget's disease is a disorder characterized by an abnormal and rapid rate of bone formation and breakdown. Calcitonin slows the rate of bone turnover, improves bone lesions on radiologic examination, and relieves bone pain. In postmenopausal osteoporosis, calcitonin prevents further bone loss and increases bone mass in the presence of adequate calcium and vitamin D.

Routes and dosage ranges

Adults: Hypercalcemia, SC, IM 4 MRC (Medical Research Council) units/kg q12h. Can be increased after 1–2 days to 8 MRC units/kg q12h. Maximal dose, 8 MRC units/kg q6h
Paget's disease, SC, IM, 50–100 MRC units daily
Postmenopausal osteoporosis, SC, IM 100 MRC units daily (along with supplemental calcium [1500 mg] and vitamin D [400 units] daily)

Etidronate (Didronel) is a nonhormonal substance, similar to calcitonin, that decreases the rate of bone turnover. Etidronate is used in the symptomatic treatment of Paget's disease and heterotopic ossification (growth of bone in abnormal locations) associated with spinal cord injury or total hip replacement. It is *not* used in the treatment of hypercalcemia. The drug is excreted by the kidneys, and dosage must be reduced in the presence of renal insufficiency.

Route and dosage ranges

Adults: Paget's disease, PO 5 mg/kg/day for periods up to 6 months. The course of therapy may be repeated if symptoms recur. Heterotopic ossification caused by spinal cord injury, PO 20 mg/kg/day for 2 weeks, then 10 mg/kg/day for 10 weeks
Heterotopic ossification associated with total hip replacement, PO 20 mg/kg/day for 1 month preoperatively and continued for 3 months postoperatively

Furosemide (Lasix) is a potent diuretic that increases calcium excretion in urine by preventing its reabsorption in renal tubules. Furosemide can be given IV for rapid effects in hypercalcemic crises or orally for nonemergency situations. (See Chapter 56 for further discussion of diuretic drug therapy.)

Route and dosage ranges

Adults: IV 80–100 mg q2h until a diuretic response is obtained or other treatment measures are initiated
Children: IV 20–40 mg q4h until a diuretic response is obtained or other treatment measures are initiated

Hydrocortisone (Solu-Cortef and others) and **prednisone** (Deltasone and others) are adrenal corticosteroid drugs that may be used to treat hypercalcemia. Since all the glucocorticoids have similar effects, others may be used. In the treatment of hypercalcemia, corticosteroid drugs antagonize effects of vitamin D and therefore decrease intestinal absorption of calcium. They are probably most useful in treating hypercalcemia resulting from excess vitamin D, sarcoidosis, and renal insufficiency. They may also be useful in treating hypercalcemia due to malignant neoplasms (*e.g.*, multiple myeloma, leukemia, lymphomas) by decreasing bone resorption. High doses or prolonged administration of corticosteroids leads to serious adverse reactions. (See Chapter 24 for further discussion of corticosteroid drug therapy.)

Routes and dosage ranges

Hydrocortisone

Adults: IM, IV 100–500 mg daily

Prednisone

Adults: PO 40–60 mg daily initially, then gradually reduced

Mithramycin (Mithracin) is an antineoplastic antibiotic drug (see Chap. 64) used primarily in cancer chemotherapy. Mithramycin probably lowers serum calcium levels by blocking calcium resorption from bone. Because of potential bone marrow depression and other toxic effects, mithramycin is not recommended for routine treatment of hypercalcemia. However, much smaller doses are used in hypercalcemia than in malignant neoplasms. Thus, adverse reactions are less likely to occur.

Route and dosage range

Adults: IV 25 μg/kg/day for 3 or 4 days, repeated at intervals of 1 week or more, if necessary

Phosphate salts (Neutra-Phos) lower serum calcium levels by increasing tissue uptake of calcium. They are effective in the treatment of hypercalcemia of any etiology. A potential adverse reaction to phosphates is calcification of soft tissues due to deposition of calcium phosphate. This can lead to severe impairment of function in the kidneys and other organs. This problem is less likely to occur with oral phosphates than with IV phosphates. Consequently, IV phosphates are no longer recommended for use in treating hypercalcemia. Phosphates should be given only when hypercalcemia is accompanied by hypophosphatemia. Neutra-Phos is a combination of sodium phosphate and potassium phosphate.

Route and dosage range

Adults: PO 1–2 tablets 3–4 times daily or contents of 1 capsule mixed with 75 ml of water 4 times daily

0.9% Sodium chloride injection (normal saline) is an IV solution containing water, sodium, and chloride. It is included here because it is the treatment of choice for hypercalcemia and, along with furosemide (Lasix), is usually effective. The sodium contained in the solution inhibits the reabsorption of calcium in renal tubules and thereby increases urinary excretion of calcium. The solution also relieves the dehydration caused by vomiting and polyuria, and it dilutes the calcium concentration of serum and urine. Saline, 4 to 6 liters/day, is given first to hydrate the client; then, furosemide is given.

Principles of therapy: drugs used in hypercalcemia

ASSESSMENT GUIDELINES

Identify clients at risk of developing hypercalcemia and assess them regularly for signs and symptoms. Check serum calcium reports when available. Although laboratories vary in normal values, hypercalcemia is usually indicated by a total serum calcium level above 10 mg/100 ml. Electrocardiographic changes indicative of hypercalcemia include a shortened QT interval and an inverted T wave.

TREATMENT OF HYPERCALCEMIA

Treatment of hypercalcemia depends largely on its cause and severity.

1. When hypercalcemia is caused by an adenoma of a parathyroid gland, surgical excision is indicated. When it is caused by malignant tumors, excision or treatment of the tumor is likely to decrease serum calcium levels. When it is caused by excessive intake of vitamin D, the vitamin D preparation should be stopped immediately.
2. Mild hypercalcemia may respond to nondrug measures aimed toward decreasing calcium intake and preventing precipitation of calcium in the kidneys (formation of renal calculi).
    a. The most effective measure to decrease dietary calcium is to avoid milk and milk products.
    b. Measures to decrease formation of renal calculi include forcing fluids to about 3000 to 4000 ml/day, having the client drink about 1 pint of cranberry juice daily to help acidify the urine (calcium tends to stay in solution in acid urine and to precipitate and form stones in alkaline urine), and taking measures to decrease urinary tract infections.
3. Acute hypercalcemia is a medical emergency and requires immediate treatment. The priority is fluid replacement and rehydration. This need can be met by IV saline infusion (0.9% or 0.45% NaCl), about 3000 to 4000 ml/day if kidney function is adequate. At the same time, calcium intake is limited. After rehydration, a diuretic such as furosemide is usually given IV to increase renal excretion of calcium further and to prevent fluid overload. Since sodium, potassium, and water are also lost in the urine, these must be replaced in the IV fluids.

    As a general rule, most clients will respond to the above treatment, and further drug therapy is not needed. Phosphates should not be used unless hypophosphatemia is present. They are also contraindicated in clients with persistent urinary tract infections and an alkaline urine because calcium phosphate kidney stones are likely to form in such cases.

4. Chronic hypercalcemia requires treatment of the underlying disease process and measures to control serum calcium levels (*e.g.*, a low-calcium diet, high fluid intake, and mobilization). Oral phosphate administration may be helpful if other measures are not effective.
5. Serum calcium levels should be measured to monitor effects of therapy. In acute hypercalcemia, these are measured frequently.
6. For clients with severely impaired renal function who develop hypercalcemia, hemodialysis or peritoneal dialysis with a calcium-free solution may be used.

NURSING ACTIONS: DRUGS USED IN HYPERCALCEMIA

Nursing Actions	*Rationale/Explanation*
1. Administer accurately	
a. With calcitonin, add the provided gelatin diluent to the powdered drug in an amount to give a dose volume of 0.5 ml. Give the reconstituted drug IM or SC. The remainder may be stored in the refrigerator up to 2 weeks.	These are the manufacturer's recommendations for administration of calcitonin in Paget's disease of bone.
b. With furosemide, give IV or orally.	
c. With hydrocortisone	
(1) Give IV or IM.	In acute hypercalcemia, IV administration (by bolus injection or by addition to 5% dextrose in water or NaCl injection, given as an IV infusion over several hours) is preferred.
(2) Be sure to have the appropriate drug preparation for the ordered route.	Several commercial preparations of hydrocortisone are available. Some are given IV, some IM, and some by either route. Do not assume that any preparation can be given by both routes of administration.
(3) Decrease dosage gradually—do not discontinue abruptly.	Abrupt discontinuance can lead to acute adrenal insufficiency.
d. With mithramycin, give IV for a limited number of doses. See package insert for specific instructions.	
e. With phosphate salts, mix powder forms with water for oral administration. See package inserts for specific instructions.	
2. Observe for therapeutic effects	
a. Decreased serum calcium level	Calcitonin lowers serum calcium levels in approximately 2 hours after injection, and effects last 6 to 8 hours. When given every 12 hours, effects last 5 to 8 days. Corticosteroids require 10 to 14 days to lower serum calcium. Mithramycin lowers serum calcium levels within 24 to 48 hours, but effects last only 3 to 4 days.
b. Decreased signs and symptoms of hypercalcemia	
c. Decreased signs and symptoms of Paget's disease	Decreased serum alkaline phosphatase and radiologic improvement of bone lesions may require several months. Neurologic improvement may require 1 year or more.

Nursing Actions	***Rationale/Explanation***
3. Observe for adverse effects	
a. Hypocalcemia	Hypocalcemia may result from overly vigorous treatment of hypercalcemia. This can be prevented by frequent determinations of serum calcium levels and appropriate adjustments in drug dosages and other treatment measures.
b. With calcitonin, observe for nausea, vomiting, tissue irritation at injection sites, and allergic reactions.	Adverse reactions are usually mild and transient.
c. With furosemide, observe for dehydration, hypokalemia, hypomagnesemia, and other fluid and electrolyte imbalances.	As furosemide exerts its therapeutic effect of removing excess calcium from the body by increased urine output, water and other electrolytes are lost as well. Adverse reactions can be prevented by avoiding overdosage of furosemide and by careful replacement of the water and electrolytes lost in the urine. Frequent measurements of serum electrolytes help determine amounts of replacement fluids and electrolytes needed.
d. With hydrocortisone and prednisone, see Chapter 24.	Adrenal corticosteroids may cause many adverse reactions, especially with high doses or prolonged administration.
e. With mithramycin, observe for bone marrow depression, nausea, vomiting, and impaired liver function.	These adverse reactions may occur but are much less likely with the small doses used for hypercalcemia than with the large doses used for malignant neoplasms.
f. With phosphates, observe for nausea, vomiting, and diarrhea.	
4. Observe for drug interactions	
a. With calcitonin, testosterone and other androgens *increase* effects; parathyroid hormone *decreases* effects.	Androgens and calcitonin have additive effects on calcium retention and inhibition of bone resorption (movement of calcium from bone to serum). Parathyroid hormone antagonizes or opposes calcitonin. Parathyroid hormone *increases* serum calcium concentration, while calcitonin *decreases* it.
b. With hydrocortisone and prednisone, see Chapter 24.	
c. With mithramycin, see Chapter 64.	
d. With phosphate salts, avoid concomitant use of antacids containing aluminum and magnesium.	Aluminum and magnesium may combine with phosphate and thereby prevent its absorption and therapeutic effect.
5. Teach clients	
a. Maintain a low-calcium diet by limiting intake of dairy products.	One serving of milk, cheese, or other dairy product plus fruits and vegetables furnish a daily calcium intake of about 400 mg.
b. Drink 3 to 4 quarts of fluid daily if able.	To keep the urine dilute. This helps to prevent formation of kidney stones and urinary tract infections.
c. Drink about 1 pint (2 glasses) of cranberry juice as part of the daily fluid intake.	This helps to keep urine acidic and decreases the likelihood of kidney stone formation.
d. Report any signs of cystitis, such as burning or discomfort with urination.	Infections in the urinary tract can increase kidney stone formation. If they occur, early treatment is needed.

Selected References

American Medical Association (AMA) Division of Drugs: AMA Drug Evaluations, 5th ed. New York, John Wiley & Sons, 1983

Facts and Comparisons. St. Louis, J B Lippincott (Updated monthly)

Guyton AC: Textbook of Medical Physiology, 7th ed. Philadelphia, W B Saunders, 1986

Haynes RC Jr, Murad F: Agents affecting calcification: Calcium, parathyroid hormone, calcitonin, vitamin D, and other compounds. In Gilman AG, Goodman LS, Rall TW, Murad F (eds): The Pharmacological Basis of Therapeutics, 7th ed., pp 1517–1543. New York, Macmillan, 1985

Hoffman JTT: Syndromes of ectopic hormone production in cancer. Nurs Clin North Am 15:499–509, September 1980

Hoffman JTT, Newby TB: Hypercalcemia in primary hyperparathyroidism. Nurs Clin North Am 15:469–480, September 1980

McFadden EA, Zaloga GP, Chernow B, et al: Hypocalcemia: A medical emergency. Am J Nurs 83:227–230, February 1983

Menzel LK: Clinical problems of electrolyte balance. Nurs Clin North Am 15:559–575, September 1980

27
ANTIDIABETIC DRUGS

Description and uses

There are two types of antidiabetic drugs: insulin and oral sulfonylurea agents. These drugs are used to lower blood glucose; hence, they are also called hypoglycemic agents. Diabetes mellitus is a common, complex disorder. To understand clinical usage of antidiabetic drugs, it is necessary to understand characteristics of endogenous insulin and diabetes mellitus as well as characteristics of the drugs.

ENDOGENOUS INSULIN

Insulin is secreted by the islets of Langerhans, which are scattered in the pancreas. They contain alpha cells, which secrete glucagon, beta cells, which secrete insulin, and other cells that secrete somatostatin. Insulin is a protein secreted into the bloodstream and transported to body cells. It is normally secreted in response to a rise in blood glucose levels. Before insulin can enter the cell and influence cell metabolism, it must become attached to the cell membrane. This attachment is accomplished by the binding of insulin to receptors. Receptors with specific binding sites for insulin are found primarily in liver, fat, and muscle cells. They are also present in placental cells, white blood cells, and fibroblasts.

Insulin plays a major role in metabolism of carbohydrate, fat and protein. These foodstuffs are broken down into molecules of glucose, lipids, and amino acids, respectively. These molecules enter the cells and are converted to energy for cellular activities. The energy can be used immediately or converted to storage forms for later use. In carrying out its metabolic functions, the overall effect of insulin is to lower blood glucose levels, primarily by the following mechanisms:

1. In the liver, insulin acts to *decrease* breakdown of glycogen (glycogenolysis), formation of new glucose from fatty acids and amino acids (gluconeogenesis), and formation of ketone bodies (ketogenesis). At the same time, it acts to *increase* synthesis and storage of glycogen and fatty acids.
2. In adipose tissue, insulin acts to *decrease* breakdown of fat (lipolysis) and to *increase* production of glycerol and fatty acids.
3. In muscle tissue, insulin acts to *decrease* protein breakdown and amino acid output and to *increase* amino acid uptake, protein synthesis and glycogen synthesis.

Effects of insulin on carbohydrate metabolism

Specific effects of insulin on carbohydrate metabolism include the following:

1. It increases glucose transport into most body cells. Complete lack of insulin allows transport of about one fourth the normal amount of glucose. Insulin facilitates glucose transport into skeletal muscle, adipose tissue, the heart, and some smooth muscle

organs such as the uterus. It does not increase glucose transport into brain cells, red blood cells, intestinal mucosal cells, or tubular epithelial cells of the kidney.

2. It regulates glucose metabolism and homeostasis. When insulin is present in adequate amounts, glucose serves as the primary fuel for production of energy. When insulin is present in excessive amounts, large amounts of glucose enter the cells to be used for energy or stored as glycogen or fat. When both insulin and glucose are present in excessive amounts, more glycogen is stored in skeletal muscle, liver, and skin. Excessive glucose and insulin also cause increased conversion of glucose to fat. Almost all the excess glucose transported into fat cells of adipose tissue is converted to fat for storage. The excess glucose transported to liver cells is converted to fat only after glycogen stores have been saturated. When insulin is absent, or when blood glucose levels are low, these stored forms of glucose can be reconverted. The liver is especially important in restoring blood sugar levels by breaking down glycogen or by forming new glucose.

Effects of insulin on fat metabolism

Specific effects of insulin on fat metabolism include the following:

1. Insulin promotes transport of glucose into fat cells. Once inside the cell, glucose is broken down. One of the breakdown products is alphaglycerophosphate, which combines with fatty acids to form triglycerides. This is the mechanism by which insulin promotes fat storage.
2. When insulin is lacking, fat is not stored in the fat cells. Instead, it is released into the bloodstream in the form of free fatty acids. Blood concentrations of other lipids (triglycerides, cholesterol, phospholipids) are also increased. The high blood lipid concentration probably accounts for the atherosclerosis that tends to develop early and progress more rapidly in people with diabetes mellitus. Also, when more fatty acids are released than the body can use as fuel, some fatty acids are converted into ketone bodies. Excessive amounts of ketones produce acidosis and coma.

Effects of insulin on protein metabolism

Effects of insulin on protein metabolism and growth include the following:

1. Insulin increases the total amount of body protein by increasing transport of amino acids into cells and synthesis of protein within the cells. The basic mechanism of these effects is unknown.
2. Insulin potentiates the effects of growth hormone.
3. Lack of insulin causes protein depletion and breakdown into amino acids. These amino acids are released into the bloodstream and transported to the liver for energy or gluconeogenesis. These proteins are not replaced by synthesis of new proteins. The overall consequences of protein wasting include abnormal functioning of many body organs, severe weakness, and weight loss.

CHARACTERISTICS OF DIABETES MELLITUS

Diabetes mellitus is a chronic systemic disease characterized by metabolic and vascular abnormalities. Metabolic problems occur early in the disease process and are related to changes in the metabolism of carbohydrate, fat, and protein. One of the primary clinical manifestations of disordered metabolism is hyperglycemia. Vascular problems include rapid development and progression of atherosclerosis throughout the body and changes in small blood vessels, which especially affect the retina and the kidneys. Clinical manifestations of vascular disorders may include hypertension, myocardial infarction, stroke, retinopathy, blindness, nephropathy, and peripheral vascular disease.

ETIOLOGY OF DIABETES MELLITUS

Etiology of diabetes mellitus is complex and probably involves many factors. Some generally accepted causative factors include the following:

1. *Obesity.* This is considered to be a major cause of type II diabetes. More insulin is required in the presence of obesity, and that which is present may be less effective.
2. *Heredity.* There is definitely a familial tendency to the development of diabetes. This condition is transmitted as a recessive genetic trait. Other hereditary mechanisms may also be involved.
3. *Destruction or damage of pancreatic tissue.* Destruction of the insulin-producing beta cells in the islets of Langerhans can result from cancer, pancreatitis, surgical excision of pancreatic tissue, and viral infections.
4. *Diabetogenic hormones.* A number of hormones can cause hyperglycemia and diabetes when present in excessive amounts, whether from endogenous

oversecretion or from excessive administration of exogenous hormones. These include growth hormone, thyroid hormone, epinephrine, adrenal corticosteroids, and glucagon.

5. *Other diabetogenic drugs.* In addition to certain hormones, some other drugs may cause or aggravate hyperglycemia without producing irreversible diabetes mellitus. These include epinephrine, diazoxide, thiazide diuretics, phenothiazines, propranolol, and phenytoin.
6. *Other factors.* These include hemochromatosis, disorders of insulin receptors, factors of immunity and autoimmunity, aging, illness, and stress.

Classifications

The two major classifications of diabetes mellitus are type I and type II. Although both types are characterized by hyperglycemia, they differ significantly in onset, course, treatment, and pathologic changes. Actually, persons with diabetes present a continuum of disease manifestations rather than separate distinct categories.

1. Type I, or insulin-dependent, diabetes mellitus (IDDM) may occur at any age but usually starts before 20 years of age. It generally has a sudden onset, produces more severe symptoms, is more difficult to control (*i.e.,* it tends to be labile or brittle), produces a high incidence of complications such as diabetic ketoacidosis (DKA) and renal failure, and requires administration of exogenous insulin. Fortunately, type I diabetes is relatively uncommon, comprising about 5% of the diabetic population.
2. Type II, or non-insulin-dependent, diabetes mellitus (NIDDM) may occur at any age but usually starts after 40 years of age. Unlike type I, type II generally has a gradual onset, produces less severe symptoms initially, is easier to control (tends to be more stable), causes less DKA and renal failure but more myocardial infarctions and strokes, and does not necessarily require exogenous insulin, since endogenous insulin is still produced by pancreatic beta cells. In fact, many people with type II diabetes have apparently adequate blood levels of insulin. Their symptoms may result from low numbers or impaired binding capacity of insulin receptors. Thus, insulin may be present but unable to act effectively to lower blood sugar. Approximately 90% of the diabetic population has type II diabetes; 20% to 30% of them require exogenous insulin.

Signs and symptoms

Most clinical signs and symptoms of diabetes mellitus stem from a relative or an absolute lack of insulin and subsequent metabolic abnormalities. The incidence and severity of signs and symptoms are correlated with the amount of effective insulin. In type I diabetes, insulin secretion is absent or severely impaired. Clinical signs and symptoms may be precipitated by infection, rapid growth, pregnancy, or other factors that increase demand for insulin. In type II diabetes, insulin is still secreted but in insufficient amounts, especially when insulin demand is increased by obesity, pregnancy, aging, or other factors. There may also be a decrease in the number or sensitivity of insulin receptors. In many people, signs and symptoms occur with obesity and are relieved when normal weight is maintained.

Most early clinical manifestations result from disordered carbohydrate metabolism, which causes excess glucose to accumulate in the blood (hyperglycemia). Hyperglycemia produces glucosuria, which in turn produces polydipsia, polyuria, dehydration, and polyphagia.

Glucosuria usually appears when blood glucose level is about twice the normal value and the kidneys receive more glucose than can be reabsorbed. There is considerable variation, though, and the amount of glucose being lost in the urine may not be an accurate indicator of blood glucose. In the very young, glucose tends to appear in urine at much lower or even normal blood glucose levels. In older people, the ability of the kidneys to excrete excess glucose from the blood is decreased. Therefore, some older people can have rather high blood glucose levels with little or no glucose appearing in the urine.

When large amounts of glucose are present in the urine, water is pulled into the renal tubule to dilute the urine. This results in a greatly increased urine output (polyuria). The excessive loss of fluid in urine (osmotic diuresis) leads to increased thirst (polydipsia) and, if fluid intake is inadequate, to dehydration. Dehydration also occurs because high blood glucose levels increase osmotic pressure in the bloodstream and fluid is pulled out of the cells in the body's attempt to regain homeostasis.

Polyphagia, or increased appetite, occurs because the body is unable to use ingested foods. Many people with diabetes lose weight because of abnormal metabolism.

Complications

Complications of diabetes mellitus are common and potentially disabling or life threatening. Although much remains to be learned, complications appear to result primarily from lack of insulin and subsequent metabolic abnormalities. These metabolic abnormalities, especially those associated with hyperglycemia, can cause early, acute complications such as DKA or nonketotic hyperosmolar coma. Eventually, metabolic abnormalities lead to changes in structure and function of blood vessels and other body tissues. Some complications of diabetes are described more specifically in the following paragraphs.

1. **Ketoacidosis.** This condition is an acute, life-threatening complication of diabetes that occurs with severe insulin deficiency. In the absence of insulin, glucose cannot be used by body cells for energy, and fat is mobilized from adipose tissue to furnish a fuel source. The mobilized fat circulates in the bloodstream, from which it is extracted by the liver and broken down into glycerol and fatty acids. The fatty acids are further changed in the liver to ketone bodies (acetoacetic acid, acetone, betahydroxybutyric acid), which then enter the bloodstream and are circulated to body cells for metabolic conversion to energy, carbon dioxide, and water.

   Owing to these metabolic abnormalities, clinical signs and symptoms develop rather rapidly because ketone bodies tend to be produced more rapidly than body cells can use them. Thus, they accumulate and produce acidemia (a drop in blood *p*H and an increase in blood hydrogen ions). The body attempts to buffer the acidic hydrogen ions by exchanging them for intracellular potassium ions. Thus, hydrogen ions enter body cells and potassium ions leave the cells, to be excreted in the urine. Another attempt to remove excess acid involves the lungs. Deep, labored respirations, called Kussmaul respirations, eliminate more carbon dioxide and prevent formation of carbonic acid. A third attempt to regain homeostasis involves the kidneys, which excrete some of the ketones, thereby producing acetone in the urine.

   DKA worsens as the compensatory mechanisms fail. Clinical signs and symptoms vary and become progressively more severe. Early ones include blurred vision, anorexia, nausea and vomiting, thirst, and polyuria. Later ones include drowsiness, which progresses to stupor and coma, Kussmaul breathing, dehydration and other signs of fluid and electrolyte imbalances, and decreased blood pressure, increased pulse, and other signs of shock.
2. **Hyperglycemic hyperosmolar nonketotic coma.** This is another type of diabetic coma that is potentially life threatening. It is a relatively rare condition with a high mortality. The term *hyperosmolar* refers to an excessive amount of glucose, electrolytes, and other solutes in the blood in relation to the amount of water.

   This condition has both similarities and differences when compared with DKA. Like DKA, hyperosmolar coma is characterized by hyperglycemia, which leads to osmotic diuresis and resultant thirst, polyuria, dehydration, and electrolyte losses as well as neurologic signs ranging from drowsiness to stupor to coma. Additional clinical problems may include hypovolemic shock, thrombosis, renal problems, or cerebrovascular accident. Hyperosmolar coma differs from DKA by occurring in people with previously unknown or mild diabetes; by lack of ketosis; by following an illness; and by occurring in other hyperglycemic conditions as well as in diabetes (*e.g.*, severe burns, corticosteroid drug therapy).
3. **Cardiovascular complications.** Diabetics develop generalized atherosclerosis that, compared to nondiabetics, occurs at an earlier age, progresses more rapidly, and becomes more severe. Changes occur in both large and small blood vessels. Reasons for vascular changes are not clear, but the sequence of events is thought to involve damage to the endothelial lining, followed by platelet aggregation, lipid deposition, plaque formation, and thrombosis in the damaged area.

   Vascular disease is a leading cause of death in people with diabetes. It is also a leading cause of morbidity, since diabetics are much more likely to have myocardial infarction, peripheral arterial insufficiency, kidney failure, and blindness than nondiabetics. Other vascular complications include angina pectoris, congestive heart failure, hypertension, and cerebral thrombosis (stroke).
4. **Nephropathy.** The several types of kidney lesions in diabetes mellitus are collectively called *diabetic nephropathy.* One such lesion is diffuse glomerulosclerosis, which is found in about 90% of people who have had diabetes more than 10 years. Another lesion is called *nodular glomerulosclerosis,* or Kimmelstiel–Wilson syndrome. It occurs in 10% to 25% of people with diabetes. A third lesion is acute or chronic pyelonephritis. Although pyelonephritis also occurs in nondiabetics, it is usually more severe in diabetics. A fourth lesion involves atherosclerosis and arteriosclerosis of renal arteries as a manifestation of generalized atherosclerosis. These disorders all produce abnormal renal function and may cause renal failure.
5. **Retinopathy.** This is the most common and most

serious ocular complication of diabetes, although cataract formation and glaucoma may develop at an earlier age in the client with diabetes. Diabetic retinopathy is related to duration of diabetes. About 50% of diabetics have some degree of retinopathy after 10 years, and about 80% to 90% do after 20 years. Occasionally the condition develops rapidly in type I diabetes and causes blindness by late adolescence. Retinopathy seems to result from vascular changes, and severity is correlated with the degree of generalized vascular disease. Hemorrhage, edema, and exudates may be visualized through the ophthalmoscope. Retinal detachment may occur.

6. **Neuropathy.** Several nonspecific neurologic disorders are often associated with diabetes mellitus. The degenerative changes in nerves that produce neuropathy have long been attributed to ischemia resulting from vascular disease. Currently, sorbitol (an alcohol produced by glucose metabolism) is thought to be a causative factor in the development of neuropathy.

   In the extremities, neuropathy causes discomfort and impairment of sensory and motor functions. Injuries often result, usually in the feet, and even minor injuries may eventually necessitate leg amputation. In the cardiovascular system, silent myocardial infarction, postural hypotension, and impaired response to sympathetic or parasympathetic stimulation may occur. Another autonomic manifestation is the absence of warning signs of hypoglycemia. In the gastrointestinal system, neuropathy may cause disturbances of motility and changes in bowel function. In the genitourinary system, bladder atony may cause urine retention and urinary tract infections. In addition, impotence and retrograde ejaculation may occur in men.
7. **Other complications.** Arthropathy and osteolysis may develop, probably from trauma and decreased ability to perceive pain. Diabetics are more susceptible to infections, especially tuberculosis, pneumonia, and urinary tract and skin infections. When infections occur, they tend to progress more rapidly and become more severe. Formerly, it was thought that infections were caused and perpetuated by hyperglycemia because microorganisms thrive on glucose. More recently, however, infections are attributed to impairment of phagocytosis and other defense mechanisms. Women with diabetes are more likely to develop toxemia and other complications of pregnancy. Babies born to diabetic mothers are more likely to be premature or stillborn.

HYPOGLYCEMIC DRUGS

Individual insulins and oral hypoglycemic drugs are listed in Tables 27-1 and 27-2, respectively.

Insulin

1. Commercially available insulin preparations are combinations of beef and pork insulins, single-component beef or pork insulin, and human insulin. Early products contained beef and pork insulins and relatively large amounts of proinsulin and other protein contaminants. These preparations caused a relatively high incidence of allergic reactions and insulin antibody formation. With newer manufacturing techniques, combination products currently available contain only small amounts of contaminants and are therefore less likely to be antigenic. Single-component insulins are even more highly purified. Beef insulin differs from human insulin by three amino acids and is more antigenic than pork insulin. Pork insulin differs from human insulin by one amino acid. Human insulin is produced in the laboratory with recombinant deoxyribonucleic acid (DNA) techniques, using strains of *Escherichia coli,* or by chemically modifying pork insulin to replace the single different amino acid. Thus, human insulin has the same number and sequence of amino acids as endogenous insulin. It is not derived from the human pancreas.
2. Insulin cannot be given orally because it is a protein that is destroyed by proteolytic enzymes in the gastrointestinal tract. It is given only by the parenteral route.
3. Insulin preparations differ primarily in onset and duration of action. They are usually categorized as short-, intermediate-, or long-acting insulins. Short-acting insulins have a rapid onset and short duration of action. Intermediate- and long-acting insulins are modified by adding protamine (a large, insoluble protein), zinc, or both to slow absorption and prolong drug action.
4. Insulin preparations are available in two concentrations, U-40 and U-100. These terms refer to the concentration or number of units of insulin per milliliter of fluid. For example, U-100 contains 100 units of insulin per milliliter. Each concentration must be given with a syringe calibrated for that concentration (*e.g.,* U-100 insulin can be accurately measured only in a U-100 syringe). Because dosage errors can have serious consequences, the current trend is to use only U-100 insulin and U-100 insulin syringes.

(Text continues on p. 253.)

TABLE 27-1. INSULINS

	Generic name	Trade name	Characteristics	Routes and dosage ranges	Action (hrs)		
					Onset	*Peak*	*Duration*
Short-acting insulins	Insulin injection	Insulin, Regular Iletin I Purified preparations: Regular Iletin II (beef or pork), Actrapid (pork), Velosulin (pork) Human insulin: Humulin R, Novolin R	1. A clear liquid solution with the appearance of water 2. The hypoglycemic drug of choice for diabetics experiencing acute or emergency situations, DKA, hyperosmolar nonketotic coma, severe infections or other illnesses, major surgery, and pregnancy 3. The only insulin preparation that can be given IV 4. Rarely used alone for long-term maintenance but may be combined with an intermediate-acting insulin (*e.g.,* NPH) for this purpose	SC, dosage individualized according to blood and urine glucose levels. For sliding scale, 5–20 units before meals and bedtime, depending on blood glucose levels or urine levels of glucose and acetone. IV, dosage individualized. For ketoacidosis, regular insulin may be given by direct injection, intermittent infusion, or continuous infusion. One regimen involves an initial bolus injection of 10–20 units followed by a continuous low-dose infusion of 2–10 units/hour, based on hourly blood and urine glucose levels	½–1	2–3	5–7
	Prompt insulin zinc suspension	Semilente Insulin, Semilente Iletin I Purified preparation: Semitard (pork)	1. Modified by chemical combination with zinc to produce small crystals, which are rapidly absorbed 2. Rarely used alone; most often used in combination with intermediate (Lente) or long-acting (Ultralente) insulins. 3. A suspension that is milky or cloudy when mixed thoroughly in the drug vial 4. Given *only* by the subcutaneous route, and is not recommended in emergencies	SC, dosage individualized. Initially, 10–20 units once or twice daily may be given.	½–1½	4–6	12–16
Intermediate acting insulins	Isophane insulin suspension	NPH Iletin I, NPH Insulin Purified preparation: Insulatard NPH, Iletin II (beef or pork), NPH purified pork Human insulin: Humulin N Novolin N	1. Commonly used for long-term administration 2. Modified by addition of protamine (a protein) and zinc 3. A suspension with a cloudy appearance when correctly mixed in the drug vial 4. Given only by the subcutaneous route 5. Not recommended for use in acute situations	SC, dosage individualized. Initially, 7–26 units may be given once or twice daily.	1–1½	8–12	18–24

TABLE 27-1. INSULINS (*Continued*)

	Generic name	Trade name	Characteristics	Routes and dosage ranges	Action (hrs) Onset	Peak	Duration
			6. Hypoglycemic reactions are more likely to occur during mid-to-late afternoon.				
	Insulin zinc suspension	Lente insulin Lente Iletin I Purified preparations: Lente Iletin II (beef or pork), Lente purified pork Human insulin: Novolin L	1. Modified by addition of zinc. 2. A mixture of 30% Semilente and 70% Ultralente. The small crystals of Semilente are rapidly absorbed, and the large crystals of Ultralente are slowly absorbed. 3. May be used interchangeably with NPH insulin 4. A suspension with a cloudy appearance when correctly mixed in the drug vial 5. Given only by the subcutaneous route	SC, dosage individualized. Initially, 7–26 units may be given once or twice daily.	1–2	8–12	18–24
Long-acting insulins	Protamine zinc insulin suspension (PZI)	Protamine, Zinc & Iletin I Purified preparation: Protamine, Zinc & Iletin II (pork or beef)	1. Contains more protamine and zinc than NPH insulin 2. Has limited clinical usefulness because its long duration of action increases risks of hypoglycemic reactions, especially during sleep 3. Cannot be combined with regular insulin 4. A suspension with a cloudy appearance when thoroughly mixed in the vial	SC, dosage individualized. Initially 7–26 units may be given once daily.	4–8	14–24	36 plus
	Extended insulin zinc suspension	Ultralente Purified preparation: Ultratard (beef)	1. Modified by addition of zinc and formation of large crystals, which are slowly absorbed 2. Hypoglycemic reactions are frequent and likely to occur during sleep 3. Rarely used alone. May be combined with Lente or Semilente. 4. Contains no protein, thus is less likely to cause allergic reactions	SC, dosage individualized. Initially, 7–26 units may be given once daily	4–8	10–30	36 plus

TABLE 27-2. ORAL HYPOGLYCEMIC AGENTS

	Generic name	Trade name	Characteristics	Routes and dosage ranges	Duration of action (hr)
First-generation sulfonylureas	Acetohexamide	Dymelor	1. Intermediate-acting agent 2. Hypoglycemic activity due to the parent drug and an active metabolite 3. Readily absorbed from the gastrointestinal tract, metabolized in the liver, and excreted in urine 4. Has uricosuric properties; therefore, is probably the preferred oral agent for diabetics with gout	PO, dosage individualized. Usual range, 250 mg–1.5 g; maximal daily dose, 1.5 g Dosages of 1 g or less daily can be given in a single dose. Dosage of 1.5 g daily should be given in 2 divided doses, before morning and evening meals.	12–24
	Chlorpropamide	Diabinese	1. Long-acting agent 2. When chlorpropamide therapy is started, therapeutic effects may not be evident for 1–2 weeks. When the drug is discontinued, several weeks are required for complete elimination of the drug from the body. These effects are due to the long half-life of the drug.	PO, dosage individualized. Initially, 100–250 mg daily in a single dose. Dosage may be increased or decreased by 50–125 mg at weekly intervals. Usual maintenance dose is 100–500 mg daily. Avoid doses greater then 750 mg daily.	Up to 60
	Tolazamide	Tolinase	1. Similar to other sulfonylurea hypoglycemic agents except it does not have an antidiuretic action. Consequently, tolazamide may be useful in diabetics with congestive heart failure, hepatic cirrhosis, or other conditions characterized by fluid retention and edema.	PO, dosage individualized. Initially, 100–250 mg daily is given in a single dose. Dosage may be adjusted every 4–6 days, as needed. If 500 mg or more is required daily, two divided doses are given.	10–16
	Tolbutamide	Orinase	1. Short-acting agent 2. One of the most frequently used oral antidiabetic drugs 3. Metabolized in the liver to inactive metabolites that are excreted in urine	PO, dosage individualized. Initially, 500 mg is given in divided doses, twice daily. Dosage is adjusted according to blood and urine glucose levels. Maintenance dose is 250 mg–3 g daily, in divided doses.	6–12
Second-generation sulfonylureas	Glipizide	Glucotrol	1. Metabolized in the liver to inactive compounds, excreted in urine and bile 2. Greater hypoglycemic effect per milligram then first-generation drugs 3. May cause less toxicity than first-generation drugs	PO 5 mg daily in a single dose	24
	Glyburide	DiaBeta, Micronase	See glipizide, above	PO 2.5–5 mg daily in a single dose	24

5. Insulin absorption is delayed or decreased when it is injected into subcutaneous tissue with lipodystrophy or other lesions, when circulatory problems (*e.g.*, edema or hypotension) are present, by insulin-binding antibodies (which develop after 2 or 3 months of insulin administration), and by injecting cold (*i.e.*, refrigerated) insulin.
6. Temperature extremes can cause loss of potency. Insulin retains potency up to 36 months under refrigeration and about 18 to 24 months at room temperature. At high temperatures (about 100°F or 37.8°C), insulin loses potency in about 2 months. If frozen, insulin remains potent but tends to clump or precipitate. This prevents withdrawal of an accurate dose, and the vial should be discarded.
7. Insulin preparations are metabolized primarily in the liver and secondarily in the kidneys and muscle tissue.

Oral hypoglycemic drugs

1. The oral hypoglycemic drugs in current clinical use are all compounds that are chemically related to sulfonamides. Older agents, sometimes called first-generation sulfonylureas, are chemically and pharmacologically similar. They are extensively metabolized in the liver; the remaining unchanged drug and its metabolites are excreted by the kidneys. Acetohexamide (Dymelor) and chlorpropamide (Diabinese) are converted to other active compounds; tolazamide (Tolinase) and tolbutamide (Orinase) are converted to inactive compounds. The major difference among first-generation agents is duration of action. Second-generation sulfonylureas produce therapeutic and adverse effects similar to the older drugs and to each other. The newer drugs are more potent on a milligram-per-milligram basis and may cause less toxicity. They are metabolized to inactive compounds, which may be advantageous in clients with impaired renal or hepatic function.
2. Oral hypoglycemic agents act to lower blood glucose by increasing secretion of insulin, increasing peripheral use of glucose, decreasing production of glucose in the liver, and possibly increasing the number of insulin receptors or altering postreceptor actions to increase tissue responsiveness to insulin. The drugs stimulate pancreatic beta cells to produce more insulin and cause insulin to be released from beta-cell storage granules. These drugs are effective only when functioning pancreatic beta cells are present. Pancreatic stimulation of insulin production has long been considered the major mechanism of action. However, insulin interactions with muscle, liver, and other target tissues (*i.e.*, insulin receptors on cell membranes and intracellular components) are receiving increased attention.
3. Oral antidiabetic drugs are not effective in all clients with type II diabetes mellitus. Even when carefully selected, a fairly large group of clients experience primary or secondary treatment failure. Primary failure involves a lack of initial response to the drugs. Secondary failure means that a therapeutic response occurs when the drugs are first given, but the drugs eventually become ineffective. The reasons for secondary failure are not clear but may include decreased compliance with diet instructions, failure to take the drugs as prescribed, or decreased ability of the pancreatic beta cells to produce more insulin in response to the drugs.
4. In addition to their hypoglycemic actions, oral antidiabetic drugs have other pharmacologic activities. For example, acetohexamide, tolazamide, glyburide (Micronase), and glipizide (Glucotrol) have mild diuretic effects, acetohexamide has uricosuric effects, and chlorpropamide may potentiate the action of antidiuretic hormone (ADH).

CLINICAL INDICATIONS

The primary clinical indication for use of insulin is diabetes mellitus. Diabetes is characterized by a lack of the natural pancreatic hormone, so insulin from a source outside the body is needed as a substitute or replacement. Insulin is the only effective treatment for type I diabetes, since little, if any, endogenous insulin is produced and metabolism is severely impaired. Insulin is required on a regular basis for the 20% to 30% of type II diabetics who are unable to control their disease with diet, weight control, and oral hypoglycemic drugs. It may be needed for all diabetics during times of stress, such as infection or surgery. Insulin is also used to control diabetes induced by chronic pancreatitis or surgical excision of pancreatic tissue. Finally, it is used to prevent or treat hyperglycemia induced by intravenous (IV) hyperalimentation solutions.

Oral hypoglycemic agents are indicated for clients with symptomatic type II diabetes that cannot be controlled by diet or weight loss. These drugs are contraindicated in clients with hypersensitivity to sulfonylureas, severe renal or hepatic impairment, and during pregnancy. They are not likely to be effective during periods of stress such as major surgery, severe illness, or infection. Insulin is usually required in these circumstances.

Principles of therapy: insulin and oral hypoglycemic drugs

ASSESSMENT GUIDELINES

Assess the client's knowledge, attitude, and condition in relation to diabetes, the prescribed treatment plan, and complications. Assessment data should include past manifestations of the disease process and the client's response to them, present status, and potential problem areas.

1. Historical data include age at onset of diabetes, prescribed control measures and their effectiveness, the ease or difficulty of complying with the prescribed treatment, occurrence of complications such as ketoacidosis, and whether other disease processes have interfered with diabetes control.
2. Assessment of the client's current status includes both subjective and objective information related to the following areas:
   a. **Diet.** How many calories are prescribed, how are they calculated (food exchanges, weighing portions, or other), who prepares the food, what factors help in following the diet, what factors interfere with following the diet, what is the present weight, and has there been a recent increase or decrease? Also, list specific foods eaten at home during a 1- to 3-day period. This information assists in evaluating the nutritional adequacy of the diet actually taken and the client's adherence to the prescribed diet.
   b. **Activity.** Ask the client to describe usual activities of daily living, including those related to work, home, and recreation.
   c. **Medication.** If the client takes insulin, ask what kind, how much, who administers it, usual time of administration, sites used for injections, if a hypoglycemic reaction to insulin has ever been experienced, and, if so, how it was handled. This information helps to assess knowledge, usual practices, and teaching needs. If the client takes an oral antidiabetic drug, ask about the name, the prescribed dosage, and the dosage actually taken.
   d. **Monitoring methods.** Blood or urine testing for glucose are the two methods of monitoring disease control and response to treatment. Try to determine the method(s) used and the frequency of testing as well as the pattern of results.
   e. **Skin and mucous membranes.** Inspect for signs of infection and any other lesions. Infections are relatively common in axillary and groin areas, since these are areas with large numbers of microorganisms. Periodontal disease, also called pyorrhea, is relatively common and may be manifested by inflammation and bleeding of the gums. Women with diabetes are susceptible to monilial vaginitis and infections underneath the breasts. Check the sites of insulin injection for atrophy (dimpling or indentation), hypertrophy (nodules or lumps), and fibrosis (hardened areas). Check the lower leg for brown spots. These are apparently caused by small hemorrhages into the skin and may indicate widespread changes in the blood vessels.

      Problems are especially likely to develop in the feet owing to infection, trauma, pressure, vascular insufficiency, and neuropathy. Therefore, inspect the feet for calluses, ulcers, and signs of infection. When such problems develop, sensory impairment from neuropathy may delay detection, and impaired circulation may delay healing. Check pedal pulses, color, and temperature in both feet to assist in evaluating the adequacy of arterial blood flow to the feet.
   f. **Eyes.** Ask if the client has experienced any changes in visual acuity or blurring of vision and if regular eye examinations are done. Clients with diabetes are prone to the development of retinopathy, cataracts, and possibly glaucoma.
   g. **Cardiovascular system.** Since atherosclerosis tends to develop in diabetics, they are susceptible to a number of cardiovascular problems such as hypertension, angina pectoris, myocardial infarction, and peripheral vascular disease. Therefore, check blood pressure, ask if chest pains ever occur, and ask about pain in the legs with exercise (intermittent claudication).
   h. **Genitourinary system.** People with diabetes are likely to have kidney and bladder problems. Assess for signs of urinary tract infection such as burning on urination, recurring urinary tract infections, albumin, white blood cells or blood in urine, edema, increased urination at night, difficulty voiding, generalized itching, easy bleeding and bruising, fatigue, and muscular weakness. Impotence may develop in male diabetics and is probably caused by neuropathy.

NURSING INTERVENTIONS

Use nondrug measures to improve control of diabetes and to help prevent complications.

1. Assist the client in maintaining the prescribed diet. Specific measures vary but may include teaching the client and family about the importance of diet, referring to a dietitian, and helping to identify and modify factors that decrease compliance with the diet. If the client is obese, assist in developing a program to lose weight and then maintain weight at a more nearly normal level.
2. Assist to develop and maintain a regular exercise program.
3. Perform and interpret blood tests for glucose accurately and teach clients and family members to do so. Self-monitoring of blood glucose levels is much more accurate than urine testing. It also allows the client to view the effects of diet, exercise, and hypoglycemic medications on blood glucose levels and may promote compliance.

   Several products are available for home glucose monitoring. All involve obtaining a drop of capillary blood from a finger with a sterile lancet. The blood is placed on a semipermeable membrane that contains a reagent. The amount of blood glucose, in milligrams/100 ml, can be read visually with Dextrostix, Chemstrip bG, and Visidex II. Dextrostix can also be read with various machines (*e.g.*, Dextrometer, Glucometer). The latter method is more accurate but less convenient and more expensive than visual reading.
4. Perform and interpret urine tests for glucose and acetone accurately and teach clients and family members to do so.
   a. Follow instructions for the particular test being used.
   b. Use double-voided urine specimens. This is done by having the client void, discard the urine, drink a glass of water and urinate about $\frac{1}{2}$ hour later. The second specimen is the one to test, since the urine is more recently produced by the kidneys and should more accurately reflect blood glucose. This procedure is preferable anytime glucose is present in the urine but especially when attempting to regulate insulin dosage or when dosage depends on urine tests (*i.e.*, sliding-scale regular insulin).
   c. Do all urine testing in a well-lighted area. If lighting is poor, ability to distinguish among the colors may be impaired and inaccurate results may be recorded.
   d. Record results as percentage amounts of glucose in the urine rather than 1+, 2+, and so on. "Pluses" have long been used and are still used in many places. However, their use may cause confusion and prevent comparison of results when different types of urine tests are used. For example, 2+ indicates $\frac{3}{4}$% glucose with Clinitest, $\frac{1}{2}$% glucose with Diastix, and $\frac{1}{4}$% glucose with Tes-Tape.
   e. Note conditions that may alter urine test results. For example, a number of drugs may cause false-positive reactions with Clinitest tablets. These include ascorbic acid (vitamin C), cephalosporin antibiotics such as Keflin, chloramphenicol (Chloromycetin), levodopa (L-dopa), methyldopa (Aldomet), nalidixic acid (Neg Gram), probenecid (Benemid), and moderate to high doses of salicylates (such as aspirin), sulfonamides, and tetracyclines. With Clinistix, false-negative reactions may occur if the client is receiving ascorbic acid, levodopa, phenazopyridine (Pyridium), moderate to high doses of salicylates, and parenteral tetracycline. With Tes-Tape, false-negative reactions occur with ascorbic acid, levodopa, methyldopa, and moderate to high doses of salicylates. With Acetest tablets, false-positive reactions may occur with levodopa, ethanol, and moderate to high doses of salicylates.
5. Promote early recognition and treatment of problems by observing for signs and symptoms of urinary tract infection, peripheral vascular disease, vision changes, ketoacidosis, hypoglycemia, and others. Teach clients and families to observe for these conditions and report their occurrence.
6. Discuss the importance of regular visits to the physician, clinic, or other facility for blood sugar measurements, weights, measurement of blood pressure, and examination of the eyes.
7. Perform and teach correct foot care. Have the client observe the following safeguards: avoid going barefoot to prevent trauma to the feet; wear correctly fitted shoes; wash the feet daily with warm water, dry well, inspect for any lesions or pressure areas, and apply lanolin if the skin is dry; wear cotton or wool socks, since they are more absorbent than synthetic materials such as nylon; cut toenails straight across and only after the feet have been soaked in warm water and washed thoroughly. Teach the client to avoid use of hot water bottles or electric heating pads, cutting toenails if vision is impaired, use of strong antiseptics on the feet, and cutting corns or calluses. Also teach the client to report any lesions on the feet to the physician.

TREATMENT REGIMENS

Once a diagnosis of diabetes mellitus is established, the physician must choose a treatment regimen that will, it is hoped, control the disease process. The goal of treatment is to maintain blood sugar at normal or near-normal levels. There is increasing evidence that strict control of blood sugar decreases complications of diabetes. Home monitoring of blood glucose and insulin infusion pumps are newer developments that may be helpful. The treatment regimen chosen for a particular diabetic depends on the type of diabetes, the client's age and general condition, and the client's ability and willingness to comply with the prescribed therapy.

In type I diabetes, the only effective treatment measures are insulin, diet, and exercise. In type II diabetes, the treatment of choice is diet therapy and weight control. If this regimen is ineffective, an oral agent or insulin may be added.

GUIDELINES FOR INSULIN THERAPY

Choice of preparation

When insulin therapy is indicated, the physician may choose from several preparations that vary in composition, onset and duration of action, and other characteristics. Some factors to be considered include the following:

1. Highly purified pork or human insulin is preferred for newly diagnosed type I diabetes, gestational diabetes, poorly controlled diabetes, and diabetics undergoing surgery or experiencing illness that requires short-term insulin therapy. These insulins are less likely to cause allergic reactions and insulin-antibody formation. However, they are more expensive than older preparations.
2. Isophane insulin (NPH) or insulin zinc suspension (Lente) is probably the insulin of choice for clients who require long-term insulin therapy.
3. Regular insulin (insulin injection) is the only preparation that has a rapid onset of action and can be given IV. Therefore, it is the insulin of choice during acute situations such as diabetic ketoacidosis, severe infection or other illness, and surgical procedures.
4. For some clients, a combination of regular insulin and an intermediate-acting insulin, most often NPH, provides more consistent control of blood glucose levels.
5. For clients with local or systemic manifestations of insulin allergy, the insulin of choice is either human insulin or purified pork insulin.

Dosage factors

Dosage of insulin must be individualized. It depends largely on symptomatic response, postprandial blood glucose levels, and the results of before-meals urine tests. However, many factors influence blood glucose response to exogenous insulin and therefore influence insulin requirements.

1. Factors that increase insulin requirements include weight gain, increased caloric intake, pregnancy, decreased activity, acute infections, hyperadrenocorticism (Cushing's disease), primary hyperparathyroidism, acromegaly, hypokalemia, and drugs such as adrenocorticosteroids, thyroid, epinephrine, and some diuretics.
2. Factors that decrease insulin requirements include weight reduction, decreased caloric intake, increased physical activity, development of renal insufficiency, stopping administration of adrenocorticosteroids, thyroid, epinephrine, and diuretics, hypothyrodism, hypopituitarism, recovery from hyperthyroidism, recovery from acute infections, and the "honeymoon period," which sometimes occurs with type I diabetes.

   This honeymoon period may occur after diabetes is first diagnosed. It is characterized by apparent recovery of islet cell function and temporary production of insulin. Insulin requirements may decrease rapidly, and, if dosage is not decreased, severe hypoglycemic reactions may result.
3. In acute situations, dosage of regular insulin needs frequent adjustments. These adjustments are usually based on measurements of blood glucose or on measurements of urine glucose and acetone. Regular insulin is often ordered on a "sliding scale" in which a double-voided urine specimen is tested at specified intervals, such as before meals and at bedtime if the client is eating or every 4 to 6 hours if allowed nothing by mouth, and a dose of insulin is given subcutaneously according to the urine test results.

   If insulin is given IV in a continuous infusion, approximately 20% to 30% of the added insulin becomes bound to the glass or plastic container of IV fluids and to the plastic infusion set. It is recommended to discard 10 to 50 ml of the solution to saturate binding sites in the glass or plastic.
4. Dosage of insulin for long-term therapy is usually

determined by a trial-and-error method. One such method involves an intermediate-acting insulin preparation such as NPH or Lente, given 30 to 60 minutes before breakfast, in an initial dose of 10 to 26 units daily. This dose may be increased by 2 to 10 units at daily to weekly intervals, depending on blood or urine glucose levels, until before-meal urine tests for glucose become negative or hypoglycemia develops. Once hyperglycemia is relatively well controlled with an insulin dose, additional changes in dosage should generally be small (1 or 2 units at a time) and no more often than every 2 or 3 days. Occasional dosage adjustments may be necessary because of illness or changes in physical activity.

A second method involves initial use of regular insulin. Five to 10 units are given 15 to 30 minutes before meals, and dosage is gradually increased according to blood or urine glucose tests. Once hyperglycemia is relatively well controlled, an intermediate-acting insulin preparation is substituted. This type of insulin is usually given once daily, in the morning, before breakfast. Initial dosage is approximately two thirds of the daily dose previously established for regular insulin. As in the above method, dosage of the intermediate-acting insulin is usually increased until before-meal urine glucose tests become negative or the client shows signs and symptoms of hypoglycemia. Using this method to achieve control of diabetes may take longer, but it is usually more effective, especially for the ketoacidosis-prone client.

A third method involves various combinations of short-acting regular insulin and an intermediate-acting insulin, most often NPH. Many physicians use this method for diabetics who do not achieve satisfactory control with a single daily dose of an intermediate-acting insulin.

Whichever method is used, regulating insulin dosage to establish and maintain control of hyperglycemia and other manifestations of diabetes may be difficult and time consuming. For example, dosage may be well regulated in a hospital, where diet can be controlled and exercise is limited. When the client leaves the hospital, however, dosage may need to be adjusted. Also, dosage may need to be decreased if the client is being switched from conventional to highly purified or human insulin.

Timing of food intake

Clients receiving insulin need food at the peak action time of the insulin preparation being used and at bedtime. The food is usually taken as a between-meal and a bedtime snack. These snacks help to prevent hypoglycemic reactions between meals and at night.

Brittle diabetes

Insulin treatment in brittle or labile diabetes must be individualized. An acceptable level of control can usually be reached only after trial-and-error use of various insulins, alone or in combination, and various frequencies of administration. Brittle diabetes is characterized by instability and wide variations in blood glucose levels, ranging from hypoglycemic levels to hyperglycemia and ketoacidosis. The cause of brittle diabetes is unknown, but several factors have been implicated. These include changes in diet and physical activity, errors in insulin administration, mild infections, emotional upsets, and changes in the concentration of insulin antibodies in the blood. Of these factors, occult infection is probably the most common. Consequently, people with brittle diabetes should be examined for sinusitis, osteomyelitis, prostatitis, and other types of infections.

As a general rule, blood sugar levels in brittle diabetes cannot be well controlled with one daily injection of insulin. Therefore, treatment programs often consist of divided doses of insulin, and perhaps more than one type of insulin as well. Divided doses are especially indicated for clients who have severe early morning hyperglycemia (*i.e.*, blood sugar above 300 mg/100 ml) when receiving a single daily dose of insulin and for clients requiring 70 or more units of insulin daily. Some specific treatment programs include the following:

1. Giving a mixture of an intermediate-acting insulin, most often NPH, and regular insulin, which is short acting.
2. Giving frequent injections of regular insulin, usually before each meal, depending on the results of urine tests for sugar. Small additional amounts may be ordered if acetone is present in the urine.
3. Splitting the dosage of an intermediate-acting insulin such as Lente or NPH so that two thirds to three fourths of the total daily dose is given in the morning and the remainder before the evening meal. If this regimen is followed, the evening dose should not be more than 20 to 25 units and should be given at the same time each day. Also, an evening snack is usually needed to avoid early morning hypoglycemia.
4. Giving a mixture of Semilente insulin (short acting) and Ultralente insulin (long acting). Propor-

tions of each type can be varied according to the client's needs.

5. Insulin pumps are devices that allow continuous subcutaneous administration of regular insulin. A basal amount of insulin is injected (*e.g.*, 1 unit/hour or a calculated fraction of the dose used previously) continuously, with bolus injections before meals. This method of insulin administration maintains more normal blood glucose levels and avoids the wide fluctuations that commonly occur with other methods. Candidates for insulin pumps include clients with diabetes that is poorly controlled with more conventional methods and those who are willing to care for the devices properly.

Diabetic ketoacidosis

Insulin therapy is a major component of any treatment program for DKA. Clients with DKA have both a deficiency in the total amount of insulin in the body and a resistance to the action of the insulin that is available, probably owing to acidosis, hyperosmolality, infection, and other factors. To be effective, insulin therapy must be individualized according to frequent measurements of blood glucose. Low doses, given by continuous IV infusion, are preferred in most circumstances.

Other measures that must usually accompany insulin to treat DKA effectively include identification and treatment of conditions that precipitate DKA, administration of IV fluids to correct hyperosmolality and dehydration, administration of potassium supplements to maintain normal serum potassium levels, and administration of sodium bicarbonate to correct metabolic acidosis.

Although other conditions may predispose a client with diabetes to the development of DKA, infection is one of the most common and important. If no obvious source of infection is identified, cultures of blood, urine, and throat swabs are recommended. When infection is identified, antibacterial drug therapy may be indicated.

Intravenous fluids, possibly the single most important first step in treating DKA, usually consist of 0.9% sodium chloride, an isotonic solution. Hypotonic solutions are usually avoided because they allow intracellular fluid shifts and may cause cerebral, pulmonary, and peripheral edema.

Although serum potassium levels may be normal at first, they fall rapidly after insulin and IV fluid therapy are begun. Decreased serum potassium levels are caused by expansion of extracellular fluid volume, movement of potassium into cells, and continued loss of potassium in the urine as long as hyperglycemia persists. For these reasons, potassium supplements are usually added to IV fluids. Since both hypokalemia and hyperkalemia can cause serious cardiovascular disturbances, dosage of potassium supplements must be based on frequent measurements of serum potassium levels. Also, continuous or frequent monitoring of the electrocardiogram is recommended.

Severe acidosis can cause serious cardiovascular disturbances. Specifically, these disturbances usually stem from peripheral vasodilation and decreased cardiac output with hypotension and shock. Acidosis can be corrected by the administration of sodium bicarbonate. However, acidosis must be corrected relatively slowly and cautiously. Rapid alkalinization can cause potassium to move into body cells faster than it can be replaced intravenously. The result may be severe hypokalemia and cardiac arrhythmias. Also, giving excessive amounts of sodium bicarbonate can produce alkalosis.

Treatment of the unconscious client

When a client with diabetes becomes unconscious and it cannot be determined whether unconsciousness is caused by DKA or by hypoglycemia from insulin, the client should be treated for hypoglycemia. If hypoglycemia is the cause of unconsciousness, giving some form of glucose may avert brain damage, which results from severe, prolonged hypoglycemia. If DKA is the cause of unconsciousness, giving glucose will not harm the client. Sudden unconsciousness in the insulin-dependent diabetic is most likely to result from an insulin reaction; DKA usually develops gradually over several days or even weeks.

Hyperosmolar nonketoacidotic diabetic coma

Treatment of hyperosmolar nonketoacidotic diabetic coma is similar to that of DKA in that insulin, IV fluids, and potassium supplements are major components. Regular insulin is given by continuous IV infusion, and dosage is individualized according to frequent measurements of blood glucose levels. Intravenous fluids are given to correct the profound dehydration and hyperosmolality, and potassium is given IV to replace the large amounts lost in urine during a hyperglycemic state.

Insulin therapy during the perioperative period

Insulin therapy for diabetics who are having surgery usually consists of regular, short-acting insulin, given

IV or subcutaneously. Dosage is determined by frequent measurements of blood and urine glucose. Quite frequently these clients are given regular insulin on a "sliding scale," in which dosage varies according to blood glucose or urine sugar and acetone tests. These urine tests are done, and insulin given if indicated, at regularly scheduled times such as before meals and at bedtime or every 6 hours.

This regimen may be used for almost all diabetics having surgery. Even those who have controlled their disease with diet alone or with diet and oral hypoglycemic drugs may need insulin during this period. Those who have been insulin dependent and well controlled with an intermediate-acting insulin need a different regimen during the operative and postoperative periods. The changes in insulin therapy are usually necessary because surgery is a stressful situation that tends to increase blood glucose levels and to increase the body's need for insulin.

The goal of insulin therapy during the operative and postoperative periods is to avoid both ketosis from inadequate insulin and hypoglycemia from excessive insulin. The specific actions to reach this goal depend largely on the severity of diabetes and the type of surgical procedure. As a general rule, minor procedures require little change in the usual treatment program. For major operations, diabetes must be well controlled before surgery. For elective procedures, this may mean a delay until a client is in optimum condition to undergo surgery. During and after the operation, the insulin-dependent diabetic may need doses approximating the usual daily requirement; the diabetic receiving oral hypoglycemic drugs will probably need only small doses of insulin.

Along with the insulin, clients need adequate sources of carbohydrate until they can resume oral intake of food and fluids. This is usually supplied by 5% or 10% glucose solutions administered IV. It is safer for the client to experience some glycosuria (2% to 3%) and a blood glucose level between 150 and 250 mg/100 ml than to try to prevent glycosuria and risk hypoglycemia.

Insulin requirements in pregnancy

Insulin requirements during pregnancy are likely to be quite variable at different phases. Therefore, the diabetic client's condition must be monitored very closely and insulin therapy individualized. At the same time, of course, careful dietary control and other treatment measures are necessary. Some general guidelines for insulin therapy during antepartal, intrapartal, and postpartal periods are as follows:

1. **Antepartal period.** Pregnancy itself has a diabetogenic effect, which is apparently produced by several factors. First, human placental lactogen (HPL), a hormone produced by the placenta, exerts an increasing diabetogenic effect throughout pregnancy. This hormone increases mobilization of free fatty acids and decreases effects of maternal insulin. Second, estrogen levels increase as pregnancy advances; estrogen is thought to be an insulin antagonist. Third, progesterone may decrease insulin effectiveness. Fourth, cortisol from the adrenal cortex is thought to increase gluconeogenesis and thus cause maternal hyperglycemia.

   Some women first show signs of diabetes during pregnancy. This is called *gestational diabetes.* These women may revert to a nondiabetic state when pregnancy ends. However, they are at higher-than-average risk of developing overt diabetes at a later time. Other women, who were previously able to control their diabetes with diet alone, may become insulin-dependent during pregnancy. Still other women, already insulin-dependent, are likely to need larger doses as pregnancy advances.

   More specifically, insulin requirements usually decrease during the first trimester of pregnancy and increase during the second and third trimesters. During the first trimester, decreased need for insulin is attributed to fetal use of maternal glucose for growth and development. This lowers maternal blood levels of glucose and may cause hypoglycemic reactions. During the second trimester, insulin requirements increase along with increasing blood levels of HPL, estrogen, progesterone, and cortisol. During the third trimester, insulin requirements increase still further, and the greatest amounts are likely to be needed near term.

   It is especially important to give sufficient insulin to prevent maternal acidosis because uncontrolled acidosis is likely to interfere with neuropsychologic development of the fetus.
2. **Intrapartal period.** Diabetic women are usually delivered at 37 to 38 weeks of gestation because of increased incidence of fetal death closer to full term. Early delivery is usually induced by oxytocin (Pitocin) or accomplished by cesarean section. Either method precipitates a high-risk situation. During labor, for example, strenuous muscular activity causes increased cell use of glucose and depletion of glycogen stores. Thus, less insulin is needed, and hypoglycemia may occur. If a cesarean section is done, the stress of surgery may increase insulin requirements. Regular, short-acting insulin and frequent blood and urine glucose tests

are used to control diabetes during labor and delivery as during other acute situations.

3. **Postpartal period.** Insulin requirements continue to fluctuate during the immediate postpartal period because stress, trauma, infection, surgery, or other factors associated with delivery tend to increase blood glucose levels and insulin requirements. At the same time, termination of the pregnancy reverses the hormonal changes, which are diabetogenic, and decreases insulin requirements. Usually, women are at higher risk of hypoglycemic reactions during the first 24 to 48 hours after delivery, and some may require no insulin during this period. As during the intrapartal period, regular, short-acting insulin is given and dosage is based on frequent measurement of blood and urine sugar levels. Once insulin requirement is stabilized, the client can return to the prepregnancy treatment program of diet alone or diet and intermediate-acting insulin. Gestational diabetes usually subsides within 6 weeks after delivery.

ORAL HYPOGLYCEMIC DRUGS

1. All the oral hypoglycemic agents must be used cautiously in clients with impaired renal or hepatic function, especially acetohexamide and chlorpropamide. Tolbutamide, glipizide, or glyburide is preferred in these situations.
2. Dosage of oral hypoglycemic drugs is usually started at lower amounts and increased gradually until symptomatic glycosuria is controlled and the fasting blood glucose level is 110 mg/100 ml or less. The lowest dose that will achieve normal levels of both fasting and postprandial (after meals) blood sugars is recommended.
3. Oral antidiabetic drugs are not recommended for use during pregnancy because some of these drugs cross the placental barrier and may cause hypoglycemia and even fetal death. Also, an increased risk of congenital anomalies is possible. A third reason is the risk that women with gestational diabetes will develop overt diabetes because the drugs stimulate an already overstimulated pancreas.

TREATMENT OF HYPOGLYCEMIA

1. When hypoglycemic reactions occur with insulin or oral agents, treatment consists of the immediate administration of a rapidly absorbed carbohydrate. If the client is awake and able to swallow, the carbohydrate is given orally. About 10 g of carbohydrate is usually sufficient and can be furnished by a variety of foods and fluids: for example, 2 sugar cubes; 1 to 2 teaspoons of sugar, syrup, honey, or jelly; 2 to 3 small pieces of candy; 5 to 6 Lifesaver candies; 4 ounces of fruit juice such as orange, apple, or grape; 4 ounces of ginger ale; coffee or tea with 2 teaspoons of sugar added. Concentrated glucose products available include gel formulations (*e.g.*, Glutose, Insta-Glucose, Monojel) and chewable tablets (*e.g.*, B-D Glucose). All these products must be swallowed to be effective.
2. If the client is unable to swallow or is unconscious, carbohydrate cannot be given orally because of the risks of aspiration. Therefore, the treatment choices involve parenteral glucose or glucagon. If the client is in a health care facility where medical help is readily available, IV glucose in a 50% concentrated solution is the treatment of choice. It acts rapidly to raise blood glucose levels and arouse the client. If the client is at home or elsewhere, glucagon may be given if available and there is someone to inject it. A family member may be taught to give glucagon subcutaneously or intramuscularly. It can also be given IV. The usual adult dose is 0.5 to 1 mg. Glucagon is a pancreatic extract that increases blood sugar by converting liver glycogen to glucose. Thus, it is effective only when liver glycogen is present. Some clients are unable to respond to glucagon because glycogen stores are depleted by such conditions as starvation, adrenal insufficiency, or chronic hypoglycemia. The hyperglycemic effect of glucagon occurs more slowly than that of IV glucose and is of relatively brief duration. If the client does not respond to one or two doses of glucagon within 20 minutes, IV glucose is indicated.
3. Once hypoglycemia is relieved, the client should take slowly absorbed carbohydrate and protein foods such as milk, cheese, and bread. These foods are needed to replace glycogen stores in the liver and to prevent secondary hypoglycemia from rapid use of the carbohydrates given earlier.
4. Although the main goal of treatment is to relieve hypoglycemia and restore the brain's supply of glucose, a secondary goal is to avoid overtreatment and excessive hyperglycemia. Thus, caution is needed in the treatment of hypoglycemia. The client having a hypoglycemic reaction should not use it as an excuse to eat large amounts of food in addition to or instead of the prescribed diet. Health care personnel caring for the client should avoid giving excessive amounts of glucose. Repeated episodes of hypoglycemia require that the therapeutic regimen and client compliance be reevaluated.

NURSING ACTIONS: ANTIDIABETIC DRUGS

Nursing Actions	*Rationale/Explanation*
1. Administer accurately	
a. With insulin	
(1) Store the insulin vial in current use and administer insulin at room temperature. Refrigerate extra vials.	Cold insulin is more likely to cause lipodystrophy, local sensitivity reactions, discomfort, and delayed absorption. Insulin preparations are stable for months at room temperature, if temperature extremes are avoided.
(2) Avoid freezing temperatures (32°F) or high temperatures (95°F or above).	Extremes of temperature decrease insulin potency and cause clumping of the suspended particles of modified insulins (all except regular insulin). This clumping phenomenon causes inaccurate dosage even if the volume is accurately measured.
(3) Use only an insulin syringe calibrated to measure the specific insulin concentration; that is, use only a U-40 insulin syringe to measure U-40 insulin and only a U-100 syringe for U-100 insulin.	For accurate measurement of the prescribed dosage. U-100 insulin and syringes are recommended and are eventually expected to be the only ones available.
(4) With modified insulin preparations, which includes all except regular, short-acting insulin, invert and rotate the vial before withdrawing the insulin. Do not shake the vial.	These insulin preparations are suspensions, and the components separate on standing. Unless the particles are resuspended in the solution and distributed evenly, dosage will be inaccurate. Shaking the vial causes air bubbles, which enter the syringe and interfere with accurate measurement of the prescribed dose.
(5) When a mixture of two insulins is prescribed, such as regular insulin and NPH or Lente, always follow the same sequence of preparation.	It is necessary to use the same sequence to avoid errors and fluctuations in dosage.
(6) Rotate injection sites systematically, and use all available sites. These include the thighs, abdomen, upper back, upper arms, and buttocks unless some of these locations are contraindicated.	Frequent injection in the same site can cause tissue fibrosis, erratic absorption, and deposits of unabsorbed insulin. Also, if insulin is usually injected into fibrotic tissue where absorption is slow, injection into healthy tissue may result in hypoglycemia because of more rapid absorption. Further, deposits of unabsorbed insulins may initially lead to hyperglycemia. If dosage is increased to control the apparent hyperglycemia, hypoglycemia may occur. In addition, a sudden increase in physical activity is likely to increase subcutaneous blood circulation, causing rapid absorption of insulin.
(7) Rotate sites within the same anatomic area (*e.g.,* abdomen) until all sites are used. Avoid random rotation between the abdomen and thigh or arm, for example.	Rates of absorption differ among anatomic sites, and random rotation increases risks of hypoglycemic reactions.
(8) Inject insulin at a 90° angle into a subcutaneous pocket created by raising subcutaneous tissue away from muscle tissue. Avoid intramuscular injection.	Injection into a subcutaneous pocket is thought to produce less tissue irritation and better absorption than injection into subcutaneous tissue. Intramuscular injection should not be used because of rapid absorption.
(9) Always aspirate.	To avoid inadvertent IV injection
2. Observe for therapeutic effects	For the most part, therapeutic effects of insulin are associated with decreased hyperglycemia and the signs and symptoms that accompany increases in blood glucose levels.
a. Decreased blood glucose levels (normal range [N] = 60–100 mg/100 ml)	The goal of most insulin therapy is normoglycemia, but only if hypoglycemia can be avoided.
b. Absent or decreased urine glucose level (N = none)	
c. Absent or decreased ketones in urine (N = none)	In diabetes, ketonuria indicates insulin deficiency and impending DKA if preventive measures are not taken. Thus, always

Nursing Actions	Rationale/Explanation
	report the presence of ketones. In addition, when adequate insulin is given, ketonuria decreases. Ketonuria does not often occur with maturity-onset, ketoacidosis-resistant diabetes.
d. Absent or decreased pruritus, polyuria, polydipsia, polyphagia, and fatigue	These signs and symptoms occur in the presence of hyperglycemia. When blood sugar levels are lowered with antidiabetic drugs, they tend to subside.
3. Observe for adverse reactions	
a. Hypoglycemia—tachycardia, cardiac palpitations, hunger, nausea, blurred vision, weakness and fatigue, confusion, inability to concentrate, muscle tremors and incoordination, sweating, delirium, convulsions, coma	Hypoglycemic reactions are more likely to occur with insulin therapy than with oral antidiabetic drugs. Also, with insulin, they are most likely to occur during the peak activity time of the particular insulin preparation being used. For example, peak activity with regular insulin occurs about 2 to 3 hours after injection. With NPH and Lente insulins, it often occurs 8 to 12 hours after injection but may occur at other times.
b. Local allergic reactions—erythema or induration at injection sites	
c. Systemic allergic reactions—urticaria, edema, nausea and vomiting, diarrhea, dyspnea, occasionally hypotension, shock, and death	
d. Lipodystrophy—atrophy and "dimpling" at injection site, hypertrophy at injection site	These changes in fatty subcutaneous tissue occur from too-frequent injections into the same site.
e. Insulin resistance—requirement of large doses of insulin in the absence of DKA, infection or other factors that serve to increase requirements for insulin	This may be caused by the development of antibodies.
f. Somogyi effect—hyperglycemia despite relatively large doses of insulin	This type of hyperglycemia is a rebound phenomenon that may occur following an insulin-induced hypoglycemic reaction. It results from increased secretion of epinephrine, adrenal corticosteroids, and growth hormone in the body's attempt to oppose the excessive insulin.
4. Observe for drug interactions	
a. Drugs that *increase* effects of insulin	
(1) Monoamine oxidase (MAO) inhibitors	These drugs may significantly potentiate and prolong insulin-induced hypoglycemia. Such a combination is hazardous and should be used very cautiously, if at all.
(2) Anabolic steroids, salicylates (*e.g.,* aspirin), sulfinpyrazone (Anturane), sulfonamides, sulfonylureas (*e.g.,* oral antidiabetic drugs)	Increased hypoglycemia
(3) Propranolol (Inderal)	May increase hypoglycemia by inhibiting the normal elevation of blood glucose levels occurring as a homeostatic mechanism in response to hypoglycemia. However, propranolol may also inhibit insulin release. Thus propranolol may increase or decrease the effects of insulin.
b. Drugs that *decrease* effects of insulin	These drugs are often called diabetogenic because of their tendencies to raise blood surgar levels.
(1) Corticosteroids (*e.g.,* hydrocortisone)	Antagonize hypoglycemic effects, produce hyperglycemia
(2) Diuretics (especially thiazide diuretics such as hydrochlorothiazide)	These drugs antagonize hypoglycemic effects of insulin and may cause hyperglycemia.
(3) Epinephrine	This adrenergic drug tends to raise blood glucose levels and thereby antagonize hypoglycemic effects of insulin.
(4) Glucagon	In small doses, glucagon is used to counteract hypoglycemia

Nursing Actions	Rationale/Explanation
	induced by insulin. Glucagon raises blood glucose levels by converting liver glycogen to glucose.
(5) Oral contraceptives	Tend to raise blood glucose levels and thereby antagonize insulin effects. Insulin dosage may need to be increased.
(6) Phenytoin (Dilantin)	Inhibits insulin secretion and may cause severe hyperglycemia
(7) Propranolol (Inderal)	May inhibit insulin release
(8) Thyroid preparations (*e.g.,* levothyroxine [Synthroid])	May cause hyperglycemia
c. Drugs that *increase* effects of oral antidiabetics	
(1) Acidifying agents (*e.g.,* ascorbic acid) and probenecid (Benemid)	Increase effects by slowing the rate of urinary excretion
(2) Alcohol	Additive hypoglycemia. If alcohol use is chronic and heavy, oral hypoglycemic agents may be metabolized more rapidly and *hyperglycemia* may occur.
(3) Allopurinol (Zyloprim), anabolic steroids, chloramphenicol (Chloromycetin), clofibrate (Atromid-S), cyclophosphamide (Cytoxan), guanethidine (Ismelin), MAO inhibitors, sulfinpyrazone (Anturane), tetracyclines	Increase hypoglycemia, mechanisms not clear
(4) Anticoagulants, oral	Increase hypoglycemia by slowing metabolism of oral antidiabetic agents and possibly by decreasing their urinary excretion
(5) Insulin	Additive hypoglycemia
(6) Salicylates (*e.g.,* aspirin) and sulfonamides	Increase hypoglycemia by displacing oral antidiabetic agents from protein-binding sites.
d. Drugs that *decrease* effects of oral antidiabetic agents	
(1) Alcohol	Heavy, chronic intake of alcohol induces metabolizing enzymes in the liver. This increases the rate of metabolism of oral antidiabetic drugs, shortens their half-lives, and may produce hyperglycemia.
(2) Beta-blocking agents	Decrease hypoglycemic effects, possibly by decreasing release of insulin in the pancreas
(3) Corticosteroids, diuretics, epinephrine, estrogens, and oral contraceptives	These drugs have hyperglycemic effects.
(4) Glucagon	Raises blood glucose levels. It is used to treat severe hypoglycemia induced by insulin or oral antidiabetic agents.
(5) Nicotinic acid	Large doses have a hyperglycemic effect.
(6) Phenytoin (Dilantin)	Inhibits insulin secretion and has hyperglycemic effects
(7) Rifampin	Increases the rate of metabolism of oral antidiabetic agents by inducing liver-metabolizing enzymes
(8) Thyroid preparations	Antagonize the hypoglycemic effects of oral antidiabetic drugs
5. Teach clients	
a. The nature and characteristics of diabetes mellitus and proposed control measures	Few diseases require as much adaptation in activities of daily living as diabetes mellitus. Thus, the client must be well informed to control the disease, minimize complications, and achieve an optimum quality of life.
(1) Signs and symptoms of hyperglycemia—increased urine glucose, excessive thirst, hunger, and urine output	Persistent hyperglycemia may indicate a need to change some aspect of the treatment program such as diet or medication.
(2) Symptoms of hypoglycemia—sweating, nervousness, hunger, weakness, tremors, mental confusion	Hypoglycemia may indicate too much medication or exercise or too little food. If it occurs, take about 4 oz of orange juice, 2 lumps of sugar, or a few bites of candy. Repeat in 10 to 15 minutes if necessary. Avoid taking so much sugar that hyperglycemia occurs.

Nursing Actions	Rationale/Explanation
(3) Importance of diet, weight control, and exercise in control of diabetes	Maintaining normal weight and avoiding excessive caloric intake decrease need for medication, decrease the work load of the pancreas, and help the body use insulin more efficiently. Exercise improves utilization of insulin and helps to promote more normal blood glucose levels.
(4) Measures to delay, prevent, or decrease severity of complications	These measures are wide ranging and include regular medical supervision, regular vision and glaucoma testing, and special foot care. The goal of such measures is to prevent complications. If they cannot be prevented, early recognition and treatment may minimize their severity.
(5) Take only those drugs prescribed by a physician who knows the client has diabetes. Avoid other prescriptions and over-the-counter drugs unless these are discussed with the physician who is treating the patient.	Adverse reactions and interactions may occur. For example, aspirin and other salicylates increase the likelihood of hypoglycemia. These drugs are often included in over-the-counter preparations for pain.
(6) Test blood or urine regularly for glucose. A frequently recommended schedule is before meals and at bedtime. When testing urine, a double-voided urine specimen is preferred.	Blood glucose levels are much preferred. Urine glucose levels help indicate the degree of control of diabetes. Persistent presence of sugar or acetone in the urine may indicate a need for changes in the treatment plan.
b. With insulin-dependent diabetes, teach	
(1) Characteristics of the prescribed insulin preparation, including the expected time of peak insulin activity	The client may be able to eat at the time of peak insulin activity and reduce the likelihood of hypoglycemia. If hypoglycemia does occur, it is important that it be recognized as early as possible so that some kind of fast-acting carbohydrate can be taken.
(2) Correct techniques for self-administration of insulin	
(a) Use sterile technique.	
(b) Draw up insulin in a good light.	
(c) Use appropriate needle and syringe.	
(d) If it is necessary to mix two insulin preparations, always draw them up in the same order.	For accurate dosage
(e) Inject at a 90° angle	To prevent local reactions
(f) Rotate injection sites.	To prevent fibrosis, loss, or enlargement of subcutaneous tissue. If these changes occur, unpredictable absorption of the insulin may lead to unstable blood sugar levels and hyperglycemia or hypoglycemia.
(g) Always aspirate.	To avoid inadvertent injection into a blood vessel
(h) Change insulin dosage only if instructed to do so and the circumstances are specified.	
(i) Keep several days' supply of insulin, syringes, and needles on hand.	To allow for weather or other conditions that might prevent replacement of insulin or other supplies when needed.
(j) Carry sugar or candy.	For immediate use if a hypoglycemic reaction occurs
(k) If illness occurs, take the usual daily dose of insulin; do not omit insulin. If possible, check blood glucose levels frequently. If unable to do so, test urine for sugar at least 4 times daily, such as before each meal and at bedtime, preferably on a double-voided urine specimen; test urine for ketones if sugar is present; if unable to test own urine, have someone else do it; rest, keep warm, do not exercise, keep someone with you if possible; drink some fluids every hour if able—broth and clear soups help.	Apparently a rather common occurrence is that diabetics who are unable to eat because of nausea, vomiting, or other difficulty omit their insulin. Such a practice increases the likelihood that DKA will occur. In fact, insulin requirements are often increased during illness, probably owing to stress, decreased activity, and other factors. The Joslin Diabetes Foundation recommends keeping a bottle of regular, short-acting insulin on hand even if it is not used ordinarily. The client's personal physician should be consulted regarding this and the circumstances in which any supplemental insulin should be taken.
(l) Reduce insulin dosage or eat extra food if expect to exercise more than usual.	Specific recommendations should be individualized and worked out with the physician in relation to the type of exercise.

Nursing Actions	***Rationale/Explanation***
c. With oral hypoglycemic agents, teach	
(1) Signs and symptoms of hypoglycemia	Hypoglycemic reactions may occur with oral antidiabetic drugs, although they are less common than with insulin.
(2) Do not skip meals and snacks.	This increases the risk of hypoglycemic reactions.
(3) More food may be needed if vigorous exercise is undertaken.	Exercise decreases the need for insulin. Thus, smaller doses of the oral drugs or larger amounts of food are needed. Specific recommendations from the physician will consider the type of exercise.
(4) Follow the same "sick day rules" as prescribed for clients taking insulin, unless otherwise instructed; that is, take the oral hypoglycemic drug; try to take fluids, such as broths and clear soups, every hour unless vomiting; rest; avoid exercise; test urine, on a double-voided urine specimen, before meals, and at bedtime.	Specific, individualized recommendations should be discussed with the physician before illness occurs. Some clients receiving oral agents need injections of regular, short-acting insulin during episodes of illness.

Selected References

American Medical Association (AMA) Division of Drugs: AMA Drug Evaluations, 5th ed. New York, John Wiley & Sons, 1983

Childs BP: Insulin infusion pumps: New solution to an old problem. Nursing 13:54–57, November 1983

Facts and Comparisons. St. Louis, J B Lippincott (Updated monthly)

Feinglos MN: When to prescribe sulfonylureas and insulin. Drug Ther 14:127–134, March 1984

Gerich JE: Sulfonylureas in the treatment of diabetes mellitus—1985. Mayo Clin Proc 60:439–443, July 1985

Glyburide and glipizide. Med Lett Drugs Ther 26:79–80, August 1984

Guyton AC: Textbook of Medical Physiology, 7th ed. Philadelphia, W B Saunders, 1986

Hansten PD: Drug Interactions: Clinical Significance of Drug–Drug Interactions, 5th ed. Philadelphia, Lea & Febiger, 1985

Knott SP, Herget MJ: Teaching self-injection to diabetics: An easier and more effective way. Nursing 14:57, January 1984

Larner J: Insulin and hypoglycemic drugs; glucagon. In Gilman AG, Goodman LS, Rall TW, Murad F (eds): The Pharmacological Basis of Therapeutics, 7th ed., pp 1490–1516. New York, Macmillan, 1985

Lindsey NM: Insights into interventions for coping with diabetes. Nursing 13:48–49, March 1983

McCarthy JA: The continuum of diabetic coma. Am J Nurs 85:878–882, August 1985

McFadden HE: The ups and downs of diabetes. Am J Nurs 85:881, August 1985

Nugent CA: Diabetes mellitus: Goals and techniques for normalizing blood glucose. Drug Ther 14:160–168, October 1984

Price MJ: Insulin and oral hypoglycemic agents. Nurs Clin North Am 18:687–706, December 1983

Rancilio N: When a pregnant woman is diabetic: Postpartal care. Am J Nurs 79:453–456, March 1979

Rodman MJ, Karch AM, Boyd EH, Smith DW: Pharmacology and Drug Therapy in Nursing, 3rd ed. Philadelphia, J B Lippincott, 1985

Schuler K: When a pregnant woman is diabetic: Antepartal care. Am J Nurs 79:448–450, March 1979

Stock-Barkman P: Confusing concepts: Is it diabetic shock or diabetic coma? Nursing 13:32–41, March 1983

Surr CW: Teaching patients to use the new blood-glucose monitoring products. Nursing 13:42–45, January 1983

Thatcher G: Insulin injection: The case against random rotation. Am J Nurs 85:690–692, June 1985

Wimberley D: When a pregnant woman is diabetic: Intrapartal care. Am J Nurs 79:451–452, March 1979

28

ESTROGENS, PROGESTINS, AND ORAL CONTRACEPTIVES

Description and uses

Estrogens and progestins are female sex hormones and are produced by the gonads and adrenal cortices of both men and women. In nonpregnant women, these hormones are produced primarily by the ovaries and secondarily by the adrenal glands. In pregnant women, large amounts of estrogens are produced by the placenta.

Estrogens and progestins are synthesized mainly from cholesterol. The ovaries and adrenal glands can manufacture cholesterol or extract it from the blood. Through a series of chemical reactions, cholesterol is converted to progesterone, then to the androgens, testosterone and androstenedione. These androgens are used by the ovaries to produce estrogens. After formation, the hormones are secreted into the bloodstream in response to stimulation by the anterior pituitary gonadotropic hormones, follicle-stimulating hormone (FSH), and luteinizing hormone (LH). In the bloodstream, the hormones combine with serum proteins and are transported to target tissues, where they enter body cells.

ESTROGENS

The main group of female sex hormones is the estrogens. Several different estrogens have been identified, but only three are secreted in significant amounts: estradiol, estrone, and estriol. Estradiol is considered the major estrogen because it usually exerts more estrogenic activity than the other two combined. The main function of the estrogens is to promote growth in tissues related to reproduction and sexual characteristics in the female. More specific effects of estrogens on body tissues include the following:

1. Effect on breasts. Estrogens stimulate growth of breast tissue at puberty by causing deposition of fat, formation of connective tissue, and construction of ducts. These ducts become part of the milk-producing apparatus after additional stimulation by progesterone.
2. Effect on sexual organs. At puberty, estrogen secretion is greatly increased. The increased estrogen produces enlargement and other changes in the sexual organs. The fallopian tubes, uterus, vagina,

and external genitalia increase in size. The endometrial lining of the uterus proliferates and develops glands that will later nourish the implanted ovum when pregnancy occurs. The epithelial lining of the vagina becomes more resistant to trauma and infection.
3. Effect on the skeleton. Estrogen stimulates skeletal growth so that, beginning at puberty, height increases rapidly for several years. Then, estrogen causes the epiphyses to unite with the shafts of the long bones, and linear growth is halted. This effect of estrogen is stronger than the similar effect of testosterone in the male. Consequently, females stop growing in height several years earlier than males and on the average are shorter than males. Estrogen also conserves calcium and phosphorus. This action promotes bone formation and decreases bone resorption. An additional skeletal effect of estrogen is to broaden the pelvis in preparation for childbirth.
4. Effect on skin and subcutaneous tissue. Estrogen increases vascularity in the skin. This leads to greater skin warmth and likelihood of bleeding in women. Estrogen also causes deposition of fat in subcutaneous tissue, especially in the breasts, thighs, and buttocks, which produces the characteristic female figure.
5. Effect on the anterior pituitary gland. Estrogens decrease pituitary secretion of FSH and increase secretion of LH when blood levels are sufficiently high. Thus, they control their own secretion, in part, by feedback mechanisms to the anterior pituitary gland.
6. Effect on metabolism. In addition to protein anabolism and skeletal effects, estrogen increases sodium and water retention, increases serum triglycerides, decreases serum cholesterol and low-density lipoproteins, and alters glucose metabolism.
7. Effect on blood coagulation. Estrogen enhances coagulation by increasing blood levels of several clotting factors, including prothrombin and factors VII, IX, and X.

In nonpregnant women, between puberty and menopause, estrogens are secreted in a monthly cycle called the menstrual cycle. During the first half of the cycle, before ovulation, estrogens are secreted in progressively larger amounts. During the second half of the cycle, both estrogens and progesterone are secreted in increasing amounts until about 2 days before the onset of menstruation. At that time, secretion of both hormones decreases abruptly. When the endometrial lining of the uterus loses its hormonal stimulation, it is discharged vaginally as menstrual flow.

During pregnancy, the placenta produces large amounts of estrogen, mainly estriol. The increased estrogen produces enlargement of the uterus and breasts, growth of glandular tissue in the breasts, and relaxation of ligaments and joints in the pelvis. All these changes are necessary for growth and birth of the fetus.

The exact mechanism of estrogen action is not clearly understood. After secretion into the bloodstream, estrogens apparently combine with serum proteins and are transported to their target tissues, where they are released. They are thought to cross cell membranes easily, probably because of their steroid molecular structure. Once inside the cells, they apparently stimulate cellular protein synthesis.

Finally, estrogens, like the other naturally occurring steroid hormones, are inactivated in the liver. They are conjugated with glucuronic acid or sulfuric acid, which makes them water soluble and readily excreted through the kidneys.

PROGESTERONE

Progesterone is a progestin concerned almost entirely with reproduction. In the nonpregnant woman, progesterone is secreted by the corpus luteum during the last half of the menstrual cycle, after ovulation. This hormone continues the changes in the endometrial lining of the uterus begun by estrogens during the first half of the menstrual cycle. These changes provide for implantation and nourishment of a fertilized ovum. When fertilization does not take place, the levels of estrogen and progesterone decrease and menstruation occurs.

If the ovum is fertilized, progesterone acts to maintain the pregnancy. The corpus luteum produces progesterone during the first few weeks of gestation. Then, the placenta produces the progesterone needed to maintain the endometrial lining of the uterus. In addition to its effects on the uterus, progesterone prepares the breasts for lactation by promoting development of milk-producing cells. Milk is not secreted, however, until the cells are further stimulated by prolactin from the anterior pituitary gland. Progesterone may also help maintain pregnancy by decreasing uterine contractility. This, in turn, decreases the risk of spontaneous abortion.

ESTROGENS AND PROGESTINS USED AS DRUGS

1. When estrogens and progestins are given from exogenous sources as drugs for therapeutic purposes,

they produce the same effects as endogenous (naturally occurring) hormones.

2. Several preparations of estrogens and progestins are available for various purposes and routes of administration.
   a. Naturally occurring, nonconjugated estrogens (estradiol, estrone) and natural progesterone are given intramuscularly (IM) because they are rapidly metabolized if given orally. There are some crystalline suspensions of estrogens and oil solutions of both estrogens and progesterone, which prolong drug action by slowing absorption.
   b. Conjugated estrogens (Premarin) and some synthetic derivatives of natural estrogens (*e.g.*, ethinyl estradiol) and natural progesterone (*e.g.*, norethindrone) are chemically modified to be effective with oral administration.
   c. Nonsteroidal, synthetic preparations are usually given orally or topically. They are chemically altered to slow their metabolism in the liver. They are also less bound to serum proteins than the naturally occurring hormones.
3. Oral contraceptives consist of a synthetic estrogen and a synthetic progestin. A commonly used estrogen component is ethinyl estradiol, and a commonly used progestin is norethindrone. Earlier contraceptives (monophasics) contain fixed amounts of both estrogen and progestin components. Because of a high incidence of adverse effects, the amount of estrogen has been reduced in newer preparations. Recent preparations, biphasics and triphasics, deliver fixed amounts of estrogen but varied amounts of progestin during different phases of the menstrual cycle. One of these, Triphasil, varies both estrogen and progestin content. These preparations mimic normal variations of hormone secretion and may decrease adverse effects. These contraceptives are dispensed in containers with color-coded tablets that must be taken in the correct sequence. Dispensers with 28 tablets contain 7 inactive or placebo tablets of a third color. A few contraceptive products contain a progestin only. These are less effective in preventing pregnancy and are more likely to cause vaginal bleeding irregularities, which makes them less acceptable to many women.

Oral contraceptive drugs act primarily by decreasing pituitary secretion of FSH and LH. When these gonadotropic hormones are absent, ovulation and therefore conception cannot occur. These drugs may also prevent conception by interfering with transport of the fertilized ovum, by making the endometrial lining of the uterus unfavorable for implantation of the fertilized ovum, and by making cervical mucus resistant to penetrations by spermatozoa. Whatever the mechanism of action, these drugs are highly effective in preventing pregnancy, although they are capable of causing serious adverse reactions as well.

Clinical indications

Estrogen is most often used as replacement therapy in deficiency states and as a component in birth control pills. Deficiency states usually result from hypofunction of the pituitary gland or the ovaries and may occur anytime during the life cycle. For example, in the adolescent girl with delayed sexual development, estrogen can be given to produce the changes that normally occur at puberty. In the woman of reproductive age (approximately 12 to 45 years), estrogens are sometimes used in menstrual disorders. These include amenorrhea and abnormal uterine bleeding due to estrogen deficiency. Estrogens are also used widely in this age group to control fertility, usually combined with a progestin. If pregnancy does occur, estrogens are contraindicated because their use during pregnancy has been associated with the occurrence of vaginal cancer in female offspring and possible harmful effects on male offspring. After pregnancy, however, during the postpartum period, estrogen may be given to suppress lactation if the mother is not going to breast-feed her baby. Estrogen apparently suppresses lactation by allowing the hypothalamus to continue secretion of prolactin-inhibiting factor (PIF). During menopause, estrogens are given to relieve atrophic vaginitis and vasomotor instability, which produces "hot flashes," and to prevent osteoporosis. They may also prevent or delay coronary atherosclerosis and subsequent myocardial infarction. Some authorities have not recommended replacement estrogen therapy during or after menopause because of a concern about endometrial cancer. Current opinion is that giving a progestin along with the estrogen negates this risk.

Other clinical uses of estrogen include treatment of metastatic breast cancer in women more than 5 years postmenopause, metastatic prostate cancer in men, acne and hirsutism in women with excessive male sex hormone secretion, and prevention of excessive height in young girls.

Progesterone and other progestins are probably used most frequently in oral contraceptive pills. They are also used in menstrual disorders such as amenorrhea, dysmenorrhea and abnormal uterine bleeding, endometriosis, threatened abortion, infertility, and endometrial cancer. The progestins are being increasingly used for conditions formerly treated with estrogens.

The primary clinical indication for use of oral contraceptives is, of course, to control fertility and prevent pregnancy. These preparations are also used to treat various menstrual disorders such as amenorrhea and dysmenorrhea.

Contraindications

Because of their widespread effects on body tissues and reported adverse reactions, estrogens, progestins, and oral contraceptives are contraindicated in the following conditions:

1. Known or suspected pregnancy, since damage to the fetus may result
2. Presence of thromboembolic disorders, such as thrombophlebitis, deep vein thrombosis, or pulmonary embolism
3. Known or suspected cancers of breast or genital tissues, since the drugs may stimulate tumor growth. An exception is use of estrogens for treatment of metastatic breast cancer in women at least 5 years postmenopause
4. Undiagnosed vaginal or uterine bleeding
5. Fibroid tumors of the uterus
6. Active liver disease or impaired liver function
7. History of cerebrovascular disease, coronary artery disease, thrombophlebitis, hypertension, or conditions predisposing to these disease processes
8. Women over 35 years of age who are heavy smokers (more than 15 cigarettes daily)
9. Family history of breast or reproductive system cancer

Individual estrogens, progestins, and oral contraceptives

Table 28-1 lists the clinical indications, routes of administration, and dosages of estrogens. Table 28-2 provides the clinical indications, routes of administration, and dosages of progestins. Oral contraceptive agents are listed in Table 28-3.

Principles of therapy: estrogens, progestins, and oral contraceptives

NEED FOR CONTINUOUS SUPERVISION

Because estrogens, progestins, and oral contraceptives are usually taken for several months or years and may cause significant adverse reactions, clients taking these drugs need continued medical supervision. Before the drugs are given, a complete medical history, a physical examination with breast and pelvic examinations plus a Papanicolaou smear, urinalysis, and weight and blood pressure measurement are recommended. These examinations should be repeated periodically, at least annually, as long as the client is taking these drugs.

DRUG SELECTION FACTORS

Choice of estrogen preparation depends on the reason for use and desired route of administration. Conjugated estrogens (*e.g.*, Premarin) are commonly used and may be associated with fewer liver problems than other preparations. Diethylstilbestrol is the only estrogen approved for use as a postcoital contraceptive. Such usage is recommended for females who are victims of rape or incest or whose physical or mental health is threatened by pregnancy. To be effective, the drug should be started within 24 hours if possible and no later than 72 hours after exposure.

DOSAGE FACTORS

Although dosage needs vary with clients and the conditions for which the drugs are prescribed, a general rule is to use the smallest effective dose for the shortest effective time. Approximately equivalent doses of estrogen preparations are estradiol 50 μg, mestranol 80 μg, diethylstilbestrol 1 mg, and conjugated estrogens 5 mg. Estrogens are given cyclically, alone or with a progestin. In one regimen, the drug is taken for 3 weeks, then omitted for 1 week. In another, it is omitted the first 5 days of each month. These regimens more closely resemble normal premenstrual secretion of estrogen and avoid prolonged stimulation of body tissues.

USE IN SPECIFIC SITUATIONS

Menopause

In treatment of menopause, estrogen replacement therapy relieves vasomotor and vaginal symptoms and

TABLE 28-1. ESTROGENS

Generic name	Trade name	Routes and dosage ranges for various indications					
		Dysfunctional uterine bleeding	*Menopausal symptoms*	*Female hypogonadism*	*Postpartum breast engorgement**	*Prostate cancer*	*Other*
Chlorotrianisene	Tace		PO 12–25 mg daily for 21 days, followed by 7 days without the drug	PO 12–25 mg daily for 21 days	PO 72 mg twice daily for 2 days; 12 mg 4 times daily for 7 days, or 50 mg q6h for 6 doses	PO 12–25 mg daily	
Conjugated estrogens	Premarin	IM or IV for emergency use, 25 mg, repeated in 6–12 hrs if necessary	PO 0.3–1.25 mg daily for 21 days followed by 7 days without the drug	PO 2.5–7.5 mg daily in divided doses, cyclically, 20 days on, 10 days off the drug	PO 1.25 mg q4h for 5 days or 3.75 mg q4h for 5 doses	PO 1.25–2.5 mg 3 times daily	Breast cancer: PO 10 mg tid for at least 3 months Atrophic vaginitis: Topically, 2.4 g of vaginal cream inserted daily Osteoporosis: PO 1.25 mg daily for 21 days, then 7 days without the drug
Dienestrol	DV						Atrophic or senile vaginitis: Topically, vaginal cream applied 2–3 times daily for about 2 weeks, then reduced to 3 times weekly
Diethylstilbestrol (DES)	Stilbestrol		PO 0.2–0.5 mg daily for 21 days, followed by 7 days without the drug	PO 0.2–0.5 mg daily for 21 days, followed by 7 days without the drug		PO 1–3 mg daily	Breast cancer: PO 15 mg daily Postcoital contraception: PO 25 mg twice daily for 5 days
Esterified estrogens	Estratab		PO 0.3–1.25 mg daily for 21 days, then 7 days without the drug	PO 2.5–7.5 mg daily, in divided doses, for 21 days, then 7 days without the drug		PO 1.25–2.5 mg 1–3 times daily	Breast cancer: PO 10 mg 3 times daily for at least 3 months
Estradiol	Estrace		PO 1–2 mg daily for 3 weeks, then 1 week off or daily Monday through			PO 1–2 mg 3 times daily for at least 3 months	Breast cancer: PO 10 mg 3 times daily for at least 3 months

TABLE 28-1. ESTROGENS (*Continued*)

Generic name	Trade name	Routes and dosage ranges for various indications: *Dysfunctional uterine bleeding*	*Menopausal symptoms*	*Female hypogonadism*	*Postpartum breast engorgement**	*Prostate cancer*	*Other*
			Friday, none on Saturday or Sunday				
Estradiol cypionate	Depo-Estradiol		IM 1–5 mg q3–4 weeks	IM 1.5–2 mg at monthly intervals			
Estradiol valerate	Delestrogen		IM 10–20 mg q4 weeks	IM 10–20 mg q4 weeks	IM 10–25 mg at end of first-stage labor	IM 30 mg q1–2 weeks	
Estrone	Theelin	IM 2–4 mg daily for several days until bleeding is controlled, followed by progestin for 1 week	IM 0.1–0.5 mg weekly in single or divided doses	IM 0.1–2 mg weekly		IM 2–4 mg q3–4 days	
Estropipate	Ogen		PO 0.625–5 mg daily, cyclically	PO 1.25–7.5 mg daily for 3 weeks, followed by an 8- to 10-day rest period. Repeat as needed			Ovarian failure: same dosage as for female hypogonadism Atrophic vaginitis: topically, 1–2 g vaginal cream daily
Ethinyl estradiol	Estinyl, Feminone		PO 0.02–0.05 mg daily, cyclically	PO 0.05 mg 1–3 times daily for 2 weeks with addition of progestin for last 2 weeks of month	PO 0.5–1 mg daily for 3 days, reduced to 0.1 mg after 7 days	PO 0.15–2 mg daily	Breast cancer: PO 1 mg 3 times daily
Quinestrol	Estrovis		PO 100 μg daily for 7 days, then 100–200 μg once weekly			Atrophic vaginitis: PO 100 μg daily for 7 days, then 100–200 μg weekly	

* When estrogens are given to prevent breast engorgement and lactation, the first dose should be given within 8 hours after delivery.

prevents osteoporosis. A commonly prescribed regimen is a conjugated estrogen such as Premarin, 0.625 mg to 1.25 mg, daily for 25 days of each month, with a progestin such as Provera, 10 mg, daily for 10 days of each month, on days 15 to 25 of the cycle. The main function of the progestin is to decrease the risk of endometrial cancer; thus, some authorities do not prescribe progestin for the hysterectomized woman. Therapy should probably be continued indefinitely to prevent osteoporosis.

TABLE 28-2. PROGESTINS

Generic name	Trade name	Routes and dosage ranges for various indications			
		Menstrual disorders	*Endometriosis*	*Endometrial cancer*	*Other*
Hydroxyprogesterone caproate	Delalutin	Amenorrhea, dysfunctional uterine bleeding: IM 375 mg. If no bleeding after 21 days, begin cyclic therapy with estradiol and repeat q4 weeks for 4 cycles.			Uterine adenocarcinoma: IM 1 g or more initially; repeat 1 or more times each week (maximum, 7 g/week). Stop when relapse occurs or after 12 weeks with no response. Test for endogenous estrogen production: IM 250 mg, repeated in 4 weeks. Bleeding 7–14 days after injection indicates endogenous estrogen.
Medroxyprogesterone acetate	Depo-Provera, Provera	Dysfunctional uterine bleeding: PO 5–10 mg daily for 5–10 days beginning on 16th or 21st day of cycle Amenorrhea: PO 5–10 mg daily for 5–10 days		IM 400–1000 mg weekly until improvement, then 400 mg monthly	
Megestrol acetate	Megace			PO 40–320 mg daily in 4 divided doses for at least 2 months	Breast cancer: PO 160 mg daily in 4 divided doses for at least 2 months
Norethindrone	Norlutin	Amenorrhea, dysfunctional uterine bleeding: PO 5–20 mg daily, starting on 5th day of menstrual cycle and ending on 25th day	PO 10 mg daily for 2 weeks, increase by 5 mg daily every 2 weeks to dose of 30 mg. Then give 20–30 mg daily for maintenance up to 6–9 months		Norethindrone is also used as a contraceptive (see Table 28-3)
Norethindrone acetate	Norlutate	Amenorrhea, dysfunctional uterine bleeding: PO 2.5–10 mg daily, starting on 5th day of menstrual cycle and ending on 25th day	PO 5 mg daily for 2 weeks, increase by 2.5 mg daily every 2 weeks to dose of 15 mg. Then give 10–15 mg daily for maintenance.		
Progesterone	Femotrone, Progelan	Amenorrhea, dysfunctional uterine bleeding: IM 5–10 mg for 6–8 consecutive days			

Cancer

When estrogens and progestins are used in the treatment of cancer, several factors must be considered. First, the goals of treatment are palliation of symptoms and shrinkage of tumor tissue rather than cure. Second, these drugs have limited effectiveness, and careful selection of recipients is essential. Estrogens are recom-

TABLE 28-3. ORAL CONTRACEPTIVE AGENTS

	Trade name	Estrogen (μg)	Progestin (mg)
Monophasics	Brevicon	Ethinyl estradiol 35	Norethindrone 0.5
	Demulen	Ethinyl estradiol 50	Ethynodiol diacetate 1
	Enovid 5 mg	Mestranol 75	Norethynodrel 5
	Enovid E	Mestranol 100	Norethynodrel 2.5
	Loestrin 1/20	Ethinyl estradiol 20	Norethindrone acetate 1
	Loestrin 1.5/30	Ethinyl estradiol 30	Norethindrone acetate 1.5
	Lo/Ovral	Ethinyl estradiol 30	Norgestrel 0.3
	Modicon	Ethinyl estradiol 35	Norethindrone 0.5
	Nordette	Ethinyl estradiol 30	Levonorgestrel 0.15
	Norinyl 1 + 35	Ethinyl estradiol 35	Norethindrone 1
	Norinyl 1 + 50	Mestranol 50	Norethindrone 1
	Norinyl 1 + 80	Mestranol 80	Norethindrone 1
	Norinyl 2 mg	Mestranol 100	Norethindrone 2
	Norlestrin 1/50	Ethinyl estradiol 50	Norethindrone acetate 1
	Norlestrin 2.5/50	Ethinyl estradiol 50	Norethindrone acetate 2.5
	Ortho-Novum 1/35	Ethinyl estradiol 35	Norethindrone 1
	Ortho-Novum 1/50	Mestranol 50	Norethindrone 1
	Ortho-Novum 1/80	Mestranol 80	Norethindrone 1
	Ortho-Novum 2 mg	Mestranol 100	Norethindrone 2
	Ovcon-35	Ethinyl estradiol 35	Norethindrone 0.4
	Ovcon-50	Ethinyl estradiol 50	Norethindrone 1
	Ovral	Ethinyl estradiol 50	Norgestrel 0.5
	Ovulen	Mestranol 100	Ethynodiol diacetate 1
Biphasics	Ortho-Novum 10/11–21 Ortho-Novum 10/11–28	Ethinyl estradiol 35	Norethindrone 0.5 (10 tablets), 1.0 (11 tablets)
Triphasics	Ortho-Novum 7/7/7	Ethinyl estradiol 35	Norethindrone 0.5 (7 tablets), 0.75 (7 tablets), 1.0 (7 tablets)
	Tri-Norinyl	Ethinyl estradiol 35	Norethindrone 0.5 (7 tablets), 1.0 (9 tablets), 0.5 (5 tablets)
	Triphasil	Ethinyl estradiol 30 (6 tablets), 40 (5 tablets), 30 (10 tablets)	Levonorgestrel 0.05 (6 tablets), 0.075 (5 tablets), 0.125 (10 tablets)
Progestin-only products	Micronor		Norethindrone 0.35
	Nor-Q.D.		Norethindrone 0.35
	Ovrette		Norgestrel 0.075

mended only for men with recurrent or metastatic cancer of the prostate gland and for postmenopausal women with recurrent or metastatic breast cancer. Progestins are used for metastatic cancer of the endometrium. Third, relatively large doses are needed for antineoplastic effects, and the drugs are given continuously rather than cyclically. This means that adverse reactions are more likely to occur and that most specific symptoms are those resulting from hormone excess. Recommended dosages may be decreased. Some studies, for example, indicate that diethylstilbestrol 1 mg daily is as effective as 5 mg daily in the treatment of prostatic cancer. Further, fewer deaths from cardiovascular disease occur with the smaller dose.

Contraception

When estrogens and progestins are used as oral contraceptives, some guidelines include the following:

1. These drugs are nearly 100% effective in preventing pregnancy. The primary difficulty associated with their use is a relatively high incidence of potentially serious adverse reactions. Clients should be informed about potential benefits and risks and participate in the decision to use or not to use these drugs. Oral contraceptives are considered safest when given to nonsmoking women under 35 years of age who do not have a history of thromboembolic problems, diabetes mellitus, hypertension, or migraine headache.
2. Assess each client's need and desire for oral contraceptive drugs as well as her willingness to comply with the prescribed regimen. Assessment information includes the client's knowledge about oral contraceptives and other methods of birth control. Compliance involves the willingness to take the drugs as prescribed, to have examinations of breasts and pelvis and blood pressure measure-

ments every 6 to 12 months, and to stop the oral contraceptive periodically (other contraceptive methods can be used during these periods). Assessment also includes identifying clients in whom oral contraceptives are contraindicated or who are at increased risk of adverse reactions.

3. The most effective and widely used oral contraceptives are estrogen–progestin combinations. Several are available. The preparation of choice for most clients is one that contains less than 50 μg of estrogen, since fewer adverse reactions occur at this dosage level. Effects of estrogen components are similar when prescribed in equipotent doses, but progestins differ in progestogenic, estrogenic, antiestrogenic, and androgenic activity. Consequently, adverse effects may differ to some extent, and a client may be able to tolerate one oral contraceptive better than another.

4. Oral contraceptives decrease effects of oral anticoagulants, insulin and oral antidiabetic agents, antihypertensive drugs, and drugs used to lower serum cholesterol. If oral contraceptives are used concurrently with these drug groups, dosage of these groups may need to be increased. If oral contraceptives are discontinued, dosage of the other drugs may need to be decreased.

NURSING ACTIONS: ESTROGENS, PROGESTINS, AND ORAL CONTRACEPTIVES

Nursing Actions	*Rationale/Explanation*
1. Administer accurately	
a. Give oral estrogens, progestins, and contraceptive preparations after meals or at bedtime.	To decrease nausea, a common adverse reaction
b. With aqueous suspensions to be given IM, roll the vial between the hands several times.	To be sure that drug particles are evenly distributed through the liquid vehicle
c. Give oil preparations deeply into a large muscle mass, preferably gluteal muscles.	
2. Observe for therapeutic effects	Therapeutic effects vary, depending on the reason for use.
a. With estrogens	
(1) When given for menopausal symptoms, observe for decrease in "hot flashes" and vaginal problems.	
(2) When given for amenorrhea, observe for menstruation.	
(3) When given for female hypogonadism, observe for menstruation, breast enlargement, axillary and pubic hair, and other secondary sexual characteristics.	
(4) When given for postpartum breast engorgement, observe for decreased tenderness and pain and absence of milk secretion.	
(5) When used in cancer of the breast or prostate gland, observe for relief of symptoms.	
b. With progestins	
(1) When given for menstrual disorders such as abnormal uterine bleeding, amenorrhea, dysmenorrhea, premenstrual discomfort, and endometriosis, observe for relief of symptoms.	
3. Observe for adverse reactions	Most adverse reactions are attributed to estrogens, although many of the same ones are listed for progestins as well. Thus,

Nursing Actions	***Rationale/Explanation***
	the nurse should observe for similar adverse reactions whether the client is receiving estrogen or progestin alone or in combination as an oral contraceptive drug.
a. Gastrointestinal system—anorexia, nausea, vomiting, diarrhea, gallbladder disease, cholestatic jaundice	Nausea is the most common adverse reaction. It usually subsides within 1 to 2 weeks of continued drug therapy.
b. Cardiovascular system	
(1) Thromboembolic conditions such as thrombophlebitis, pulmonary embolism, cerebral thrombosis, and coronary thrombosis	A greater incidence of blood clotting disorders has been well documented in women taking these drugs, especially the oral contraceptives.
(2) Hypertension	
(3) Edema, weight gain	These are caused by drug-induced fluid retention.
c. Central nervous system—headache, mental depression, insomnia, nervousness, anxiety	
d. Genitourinary system—vaginal bleeding or spotting, breast engorgement, endometrial cancer, vaginitis due to fungus (*Candida albicans*)	With oral contraceptives, breakthrough bleeding early in the cycle indicates an estrogen deficiency, and bleeding after midcycle indicates a progestin deficiency. Treatment involves altering estrogen or progestin dosage.
e. Integumentary system—skin rash, pruritus, acne, hirsutism	
f. When estrogens are given to men, adverse reactions include gynecomastia, feminizing effects, impotence, atrophy of testicles, and thromboembolic complications	
g. Decreased glucose tolerance and increased blood and urine sugar levels	
4. Observe for drug interactions	
a. Drugs that *decrease* effects of estrogens, progestins, and oral contraceptives	
(1) Anticonvulsants, barbiturates, rifampin	Decrease effects by inducing enzymes that accelerate metabolism of estrogens and progestins.
(2) Antimicrobials—ampicillin, chloramphenicol, neomycin, nitrofurantoin, penicillin V, sulfonamides, tetracyclines	By disrupting the normal bacterial flora of the gastrointestinal tract, antimicrobial drugs may decrease or eliminate enterohepatic circulation of estrogens and their conjugates. This action may decrease effectiveness of the contraceptive or cause breakthrough bleeding.
5. Teach clients	
a. Take estrogens, progestins, or oral contraceptives with meals or food or at bedtime.	To decrease nausea, which is a common adverse reaction
b. If cyclic therapy is prescribed, take the drug for 3 weeks and then omit it for 1 week. Explain that menstruation occurs but pregnancy does not, since ovulation has been prevented. With oral contraceptives, consult the physician about what to do if one or more daily doses is omitted for any reason. Another method of contraception may be needed temporarily; since ovulation may have occurred.	
c. Medical supervision, usually every 6 to 12 months, is necessary when these drugs are taken for long periods.	To check blood pressure, breasts, pelvis, and other areas for possible adverse reactions
d. To weigh themselves at least weekly and to report sudden weight gain.	Fluid retention and edema may occur and produce weight gain.
e. To report any unusual vaginal bleeding.	This may be caused by excessive amounts of estrogen.

Nursing Actions	Rationale/Explanation
f. To observe for and report adverse reactions such as calf tenderness, redness, or swelling, which are signs of thrombophlebitis.	
g. Teach women with diabetes to check urine for sugar and report if present in increased amounts.	Estrogens increase blood and urine glucose levels.
h. Teach women receiving vaginal suppositories of estrogen how to insert them correctly.	
i. When diethylstilbestrol is used as a postcoital contraceptive, teach clients to take the drug despite the nausea that often occurs.	This drug must be taken as prescribed to be effective in preventing pregnancy.
j. Teach men who receive estrogens that feminizing effects and impotence are temporary and subside when drug therapy is discontinued.	
k. Advise women who take oral contraceptives not to smoke cigarettes.	Cigarette smoking increases risks of thromboembolic disorders in women taking birth control pills.

Selected References

Aloia JF, Cohn SH, Vaswani A, et al: Risk factors for postmenopausal osteoporosis. Am J Med 78:95–100, January 1985

American Medical Association (AMA) Division of Drugs: AMA Drug Evaluations, 5th ed. New York, John Wiley & Sons, 1983

Babington MA: Adolescent use of oral contraceptives. Pediatr Nurs 10:111–114, March–April 1984

Brinton LA: The relationship of exogenous estrogens to cancer risk. Cancer Detect Prevent 7:159–171, 1984

Facts and Comparisons. St. Louis, J B Lippincott (Updated monthly)

Hansten PD: Drug Interactions: Clinical Significance of Drug–Drug Interactions, 5th ed. Philadelphia, Lea & Febiger, 1985

Horsman A, Jones M, Francis R, et al: The effect of estrogen dose on postmenopausal bone loss. N Engl J Med 309:1405–1407, December 1983

Judd HL, Meldrum DR, Deftos LJ, Henderson BE: Estrogen replacement therapy: Indications and complications. Ann Intern Med 98:195–205, February 1983

Malseed RT: Pharmacology: Drug Therapy and Nursing Considerations, 2d ed. Philadelphia, J B Lippincott, 1985

Murad F, Haynes RC Jr: Estrogens and progestins. In Gilman AG, Goodman LS, Rall TW, Murad F (eds): The Pharmacological Basis of Therapeutics, 7th ed., pp 1412–1439. New York, Macmillan, 1985

Rodman MJ, Karch AM, Boyd EH, Smith DW: Pharmacology and Drug Therapy in Nursing, 3rd ed. Philadelphia, J B Lippincott, 1985

Tri Norinyl and Ortho-Novum 7/7/7—two triphasic oral contraceptives. Med Lett Drugs Ther 26:93–94, October 1984

Triphasil—a new triphasic oral contraceptive. Med Lett Drugs Ther 27:48, May 1985

29

ANDROGENS AND ANABOLIC STEROIDS

Description and uses

Androgens are a group of male sex hormones secreted by the testes in men, the ovaries in women, and the adrenal glands of both sexes. Like the female sex hormones, the naturally occurring male sex hormones are steroids synthesized from cholesterol. The sex organs and adrenal glands can produce cholesterol or remove it from the blood. Cholesterol then undergoes a series of conversions to progesterone, androgenic prehormones, and finally to testosterone. The androgens produced by the ovaries have little androgenic activity and are used mainly as precursor substances for the production of naturally occurring estrogens. The adrenal glands produce about five androgens, including androstenedione and dehydroepiandrosterone, but these ordinarily have little masculinizing effect.

Anabolic steroids are synthetic drugs with increased anabolic activity and decreased androgenic activity when compared to testosterone. They were developed during attempts to modify testosterone so that its tissue-building and growth-stimulating effects could be retained while its masculinizing effects could be eliminated or reduced. These attempts have not been entirely successful because all the anabolic steroids still have androgenic activity, although it is weaker than that of testosterone.

Testosterone is normally the only important male sex hormone. It is secreted by the Leydig cells in the testes in response to stimulation by luteinizing hormone (LH) or interstitial cell-stimulating hormone (ICSH) from the anterior pituitary gland. The main functions of testosterone are related to the development of male sexual characteristics, reproduction, and metabolism. Specific effects of testosterone on body tissues include the following:

1. Effect on fetal development. Large amounts of chorionic gonadotropin are produced by the placenta during pregnancy. Chorionic gonadotropin is similar to LH from the anterior pituitary gland. It promotes development of the interstitial or Leydig cells in fetal testes, which then secrete testosterone. Testosterone production begins about the second month of fetal life. When present, testosterone promotes development of male sexual characteristics such as the penis, scrotum, prostate gland, seminal vesicles, and seminiferous tubules and suppresses development of female sexual characteristics. In the absence of testosterone, the fetus develops female sexual characteristics.

   Testosterone also provides the stimulus for the descent of the testes into the scrotum. This normally occurs after the seventh month of pregnancy, when the fetal testes are secreting relatively large amounts of testosterone. If the testes do not descend before birth, administration of testosterone or gonadotropic hormone, which stimulates testosterone secretion, will produce descent in most cases.

2. Effect on adult development. Little testosterone is secreted in male children until the age of approximately 11 to 13 years. At the onset of puberty, testosterone secretion increases rapidly and remains at a relatively high level until about 40 years of age, after which it gradually declines.
   a. The testosterone secreted at puberty acts as a growth hormone to produce enlargement of the penis, testes, and scrotum until about 20 years of age. The prostate gland, seminal vesicles, seminiferous tubules, and vas deferens also increase in size and functional ability. Under the combined influence of testosterone and follicle-stimulating hormone (FSH) from the anterior pituitary gland, sperm production is initiated and maintained throughout the man's reproductive life.
   b. Effect on skin. Testosterone increases skin thickness and activity of the sebaceous glands. Acne in the adolescent male is attributed to the increased production of testosterone.
   c. Effect on the voice. The larynx enlarges and deepens the voice of the adult male.
   d. Effect on body hair. Testosterone produces the distribution of hair growth on the face, limbs, and trunk typical of the adult male. In men with a genetic trait toward baldness, large amounts of testosterone cause alopecia (baldness) of the scalp.
   e. Effect on skeletal muscles. Testosterone is largely responsible for the larger, more powerful muscles of men. This characteristic is caused by the effects of testosterone on protein metabolism. Testosterone helps the body retain nitrogen, form new amino acids, and build new muscle protein. At the same time, it slows the loss of nitrogen and amino acids formed by the constant breakdown of body tissues. Overall, then, testosterone increases protein anabolism (build-up) and decreases protein catabolism (breakdown).
   f. Effects on bone. Testosterone makes bones both thicker and longer. After puberty, more protein and calcium are deposited and retained in bone matrix. This causes a rapid rate of bone growth. The height of a male adolescent increases rapidly for a time, then stops as epiphyseal closure occurs. This happens when the cartilage at the end of the long bones in the arms and legs becomes bone. Further lengthening of the bones is then prevented.
   g. Effect on anterior pituitary function. High blood levels of testosterone decrease secretion of FSH and of LH or ICSH from the anterior pituitary gland. This, in turn, decreases testosterone production.

The exact mechanisms by which testosterone produces the effects noted above are not completely understood. Most effects, however, are attributed to increased protein production in most body cells, especially those related to male sexual characteristics. After testosterone is secreted by the testes, most of it binds reversibly to plasma proteins. It then circulates in the bloodstream for a half hour or less before it becomes attached to tissues or is broken down into inactive products. The portion that is attached to tissues enters the cells and is changed to dihydrotestosterone. The dihydrotestosterone binds with receptors within the cell and stimulates increased production of protein by the cell. The portion that does not become attached to tissues is converted into androsterone and dehydroepiandrosterone by the liver. These are conjugated with glucuronic or sulfuric acid and excreted in the bile or urine.

CHARACTERISTICS OF ANDROGENIC AND ANABOLIC STEROID DRUGS

Individual androgens and anabolic steroids are listed in Table 29-1.

1. When male sex hormones or androgens are given from exogenous sources for therapeutic purposes, they produce the same effects as the naturally occuring hormones.
2. Male sex hormones given to women antagonize or reduce the effects of female sex hormones. Thus, administration of testosterone to women can suppress menstruation and cause atrophy of the endometrial lining of the uterus.
3. Exogenous androgens are given intramuscularly or orally. Naturally occurring androgens are given by injection because they are rapidly metabolized by the liver if given orally. There are some esters of testosterone that have been modified to slow the rate of metabolism and thus prolong action.
4. All synthetic anabolic steroids are weak androgens. Consequently, giving these drugs for anabolic effects also produces masculinizing effects. This characteristic tends to limit the clinical usefulness of these drugs in women and children. Profound changes in growth and sexual development may occur if these drugs are given to young children.

CLINICAL INDICATIONS

Male sex hormones are used clinically in a variety of conditions to increase or change hormonal effects on body tissues. They are used in both males and females.

(Text continues on p. 281.)

TABLE 29-1. ANDROGENS AND ANABOLIC STEROIDS

	Generic name	Trade name	Routes and dosage ranges for various indications			
			Hypogonadism	*Anabolic effects*	*Breast cancer*	*Other*
Androgens	Testosterone	Android-T Testoject Testaqua Oreton (pellets)	IM 10–25 mg 2–3 times weekly SC (75-mg pellets) 150–450 mg every 3–6 months; not implanted until dose has been stabilized orally or parenterally		IM 100 mg 3 times weekly	Postpartum breast engorgement: IM 25–50 mg daily for 3–4 days, starting at time of delivery
	Testosterone cypionate	Depo-testosterone	IM 200–400 mg every 4 weeks			Osteoporosis: IM 200–400 mg every 4 weeks Oligospermia: IM 100–200 mg every 4–6 weeks
	Testosterone enanthate	Delatestryl	IM 200–400 mg every 4 weeks			See Testosterone cypionate
	Testosterone propionate	Various	IM 10–25 mg 3–4 times weekly		IM 100 mg 3 times weekly	
	Fluoxymesterone	Halotestin	PO 2–10 mg daily		PO 15–30 mg daily in divided doses	Delayed puberty: PO 2 mg daily initially. Increase gradually as necessary Postpartum breast engorgement: 2.5 mg when active labor begins, then 5–10 mg daily in divided doses for 4–5 days
	Methyltestosterone	Metandren	PO 10–40 mg daily initially, reduced for maintenance Buccal tablets, half the oral dose		PO 200 mg daily in divided doses Buccal tablets, 100 mg daily	Cryptorchidism: PO 30 mg daily; buccal tablets, 15 mg daily Postpartum breast engorgement: PO 80 mg daily for 3–5 days; buccal tablets, 40 mg daily for 3–5 days
	Danazol	Danocrine				Endometriosis: PO 800 mg daily in 2 divided doses for 6–9 months Fibrocystic breast disease; PO 100–400 mg daily in 2 divided doses for 3–6 months
Anabolic steroids	Dromostanolone	Drolban			IM 100 mg 3 times weekly for 8–12 weeks	

TABLE 29-1. ANDROGENS AND ANABOLIC STEROIDS (*Continued*)

Generic name	Trade name	Routes and dosage ranges for various indications			
		Hypogonadism	*Anabolic effects*	*Breast cancer*	*Other*
Ethylestrenol	Maxibolin		Adults: PO 4–8 mg daily Children: PO 1–3 mg daily		
Methandriol	Anabol		Children: IM 5–10 mg daily		Senile and post-menopausal osteoporosis: IM 50–100 mg 1–2 times weekly or 10–40 mg daily
Methandrostenolone	Dianabol				Senile and post-menopausal osteoporosis: PO 5 mg daily initially. Usual maintenance dose, 2.5–5 mg daily Pituitary dwarfism in children: 0.05 mg/kg/day
Nandrolone decanoate	Deca-Durabolin		Adults: IM 50–100 mg every 3–4 weeks Children: IM 25–50 mg every 3–4 weeks	IM 100–200 mg weekly	Osteoporosis (adults): IM 50–100 mg every 3–4 weeks Erythropoiesis: IM up to 200 mg every 3–4 weeks
Nandrolone phenpropionate	Durabolin		Adults: IM 25–50 mg weekly Children: IM 12.5–25 mg every 2–4 weeks	IM 25–100 mg weekly	Osteoporosis (adults): IM 25–50 mg weekly Erythropoiesis: IM up to 100 mg weekly
Oxandrolone	Anavar		Adults: PO 5–10 mg daily in divided doses (up to 20 mg daily) for 2–4 weeks Children: PO 0.25 mg/kg/day		Osteoporosis (adults): PO 5–10 mg daily in divided doses (up to 20 mg daily)
Oxymetholone	Adroyd				Osteoporosis (adults): PO 5–10 mg daily (up to 30 mg daily) for 7–21 days Erythropoiesis: PO 1–4 mg/kg/day (maximal daily dose, 100 mg)
Stanazolol	Winstrol		Adults: PO 6 mg daily in divided doses Children ages 6–12: PO 2–6 mg daily in divided doses Children under 6: PO 2 mg daily in divided doses		
Testolactone	Teslac			PO 250 mg 4 times daily	

In boys and men, androgens are used mainly to treat androgen deficiency states such as hypogonadism. Hypogonadism may result from either hypothalamic–pituitary or testicular problems. In prepubertal boys, administration of male sex hormones stimulates the development of masculine characteristics. In postpubertal men who become androgen deficient, the hormones reestablish and maintain masculine characteristics and functions.

In women, male sex hormones are sometimes used in the palliative treatment of metastatic breast cancer. These women are usually premenopausal or menopausal and have breast tumors whose growth is stimulated by estrogen, the major female sex hormone. The male sex hormones apparently inhibit the stimulating effects of estrogen. In addition, danazol (Danocrine) may be used to treat endometriosis when other treatment measures are ineffective or contraindicated.

Other clinical uses of androgens include treatment of cryptorchidism, impotence, oligospermia, and some severe anemias in which androgens stimulate the production of red blood cells.

Anabolic steroids are used to prevent or treat tissue wasting associated with severe illnesses, burns, trauma, and long-term use of adrenal corticosteroids. All these conditions produce catabolism and negative nitrogen balance. The anabolic steroids can promote tissue buildup (anabolism) and a positive nitrogen balance.

CONTRAINDICATIONS

Androgens and anabolic steroids are contraindicated during pregnancy (because of possible masculinizing effects on a female fetus), in clients with preexisting liver disease, and in men with prostate gland disorders. Men with enlarged prostates may develop additional enlargement, and men with prostatic cancer may experience tumor growth. Although not contraindicated in children, these drugs must be used very cautiously and with roentgenograms about every 6 months to evaluate bone growth.

Principles of therapy: androgens and anabolic steroids

1. When androgens or anabolic steroids are given to adults, liver function tests and serum electrolytes must be done before drug therapy and periodically during treatment. Liver function tests are needed because one of the adverse reactions to these drugs is cholestatic jaundice. The serum electrolytes should be measured because the drugs may cause retention of sodium chloride, potassium, phosphates, and water.
2. When these drugs are given to children, roentgenograms to determine bone maturation are needed about every 6 months to prevent early epiphyseal closure and loss of adult height. Stimulation of skeletal growth continues for about 6 months after drug therapy is stopped.
3. When androgen or anabolic steroids are used in the treatment of metastatic breast cancer or refractory anemia, required dosage may be 2 to 3 times the amount needed for androgen replacement therapy. These high dosages increase the incidence of adverse reactions.
4. When these drugs are given to women and prepubertal males, good skin care is indicated to decrease the incidence and severity of acne.
5. When these drugs are given for anabolic effects, an adequate intake of protein and calories is necessary to achieve maximum benefit. Similarly, if they are given for anemia, an adequate amount of iron must be available.
6. Drug therapy with androgens and anabolic steroids may be short or long term, depending on the condition in question, the client's response to treatment, and the incidence of adverse reactions. If feasible, intermittent rather than continuous therapy is recommended.
7. Androgens generally potentiate oral anticoagulants, oral antidiabetic agents, and insulin. Dosage of these drugs may need to be decreased during concurrent therapy with androgens or anabolic drugs.

NURSING ACTIONS: ANDROGENS AND ANABOLIC STEROIDS

Nursing Actions	*Rationale/Explanation*
1. Administer accurately	
a. Give intramuscular preparations of testosterone, other androgens and anabolic steroids deeply, preferably in the gluteal muscle.	

Nursing Actions	***Rationale/Explanation***
b. Give oral preparations before or with meals, in divided doses	To decrease gastrointestinal disturbances
c. For buccal preparations	
(1) Give in divided doses	
(2) Place the tablet between the cheek and gum	Buccal preparations must be absorbed through the mucous membranes.
(3) Instruct the client not to swallow the tablet and not to drink, chew, or smoke until the tablet is completely absorbed.	
(4) Maintain oral hygiene	To decrease irritation and risk of infection
2. Observe for therapeutic effects	
a. When the drug is given for hypogonadism, observe for masculinizing effects such as growth of sexual organs, deepening of voice, growth of body hair, acne.	
b. When the drug is given for anabolic effects, observe for increased appetite, euphoria, or statements of feeling better.	
c. When the drug is given for cancer, observe for decreased pain and increased reports of feeling better.	
d. When the drug is given for anemia, observe complete blood count reports for increased red blood cells, hematocrit, and hemoglobin.	
3. Observe for adverse reactions	
a. Virilism or masculinizing effects	
(1) In adult men with adequate secretion of testosterone—priapism, increased sexual desire, reduced sperm count, and prostate enlargement	
(2) In prepubertal boys—premature development of sex organs and secondary sexual characteristics such as enlargement of the penis, priapism, pubic hair	
(3) In women—masculinizing effects include hirsutism, deepening of the voice, menstrual irregularities	
b. Jaundice—dark urine, yellow skin and sclera, itching	
c. Edema	Edema is more likely to occur in clients who are elderly or who have heart or kidney disease.
d. Hypercalcemia	This is more likely to occur in women with advanced breast cancer.
e. Difficulty voiding due to prostate enlargement	This is more likely to occur in middle-aged or elderly men.
f. Inadequate growth in height of children	
4. Observe for drug interactions	
a. Drugs that *decrease* effects of androgens and anabolic agents	
(1) Aminopyrine	Increases the rate of metabolism
(2) Antihistamines	Increase enzyme induction
(3) Barbiturates	Increase enzyme induction and rate of metabolism
(4) Calcitonin	Decreases calcium retention and thus antagonizes calcium-retaining effects of androgens

Nursing Actions	Rationale/Explanation
(5) Chlorcyclizine (Perazil), phenylbutazone (Butazolidin)	Increase metabolism
(6) Estrogens	Antagonize the anticancer effects of androgens
5. Teach clients	
a. Correct use of buccal tablets when these are prescribed	
b. Report adverse reactions such as jaundice, edema, masculinizing effects.	
c. Weigh weekly and report gains.	May indicate fluid retention and edema or a therapeutic effect of anabolic drugs
d. Practice frequent and thorough skin cleansing.	To decrease acne, which is most likely to occur in women and children
e. With anabolic drugs, eat a well-balanced diet.	Adequate protein and calories are necessary for full anabolic effects. Folic acid is necessary when these drugs are given for anemia.

Selected References

American Medical Association (AMA) Division of Drugs: AMA Drug Evaluations, 5th ed. New York, John Wiley & Sons, 1983

Facts and Comparisons. St. Louis, J B Lippincott (Updated monthly)

Malseed RT: Pharmacology: Drug Therapy and Nursing Considerations, 2d ed. Philadelphia, J B Lippincott, 1985

Murad F, Haynes RC Jr: Androgens. In Gilman AG, Goodman LS, Rall TW, Murad F (eds): The Pharmacological Basis of Therapeutics, 7th ed., pp 1440–1458. New York, Macmillan, 1985

Perlmutter G, Lowenthal DT: Use of anabolic steroids by athletes. An Fam Physician 32:203–210, October 1985

Rodman MJ, Karch AM, Boyd EH, Smith DW: Pharmacology and Drug Therapy in Nursing, 3rd ed. Philadelphia, J B Lippincott, 1985

V

NUTRIENTS, FLUIDS, AND ELECTROLYTES

30

NUTRITIONAL PRODUCTS, ANOREXIANTS, AND DIGESTANTS

Water, carbohydrates, proteins, fats, vitamins, and minerals are required for human nutrition. These substances are necessary for promotion or maintenance of health, prevention of illness, and promotion of recovery from illness. The first four nutrients are discussed in this chapter; vitamins and minerals are discussed in the following chapters.

Water, carbohydrates, proteins, and fats are necessary for life. Water is second only to oxygen in importance, since a person can live only a few days without water intake. Proteins are basic anatomic and physiologic components of all body cells and tissues. Carbohydrates and fats serve primarily as sources of energy for cell metabolism.

Energy is measured in terms of kilocalories per gram of food oxidized in the body. The term *calorie* is often used instead of *kilocalorie.* Carbohydrates are oxidized first and provide an immediate source of energy; fats are used second and provide a long-term or reserve supply of energy; and proteins are used last. Undernutrition, starvation, and death occur within a few weeks when there is no intake of carbohydrates, proteins, and fats. Table 30-1 lists more specific characteristics of water, carbohydrates, proteins, and fats in relation to normal nutrition.

When inadequate or excessive amounts of these nutrients are ingested, nutritional disorders result. These disorders include water deficit (also called dehydration or fluid volume deficit), water excess (also called water intoxication or fluid volume excess), undernutrition, and obesity. Causes and clinical manifestations of water imbalances are listed in Table 30-2; protein–calorie imbalances are described in Table 30-3.

Numerous products are available to supplement or substitute for dietary intake in clients who are unable to ingest, digest, absorb, or utilize nutrients. For example, liquid formulas are available for oral or tube feedings. Many liquid formulas are nutritionally complete, except for water, when given in sufficient quantities. Others are nutritionally incomplete but useful in certain circumstances. Additional water is given to meet fluid needs. A variety of intravenous fluids is also available. Most intravenous fluids are nutritionally incomplete and are designed for short-term use when oral or tube feedings are contraindicated. They are most useful in meeting fluid and electrolyte needs. A special intravenous formula, called intravenous nutritional formula (INF), total parenteral nutrition (TPN), or parenteral hyperalimentation, can be prepared to meet long-term nutritional needs. These formulas vary but

(Text continues on p. 290.)

TABLE 30-1. WATER, CARBOHYDRATES, PROTEINS, AND FATS

Nutrient	Characteristics	Functions	Requirements	Normal sources	Normal losses
Water	1. Major chemical constituent of the body 2. Intracellular fluid includes the water inside body cells 3. Extracellular fluid includes the water or liquid portion of blood, lymph, spinal fluid, saliva, gastrointestinal secretions, bile, sweat, urine, and the tissue fluid that surrounds body cells	1. Serves as a solvent or medium in which all cell metabolism occurs. 2. Maintains blood volume. 3. Transports nutrients to body cells. 4. Assists in maintaining electrolyte balance in blood and cells. 5. Assists in maintaining body temperature.	Approximately 2000–3000 ml daily, depending on activity, environmental temperature, and other factors	1. Drinking water and other beverages (about 1200 ml/day) 2. Water in foods (about 1000 ml/day) 3. Water produced by oxidation of foods in the body (about 300 ml/day)	1. Urine (about 1500 ml/day) 2. Insensible losses from skin and lungs (about 900 ml/day) 3. Feces (about 100 ml/day)
Carbohydrates	1. Chemical substances composed of carbon, hydrogen, and oxygen 2. The major source of energy for body activities. When oxidized in the body, carbohydrates furnish 4 kcal of energy per gram. 3. They must be broken down into glucose, galactose, or fructose before they can be absorbed. The simple sugars can then be used for energy or stored as glycogen.	1. Provide glucose, which is necessary for normal cellular metabolism 2. Conserve body proteins for tissue building and repair by preventing use of proteins for energy 3. Promote normal fat metabolism 4. Promote normal function of nerve cells. Glucose is the only source of energy which can be used by the brain. 5. Promote growth of normal intestinal bacteria by providing lactose. These bacteria synthesize certain vitamins, mainly vitamin K. 6. Promote normal bowel elimination by stimulating peristalsis, absorbing water and increasing the bulk of intestinal contents. This function is fulfilled by complex or indigestible carbohydrates.	Approximately 2000 kcal daily for the average adult female (58 kg or 127 lb) and 2700 kcal for the average adult male (70 kg or 154 lb) Requirements vary, depending on age, size, activity, and other factors. They increase in pregnancy and lactation; rapid growth periods of infancy, early childhood and adolescence; periods of strenuous activity; and in disorders such as fever, hyperthyroidism, severe burns, trauma, or surgery. They decrease with sedentary activities and in elderly people.	Grains, fruits and vegetables are good sources of carbohydrate and other essential nutrients. Candy and carbonated beverages contain kilocalories but lack other nutrients. Glycogen is a reserve supply of glucose that can be mobilized to meet energy needs. The amount available is relatively small—approximately 110 g in the liver and 225 g in muscle. For some people, this amount would not meet requirements for 24 hours during a fasting state.	Waste products from carbohydrate metabolism are mainly carbon dioxide and water. Carbon dioxide is mainly excreted through the lungs, and water may be excreted in urine or used for other metabolic processes.
Proteins	1. Chemical substances composed of carbon, hydrogen, water, nitrogen, phosphorus, sulfur, and iron. 2. When broken down in the body, proteins yield 4 kcal of energy per gram. They are used for energy only when intake of carbohydrates and fats is inadequate.	1. Furnish amino acids for growth of new tissue and repair of damaged or worn-out tissue. Amino acids are the basic constituents or building blocks of all body cells. 2. Serve as components of numerous body fluids and secretions, including enzymes, many hormones, milk, mucus, and sperm. (Sweat, bile and	Approximately 0.8 g/kg of body weight daily. This amount maintains normal nitrogen balance and tissue growth and repair. An average adult female (58 kg) requires about 46 g; an average adult male (70 kg) requires about 56 g. Requirements increase during growth periods of	Animal foods such as meat, fish, poultry, milk, eggs, and cheese provide "complete" proteins, which contain all the essential amino acids. Proteins from beans, breads, and cereals are incomplete, but they can be combined in ways that provide adequate intake.	Nitrogenous waste products, ammonia, urea, and uric acid are excreted in the urine.

TABLE 30-1. WATER, CARBOHYDRATES, PROTEINS, AND FATS (*Continued*)

Nutrient	Characteristics	Functions	Requirements	Normal sources	Normal losses
	3. Most proteins are found in muscle tissue; others are found in soft tissues, bones, teeth, and blood and other body fluids.	urine are normally protein free.) 3. Assist in maintaining normal osmotic pressure in the blood. Albumin is especially important in fulfilling this function. 4. Transport various substances in the blood. Lipid-carrying plasma proteins transport fat-soluble vitamins, cholesterol, triglycerides, and phospholipids. Transferrin carries iron and another protein carries calcium. Albumin transports free fatty acids, bilirubin, and many drugs. 5. Provide immunoglobulins or antibodies, which are important in resistance to disease.	children; pregnancy and lactation; fever; burn injuries; surgery; hyperthyroidism and stress. Elderly adults need the same amount of protein (0.8 g/kg) as younger adults.		
Fats (lipids)	1. Several different chemical substances of which the major ones are triglycerides, phospholipids, and cholesterol. More than 98% of natural fats are triglycerides. 2. Second choice as energy source, after carbohydrates. They furnish 9 kcal of energy per gram. 3. Excess dietary fats are stored; excess carbohydrates and proteins are converted to fat and stored in adipose tissue.	1. Provide energy for body metabolism. 2. Conserve proteins for tissue synthesis by preventing use of proteins for energy. 3. Protect organs from injury. 4. Conserve body heat and help maintain normal body temperature. 5. Conserve thiamine. Thiamine is a vitamin that is required for carbohydrate metabolism but not fat metabolism. 6. Promote intestinal absorption of fat-soluble vitamins. 7. Increase palatability of foods. 8. Slow gastric emptying, thereby increasing and prolonging satiety. 9. Promote normal growth and development. 10. Serve as essential components of cells and cell membranes. 11. Protect against entry of foreign substances and loss of water through the skin.	Approximately 50–130 g daily (900–1200 kilocalories in a 3000 kcal diet). Requirements depend on weight, size, amount of carbohydrate ingested, physical activity, and other factors.	High amounts of fat are contained in meat, egg yolk, cheese, butter, whole milk, salad dressings, cream, and ice cream. In addition to food sources, triglycerides and cholesterol are formed in the liver. Cholesterol in foods is only about 50% absorbed.	Fats are excreted in sweat, bile, and feces or are oxidized to carbon dioxide and water, which are excreted.

TABLE 30-2. WATER IMBALANCES

Water deficit		Water excess	
Causes	*Signs and symptoms*	*Causes*	*Signs and symptoms*
1. Inadequate fluid intake, most likely to occur in people who are comatose, unable to swallow, or otherwise incapacitated 2. Excessive fluid loss due to vomiting, diarrhea, fever, diuretic drug therapy, high environmental temperatures, strenuous physical activity, or excessive sweating 3. A combination of 1 and 2	1. Thirst 2. Oliguria and concentrated urine 3. Weakness 4. Dry tongue and oral mucous membranes 5. Flushed skin 6. Weight loss 7. Fever 8. Increased hematocrit 9. Mental disturbances ranging from mild confusion to delirium, convulsions, and coma 10. Hypovolemic shock if the deficiency is severe or develops rapidly	1. Excessive intake, most likely to occur with excessive amounts or rapid infusion of intravenous fluids 2. Impaired excretion of fluids due to endocrine, renal, cardiovascular, or CNS disorders	1. Drowsiness 2. Weakness and lethargy 3. Weight gain 4. Edema 5. Low serum sodium and hematocrit 6. Disorientation 7. Circulatory overload and pulmonary edema if water excess is severe or develops rapidly

usually include sufficient amounts of water, carbohydrate, protein, vitamins, and minerals. Fat emulsions are administered separately to supply additional calories and essential fatty acids. For nutritional deficiencies due to malabsorption of carbohydrate, protein, and fat, pancreatic enzymes may be given. Other so-called digestants (*e.g.*, hydrochloric acid, bile salts) are available alone and in combination with other drugs. These products are ineffective, obsolete, and not recommended for use.

In nutritional excesses or obesity, anorexiant drugs are sometimes given to decrease appetite (Table 30-4). Amphetamines (see Chap. 16) have been used for this purpose, but they can no longer be legally prescribed because of their high potential for abuse and dependence. The other anorexiant drugs that have been developed are similar to amphetamines but are promoted for use only in appetite control. These drugs are of limited effectiveness in obesity and lose their appetite-suppressant effects in about 4 to 6 weeks. They are useful only for short-term therapy and as part of a weight reduction program that also includes calorie restriction, exercise, medical supervision, and psychologic support. These drugs may lead to abuse and dependence of the amphetamine type. Their use is regulated by the Controlled Substances Act. Anorexiant drugs are contraindicated in cardiovascular disease, hyperthyroidism, glaucoma, and agitated psychologic disturbances.

Phenylpropanolamine is an adrenergic drug commonly used as a nasal decongestant in over-the-

TABLE 30-3. CARBOHYDRATE, PROTEIN, AND FAT IMBALANCES

Protein–calorie deficit		Protein–calorie excess	
Causes	*Signs and symptoms*	*Causes*	*Signs and symptoms*
1. Inadequate intake of protein, carbohydrate, and fat 2. Impaired ability to digest, absorb, or utilize nutrients 3. Excessive losses	1. Weight loss with eventual loss of subcutaneous fat and muscle mass 2. Increased susceptibility to infection 3. Weakness and fatigability 4. Dry, scaly skin 5. Impaired healing 6. Impaired growth and development in children 7. Edema 8. Decreased hemoglobin 9. Acidosis 10. Disordered brain function 11. Coma 12. Starvation	1. Excessive intake, especially of carbohydrates and fats	1. Weight gain 2. Obesity

TABLE 30-4. ANOREXIANTS

Generic name	Trade name	Route and dosage range (adults)	Status under Controlled Substances Act	Remarks
Benzphetamine	Didrex	PO 25–50 mg 1–3 times daily	Schedule III	Dosages have not been established for children under 12 years of age.
Diethylpropion	Tenuate	PO 25 mg 3 times daily	Schedule IV	
Fenfluramine	Pondimin	PO 20–40 mg 3 times daily; maximal daily dose, 120 mg	Schedule IV	Fenfluramine generally has the same actions, uses, and characteristics as the other nonamphetamine anorexiant drugs. An important difference, however, is that fenfluramine depresses, rather than stimulates, the CNS.
Mazindol	Sanorex	PO 1 mg 3 times daily	Schedule III	
Phendimetrazine	Plegine	PO 35 mg 2–3 times daily or 105 mg once daily	Schedule III	
Phentermine hydrochloride	Fastin	PO 8.0 mg 3 times daily or 15–37.5 mg daily in the morning	Schedule IV	
Phentermine resin	Ionamin	PO 15–30 mg once daily	Schedule IV	

counter cold remedies. It is also the active ingredient in over-the-counter appetite suppressants (*e.g.,* Dexatrim, Acutrim). Effectiveness of the drug in weight reduction is limited, and its use has been associated with psychosis, hypertension, stroke, renal failure, cardiac arrhythmias, and death. These adverse effects have apparently occurred with recommended doses but are especially likely with overdoses or concomitant use of other drugs, such as caffeine.

Individual nutritional products for oral or tube feeding

NUTRITIONALLY COMPLETE LIQUID FORMULAS FOR GENERAL USE

Compleat B (TF 1600 ml), **Ensure** (PO or TF 2000 ml), **Isocal** (PO or TF 2000 ml), **Meritene** (PO or TF 1200 ml), **Osmolite** (TF 2000 ml), **Sustacal** (PO or TF 1080 ml), and **Sustagen** (PO or TF 1000 ml) are formulas that provide the United States Recommended Daily Allowances (USRDAs) for protein, vitamins, and minerals. Most of the formulas provide one calorie per milliliter (1 cal/ml); Sustagen provides 1.84 cal/ml. When given in the designated amounts, these formulas meet basic nutritional needs. However, amounts should be individualized according to nutritional needs and whether the formula is being used to supplement or substitute for other sources of food and fluids.

NUTRITIONAL AGENTS FOR LIMITED USE (DEFINED FORMULA OR ELEMENTAL DIETS)

Flexical is a nutritionally complete diet that contains easily digested forms of protein, carbohydrate, and fat. It produces minimal stimulation of gastrointestinal secretions and motility and leaves little fecal residue. It is especially useful in clients who are critically ill, who have various gastrointestinal problems or malabsorption syndromes, or who have had bowel surgery. It may also be used as an alternative to a clear liquid diet, which is nutritionally inadequate.

Lofenalac is a low-phenylalanine preparation used only in infants and children with phenylketonuria (PKU), a metabolic disorder in which phenylalanine cannot be normally metabolized. Lofenalac is not adequate for complete nutrition and growth, although it meets Food and Drug Administration (FDA) requirements for infant formulas. For growth needs, it is recommended that about 85% of the child's protein needs be supplied with Lofenalac and the remaining 10% to 15% be supplied with foods containing phenylalanine, which is an essential amino acid.

MBF (Meat Base Formula) is a hypoallergenic infant formula designed for use in infants who are allergic to milk or who have galactosemia. It is nutritionally adequate and meets FDA standards for infant formulas.

Neo-Mull-Soy, Nursoy, Pro Sobee, Isomil, and **Soyalac** are hypoallergenic, milk-free formulas. They derive their protein from soybean products rather than milk. They provide 20 cal/oz when mixed or diluted as directed and provide all other essential nutrients for normal growth and development. They are used as milk substitutes for clients who are allergic to milk, most often infants.

Nutramigen is a nutritionally complete hypoallergenic formula containing predigested protein. It is used for infants and children who are allergic to ordinary food proteins or who have diarrhea or other gastrointestinal problems.

Portagen is a nutritionally complete formula that contains medium chain triglycerides, an easily digested form of fat. It is used primarily in clients with fat malabsorption problems. It may be used as the complete diet, as a beverage with meals, or as an addition to various recipes. It may induce coma in clients with severe hepatic cirrhosis.

Precision diets are nutritionally complete, low-residue formulas for oral or tube feedings. The **high-nitrogen** diet provides 125 g of protein or 20 g of nitrogen, 3000 kcal, and recommended amounts of essential vitamins and minerals in ten 3-oz servings. The **low-residue** formula contains 45 g of protein or 7.2 g of nitrogen (a maintenance amount of protein), 1900 kcal, and essential vitamins and minerals in six 3-oz servings. The **isotonic** diet contains the same amounts of protein, vitamins, and minerals as the **low-residue** formula but is isotonic rather than hypertonic and provides 1500 kcal in six 2-oz servings.

These preparations are ingested or given by tube slowly over 4 hours. The carbohydrate content may produce elevated blood sugar levels; therefore, they should not be used in clients with diabetes mellitus. These formulas can be administered to children if the amount is calculated to provide recommended amounts of nutrients for the particular age group.

Pregestimil is an infant formula that contains easily digested protein, fat, and carbohydrate. It is used in infants with diarrhea, dietary intolerances, or malabsorption syndromes.

Vivonex is a nutritionally complete diet that contains crystalline amino acids as its protein or nitrogen source. It can be used for oral or tube feedings. It requires virtually no digestion and leaves virtually no fecal residue, so it is especially useful in gastrointestinal disorders. The amount, concentration, and rate of administration can be adjusted to meet nutritional needs and tolerance in both adults and children.

NUTRITIONALLY INCOMPLETE SUPPLEMENTS

Amin-Aid is used as a source of protein for clients with acute and chronic renal insufficiency in whom dietary protein must be restricted. Amin-Aid supplies amino acids, carbohydrate, and a few electrolytes.

Cal-Power is a supplement used to increase carbohydrate calories in the diet.

Casec is an oral protein supplement for use in infants, children, or adults.

Citrotein is an oral dietary supplement that provides protein, vitamins, and minerals. It is especially useful when appetite and food intake are decreased or during rapid growth periods when intake does not meet nutritional needs.

Controlyte is a supplement that supplies a concentrated source of calories and limited amounts of protein and electrolytes. It may be given orally or by tube feeding.

Gevral Protein is an oral supplement used to increase intake of protein, vitamins, and minerals. The powder can be mixed with water, milk, or other cold liquids, added to cereals, or mixed into desserts.

Hycal is an oral supplement that provides a concentrated source of calories for clients on diets restricted in protein and electrolytes. Sixteen ounces provide 1180 calories.

Lipomul is a fat supplement. It contains corn oil and thus provides unsaturated fats.

Liprotein is an oral supplement that provides high amounts of calories and protein for use with burn victims or other debilitated persons.

Lonalac is an oral supplement that is used as a milk substitute in sodium-restricted diets or to increase protein intake when sodium must be restricted.

MCT Oil is a preparation of medium-chain triglycerides derived from coconut oil. MCT Oil is more easily digested than fats contained in most foods, which are mainly long-chain triglycerides. The medium-chain triglycerides are water soluble, are absorbed into the portal vein rather than lymphatic channels, and do not require the presence of bile salts for absorption. Thus, they are useful in children or adults with fat malabsorption syndromes. Although they are useful as a caloric substitute for dietary fat (1 tablespoon provides 115 kcal), they do not promote absorption of fat-soluble vitamins or provide essential fatty acids as the long-chain triglycerides do. MCT Oil can be mixed with fruit juices, used with salads or vegetables, or used in cooking and baking. Limited amounts of this product should be used in clients with severe hepatic cirrhosis owing to a risk of precipitating encephalopathy and coma.

Polycose is an oral supplement used to increase caloric intake. Derived from carbohydrate, Polycose may be used by clients on protein-, electrolyte-, or fat-restricted diets. Available in liquid and powder, Polycose may be mixed with water or other beverages and with foods. Amounts taken should be determined by taste, calories needed, and tolerance.

Probana is a high-protein formula for infants and children with diarrhea or various malabsorption disorders. It contains most vitamins and minerals; it does not contain iron.

COMPLETE INFANT FORMULAS

Enfamil, Similac and **SMA** are commonly used complete nutritional formulas for full-term infants or premature infants who are able to bottle-feed. Either may be used alone for bottle-fed infants or as a supplement for breast-fed infants. These preparations are quite similar to human breast milk. Their only deficiency is in iron, which may be given separately or in a formula preparation containing iron.

Intravenous fluids

Dextrose injection is available in preparations containing 2.5%, 5%, 10%, 20%, 40%, 50%, 60%, and 70% dextrose. The most frequently used concentration is 5% dextrose in water or sodium chloride injection. A concentration of 5% dextrose in water is approximately isotonic with blood. It provides water and 170 kcal/liter. The dextrose is rapidly utilized, leaving "free" water for excreting waste products, maintaining renal function, and maintaining urine output. The 10% dextrose solution provides a double amount of calories in the same volume of fluid but is hypertonic and therefore may cause phlebitis. The 20% to 50% solutions are used primarily to provide calories in total parenteral nutrition. They are hypertonic and must be administered through a central or subclavian catheter.

Dextrose and sodium chloride injection is available in various concentrations. The most frequently used are 5% dextrose in 0.2% or 0.45% sodium chloride (also called $D_5\frac{1}{4}$ and $D_5\frac{1}{2}$ normal saline, respectively). These provide approximately 170 kcal/liter, water, sodium, and chloride. They are frequently used for maintenance therapy, usually with added potassium chloride, in clients who are unable to eat or drink. They are also used for replacement therapy when large amounts of fluid are lost, for keeping intravenous lines open, and for administering medications.

Crystalline amino acid solution (Aminosyn, Freamine) contains essential and nonessential amino acids. These solutions differ from protein hydrolysates by not containing peptides. They are most often used with concentrated dextrose injection in total parenteral nutrition.

Fat emulsion (Intralipid, Liposyn) provides a source of concentrated calories and essential fatty acids. The emulsion is usually given as part of total parenteral nutrition. More calories can be supplied with fat emulsion than with dextrose–protein solutions alone. It is available in 10% and 20% emulsions; 500 ml of 10% emulsion provides 550 calories. Fat emulsions should not provide more than 60% of total caloric intake. These preparations are given separately from dextrose–protein hyperalimentation solutions.

Pancreatic enzymes

Pancreatin is an oral preparation of pancreatic enzymes usually obtained from pork pancreas. It is used to aid digestion and absorption of dietary carbohydrate, protein, and fat in conditions characterized by pancreatic enzyme deficiency. These conditions include cystic fibrosis, chronic pancreatitis, pancreatectomy, and pancreatic obstruction. **Pancrelipase** (Viokase) is essentially the same as pancreatin except that it may be more effective in steatorrhea (excess fat in the feces).

Route and dosage ranges

Pancreatin

Adults: PO 1–3 capsules or tablets after meals or snacks

Children: PO 1–2 capsules or tablets with each meal initially, increased in amount or frequency if necessary and adverse effects do not occur

Pancrelipase

Adults: PO 1–3 capsules or tablets before or with meals or snacks; or 1 or 2 packets of powder with meals or snacks

Principles of therapy: nutritional agents and anorexiants

ASSESSMENT GUIDELINES

Assess each client for current or potential nutritional disorders. Some specific assessment factors include the following:

1. What are usual drinking and eating patterns? Does fluid intake seem adequate? Does food intake seem adequate in terms of normal nutrition? Is the client financially able to purchase sufficient quality and quantity of foods? What are fluid and food likes and dislikes?
2. Does the client know the basic foods for normal nutrition? Does the client view nutrition as important in maintaining health?
3. Does the client appear overweight or underweight? How does current weight compare with the ideal weight for age and height?
4. Does the client have symptoms, disease processes, treatment measures, medications, or diagnostic tests that are likely to interfere with nutrition? For example, many illnesses and oral medications cause anorexia, nausea, vomiting, and diarrhea.
5. Are there conditions present that increase or decrease nutritional requirements?
6. Check available reports of laboratory tests such as serum proteins, complete blood count, blood glucose, urine glucose, and acetone. Nutritional disorders, as well as many other disorders, may cause abnormal values.

NURSING INTERVENTIONS

Implement measures to prevent nutritional disorders by promoting a well-balanced diet for all clients. Depending on the client's condition, diet orders, food preferences, knowledge and attitudes about nutrition, and other factors, specific activities may include the following:

1. Providing food and fluid the client is willing and able to take, at preferred times when possible
2. Assisting the client to a sitting position, cutting meat, opening containers, feeding, and other actions if indicated
3. Treating symptoms or disorders that are likely to interfere with nutrition such as pain, nausea, vomiting, or diarrhea
4. Consulting with the physician or dietitian when needed, especially when special diets are ordered. Compliance is improved when the ordered diet differs as little as possible from the usual diet. Also, preferred foods may often be substituted for disliked ones.
5. Promoting exercise and activity. For the undernourished client, this may increase appetite, improve digestion, and aid bowel elimination. For the overweight or obese client, exercise may distract from hunger.
6. Minimizing the use of sedative-type drugs when appropriate. Although no one should be denied pain relief, strong analgesics and other sedatives may cause drowsiness and decreased desire or ability to eat and drink.
7. Teaching about normal nutritional needs, the importance of nutrition in maintaining health or promoting recovery from illness, the value of a varied diet, benefits and techniques of weight control, and other topics. This activity may be shared with a dietitian.

PRINCIPLES OF MANAGING FLUID DISORDERS

Fluid deficiency

Treatment of fluid deficiency is aimed toward increasing intake or decreasing loss, depending on causative factors. The safest and most effective way of replacing body fluids is to give oral fluids, when possible. Water is probably best, at least initially. Fluids containing large amounts of carbohydrate, fat, or protein are hypertonic and may increase dehydration if taken without sufficient water. If the client cannot take oral food or fluids for a few days or is able to take only limited amounts, intravenous fluids can be used to provide complete or supplemental amounts of fluids. Frequently used solutions include 5% dextrose in water or sodium chloride.

To meet fluid needs over a longer period, a nasogastric or other gastrointestinal tube may be used to administer fluids. For a person receiving food and fluid only by tube, fluid needs must be carefully assessed. Additional water is almost always needed after or between administrations of commercial tube feeding formulas. Most of these formulas are hypertonic and will intensify fluid deficit if an inadequate amount of water accompanies them. For some reason, many nurses are reluctant to give additional water or other fluids when tube feeding formulas are used. They may give only 50 to 100 ml of water to rinse the tube even when obvious signs of fluid deficit are present (*e.g.*, concentrated urine, poor skin turgor, dry mucous membranes).

Another way of meeting long-term fluid needs when the gastrointestinal tract cannot be used is intravenous hyperalimentation. These solutions provide protein and calories as well as fluids.

Optimal amounts of fluid may vary greatly. For most clients, 2000 to 3000 ml daily is adequate. A person with severe heart failure or oliguric kidney disease needs smaller amounts, but one with extra losses (*e.g.*, vomiting, diarrhea) needs more.

Fluid excess

Treatment of fluid excess is aimed toward decreasing intake and increasing loss. In acute circulatory overload or pulmonary edema, the usual treatment is to stop fluid intake (if the client is receiving intravenous fluids, slow the rate but keep the vein open for medication) and administer diuretics. Since this is an emergency, prevention is better than treatment.

PRINCIPLES OF MANAGING PROTEIN–CALORIE DEFICIENCY (UNDERNUTRITION)

Goal of treatment

The goal of treatment is to provide an adequate quantity and quality of nutrients to meet tissue needs. Requirements for nutrients vary with age, level of activity, level of health or illness, and other factors that must be considered in designing appropriate therapy.

Oral feedings

The safest and most effective way of increasing nutritional intake is by oral feedings, when feasible. High-protein, high-calorie foods can be included in many diets and given as between-meal or bedtime snacks. Milkshakes, ice cream, and eggnog are good choices for increasing fluid intake as well.

If the client is unable to ingest enough food and fluid, many of the commercial nutritional preparations can be given as between-meal supplements to increase intake of protein and calories. These preparations vary in taste and acceptability. Measures to improve taste may include chilling, serving over ice, or mixing with fruit juice or other beverage. Specific methods depend on the client's taste preferences and the available formula. Refer to instructions, usually on the labels, for appropriate diluting and mixing beverages.

Tube feedings

When oral feeding is not possible but the gastrointestinal tract is functioning, tube feeding may be more convenient, safer, and more effective than intravenous fluids, especially if long-term feeding is required. When tube feedings are the client's only source of nutrients, they should be nutritionally complete and given in amounts calculated to provide adequate water, protein, calories, vitamins, and minerals. Although tube feeding formulas vary in osmolality and volume needed for adequate intake of protein, vitamins, and minerals, any of the complete formulas can be used effectively. Other guidelines include the following:

1. Once the kind and amount of formula are chosen, continuous or intermittent feedings must be chosen. The continuous drip method is probably better tolerated by most clients because it decreases both the amount and the hypertonicity of fluids in the gastrointestinal tract at any one time. This method decreases diarrhea, gastric distention, and possibly the risks of aspiration into the lungs. Intermittent bolus feedings are more convenient for the ambulatory client.
2. As a general rule, tube feeding formulas are better tolerated if initiated as small amounts of diluted solution (*i.e.*, half strength), then increased to full strength if desired. Isocal and Osmolite are exceptions. These preparations are isotonic and should be given full strength. Most formulas provide 1 kcal/ml so that caloric intake can be quickly calculated. Additional water is required with most formulas. The amount should be based on fluid needs. Water can be given with, after, or between regular feedings and with medications.
3. Other than problems resulting from hypertonic solutions and inadequate fluid intake (diarrhea, dehydration, hypernatremia), a major complication of tube feeding is aspiration of the formula into the lungs. This is more likely to occur with unconscious clients. It can be prevented by correct techniques of positioning clients, checking tube placement, and administering feedings slowly.

Parenteral feedings

Parenteral feedings are usually preferred only when the gastrointestinal tract cannot be used. For short-term use (about 3 to 5 days) of intravenous fluids, the goal is to provide adequate amounts of fluids and electrolytes and enough carbohydrate to minimize oxidation of body protein and fat for energy. Choice of specific solution depends on individual needs but probably should contain at least 5% dextrose. A frequently used solution is 5% dextrose in 0.22% sodium chloride, 2000 to 3000 ml/24 hours. Potassium chloride is often added, and vitamins may be added. These solutions are nutritionally inadequate.

Total parenteral nutrition

For long-term intravenous feedings (weeks to months), the goal is to provide all nutrients required for normal body functioning, including tissue growth. This goal can be met with a regimen called total parenteral nutrition (TPN), or intravenous hyperalimentation. Basic hyperalimentation solutions provide water, carbohydrate, protein, vitamins, and minerals. Originally, calories were supplied primarily by 25% to 50% glucose. This resulted in a hypertonic solution that had to be given in a central vein so it could be rapidly diluted. Later, intravenous fat emulsions were developed and given two or three times weekly to provide additional calories (in a small fluid volume) as well as essential fatty acids. These solutions are isotonic and may be given centrally or peripherally.

Although effective, central TPN requires special techniques to increase safety and decrease complications. For example, a physician must insert the central intravenous catheter, and placement must be verified by a chest x-ray film. Complications include air embolism and pneumothorax. More recently, peripheral TPN has been developed. This method uses 5% or 10% glucose and constant coinfusion of fat emulsion. The fat emulsion is thought to protect the vein and decrease or delay phlebitis. Guidelines for both methods include the following:

1. Administer with an infusion pump to control the flow rate accurately. The solution must be given at a consistent rate so nutrients can be utilized and complications prevented. The initial flow rate is usually 50 ml/hour; then, flow rate is increased as tolerated to meet nutritional requirements (approximately 2000 to 3000 ml daily).
2. To prevent infection, several measures are indicated. First, the intravenous catheter must be inserted with aseptic technique. Second, all solutions must be prepared aseptically in the pharmacy under a laminar flow hood. Third, use an 0.45 to 0.22 μm in-line filter. Fourth, change solution containers and tubing every 24 hours. Fifth, change the dressing at the venipuncture site at least every 48 hours. Most hospitals have established protocols regarding dressing changes. These usually include "defatting" the skin with alcohol, cleansing around the catheter with povidone–iodine solution (Betadine), applying povidone–iodine ointment, and reapplying an occlusive dressing. Sterile technique is used throughout.
3. "Piggyback" fat emulsions into the intravenous line beyond the filter.

PRINCIPLES OF MANAGING PROTEIN-CALORIE EXCESS (OVERWEIGHT OR OBESITY)

1. For effective weight loss and continued weight control the main elements are decreasing caloric intake and increasing exercise (caloric output). This largely depends on the client's motivation and self-discipline in changing eating habits. This is very difficult for most people to do.
2. Many reduction diets and regimens have been proposed. Among the more successful programs are groups that meet regularly and offer psychologic support as well as diet plans. Among the more radical treatments are surgical procedures that limit the amount of food and fluid that can be ingested.
3. Drug therapy has a limited role in weight control. Anorexiant drugs are effective for only a few weeks, so they may be helpful in initiating a weight reduction program. Many clients regain weight, however, when the drugs are stopped.
4. The role of the nurse may involve counseling about benefits to be gained from weight loss, about the undesirability and hazards of some "fad" diets, and about specific ways of decreasing caloric intake such as low-calorie snacks, participating in noneating activities, and not buying favorite high-calorie foods. Any program for weight control must be individualized, and continued support must be available.

NURSING ACTIONS: NUTRITIONAL PRODUCTS AND ANOREXIANTS

Nursing Actions	*Rationale/Explanation*
1. Administer accurately	
a. For oral supplemental feedings	
(1) Give at the preferred time and temperature, when possible.	To increase the likelihood the feeding will be taken. Chilling the formula may increase palatability.

Nursing Actions	*Rationale/Explanation*
(2) Mix powders or concentrated liquid preparations in preferred beverages if not contraindicated.	Some can be mixed with fruit juice, milk, tea, or coffee, which may improve taste and acceptability.
(3) Provide flavoring packets when available and preferred by the client.	To improve taste and add variety
b. For intravenous feedings	
(1) Administer fluids at the prescribed flow rate. Use an infusion control device for hyperalimentation solutions.	To administer sufficient fluids without a rapid flow rate. Rapid flow rates or large amounts of intravenous fluids can cause circulatory overload and pulmonary edema. In addition, hyperglycemia and osmotic diuresis may occur with hyperalimentation solutions.
(2) Use sterile technique when changing containers, tubings, or dressings.	To prevent infection
(3) When adding drugs, use sterile technique and add only those drugs known to be compatible with the intravenous solution.	To avoid physical or chemical incompatibility
(4) Do not administer antibiotics or other drugs through central venous catheters.	To avoid incompatibilities and possible precipitation or inactivation of the drug or fluid components
c. For tube feedings	
(1) Have the client sitting, if possible.	To decrease risks of aspirating formula into lungs
(2) Check tube placement before each feeding by aspirating stomach contents or instilling air into the tube while listening over the stomach with a stethoscope.	To prevent aspiration or accidental instillation of feedings into lungs
(3) Give the solution at room temperature.	Cold formulas may cause abdominal cramping.
(4) If giving by intermittent bolus instillation, do not give more than 500 ml per feeding, including water for rinsing the tube.	To avoid gastric distention, possible vomiting, and aspiration into lungs
(5) Give by gravity flow or infusion pump.	Rapid administration may cause nausea, vomiting, and other symptoms.
(6) With continuous or prolonged drip feedings, change containers and tubing daily. With intermittent bolus feedings, rinse all equipment after each use and change at least every 24 hours.	Most tube feeding formulas are milk based and provide a good culture medium for bacterial growth. Clean technique, not sterile technique, is required.
(7) Give an adequate amount of water, based on assessment of fluid needs. This may be done by mixing water with the tube feeding formula, giving it after the tube feeding, or giving it between feedings.	To avoid dehydration and promote fluid balance. Most clients receiving 1500 to 2000 ml of tube feeding formula daily will need 1000 ml or more of water daily.
(8) Rinse nasogastric tubes with at least 50 to 100 ml water after each bolus feeding or administration of medications through the tube.	To keep the tube patent and functioning. This water is included in calculation of fluid intake.
(9) When medications are ordered by tube, liquid preparations are preferred over crushed tablets or powders emptied from capsules.	Tablets or powders may stick in the tube lumen. This may mean the full dose of the medication does not reach the stomach. Also, the tube is likely to become obstructed.
d. With pancreatic enzymes, give with meals or food.	To obtain therapeutic effects, these agents must be in the small intestine when food is present.
e. With anorexiant drugs	
(1) Give single-dose drugs in the early morning.	For maximum appetite-suppressant effects during the day
(2) Give multiple-dose preparations 30 to 60 minutes before meals and the last dose of the day about 6 hours before bedtime.	For maximum appetite-suppressant effects at mealtime and to avoid interference with sleep from the drug's stimulating effects on the central nervous system (CNS)
2. Observe for therapeutic effects	
a. With water and other fluids, observe for fluid balance (amber-colored urine, about 1500 ml daily; moist mucous membranes in the oral cavity; adequate skin turgor).	

Nursing Actions	Rationale/Explanation
b. With nutritional formulas given orally or by tube feeding, observe for weight gain and increased serum albumin. For infants and children receiving milk substitutes, observe for decreased diarrhea and weight gain.	Therapeutic effects depend on the reason for use, that is, prevention or treatment of undernutrition.
c. With parenteral hyperalimentation, observe for weight maintenance or gain and normal serum levels of glucose, electrolytes, and protein.	These are indications of improved metabolism, nitrogen balance, and nutritional status. When parenteral hyperalimentation is used for gastrointestinal malabsorption syndromes, diarrhea and other symptoms are usually relieved when oral feedings are stopped.
d. With pancreatic enzymes, observe for decreased diarrhea and steatorrhea.	The pancreatic enzymes function the same way as endogenous enzymes to aid digestion of carbohydrate, protein, and fat.
e. With anorexiant drugs, observe for decreased caloric intake and weight loss.	The recommended rate of weight loss is approximately 2 to 3 pounds weekly.
3. Observe for adverse effects	
a. With fluids, observe for peripheral edema, circulatory overload, and pulmonary edema (severe dyspnea, rales).	Fluid excess is most likely to occur with rapid administration or large amounts of intravenous fluids, especially in people who are elderly or have congestive heart failure.
b. With commercial nutritional formulas (except Osmolite and Isocal), observe for hypotension, tachycardia, increased urine output, dehydration, nausea, vomiting, or diarrhea.	These adverse reactions are usually attributed to the hyperosmolality or hypertonicity of the preparations. They can be prevented or minimized by starting with small amounts of dilute solutions and gradually increasing to full-strength solutions. All such products require that additional water be given to meet fluid needs.
c. With parenteral hyperalimentation, observe for elevated blood and urine glucose levels, signs of infection (fever, inflammation at the venipuncture site), concentrated urine of high specific gravity (1.035 or above), hypertension, dyspnea.	These signs and symptoms indicate complications of therapy. Except for infection, they are likely to occur when the solution is given in a concentration or at a rate that delivers more glucose than can be utilized. This produces hyperglycemia, which in turn causes excessive amounts of fluid to be excreted in the urine (osmotic diuresis). Hyperglycemic, hyperosmolar, nonketotic coma may also occur.
d. With anorexiant drugs, observe for	
(1) Nervousness, insomnia, hyperactivity	These adverse effects are caused by excessive stimulation of the CNS. They are more likely to occur with large doses or too frequent administration.
(2) Hypertension	Anorexiant drugs stimulate the sympathetic nervous system and may cause or aggravate hypertension.
(3) Development of tolerance to appetite-suppressant effects	This usually occurs within 4 to 6 weeks and is an indication for discontinuing drug adminstration. Continued administration does not maintain appetite-suppressant effects but increases incidence of adverse effects. In addition, taking larger doses of the drug does not restore appetite-suppressant effects.
(4) Signs of psychologic drug dependence	This is more likely to occur with large doses or long-term use.
(5) With fenfluramine, observe for drowsiness during use and mental depression when the drug is discontinued.	Fenfluramine causes CNS depression rather than the stimulation that occurs with other anorexiant drugs.
4. Observe for drug interactions with anorexiants	
a. Drugs that *increase* effects	
(1) Alkalinizing agents (*e.g.,* sodium bicarbonate)	Potentiate anorexiants by increasing gastrointestinal absorption and decreasing urinary excretion
(2) Antidepressants, tricyclic	May increase hypertensive effects of anorexiants
(3) Monoamine oxidase (MAO) inhibitors	Increase hypertensive effects. Anorexiants should not be given within 2 weeks of MAO inhibitors because of possible hypertensive crisis.

Nursing Actions	***Rationale/Explanation***
(4) Other CNS stimulants	Additive stimulant effects
(5) Other sympathomimetic drugs (*e.g.*, epinephrine, isoproterenol)	Additive hypertensive and other cardiovascular effects
b. Drugs that *decrease* effects	
(1) Acidifying agents (*e.g.*, ascorbic acid)	Decrease gastrointestinal absorption and increase urinary excretion.
(2) Antihypertensive drugs	Anorexiants have blood pressure-raising effects that antagonize blood pressure-lowering effects of drugs used for hypertension
(3) CNS depressants (*e.g.*, alcohol, chlorpromazine)	Antagonize or decrease effects
5. Teach clients	
a. The importance of nutrition in maintaining or promoting health	
b. Kinds and amounts of foods and fluids needed for normal nutrition	
c. Ways of adapting restricted diets to increase their acceptability	
d. Benefits to be gained from nutritional agents, whether given orally, intravenously, or by tube feeding	
e. That most intravenous fluids are nutritionally inadequate and useful only for short-term treatment. Thus, return to oral feedings is desirable as soon as tolerated after surgery or illness.	
f. Take pancreatic enzymes with food.	To obtain the therapeutic benefit of increased digestion and absorption of foods
g. Take anorexiants in the dosage and for the length of time prescribed.	Excessive dosage will cause potentially serious adverse reactions. These drugs lose their appetite-depressant effects in 4 to 6 weeks. Prolonged use may lead to psychologic dependence.
h. Anorexiants are ineffective unless combined with restricted calorie intake and increased exercise.	

Selected References

Ball M, Phillips LJ: Nutritional disorders. In Wiener MB, Pepper GA (eds): Clinical Pharmacology and Therapeutics in Nursing, 2d ed., pp 353–388. New York, McGraw-Hill, 1985

Barnes LA: Infant feeding: Formula, solids. Pediatr Clin North Am 32:355–362, April 1985

Facts and Comparisons: St. Louis, J B Lippincott (Updated monthly)

Hansten PD: Drug Interactions: Clinical Significance of Drug–Drug Interactions, 5th ed. Philadelphia, Lea & Febiger, 1985

Metheny NM: 20 ways to prevent tube-feeding complications. Nursing 15:47–50, January 1985

Solomons NW: Assessment of nutritional status: Functional indicators of pediatric nutriture. Pediatr Clin North Am 32:319–334, April 1985

Van Itallie TB: Health implications of overweight and obesity in the United States. Ann Intern Med 103:983–988, December 1985

Weiner N: Norepinephrine, epinephrine, and the sympathomimetic amines. In Gilman AG, Goodman LS, Rall TW, Murad F (eds): The Pharmacological Basis of Therapeutics, 7th ed, pp 145–180. New York, Macmillan, 1985

Wilhelm L: Helping your patient "settle in" with TPN. Nursing 15:60–64, April 1985

Wink DM: Getting through the maze of infant formulas. Am J Nurs 85:388–392, April 1985

Zlotkin SH, Stallings VA, Pencharz PB: Total parenteral nutrition in children. Pediatr Clin North Am 32:381–400, April 1985

31 VITAMINS

Description and uses

Vitamins are a group of substances that are necessary for normal body metabolism of fat, carbohydrate, and protein. They act mainly as coenzymes to help convert carbohydrate and fat into energy and form bones and tissues. These compounds vary greatly in chemical structure and function. They are effective in small amounts and are normally obtained from foods. Vitamins are usually subclassified as fat soluble (A, D, E, K) and water soluble (B complex, C). Fat-soluble vitamins are absorbed from the intestine with dietary fat, and absorption requires that bile salts and pancreatic lipase be present. These vitamins are relatively stable to cooking. Water-soluble vitamins are readily absorbed but are also readily lost by improper cooking and storage. Vitamin D is discussed in Chapter 26 because of its major role in bone metabolism. Table 31-1 summarizes characteristics, functions, requirements, and food sources of vitamins. Requirements are stated in terms of the United States Recommended Daily Allowances (USRDAs) established by the Food and Drug Administration. These were established as guidelines for the healthy adult or child.

When inadequate amounts of vitamins are ingested, vitamin deficiencies result. Deficiency states are uncommon in people who are able to eat and are generally healthy. They are more likely to occur with disease processes that interfere with absorption or use of vitamins. When excessive amounts of fat-soluble vitamins are taken, excess states may occur because fat-soluble vitamins accumulate in the body. Excess states do not occur with dietary intake of water-soluble vitamins because these vitamins are rapidly excreted in the urine. Occasionally, therapeutic doses of water-soluble vitamins produce brief but rarely significant reactions. Causes and clinical manifestations of vitamin disorders are listed in Table 31-2.

There are many commercially available vitamin preparations; some contain a single vitamin, and some contain multiple vitamins. The only clear-cut indications for use of these products are prevention and treatment of vitamin deficiencies. Since vitamins are essential nutrients, some people believe that large doses (megadoses) promote health and provide other beneficial effects. There is no evidence that amounts beyond those needed for normal body functioning serve any beneficial effects; excessive intake of fat-soluble vitamins causes harmful effects. Thus, "megavitamins" should never be self-prescribed.

When vitamins are prescribed by a physician to prevent or treat deficiencies, they exert the same physiologic effects as those obtained from foods. Also, synthetic vitamins have the same structure and function as natural vitamins derived from plant and animal sources. There is no evidence that natural vitamins are superior to synthetic vitamins. Natural vitamins are usually much more expensive.

Many multivitamin preparations do not require a physician's prescription. These preparations vary widely in number, type, and amount of specific ingredients. Although useful in certain situations, they can-

(Text continues on p. 303.)

TABLE 31-1. VITAMINS AS NUTRIENTS

		Characteristics	Functions	Recommended daily allowances (USRDAs)	Dietary sources
Fat-soluble vitamins	Vitamin A	1. Obtained from animal foods and plant foods which contain carotenoids (precursors of vitamin A) 2. About one third of carotenoids are absorbed, and they become active in body functioning only after conversion to retinol in the wall of the small intestine. Retinol, another name for preformed vitamin A, is the physiologically active form. 3. Vitamin A activity has been designated in units. A recent recommendation has been that calculations include beta-carotene and other carotenoids as well as preformed vitamin A. Now, vitamin A activity may be expressed in terms of retinol equivalents (RE).	Required for normal vision, growth, bone development, skin, and mucous membrane	Nonpregnant women—4000 units or 800 RE Men and pregnant women—5000 units or 1000 RE Lactating women—6000 units or 1200 RE Children—400–5000 units or 420–1000 RE	Preformed vitamin A—meat, butter and fortified margarine, egg yolk, whole milk, and cheese made from whole milk Carotenoids—turnip and collard greens, carrots, sweet potatoes, squash, apricots, peaches, and cantaloupe
	Vitamin E	1. A group of substances called tocopherols, of which alpha-tocopherol is most biologically active 2. Not clearly established as an essential nutrient for people	Undetermined. It is thought to act as an antioxidant in preventing destruction of certain fats, including the lipid portion of cell membranes. It may also increase absorption, hepatic storage, and utilization of vitamin A.	Adults: 12–15 units Children: 7–10 units Infants: 4–6 units	Cereals, green vegetables, egg yolk, milk fat, butter, meat, and vegetable oils
	Vitamin K	1. Occurs naturally in two forms: phytonadione (K_1), which is found in plant foods, and menaquinone (K_2), which is synthesized in the intestine by bacteria 2. Absorbed mainly from the upper small intestine in the presence of bile and dietary fats	Essential for normal blood clotting. Activates precursor proteins, found in the liver, into clotting factors: prothrombin (Factor II), proconvertin (Factor VII), plasma thromboplastin component (Factor IX) and Stuart factor (Factor X)	Not established. Estimated to be very small and readily met by dietary and intestinal bacterial sources under normal circumstances	Green, leafy vegetables (spinach, kale, cabbage, lettuce), cauliflower, tomatoes, wheat bran, cheese, egg yolk, and liver
	Vitamin D	See Chapter 26			
Water-soluble vitamins					
B-complex vitamins	Biotin	Must be obtained from dietary intake. There is also some synthesis by intestinal bacteria,	Essential in fat and carbohydrate metabolism	Not established; provisionally set at 100–200 μg	Meat, especially liver, egg yolk, nuts, cereals, and most vegetables

TABLE 31-1. VITAMINS AS NUTRIENTS (*Continued*)

	Characteristics	Functions	Recommended daily allowances (USRDAs)	Dietary sources
	and a portion is absorbed.			
Cyanocobalamin (vitamin B_{12})	In addition to food sources, some is also obtained from tissue storage in the liver and from recovery of cyanocobalamin secreted in bile and reabsorbed in the small intestine.	Essential for normal metabolism of all body cells (especially those of the bone marrow, nervous tissue, and gastrointestinal tract); for normal red blood cells; for growth; and for metabolism of carbohydrate, protein, and fat	Adults: 3–5 μg Children: 2–3 μg Infants: 0.5–1.5 μg	Meat, especially liver, eggs, fish, cheese
Folic acid (folate)	1. Obtained from foods and the enterohepatic cycle. The latter provides an endogenous source, since folate is excreted in bile, reabsorbed in the small bowel, and reused. 2. May be lost from vegetables stored at room temperature or cooked at high temperatures	Essential for normal metabolism of all body cells, for normal red blood cells, and for growth	50 μg for adults, with larger amounts during pregnancy and lactation	Liver, kidney beans, fresh green vegetables (spinach, broccoli, asparagus)
Niacin (vitamin B_3)		Essential for glycolysis, fat synthesis, and tissue respiration. It functions as a coenzyme in many metabolic processes (after conversion to nicotinamide, the physiologically active form).	Adults: 14–18 mg. This includes intake of niacin and tryptophan, an amino acid precursor of niacin. Children: 9–16 mg Infants: 6–8 mg	Meat, poultry, fish, peanuts
Pantothenic acid (vitamin B_5)		A component of coenzyme A and essential for cellular metabolism (intermediary metabolism of carbohydrate, fat and protein; release of energy from carbohydrate; fatty acid metabolism; synthesis of cholesterol, steroid hormones, phospholipids and porphyrin)	Not established. Estimated at 5–10 mg	Eggs, liver, salmon, yeast, cauliflower, broccoli, lean beef, potatoes, and tomatoes
Pyridoxine (vitamin B_6)	1. Occurs in three forms (pyridoxal, pyridoxine, and pyridoxamine), all of which are converted in the body to pyridoxal phosphate, the physiologically active form.	1. Serves as a coenzyme in many metabolic processes 2. Functions in metabolism of carbohydrate, protein, and fat 3. Required for formation of tryptophan and conver-	Adults: 1.8–2.2 mg Children: 0.9–1.6 mg Infants: 0.3–0.6 mg Requirements increase with dietary intake of protein	Yeast, wheat germ, liver and other glandular meats, whole grain cereals, potatoes, legumes

TABLE 31-1. VITAMINS AS NUTRIENTS (*Continued*)

		Characteristics	Functions	Recommended daily allowances (USRDAs)	Dietary sources
			sion of tryptophan to niacin 4. As part of the enzyme phosphorylase, helps release glycogen from the liver and muscle tissue 5. Functions in metabolism of the central nervous system 6. Helps maintain cellular immunity		
	Riboflavin (vitamin B_2)		1. Serves as a coenzyme in metabolism 2. Necessary for growth 3. May function in production of corticosteroids and red blood cells and in gluconeogenesis	Adults: 1.0–1.5 mg Children: 0.8–1.4 mg Infants: 0.4–0.6 mg	Milk, cheddar and cottage cheese, meat, eggs, green leafy vegetables
	Thiamine (vitamin B_1)		A coenzyme in carbohydrate metabolism and essential for energy production	Adults: 1–1.5 mg, increased with high carbohydrate intake, hyperthyroidism, strenuous physical activity, malabsorption disorders, prolonged diarrhea, and liver disease that decreases utilization Children: 0.7–1.2 mg Infants: 0.3–0.5 mg	Meat, poultry, fish, egg yolk, dried beans, whole grain cereal products, and peanuts
Vitamin C	Vitamin C (ascorbic acid)	1. Dietary vitamin C is well absorbed from the intestinal tract and distributed widely in body tissues. 2. Not stored in body to a significant extent. Once tissues are saturated with about 1500 mg, any excess is excreted in the urine.	1. Essential for collagen formation (collagen is a fibrous protein found in connective tissue throughout the body, including skin, ligaments, cartilage, bone, and teeth) 2. Required for wound healing and tissue repair; metabolism of iron and folic acid; synthesis of fats and proteins; preservation of blood vessel integrity; and resistance to infection	Adults: 50–60 mg Children: 45 mg Infants: 35 mg	Fruits and vegetables, especially citrus fruits and juices

not be used interchangeably or indiscriminately with safety. More specific characteristics include the following:

1. Some preparations contain ingredients that are not considered essential nutrients and are of no apparent value in prevention or treatment of vitamin

(Text continues on p. 307.)

TABLE 31-2. VITAMIN IMBALANCES

		Deficiency states		Excess states	
		Causes	***Signs and symptoms***	***Causes***	***Signs and symptoms***
Fat-soluble vitamins	Vitamin A	Rarely caused by inadequate dietary intake in the United States; usually occurs with disease processes that interfere with intake, absorption, or use Absorption is decreased with a lack of dietary fat or bile salts (from biliary tract obstruction), inflammatory gastrointestinal conditions, and other conditions characterized by malabsorption and diarrhea. Hepatitis or hepatic cirrhosis may prevent liver storage of vitamin A.	Night blindness Xerophthalmia, which may progress to corneal ulceration and blindness Changes in skin and mucous membranes which lead to skin lesions and infections, respiratory tract infections, and urinary calculi	Excessive intake of vitamin A, which is unlikely with dietary intake but can occur with vitamin abuse	Anorexia Vomiting Irritability Headache Skin changes (dryness, itching, desquamation, and dermatitis) Later manifestations may include fatigue, pain in muscles, bones and joints, gingivitis, enlargement of spleen and liver, altered liver function, increased intracranial pressure, and other neurological signs. Congenital abnormalities may occur in newborns whose mothers took excessive vitamin A during pregnancy. Acute toxicity, with increased intracranial pressure, bulging fontanels, and vomiting may occur in infants who are given vitamin A.
	Vitamin E	Deficiency not established in humans		Excess state not established in humans	
	Vitamin K	Inadequate intake, absorption, or use. Rarely caused by inadequate intake after infancy. Occurs commonly in newborns owing to lack of dietary intake of vitamin K and lack of intestinal synthesis of the vitamin during the first week of life. After infancy, deficiency usually results from diseases that interfere with absorption (biliary tract and gastrointestinal disorders) or utilization (hepatic cirrhosis and hepatitis). In alcoholics, deficiency commonly occurs and probably results from both decreased intake and impaired utilization. Drug-induced deficiency occurs with oral coumarin anticoagulants and some other drugs that act as vitamin K antagonists. Also, antibiotics reduce bacterial synthesis of vitamin K in the intestine, but this is a rare cause of deficiency.	Abnormal bleeding (melena, hematemesis, hematuria, epistaxis, petechiae, ecchymoses, hypovolemic shock)	Unlikely to occur from dietary intake; may occur when vitamin K is given as an antidote for oral anticoagulants	Clinical manifestations rarely occur. However, when vitamin K is given to someone who is receiving warfarin (Coumadin), the client can be made "warfarin-resistant" for 2–3 weeks.
	Vitamin D	See Chapter 26			

TABLE 31-2. VITAMIN IMBALANCES (*Continued*)

		Deficiency states		Excess states	
		Causes	***Signs and symptoms***	***Causes***	***Signs and symptoms***
Water-soluble vitamins				Excess states do not occur with dietary intake of water-soluble vitamins but may occur with megadoses. Megadoses should be avoided.	
	Biotin	Inadequate intake or impaired absorption. Biotin deficiency is rare.	Anorexia Nausea Depression Muscle pain Dermatitis		
	Cyanocobalamin (vitamin B_{12})	Usually impaired absorption from a lack of hydrochloric acid or intrinsic factor in the stomach	Megaloblastic or pernicious anemia 1. Decreased numbers of red blood cells (RBCs) 2. Abnormally large, immature RBC's 3. Fatigue 4. Dyspnea 5. With severe deficiency, leukopenia, thrombocytopenia, cardiac arrhythmias, heart failure, or infections may occur Neurologic signs and symptoms 1. Paresthesias in hands and feet 2. Unsteady gait 3. Depressed deep-tendon reflexes 4. With severe deficiency, loss of memory, confusion, delusions, hallucinations, and psychosis may occur. Nerve damage may be irreversible.		
	Folic acid	Inadequate diet Impaired absorption (intestinal disorders) Greatly increased requirements (pregnancy, lactation, hemolytic anemias) Ingestion of folate antagonist drugs (*e.g.,* methotrexate) Alcoholism is a common cause. It interferes with both intake and absorption.	Megaloblastic anemia that cannot be distinguished from the anemia produced by B_{12} deficiency Impaired growth in children Glossitis Gastrointestinal problems (folic acid deficiency does not produce neurologic signs and symptoms as B_{12} deficiency does).		
	Niacin (vitamin B_3)	Inadequate diet or impaired absorption	Pellagra 1. Erythematous skin lesions 2. Gastrointestinal problems (stomatitis, glossitis, enteritis, diarrhea) 3. Central nervous system problems (headache, dizzi-		

TABLE 31-2. VITAMIN IMBALANCES (*Continued*)

	Deficiency states		Excess states	
	Causes	***Signs and symptoms***	***Causes***	***Signs and symptoms***
		ness, insomnia, depression, memory loss) 4. With severe deficiency, delusions, hallucinations, and impairment of peripheral motor and sensory nerves may occur.		
Pantothenic acid (vitamin B_5)	No deficiency state established			
Pyridoxine (vitamin B_6)	Inadequate intake or impaired absorption	1. Skin and mucous membrane lesions (seborrheic dermatitis, intertrigo, glossitis, and stomatitis) 2. Neurologic problems (convulsions, peripheral neuritis, and mental depression)		
Riboflavin (vitamin B_2)	Inadequate intake or impaired absorption. Uncommon and usually occurs with deficiencies of other B-complex vitamins.	Glossitis and stomatitis Seborrheic dermatitis Eye disorders (burning, itching, lacrimation, photophobia, and vascularization of the cornea)		
Thiamine (vitamin B_1)	Inadequate diet, especially among pregnant women and infants. Impaired absorption due to gastrointestinal disorders Alcoholism	Mild deficiency—fatigue, anorexia, retarded growth, mental depression, irritability, apathy, and lethargy Severe deficiency (beriberi)—peripheral neuritis, personality disturbances, heart failure, edema, Wernicke–Korsakoff syndrome in alcoholics		
Vitamin C (ascorbic acid)	Inadequate dietary intake (most likely in infants, elderly, indigent, and alcoholics) Increased requirements (people who smoke cigarettes, take oral contraceptives or have acute or chronic illness) Megadoses that are abruptly discontinued may cause a rebound deficiency. Deficiency may also occur in infants whose mothers took megadoses during pregnancy.	1. Mild deficiency—irritability, malaise, arthralgia, and increased tendency to bleed 2. Severe deficiency—scurvy and adverse effects on most body tissues (gingivitis; bleeding of gums, skin, joints, and other areas; disturbances of bone growth, anemia; and loosening of teeth). If not treated, coma, and death may occur.	Megadoses may produce excessive amounts of oxalate in the urine.	Renal calculi

deficiency states. These include choline, inositol, betamine, lecithin, and methionine.

2. Preparations promoted for use as dietary supplements may contain 50% of the amounts recommended for daily intake. In healthy people who eat a well-balanced diet, nutrient needs may be greatly exceeded.
3. Preparations for therapeutic use may contain 300% to 500% of the amounts recommended for daily intake in normal circumstances. These should not contain more than recommended amounts of vitamin D, folic acid, and vitamin A.
4. Multivitamin preparations often contain minerals as well, usually in amounts much smaller than those recommended for daily intake.

Individual vitamin preparations are listed in Table 31-3.

TABLE 31-3. VITAMIN DRUG PREPARATIONS

	Generic name	Trade name	Routes and dosage ranges
Fat-soluble vitamins	Vitamin A	Alphalin Aquasol A	Adults with severe deficiency: PO 100,000–500,000 units daily for 3 days, then 50,000 units daily for 2 weeks, then 10,000–20,000 units daily for another 2 months; IM 50,000–100,000 units daily for 3 days, then 50,000 units daily for 2 weeks Children over 8 years with severe deficiency: PO, IM, same as adults Infants and children under 8 years: 10,000–15,000 units daily for 10 days
	Vitamin E	Tocopherol Aquasol E	Adults: PO, IM 60–1000 units daily Children: PO, IM 25–60 units daily
	Vitamin K		Adults and children: PO, IM 5–10 mg daily
	Menadione		Adults: PO 5–10 mg daily; SC, IM, IV 5–15 mg daily
	Menadione sodium diphosphate	Synkayvite	Children: PO, SC, IM, IV 5–10 mg daily Adults and children: PO, SC, IM 2.5–25 mg daily
	Phytonadione	Mephyton Aqua-Mephyton	Newborns: IV, IM 0.5–2 mg immediately after birth to *prevent* hemorrhagic disease of neonates; 1–2 mg daily to *treat* hemorrhagic disease
Water-soluble vitamins			
B-complex vitamins	Calcium pantothenate (B_5)	Pantholin	Adults: PO 10–20 mg daily
	Cyanocobalamin (B_{12})	Kaybovite Redisol Rubramin Betalin 12	Adults and children: PO 10–250 μg daily for 1 month in an oral therapeutic multivitamin preparation when deficiency is due to increased requirements and gastrointestinal absorption is normal IM, SC, IV 30 μg daily for 5–10 days, then 100–200 μg monthly
	Folic acid	Folvite	Adults and children: PO, SC, IM, IV up to 1 mg daily until symptoms decrease and blood tests are normal, then maintenance dose of 0.1–0.25 mg daily
	Niacin (nicotinic acid), niacinamide (nicotinamide)		Deficiency, PO, IM, IV 50–100 mg daily Pellagra, 500 mg daily Hyperlipidemia, 1–2 g daily
	Pyridoxine (B_6)	Hexa-Betalin	Deficiency, PO, IM, IV 10–20 mg daily for 3 weeks, then 2–5 mg daily Anemia, peripheral neuritis, 100–200 mg daily Pyridoxine dependency syndrome, up to 600 mg daily
	Riboflavin	Riobin-50	PO 5–10 mg daily; IM 50 mg
	Thiamine (B_1)	Betalin S	PO 10–30 mg daily; IM 10–20 mg 3 times daily for 2 weeks, supplemented with 5–10 mg orally; IV 100–200 mg
Vitamin C	Vitamin C (ascorbic acid)		Deficiency, PO, IM, IV 100–500 mg daily Scurvy, 300–1000 mg daily for at least 2 weeks Infants receiving formula, 35–50 mg daily for first few weeks of life Urinary acidification, 4–12 g daily in divided doses every 4 hours Prophylaxis, 50–100 mg daily

Principles of therapy: vitamins

ASSESSMENT GUIDELINES

Assess each client for current or potential vitamin disorders. This is generally done in an overall assessment of nutritional status. Specific assessment factors related to vitamins include the following:

1. Deficiency states are more common than excess states.
2. People with other nutritional deficiencies are likely to have vitamin deficiency as well.
3. Deficiencies of water-soluble vitamins (B complex and C) are more common than those of fat-soluble vitamins.
4. Vitamin deficiencies are usually multiple, and signs and symptoms frequently overlap, especially with B-complex deficiency states.
5. Vitamin requirements are generally increased during infancy, pregnancy, lactation, fever, hyperthyroidism, and probably most illnesses. Thus, a vitamin intake that is normally adequate may become inadequate in certain circumstances.
6. Vitamin deficiencies are likely to occur in people who are very poor, elderly, chronically ill, alcoholic, or severely ill.
7. Vitamin excess states are uncommonly caused by excessive dietary intake but may occur with use of vitamin drug preparations, especially if megadoses are taken.

NURSING INTERVENTIONS

Implement measures to prevent vitamin disorders.

1. The safest and most effective way to prevent vitamin deficiencies is by increasing dietary intake of vitamins.
   a. A well-balanced, varied diet that is adequate in proteins and calories is adequate in vitamins for most people. Exceptions are those who have increased requirements or conditions that interfere with absorption or use of vitamins.
   b. Water-soluble vitamins are often destroyed by cooking or discarded in cooking water. Eating raw fruits and vegetables prevents loss of vitamins during cooking. When fruits and vegetables are cooked, vitamin losses can be minimized by using small amounts of water, steaming or pressure cooking for the shortest effective time, and keeping cooking utensils covered.

      In addition to cooking losses, vitamin C is lost with exposure of foods to air. Consequently, fruits and vegetables, including juices, should be kept covered during storage.
   c. When vitamin deficiency stems from inadequate dietary intake, correcting the diet is preferred over administering supplemental vitamins, when feasible. For vitamin A deficiency, increasing daily intake of plant and animal sources may be sufficient. For vitamin C deficiency, citrus juices can be used therapeutically. Since about 4 ounces of orange juice daily meets requirements, larger amounts can relieve deficiency. When folic acid deficiency anemia stems from dietary lack, one fresh, uncooked fruit or vegetable or one glass of fruit juice added to the daily diet will probably correct the deficiency, except during pregnancy, when folate requirements are increased.
   d. Even when vitamin supplements are considered necessary, dietary sources should be increased for both immediate and long-term benefit.
   e. Clients receiving only intravenous fluids or a clear liquid diet for more than 2 or 3 days probably need replacement vitamins.
   f. Teach clients which foods are good sources of vitamins and ways of cooking and storing foods to preserve vitamin content.
2. When vitamin requirements are increased or interferences with vitamin absorption or use are present, vitamins may be needed as dietary supplements to prevent deficiencies. Vitamin preparations must be chosen carefully because they differ widely in the specific vitamins contained and in the amounts of each. Their use should be based on recommended requirements after eating habits and the usual dietary supply of vitamins are assessed.

   Some oral multivitamin preparations considered appropriate for supplemental use include Adeflor, Poly-Vi-Flor, Poly-Vi-Sol, Tri-Vi-Flor, Tri-Vi-Sol, and Vi-Daylin for children and Dayalets for adults. These contain less than 150% of the USRDA for all ingredients. Preparations containing fluoride require a prescription.
3. To prevent vitamin excess, teach clients to avoid excessive intake of any vitamin preparation. Although the dangers of overdosage of fat-soluble vitamins have long been known, overdosage of water-soluble vitamins has been considered wasteful and expensive but not dangerous because these vitamins are rapidly excreted in the urine. Recent evidence, however, indicates that prolonged intake

of excessive amounts of certain water-soluble vitamins can cause serious adverse effects. More specifically, large amounts of niacin may cause gastrointestinal problems, flushing, skin rashes, and pruritus and may exacerbate asthma, uricosuria, and gouty arthritis. Long-term ingestion of high doses of pyridoxine has been associated with peripheral neuropathies characterized by decreased sensation in limbs, perioral numbness, and ataxia. These symptoms improved after pyridoxine was withdrawn but were not completely eliminated. Large amounts of vitamin C (1 g or more) may cause diarrhea, uricosuria, and oxalate kidney stones. They also increase estrogen levels, decrease activity of oral anticoagulants, and, when taken by pregnant women, have caused scurvy in infants when they no longer received the large amounts to which they were exposed *in utero.*

PRINCIPLES OF MANAGING VITAMIN DISORDERS

When vitamin disorders are present, they should be recognized as early as possible and appropriate treatment initiated. Early recognition and treatment can prevent a mild deficiency or excess from becoming severe. Some guidelines include the following:

1. **Vitamin deficiency.** For deficiency states, oral vitamin preparations are preferred, when possible. They are usually effective (except in malabsorption syndromes), safe, convenient to administer, and relatively inexpensive. If the deficiency involves only a single vitamin, then that vitamin alone is indicated. However, multiple deficiencies are common, and a multivitamin preparation may be needed. Although dosages for deficiencies are generally higher than those for dietary supplements, dosages should be titrated as nearly as possible to the amounts needed by the body.

   Multivitamin preparations for treating deficiencies contain more than 150% of the USRDA. They should be used only for therapeutic purposes and for limited periods. Some oral preparations considered appropriate for therapeutic use include Abdec, Abdol, Adeflor, Betalin Complex Elixir, Multicebrin, Natalins, Surbex, Tri-Vi-Sol, and Vi-Daylin. Several of these may be used for adults or children. Other preparations are available for use during pregnancy and lactation or for parenteral use.

   When fat-soluble vitamins are given to correct deficiency, there is risk of producing excess states. When water-soluble vitamins are given, excesses are less likely but may occur with large doses. These factors must be considered in determining vitamin dosage.
2. **Vitamin excess.** For excess states, the usual treatment is to stop administration of the vitamin preparation. There are no specific antidotes or antagonists.

Principles of treating disorders of fat-soluble vitamins A and K

1. With vitamin A deficiency, increase intake of foods containing vitamin A or carotene when feasible. Use a single, pure form of vitamin A rather than a multivitamin unless multiple deficiencies are present. Give doses no larger than 25,000 units daily unless a severe deficiency is present. Give orally if not contraindicated. Give intramuscularly if gastrointestinal absorption is severely impaired or ocular symptoms are severe. With vitamin A excess, immediately stop known sources of the vitamin.
2. With vitamin K deficiency or hypoprothrombinemia, bleeding may occur spontaneously or in response to trauma. Thus, administration of vitamin K and measures to prevent bleeding are indicated. If the deficiency is not severe, oral vitamin K may be given for a few days until serum prothrombin activity returns to a normal range. In obstructive jaundice, bile salts must be given at the same time as oral vitamin K, or vitamin K must be given parenterally. In malabsorption syndromes or diarrhea, parenteral administration is probably necessary. A single dose of vitamin K may be sufficient. With severe bleeding, vitamin K may be given intravenously. Intravenous vitamin K must be given very slowly to decrease risks of hypotension and shock. Unfortunately, a therapeutic response does not occur for at least 4 hours. For more rapid control of bleeding, transfusions of plasma or whole blood are needed. When bleeding is caused by oral anticoagulant drugs, avoid overdoses of vitamin K. Oral anticoagulants are usually given for thromboembolic disorders. Giving vitamin K as an antidote to control bleeding reestablishes the risks of thrombi. Measures to prevent bleeding include avoiding trauma, injections, and drugs that may cause bleeding.

Principles of treating disorders of B-complex vitamins

1. Most deficiencies of B-complex vitamins are multiple rather than single. Also, many of these vita-

mins are obtained from the same foods. Treating deficiencies consists of increasing intake of foods containing B-complex vitamins or giving multivitamin preparations. Multivitamin preparations vary greatly in composition and therefore must be carefully chosen. Most preparations contain thiamine, riboflavin, niacin, pyridoxine, and cyanocobalamin. Other vitamins may be included in the formulations.

If a single deficiency seems predominant, that vitamin may be given alone or in conjunction with a multiple vitamin preparation. For example, thiamine deficiency is common in alcoholic clients, apparently because large amounts of thiamine are used to metabolize alcohol.

2. Some relatively rare types of anemia occur with deficiencies of certain B-complex vitamins. One type of anemia occurs with pyridoxine deficiency and is relieved by administration of pyridoxine. Megaloblastic anemias, characterized by abnormally large, immature red blood cells, occur with deficiency of folic acid or vitamin B_{12}. If megaloblastic anemia is severe, treatment is usually instituted with both folic acid and vitamin B_{12}.
   a. In pernicious anemia, vitamin B_{12} must be given by intramuscular or subcutaneous injection because oral forms are not absorbed from the gastrointestinal tract. Vitamin B_{12} injections are specific therapy for pernicious anemia and must be continued for life. Vitamin B_{12} is sometimes given to prevent pernicious anemia in clients who are strict vegetarians, who have had gastrectomy, or who have chronic small bowel disease. Pernicious anemia must be differentiated from other megaloblastic anemias for appropriate therapy. Pernicious anemia and other megaloblastic anemias respond to administration of folic acid. However, if folic acid alone is given to the client with pernicious anemia, hematologic abnormalities disappear but neurologic deterioration continues.
   b. In other types of megaloblastic anemias, vitamin B_{12} or folic acid is indicated. Although both of these are included in many multivitamin preparations, they usually must be given separately for therapeutic purposes. With vitamin B_{12}, doses of more than 100 μg are not useful because any excess of that amount is rapidly excreted in urine. It may be given as a single dose of 1000 μg in performing the Schilling test for pernicious anemia. With folic acid, oral administration is indicated for most clients. Daily doses in excess of 1 mg are not useful because any excess is excreted in the urine.

Principles of treating vitamin C disorders

Treatment of vitamin C deficiency involves increased intake of vitamin C from dietary or pharmaceutical sources. Vitamin C (ascorbic acid) is available alone for oral, intramuscular, or intravenous administration. It is also an ingredient in most multiple vitamin preparations for oral or parenteral use.

NURSING ACTIONS: VITAMINS

Nursing Actions	*Rationale/Explanation*
1. Administer accurately	
a. With fat-soluble vitamins	
(1) Give as directed.	To increase therapeutic effects and avoid adverse reactions
(2) Do not give oral preparations at the same time as mineral oil.	Mineral oil absorbs the vitamins and thus prevents their systemic absorption.
(3) For subcutaneous or intramuscular administration of vitamin K, aspirate carefully to avoid intravenous injection, apply gentle pressure to the injection site, and inspect the site frequently. For intravenous injection, vitamin K may be given by direct injection or diluted in intravenous fluids (*e.g.,* 5% dextrose in water or saline).	Vitamin K is given to clients with hypoprothrombinemia, which causes a bleeding tendency. Thus, any injection may cause trauma and bleeding at the injection site.
(4) Administer intravenous vitamin K slowly, at a rate not to exceed 1 mg/minute, whether diluted or undiluted.	Intravenous phytonadione may cause hypotension and shock from an anaphylactic type of reaction.

Nursing Actions	*Rationale/Explanation*
b. With B-complex vitamins	
(1) Give parenteral cyanocobalamin (vitamin B_{12}) intramuscularly or deep subcutaneously.	
(2) Give oral niacin preparations, except for timed-release forms, with or after meals. Have the client sit or lie down for about ½ hour after administration.	To decrease anorexia, nausea, vomiting, diarrhea, and flatulence. Niacin causes vasodilation, which may result in dizziness, hypotension, and possibly injury from falls. Vasodilation occurs within a few minutes and may last an hour.
(3) Give intramuscular thiamine deeply into a large muscle mass. Avoid the intravenous route.	To decrease pain at the injection site. Hypotension and anaphylactic shock have occurred with rapid intravenous administration and large doses.
2. Observe for therapeutic effects (mainly decreased signs and symptoms of deficiency)	
a. With vitamin A, observe for improved vision, especially in dim light or at night, less dryness in eyes and conjunctiva (xerophthalmia), improvement in skin lesions.	Night blindness is usually relieved within a few days. Skin lesions may not completely disappear for several weeks.
b. With vitamin K, observe for decreased bleeding and more nearly normal blood coagulation tests (*e.g.,* prothrombin time).	Blood coagulation tests usually improve within 4 to 12 hours.
c. With B-complex vitamins, observe for decreased or absent stomatitis, glossitis, cheilosis, seborrheic dermatitis, neurologic problems (neuritis, convulsions, mental deterioration, psychotic symptoms), cardiovascular problems (edema, heart failure), and eye problems (itching, burning, photophobia).	Deficiencies of B-complex vitamins commonly occur together and produce many similar manifestations.
d. With vitamin B_{12} and folic acid, observe for increased appetite, strength and feeling of well being, increased reticulocyte counts, and increased numbers of normal red blood cells, hemoglobin, and hematocrit.	Therapeutic effects may be quite rapid and dramatic. The client usually feels better within 24 to 48 hours, and normal red blood cells begin to appear. Anemia is decreased within about 2 weeks, but 4 to 8 weeks may be needed for complete blood count to return to normal.
e. With vitamin C, observe for decreased or absent malaise, irritability, and bleeding tendencies (easy bruising of skin, bleeding gums, nosebleeds, and so on).	
3. Observe for adverse reactions	
a. With vitamin A, observe for signs of hypervitaminosis A (anorexia, vomiting, irritability, headache, skin changes [dryness, dermatitis, itching, desquamation], fatigue, pain in muscles, bones, and joints, and other clinical manifestations; and serum levels of vitamin A above 1200 units/100 ml).	Severity of manifestations depends largely on dose and duration of excess vitamin A intake. Very severe states produce additional clinical signs, including enlargement of liver and spleen, altered liver function, increased intracranial pressure, and other neurologic manifestations.
b. With vitamin K, observe for hypotension and signs of anaphylactic shock with intravenous phytonadione.	Vitamin K rarely produces adverse reactions. Giving intravenous phytonadione very slowly may prevent adverse reactions.
c. With B-complex vitamins, observe for hypotension and anaphylactic shock with parenteral niacin, thiamine, cyanocobalamin, and folic acid; anorexia, nausea, vomiting and diarrhea, and postural hypotension with oral niacin.	Adverse reactions are generally rare. They are unlikely with B-complex multivitamin preparations. They are most likely to occur with large intravenous doses and rapid administration.
d. With vitamin C megadoses, observe for diarrhea and rebound deficiency if stopped abruptly.	Adverse reactions are rare with usual doses and methods of administration.

Nursing Actions	Rationale/Explanation
4. Observe for drug interactions	
a. Fat-soluble vitamins	
(1) Bile salts *increase* effects.	Increase intestinal absorption
(2) Laxatives, especially mineral oil, *decrease* effects.	Mineral oil combines with fat-soluble vitamins and prevents their absorption if both are taken at the same time. Excessive or chronic laxative use decreases intestinal absorption.
(3) Antibiotics may *decrease* effects.	With vitamin K, antibiotics decrease production by decreasing intestinal bacteria. With others, antibiotics may cause diarrhea and subsequent malabsorption.
b. B-complex vitamins	
(1) Cycloserine (antituberculosis drug) *decreases* effect.	By increasing urinary excretion of vitamin B-complex
(2) Isoniazid (INH) *decreases* effect.	INH has an antipyridoxine effect. When INH is given for prevention or treatment of tuberculosis, pyridoxine is usually given also.
(3) With folic acid: alcohol, methotrexate, oral contraceptives, phenytoin and triamterene *decrease* effects.	Alcohol alters liver function and leads to poor hepatic storage of folic acid. Methotrexate and phenytoin act as antagonists to folic acid and may cause folic acid deficiency. Oral contraceptives decrease absorption of folic acid.
5. Teach clients	
a. For most clients, the safest and most effective way of obtaining an adequate amount of needed vitamins is to eat a well-balanced diet.	The nurse or dietitian can instruct the client regarding a well-balanced diet and food sources of required vitamins.
b. Avoid large doses of vitamins unless specifically prescribed by the physician.	Excessive amounts of vitamins do not promote health, strength, or youth. Excessive vitamins may cause serious adverse reactions.
c. If supplementary vitamins are taken, it is probably advisable to consult a physician.	Available preparations differ widely in amounts and types of vitamin content.
d. Take prescribed vitamins as directed and for the appropriate time.	In pernicious anemia, vitamin B_{12} injections must be taken for the remainder of life. In pregnancy and lactation, vitamins are usually taken only during this period of increased need.

Selected References

American Medical Association (AMA) Division of Drugs: AMA Drug Evaluations, 5th ed. New York, John Wiley & Sons, 1983

Ball M, Phillips LJ: Nutritional disorders. In Wiener MB, Pepper GA: Clinical Pharmacology and Therapeutics in Nursing, 2d ed, pp 353–388. New York, McGraw-Hill, 1985

Hansten PD: Drug Interactions: Clinical Significance of Drug–Drug Interactions, 5th ed. Philadelphia, Lea & Febiger, 1985

Mandel HG, Cohn VH: Fat-soluble vitamins. In Gilman AG, Goodman LS, Rall TW, Murad F (eds): The Pharmacological Basis of Therapeutics, 7th ed, pp 1573–1591. New York, Macmillan, 1985

Marcus R, Coulston AM: Water-soluble vitamins. In Gilman AG, Goodman LS, Rall TW, Murad F (eds): The Pharmacological Basis of Therapeutics, 7th ed, pp 1551–1572. New York, Macmillan, 1985

Rodman MJ, Karch AM, Boyd EH, Smith DW: Pharmacology and Drug Therapy in Nursing, 3rd ed. Philadelphia, J B Lippincott, 1985

Toxic effects of vitamin overdosage. Med Lett Drugs Ther 26:66–68, August 1984

Vitamin supplements. Med Lett Drugs Ther 27:66–68, August 1985

32 MINERALS AND ELECTROLYTES

Description and uses

Minerals and electrolytes are essential constituents of all living tissues. They are also components of many essential enzymes. In general, they function to maintain fluid, electrolyte, and acid–base balance; maintain osmotic pressure; maintain nerve and muscle function; assist in transfer of essential compounds across cell membranes; and influence the growth process.

Minerals occur in the body and foods mainly in ionic form. Ions are electrically charged particles. Metals (*e.g.*, sodium, potassium, calcium, magnesium) form positive ions or cations; nonmetals (*e.g.*, chlorine, phosphorus, sulfur) form negative ions or anions. These cations and anions combine to form salts or compounds that are physiologically inactive and electrically neutral. When placed in solution, such as a body fluid, the components separate into electrically charged particles called *electrolytes.* For example, sodium and chlorine combine to form sodium chloride (NaCl). (Table salt is composed of NaCl.) In a solution, NaCl separates into Na^+ and Cl^- ions. (The + following Na indicates that Na is a cation. The − following Cl indicates that Cl is an anion.) At any given time the body must maintain an equal number of positive and negative charges. Therefore, the ions are constantly combining and separating to maintain electrical neutrality or electrolyte balance.

These electrolytes also maintain acid–base balance of body fluids, which is necessary for normal body functioning. When foods are digested in the body, they produce mineral residues that react chemically as acids or bases. Acids are usually anions such as chloride, bicarbonate, sulfate, and phosphate. Bases are usually cations such as sodium, potassium, calcium, and magnesium. If approximately equal amounts of cations and anions are present in the mineral residue, the residue is essentially neutral and the *p*H of body fluids does not require adjustment. If there is an excess of cations (base), the body must draw on its anions (acid) to combine with the cations, render them physiologically inactive, and restore the normal *p*H of the blood. Excess cations are excreted in the urine, mainly in combination with the anion phosphate. If there is an excess of anions (acid), usually sulfate or phosphate, they combine with hydrogen ions or other cations and are excreted in the urine.

There are 21 minerals thought to be necessary for human nutrition. Some of these (calcium, phosphorus, sodium, potassium, magnesium, chlorine, sulfur) are required in relatively large amounts and thus are sometimes called macronutrients. Calcium and phosphorus are discussed in Chapter 26. The other macronutrients are described here in terms of characteristics, functions, recommended daily allowances, and food sources (see Table 32-1). Imbalances of macronutrients are classified as deficiency states and excess states. So-

TABLE 32-1. MINERALS AND ELECTROLYTES

	Characteristics	Functions	Recommended daily allowance (USRDA)	Food sources
Sodium	1. Major cation in extracellular body fluids (blood, lymph, tissue fluid) 2. Small amount in intracellular fluid 3. Large amounts of sodium in saliva, gastric secretions, bile, pancreatic and intestinal secretions	1. Assists in regulating osmotic pressure, water balance, conduction of electrical impulses in nerves and muscles, electrolyte and acid–base balance 2. Influences permeability of cell membranes and assists in movement of substances across cell membranes 3. Participates in many intracellular chemical reactions	Estimated to be approximately 2 g	1. Present in most foods. Proteins contain relatively large amounts, vegetables and cereals contain moderate to small amounts, fruits contain little or no sodium. 2. Major source of sodium in the diet is table salt added to food in cooking, processing or seasoning. One teaspoon contains 2.3 g of sodium. 3. Water in some geographic areas may contain significant amounts of sodium.
Potassium	1. Major cation in intracellular body fluids 2. Present in all body fluids 3. Eliminated from the body primarily in urine. Normally functioning kidneys excrete excessive amounts of potassium, but they are unable to conserve potassium when intake is low or absent. The kidneys excrete 10 mEq or more daily in the absence of intake. Potassium excretion is influenced by acid–base balance and aldosterone secretion. 4. A small amount of potassium is normally lost in feces and sweat.	1. Within cells, helps to maintain osmotic pressure, fluid and electrolyte balance, and acid–base balance. 2. In extracellular fluid, functions with sodium and calcium to regulate neuromuscular excitability. Potassium is required for conduction of nerve impulses and contraction of both skeletal and smooth muscle. It is especially important in activity of the myocardium. 3. Participates in carbohydrate and protein metabolism. Helps transport glucose into cells and is required for glycogen formation and storage. Required for synthesis of muscle proteins from amino acids and other components.	Approximately 40 mEq	Present in most foods, including meat, whole grain breads or cereals, bananas, citrus fruits, tomatoes, and broccoli
Magnesium	1. A cation occuring primarily in intracellular fluid 2. Widely distributed in the body, about half in bone tissue and the remainder in soft tissue and body fluids 3. Most dietary magnesium is not absorbed from the gastrointestinal tract and is excreted in feces.	1. Required for conduction of nerve impulses and contraction of muscle 2. Especially important in functions of cardiac and skeletal muscles 3. Serves as a component of many enzymes 4. Essential for metabolism of carbohydrate and protein	Approximately 300 mg for adults. Increased amounts recommended for pregnant or lactating women and children.	Present in many foods; diet adequate in other respects contains adequate magnesium. Good food sources include nuts, cereal grains, dark green vegetables, and seafoods.
Chloride	1. Ionized form of the element chlorine 2. The main anion of extracellular fluid 3. Almost all chloride is normally excreted by the kidneys.	1. Functions with sodium to help maintain osmotic pressure and water balance. 2. Forms hydrochloric acid (HCl) in gastric mucosal cells	80–110 mEq	Most dietary chloride is ingested as sodium chloride (NaCl), and foods high in sodium are also high in chloride.

TABLE 32-1. MINERALS AND ELECTROLYTES (*Continued*)

	Characteristics	Functions	Recommended daily allowance (USRDA)	Food sources
		3. Helps regulate electrolyte and acid–base balance by competing with bicarbonate ions for sodium 4. Participates in a homeostatic buffering mechanism in which chloride shifts in and out of red blood cells in exchange for bicarbonate		

dium imbalances (hyponatremia and hypernatremia) are described in Table 32-2, potassium imbalances (hypokalemia and hyperkalemia) in Table 32-3, magnesium imbalances (hypomagnesemia and hypermagnesemia) in Table 32-4, and chlorine imbalances (hypochloremic metabolic alkalosis and hyperchloremic metabolic acidosis) in Table 32-5. Each imbalance is described in terms of causes, pathophysiology, and clinical signs and symptoms.

The other 14 minerals are required in small amounts and are often called *micronutrients* or *trace elements.* Seven trace elements (chromium, cobalt, copper, fluoride, iodine, iron, zinc) have relatively well-defined roles in human nutrition. These are further described in Table 32-6. Because of their clinical importance, iron imbalances are discussed separately, in Table 32-7. Other trace elements (manganese, molybdenum, nickel, selenium, silicon, tin, vanadium) are present in

TABLE 32-2. SODIUM IMBALANCES

	Causes	Pathophysiology	Signs and symptoms
Hyponatremia	1. Inadequate intake. Unusual but may occur with sodium-restricted diets and diuretic drug therapy, or when water only is ingested after both water and sodium are lost (*e.g.,* excessive sweating). 2. Excessive losses. More common and occur with vomiting, gastrointestinal suction, diarrhea, excessive water enemas, excessive perspiration, burn wounds, and adrenal insufficiency states (*e.g.,* Addison's disease). 3. Excessive dilution of body fluids with water	1. Decreased serum sodium 2. Decreased plasma volume and cardiac output 3. Decreased blood flow to kidneys, decreased glomerular filtration rate, and decreased ability of kidneys to excrete water 4. Overhydration and swelling of brain cells (cerebral edema). Leads to impaired neurologic and muscular functions. 5. Gastrointestinal changes	1. Serum sodium below 135 mEq/liter 2. Hypotension and tachycardia 3. Oliguria and increased blood urea nitrogen (BUN) 4. Headache, dizziness, weakness, lethargy, restlessness, confusion, delirium, muscle tremors, convulsions, ataxia and aphasia 5. Anorexia, nausea, and vomiting are common; abdominal cramps and paralytic ileus may develop.
Hypernatremia	1. Deficiency of water in proportion to the amount of sodium present. Water deficiency results from lack of intake or excessive losses (diarrhea, diuretic drugs, excessive sweating). 2. Excessive intake of sodium. An uncommon cause of hypernatremia because the thirst mechanism is normally activated and water intake is increased. 3. Sodium retention due to hyperaldosteronism and Cushing's disease.	1. Increased serum sodium 2. Hypernatremia due to water deficiency decreases fluid volume in both extracellular fluid and intracellular fluid compartments (dehydration). 3. Hypernatremia due to sodium gain increases extracellular fluid volume and decreases intracellular fluid volume as water is pulled out of cells.	1. Serum sodium above 145 mEq/liter 2. Lethargy; disorientation, hyperactive reflexes; muscle rigidity, tremors and spasms; irritability; coma; cerebral hemorrhage; subdural hematoma 3. Hypotension 4. Fever, dry skin and mucous membranes 5. Oliguria, concentrated urine with a high specific gravity, and increased BUN

TABLE 32-3. POTASSIUM IMBALANCES

	Causes	Pathophysiology	Signs and symptoms
Hypokalemia	1. Inadequate intake. Uncommon in clients who are able to eat; may occur in those unable to eat or receiving only potassium-free intravenous fluids for several days. 2. Excessive losses from the gastrointestinal tract (vomiting, gastric suction, diarrhea, overuse of laxatives and enemas) or urinary tract (polyuria from diuretic drugs, renal disease, excessive aldosterone) 3. Movement of potassium out of serum and into cells. This occurs with administration of insulin and glucose in treatment of diabetic ketoacidosis and in metabolic alkalosis.	1. Decreased serum potassium 2. Impaired cardiac conduction 3. Decreased strength of myocardial contraction and decreased cardiac output. Decreased response to catecholamines and other substances that normally raise blood pressure. 4. Neurologic changes due to impaired conduction of nerve impulses 5. Impaired function of skeletal, smooth, and cardiac muscle, most likely with serum potassium below 2.5 mEq/liter. Electrical impulses are slowed until muscle contraction cannot occur. 6. Slowed gastric emptying and decreased intestinal motility, probably caused by muscle weakness 7. Decreased ability of kidney to concentrate urine and excrete acid. Decreased glomerular filtration rate with prolonged potassium deficiency. 8. Impaired carbohydrate metabolism and decreased secretion of insulin.	1. Serum potassium below 3.5 mEq/liter 2. Arrhythmias and changes in the ECG (depressed ST segment; flattened or inverted T wave; increased amplitude of P wave; prolonged PR interval; prolonged QRS complex with normal shape and size). Premature atrial and ventricular beats or atrioventricular block may occur, usually in people taking digitalis. Death from cardiac arrest may occur. 3. Postural hypotension 4. Confusion, memory impairment, lethargy, apathy, drowsiness, irritability, delirium 5. Muscle weakness and possibly paralysis. Weakness of leg muscles usually occurs first. Then, weakness ascends to include respiratory muscles and cause respiratory insufficiency. 6. Abdominal distention, constipation, and paralytic ileus 7. Polyuria, polydipsia, nocturia. Prolonged deficiency may increase serum creatinine and BUN. 8. Hyperglycemia
Hyperkalemia	1. Excess intake. Uncommon with normal kidney function. 2. Impaired excretion due to renal insufficiency, oliguria, potassium-saving diuretics, aldosterone deficiency, or adrenocortical deficiency 3. Combination of the above factors. Nonfood sources of potassium include potassium supplements, salt substitutes, transfusions of old blood, and potassium salts of penicillin (penicillin G potassium contains 1.7 mEq potassium per 1 million units). 4. Movement of potassium from cells into serum with burns, crushing injuries, and acidosis	1. Increased serum potassium 2. Impaired conduction of nerve impulses and muscle contraction 3. Impaired cardiac conduction. Hyperkalemia "anesthetizes" nerve and muscle cells so that electrical current cannot be built up to a sufficient level (repolarization) for an electrical impulse to be initiated and conducted.	1. Serum potassium above 5 mEq/liter 2. Muscle weakness, possibly paralysis and respiratory insufficiency 3. Cardiotoxicity, with arrhythmias or cardiac arrest. Cardiac effects are not usually severe until serum levels are 7 mEq or above. ECG changes include a high, peaked T wave, prolonged P-R interval, absence of P waves, and prolonged QRS complex.

many body tissues. Some are components of enzymes and may be necessary for normal growth, structure, and function of connective tissue. For most of these, requirements are unknown and states of deficiency or excess have not been identified in humans.

A variety of pharmacologic agents is used to prevent or treat mineral–electrolyte imbalances. Usually, neutral salts of minerals (*e.g.*, potassium chloride) are used in deficiency states, and nonmineral drug preparations are used in excess states.

Individual agents used in mineral–electrolyte and acid–base imbalances

ACIDIFYING AGENT

Ammonium chloride (NH_4Cl) is a systemic acidifying agent that is occasionally used in the treatment of hypochloremic metabolic alkalosis. As a general rule,

TABLE 32-4. MAGNESIUM IMBALANCES

	Causes	Pathophysiology	Signs and symptoms
Hypomagnesemia	1. Inadequate dietary intake or prolonged administration of magnesium-free intravenous fluids 2. Decreased absorption, as occurs with alcoholism 3. Excessive losses with diuretic drugs, diarrhea, or diabetic acidosis	1. Decreased serum magnesium 2. Impaired conduction of nerve impulses and muscle contraction	1. Serum magnesium below 1.5 mEq/liter 2. Confusion, restlessness, irritability, vertigo, ataxia, and seizures 3. Muscle tremors, carpopedal spasm, nystagmus, generalized spasticity 4. Tachycardia, hypotension, premature atrial and ventricular beats
Hypermagnesemia	1. Renal failure 2. Impaired renal function accompanied by excessive intake of magnesium salts in antacids or cathartics 3. Overtreatment of magnesium deficiency	1. Increased serum magnesium 2. Depressant effects on central nervous and neuromuscular systems, which block transmission of electrical impulses	1. Serum magnesium above 2.5 mEq/liter 2. Skeletal muscle weakness and paralysis, cardiac arrhythmias, hypotension, respiratory insufficiency, drowsiness, lethargy, coma

chloride is preferably replaced with sodium chloride or potassium chloride rather than ammonium chloride. However, sodium chloride may be contraindicated in an edematous client, or the alkalosis may be unresponsive to sodium or potassium chloride. Ammonium chloride is also sometimes used as a urinary acidifier to

(Text continues on p. 321.)

TABLE 32-5. CHLORIDE IMBALANCES

	Causes	Pathophysiology	Signs and symptoms
Hypochloremic metabolic alkalosis	1. Excessive losses of chloride from vomiting, gastric suctioning, diuretic drug therapy, diabetic ketoacidosis, excessive perspiration, or adrenocortical insufficiency 2. Excessive ingestion of bicarbonate or base	1. Decreased serum chloride 2. When chloride is lost, the body retains bicarbonate in order to maintain electroneutrality in extracellular fluids. The result is metabolic alkalosis, a relative deficiency of acid, and a relative excess of base. Hypokalemia is often present as well. 3. Hyperexcitability of the nervous system. 4. Retention of carbon dioxide (acid) as a compensatory attempt to restore acid–base balance 5. Fluid loss and decreased plasma volume	1. Serum chloride below 95 mEq/liter; arterial blood *p*H above 7.45 2. Paresthesias of face and extremities 3. Muscle spasms and tetany, which cannot be distinguished from the tetany produced by hypocalcemia 4. Slow, shallow respirations 5. Dehydration 6. Hypotension
Hyperchloremic metabolic acidosis	1. Most often caused by dehydration 2. Deficient bicarbonate 3. Hyperparathyroidism 4. Respiratory alkalosis 5. Excessive administration of sodium chloride or ammonium chloride	1. Increased serum chloride 2. In dehydration, the kidneys reabsorb water in an attempt to relieve the fluid deficit. Large amounts of chloride are reabsorbed along with the water. The result is metabolic acidosis, a relative excess of acid and a relative deficiency of base. 3. Central nervous system depression 4. Increased exhalation of carbon dioxide as a compensatory attempt to restore acid–base balance	1. Serum chloride above 103 mEq/liter, arterial blood *p*H below 7.35 2. Lethargy, stupor, disorientation, and coma if acidosis is not treated 3. Increased rate and depth of respiration

TABLE 32-6. SELECTED TRACE ELEMENTS

	Characteristics	Functions	Recommended daily allowances (USRDAs)	Food sources
Chromium	1. Deficiency state identified in humans and several animal species 2. Deficiency produces impaired glucose tolerance (hyperglycemia, glycosuria), impaired growth and reproduction, and decreased life span.	Aids glucose utilization by increasing effectiveness of insulin and facilitating transport of glucose across cell membranes	Not established	Brewer's yeast and whole wheat products
Cobalt	1. Most body cobalt is stored in the liver; some is stored in the spleen, kidneys, and pancreas. 2. Excreted mainly in urine with smaller amounts excreted in feces and perspiration. 3. In humans, deficiency of vitamin B_{12} produces pernicious anemia. 4. Excess state not established for humans. In animals, excess cobalt produces polycythemia, bone marrow hyperplasia, and increased blood volume.	A component of vitamin B_{12}, which is required for normal function of all body cells and for maturation of red blood cells	Approximately 1 mg in the form of vitamin B_{12}	Animal foods, including liver, muscle meats, and shell fish. Fruits, vegetables, and cereals contain no cobalt as vitamin B_{12}.
Copper	1. Found in many body tissues including the brain, liver, heart, kidneys, bone, and muscle 2. Eliminated from the body in urine, sweat, feces, and menstrual flow 3. Human deficiency occurs with lack of food intake, malabsorption syndromes, and prolonged administration of copper-free intravenous hyperalimentation solutions 4. Signs and symptoms of deficiency include decreased serum levels of copper and ceruloplasmin (a plasma protein that transports copper); decreased iron absorption; anemia from impaired erythropoiesis; leukopenia. Death can occur. In infants, three deficiency syndromes have been identified. One is characterized by anemia, a second by chronic malnutrition and diarrhea, and a third (Menke's syndrome) by retarded growth and progressive mental deterioration. 5. Copper excess (hypercupremia) may occur in women who take oral contraceptives or who are pregnant and in clients with infections or liver disease. Wilson's disease is a rare hereditary disorder characterized by accumulation of copper in vital organs (brain, liver, kidneys). Signs and symptoms vary according to affected organs.	1. A component of many enzymes 2. Essential for correct functioning of the central nervous, cardiovascular, and skeletal systems 3. Important in formation of red blood cells, apparently by regulating storage and release of iron for hemoglobin	Not established. Estimated at approximately 2 mg.	Many foods including liver, shell fish, nuts, cereals, poultry, dried fruits.
Fluoride	1. Present in water, soil, plants, and animals in small amounts. Often added to community supplies of drinking water. 2. Accumulates in the body until about 50–60 years of age	1. A component of tooth enamel 2. Strengthens bones, probably by promoting calcium retention in bones	Not established. Average daily intake estimated at approximately 4 mg.	Beef, canned salmon, eggs. Very little in milk, cereal grains, fruits, and vegetables. Fluoride content of foods de-

TABLE 32-6. SELECTED TRACE ELEMENTS (*Continued*)

	Characteristics	Functions	Recommended daily allowances (USRDAs)	Food sources
	3. Fluoride deficiency is indicated by dental caries and possibly a greater incidence of osteoporosis. 4. Fluoride excess results in mottling of teeth and osteosclerosis.	3. Adequate intake before ages 50–60 years may decrease osteoporosis and fractures during later years.		pends on fluoride content of soil where they are grown.
Iodine	1. Iodine deficiency causes thyroid gland enlargement and may cause hypothyroidism. 2. Iodine excess (iodism) produces edema, fever, conjunctivitis, lymphadenopathy, stomatitis, vomiting, and coryza. Iodism is unlikely with dietary intake but may occur with excessive intake of drugs containing iodine.	Essential component of thyroid hormones	100–300 mg for adults, larger amounts for children and pregnant or lactating women	Seafoods best source. In vegetables, iodine content varies with the amount of iodine in soil where they are grown. In milk and eggs, content depends on the amount present in animal feed.
Iron	1. Nearly three fourths of body iron is in hemoglobin in red blood cells; about one fourth is stored in the liver, bone marrow, and spleen as ferritin and hemosiderin; the remaining small amount is in myoglobin and enzymes or bound to transferrin in plasma. 2. Absorption of iron from foods varies widely and is estimated to be about 10% under normal circumstances. It is influenced by several factors, as follows: A. Factors that increase absorption (1) Presence of dietary ascorbic acid (2) Acidity of gastric fluids increases solubility of dietary iron. (3) Presence of calcium. Calcium combines with phosphate, oxalate, and phytate. If this reaction does not occur, iron combines with these substances and produces nonabsorbable compounds. (4) Physiologic states that increase iron absorption include periods of increased blood formation such as pregnancy and growth. Also, more iron is absorbed when iron deficiency is present. B. Factors that decrease absorption (1) Lack of hydrochloric acid in the stomach or administration of antacids, which produces an alkaline environment (2) Combination of iron with phosphates, oxalates, or phytates in the intestine. This results in insoluble	1. Essential component of hemoglobin, myoglobin, and several enzymes 2. Hemoglobin is required for transport and utilization of oxygen by body cells; myoglobin aids oxygen transport and use by muscle cells; and enzymes are important for cellular respiration.	10 mg for men and older women 18 mg for women during childbearing years and children during periods of rapid growth	Liver and other organ meats, lean meat, shellfish, dried beans and vegetables, egg yolks, dried fruit, molasses, whole grain and enriched breads. Milk and milk products contan essentially no iron.

TABLE 32-6. SELECTED TRACE ELEMENTS *(Continued)*

	Characteristics	Functions	Recommended daily allowances (USRDAs)	Food sources
	and nonabsorbable compounds. (3) Increased motility of the intestines, which decreases absorption of iron by decreasing contact time with the mucosa (4) Steatorrhea or any malabsorption disorder			
Zinc	1. Deficiency may occur in liver cirrhosis, hepatitis, nephrosis, malabsorption syndromes, chronic infections, malignant diseases, myocardial infarction, hypothyroidism, and prolonged administraton of zinc-free intravenous hyperalimentation solutions. Signs and symptoms are most evident in growing children and include impaired growth, hypogonadism in males, anorexia, and sensory impairment (loss of taste and smell). Also, if the client has had surgery, wound healing may be delayed. 2. Zinc excess is unlikely with dietary intake but may develop with excessive ingestion or inhalation of zinc. Ingestion may cause nausea, vomiting and diarrhea; inhalation may cause vomiting, headache, and fever.	1. A component of many enzymes that are essential for normal metabolism (*e.g.,* carbonic anhydrase, lactic dehydrogenase (LDH), alkaline phosphatase). 2. Necessary for normal cell growth, synthesis of nucleic acids (RNA and DNA), and synthesis of carbohydrates and proteins 3. May be essential for utilization of vitamin A	15 mg for adolescents and adults 10 mg for preadolescents 25–30 mg for pregnant and lactating women	Animal proteins such as meat, liver, eggs, and seafood. Wheat germ is also a good source.

TABLE 32-7. IRON IMBALANCES

	Causes	Pathophysiology	Signs and symptoms
Deficiency state	1. Inadequate intake of iron in the diet 2. Faulty absorption of iron 3. Blood loss in gastrointestinal bleeding, heavy or prolonged menstrual flow, traumatic injury, and other conditions	1. Impaired erythropoiesis 2. Inadequate hemoglobin to transport sufficient oxygen to body tissues 3. Iron deficiency increases absorption of other minerals (*e.g.,* lead, cobalt, manganese) and may produce signs of excess.	1. Anemia (decrease in red blood cells, hemoglobin, and hematocrit) 2. With gradual development of anemia, minimal symptoms occur. 3. With rapid development of anemia or severe anemia, dyspnea, fatigue, tachycardia, malaise, and drowsiness occur.
Acute excess state	Acute iron poisoning usually occurs in small children who take several tablets of an iron preparation.	Acute toxicity	Vomiting, diarrhea, melena, abdominal pain, shock, convulsions, and metabolic acidosis. Death may occur within 24 hours if treatment is not prompt.
Chronic excess state	Chronic iron excess (hemochromatosis) is rare but may be caused by long-term ingestion of excessive iron salts (*e.g.,* ferrous sulfate), large numbers of blood transfusions, or a rare genetic trait that promotes iron absorption.	Excess iron is deposited in the heart, pancreas, kidney, liver and other organs. It impairs cell function and eventually destroys cells.	Cardiac arrhythmias, heart failure, diabetes mellitus, bronze pigmentation of skin, liver enlargement, arthropathy, and others

facilitate the action or excretion of other drugs. Although it has been used as an expectorant and antitussive, its effectiveness for these purposes is questionable.

Routes and dosage ranges

Adults: PO 1–3 g 2 or 4 times daily
IV 100–500 ml of a 2% solution, infused over a 3-hour period
Dosage depends on client's status and on serum chloride concentration

ALKALINIZING AGENTS

Sodium bicarbonate is the alkalinizing drug of choice for treatment of metabolic acidosis in adults. In solution, the drug dissociates into sodium and bicarbonate ions. The bicarbonate ions combine with free hydrogen ions to form carbonic acid. This reduces the number of free hydrogen ions and thereby raises blood *p*H toward normal (7.35 to 7.45). Sodium bicarbonate is often used in cardiopulmonary arrest to combat the acidosis that rapidly develops. It is also used to alkalinize the urine. Alkalinization increases solubility of some urine constituents (*e.g.,* uric acid) and increases excretion of some acids (*e.g.,* salicylates or phenobarbital, when taken in overdoses).

Routes and dosage ranges

Adults: IV 1 mEq/kg initially, repeated as necessary until effective respiration and circulation are restored or arterial blood gas analysis indicates otherwise
Children: IV 0.9 mEq/kg initially, repeated as necessary, based on arterial blood gases. Children weighing more than 15 kg (33 lb) may be given the adult dose.

Tromethamine (Tham) is a strong alkalinizing agent that has been advocated for treatment of metabolic acidosis in clients with edema and sodium retention because it contains no sodium. However, tromethamine is generally less effective, more expensive, and more hazardous than sodium bicarbonate. For instructions regarding preparation and dosage, see the manufacturer's literature.

CATION EXCHANGE RESIN

Sodium polystyrene sulfonate (Kayexelate) is a cation exchange resin used clinically only in treatment of hyperkalemia. Given orally or rectally, the resin acts in the colon to release sodium and combine with potassium. Potassium is then eliminated from the body in the feces. Each gram of resin removes about 1 mEq of potassium. This drug is not effective in severe, acute hyperkalemia because several hours are required to lower serum potassium levels. Thus, the resin is more likely to be used after other measures (*e.g.,* calcium gluconate, sodium bicarbonate, insulin, and glucose infusions) have lowered dangerously high serum potassium levels. Sodium bicarbonate, insulin, and glucose lower serum potassium levels by driving potassium into the cells. They do not remove potassium from the body.

Routes and dosage ranges

Adults: PO 15 g in 100–200 ml of water and 70% sorbitol, 1–4 times daily
Rectally (retention enema) 30–50 g in 100–200 ml of water and 70% sorbitol q6h

CHELATING AGENTS (METAL ANTAGONISTS)

Deferoxamine (Desferal mesylate) is a chelating agent for iron and is the only drug available for removing excess iron from the body. When given orally within a few hours after oral ingestion of iron preparations, deferoxamine combines with the iron in the bowel lumen and prevents its absorption. When given parenterally, it removes iron from storage sites (*e.g.,* ferrin, hemosiderin, transferrin) and combines with the iron to produce a water-soluble compound that can be excreted by the kidneys. The drug can remove about 10 to 50 mg of iron per day. The urine becomes reddish brown owing to the iron content.

The major indication for use of deferoxamine is acute iron intoxication. It is also used in hemochromatosis due to blood transfusions or hemosiderosis due to certain hemolytic anemias. In these chronic conditions characterized by accumulation of iron in tissues, phlebotomy may be more effective in removing iron. Deferoxamine is more likely to be used in clients who are too anemic or hypoproteinemic to tolerate the blood loss.

Routes and dosage ranges

Adults: PO 4–8 g, given within a few hours of oral ingestion of iron preparations.
IM 1 g initially, then 500 mg q4h for 2 doses, then 500 mg q4–12h if needed. Maximal dose, 6 g/24 hours
IV 1 g slowly (not to exceed 15 mg/kg/hour), then 500 mg q4h for 2 doses, then 500 mg q4–12h if necessary. Maximal dose, 6 g/24 hours. This route is used only in the client in shock.
Children: PO, IM, IV, same as for adults

Penicillamine (Cuprimine) is a drug that chelates copper, zinc, mercury, and lead to form soluble complexes that are excreted in the urine. The main therapeutic use of penicillamine is to remove excess copper in clients with Wilson's disease (see Table 32-6). It can also be used prophylactically, before clinical manifestations occur, in persons likely to develop this hereditary condition. Penicillamine may be used to treat cystinuria, a hereditary metabolic disorder characterized by large amounts of cystine in the urine and renal calculi. It may be used in lead poisoning and severe rheumatoid arthritis that does not respond to conventional treatment measures.

Route and dosage ranges

Adults and older children: Wilson's disease, PO 250 mg 4 times daily, increased gradually if necessary up to 2 g daily
Lead poisoning, PO 250–500 mg 2 times daily
Rheumatoid arthritis, PO 125–250 mg daily for 4 weeks, increase by 125–250 mg daily at 1- to 3-month intervals if necessary. Usual maintenance dose, 500–750 mg daily; maximal dose, 1000–1500 mg daily

Infants over 6 months and young children: Wilson's disease, PO 250 mg daily, dissolved in fruit juice
Lead poisoning, PO 125 mg 3 times daily

IRON PREPARATIONS

Ferrous gluconate (Fergon) is an oral iron preparation that is effective in treating iron deficiency anemia. It is claimed to be less irritating to gastrointestinal mucosa and therefore better tolerated than ferrous sulfate. Ferrous gluconate contains about 12% elemental iron, so that each 320-mg tablet contains about 38 mg iron. Indications for use, adverse reactions, and contraindications are the same as for ferrous sulfate.

Route and dosage ranges

Adults: PO 320–640 mg (40–80 mg elemental iron) 3 times daily

Children: PO 100–300 mg (12.5–37.5 mg elemental iron) 3 times daily

Infants: PO 100 mg or 30 drops of elixir initially, gradually increased to 300 mg or 5 ml of elixir daily (15–37.5 mg elemental iron) in divided doses

Ferrous sulfate (Feosol), which contains 20% elemental iron, is the prototype of oral iron preparations and the preparation of choice for prevention or treatment of iron deficiency anemia. It may be used as an iron supplement during periods of increased requirements (*e.g.*, childhood, pregnancy). Nausea and other gastrointestinal symptoms may result from gastric irritation. Ferrous sulfate and other oral iron preparations discolor feces, producing a black–green color that may be mistaken for blood in the stool. Contraindications to oral iron preparations include peptic ulcer disease, inflammatory intestinal disorders, anemias other than iron deficiency anemia, multiple blood transfusions, hemochromatosis, and hemosiderosis.

Route and dosage range

Adults: PO 300 mg–1.2 g (60–240 mg elemental iron) daily in 3–4 divided doses

Children 6–12 years: PO 120–600 mg (24–120 mg elemental iron) daily, in divided doses

Infants and children under 6 years: 300 mg (60 mg elemental iron) daily, in divided doses

Iron dextran injection (Imferon) is a parenteral form of iron useful in treating confirmed iron deficiency anemia when oral supplements are not feasible. One ml equals 50 mg of elemental iron. Reasons for using iron dextran injection include peptic ulcer or inflammatory bowel disease that is likely to be aggravated by oral iron preparations, the client's inability or unwillingness to take oral preparations, and a shortage of time for correcting the iron deficiency (*e.g.*, late pregnancy or preoperative status). One of the major advantages of parenteral iron is that body iron stores can be rapidly replenished.

Routes and dosage ranges

Adults: IM (all doses indicate elemental iron), up to 250 mg daily for adults weighing over 50 kg or 110 lb; 100 mg daily for adults weighing up to 110 lb
IV no more than 100 mg/day. With direct injection, give no faster than 1 ml/min. With infusion in 500–1000 ml dextrose or sodium chloride injection, give over several hours

Children: IM, no more than 100 mg daily for children weighing 9–50 kg (20–110 lb)
IV Same as adult dosage

Infants: IM, no more than 50 mg daily for infants weighing 4.5–9 kg; no more than 25 mg daily for infants weighing under 4.5 kg

MAGNESIUM PREPARATION

Magnesium sulfate is given parenterally in hypomagnesemia, convulsions associated with toxemia of pregnancy (eclampsia), and prevention of hypomagnesemia in total parenteral nutrition. Therapeutic effects in these conditions are attributed to the drug's depressant effects on the central nervous system and smooth, skeletal, and cardiac muscle. Therapeutic uses of magnesium salts as antacids and cathartics are discussed in Chapters 60 and 61, respectively. Magnesium preparations are contraindicated in clients who have impaired renal function or who are comatose.

Routes and dosage ranges

Adults: Hypomagnesemia, IM 1–2 g (2–4 ml of 50% solution) once or twice daily based on serum magnesium levels
Eclampsia, IM 1–2 g (2–4 ml of 50% solution) initially, then 1 g every 30 minutes until seizures stop
Convulsive seizures, IM 1 g (2 ml of 50% solution) repeated as necessary
IV, do not exceed 150 mg/min (1.5 ml/min of a 10% solution, 3 ml/min of a 5% solution)

Older children: IM, same dosage as adults

POTASSIUM PREPARATIONS

Potassium chloride is usually the drug of choice for preventing or treating hypokalemia, since deficiencies of potassium and chloride often occur together. It is frequently prescribed for clients who are receiving potassium-losing diuretics (*e.g.,* hydrochlorothiazide, furosemide), those who are receiving digitalis preparations (hypokalemia increases risks of digitalis toxicity), and those who are receiving only intravenous fluids because of surgical procedures, gastrointestinal disease, or other conditions. Potassium chloride may also be used to replace chloride in hypochloremic metabolic alkalosis.

Potassium chloride can be given orally or intravenously. Oral preparations are recommended when feasible. One disadvantage of oral liquid preparations is an unpleasant taste. This has led to production of various flavored powders, liquids, and effervescent tablets (*e.g.,* Kay-Ciel Elixir, K-Lor, Klorvess). Enteric-coated tablets were developed but abandoned when they produced intestinal ulcerations in some people. More recently, tablets containing a wax matrix (*e.g.,* Slow-K) have been developed. These are apparently safe and effective and may be better tolerated by most clients than liquid formulations. Intravenous preparations of potassium chloride must be diluted before administration to prevent hyperkalemia and cardiotoxicity as well as severe pain at the injection site.

Potassium chloride is contraindicated in renal failure and in clients receiving potassium-saving diuretics such as triamterene, spironolactone, or amiloride.

Potassium gluconate (Kaon), **potassium bicarbonate and citrate** (K-Lyte), and **potassium triplex** are oral preparations of potassium salts other than chloride. They are supposedly more palatable and therefore more likely to be taken than oral potassium chloride preparations. The major indication for their use is the occasional hypokalemia associated with hyperchloremia. If given to a client with hypokalemia and hypochloremia, these preparations do not replace chloride, and another source of chloride must be given. Adverse reactions and contraindications are the same as for potassium chloride.

Routes and dosage ranges

Adults: PO 15–20 mEq 2–4 times daily
IV (potassium chloride injection) approximately 40–100 mEq/24 hours. Dosage must be individualized and depends on serum potassium levels and total potassium body stores. Potassium chloride (KCl) must be diluted. A generally safe dosage range is 20–60 mEq, diluted in 1000 ml of dextrose or sodium chloride intravenous solution, and given no faster than 10–15 mEq/hour or 60–120 mEq/24 hours.

SODIUM PREPARATIONS

Sodium chloride injection is available in several concentrations and sizes for intravenous use. Concentrations are 0.45% (hypotonic solution), 0.9% (isotonic), and 3% and 5% (hypertonic). Sodium chloride is also available in combination with dextrose. Five percent dextrose in 0.22% sodium chloride and 5% dextrose in 0.45% sodium chloride are among the most frequently used solutions for intravenous fluid therapy. They contain 38.5 mEq and 77 mEq/liter, respectively, of sodium and chloride. Isotonic or 0.9% sodium chloride contains 154 mEq of both sodium and chloride. This solution may be used to treat hyponatremia. The 3% and 5% solutions contain 513 mEq and 855 mEq of sodium and chloride per liter, respectively. They may be used in severe hyponatremia but are rarely necessary. If used at all, they must be given in small amounts (200 to 400 ml) and administered slowly to prevent circulatory overload and pulmonary edema. Most of these solutions are available in 250 ml, 500 ml, and 1000 ml sizes for intravenous infusions.

Route and dosage ranges

Adults: IV 1500–3000 ml of 0.22%, 0.45% solution/24 hours depending on client's fluid needs; approximately 50 ml/hour to keep intravenous lines open

ZINC PREPARATION

Zinc sulfate is available in tablets containing 66, 110, 200, or 220 mg of zinc sulfate (equivalent to 15, 25, 45, and 50 mg of elemental zinc, respectively) and in capsules containing 220 mg of zinc sulfate (equivalent to 80 mg of elemental zinc). It is also an ingredient in several vitamin–mineral combination products. Zinc sulfate is given orally as a dietary supplement to prevent or treat zinc deficiency. In malnourished clients, it may be used to promote wound healing after surgery. There is no evidence, though, that zinc promotes wound healing or has any other beneficial effect in the absence of zinc deficiency.

Route and dosage range

Adults: PO 15–80 mg elemental zinc daily

MULTIPLE MINERAL–ELECTROLYTE PREPARATIONS

There are numerous commercially prepared electrolyte solutions for intravenous use. One group provides maintenance amounts of fluids and electrolytes when oral intake of food and fluids is restricted or contraindicated. These solutions differ slightly in the number and amount of particular electrolytes. Specific preparations and their manufacturers include Plasma-Lyte 56 (Travenol) and Polysal-M (Cutter). A second group provides replacement amounts of electrolytes (mainly sodium and chloride) when electrolytes are being lost from the body in abnormal amounts. This group includes Normosol-R (Abbott), Plasma-Lyte 148 (Travenol), and Polysal (Cutter). These electrolyte preparations are available with dextrose 2.5% to 10%. Ringer's lactate is another replacement fluid that is used fairly often. It is manufactured by several different companies. Health care agencies use one manufacturer's products for the most part.

There are two *oral* electrolyte solutions (Lytren and Pedialyte), which contain sodium, chloride, potassium, calcium, magnesium, and other electrolytes along with a small amount of dextrose. They are used to supply maintenance amounts of fluids and electrolytes when oral intake is restricted. They are especially useful in children for treatment of diarrhea and may prevent severe fluid and electrolyte depletion. The amount given must be carefully prescribed and calculated to avoid excessive intake. They should not be used in severe circumstances in which intravenous fluid and electrolyte therapy is indicated. They must be cautiously used with impaired renal function. They should not be mixed with other electrolyte-containing fluids such as milk or fruit juices.

Routes and dosage ranges

Adults: IV 2000–3000 ml/24 hours, depending on individual fluid and electrolyte needs
Children: IV, PO, amount individualized according to fluid and electrolyte needs

Principles of therapy: mineral–electrolyte and acid–base disorders

ASSESSMENT GUIDELINES

Assess each client for current or potential mineral–electrolyte or acid–base disorders. This is usually done in an overall assessment of nutritional status. Specific assessment factors related to minerals and electrolytes include the following:

1. Deficiency states are probably more common than excess states unless a mineral–electrolyte supplement is being taken. However, deficiencies and excesses may be equally harmful, and both must be assessed.
2. Clients with other nutritional deficiencies are likely to have mineral–electrolyte deficiencies as well. Moreover, deficiencies are likely to be multiple, with overlapping signs and symptoms.
3. Many drugs influence gains and losses of minerals and electrolytes, including diuretics and laxatives.
4. Minerals and electrolytes are lost with gastric suction, polyuria, diarrhea, excessive perspiration, and other conditions.
5. Assess laboratory reports, when available.
   a. Check the complete blood count (CBC) for decreased red blood cells (RBCs), hemoglobin, and hematocrit. Reduced values may indicate iron deficiency anemia, and further assessment is needed.
   b. Check serum electrolyte reports for increases or decreases. All major minerals can be measured in clinical laboratories. The ones usually measured are sodium, chloride, and potassium; carbon dioxide content, a measure of bicarbonate, is also assessed. Normal values vary to some extent with the laboratory and the method of measurement. A general range of normal values is sodium, 135–145 mEq/liter; chloride, 95–105 mEq/liter; potassium, 3.5–5 mEq/liter; and carbon dioxide, 22–26 mEq/liter. Minor differences in these values are not significant.

NURSING INTERVENTIONS

Implement measures to prevent mineral–electrolyte disorders:

1. Promote a varied diet. A diet that is adequate in protein and calories generally provides adequate minerals and electrolytes.
2. If assessment data reveal potential development of a disorder, start preventive measures as soon as possible. For clients able to eat, foods high in iron may at least delay onset of iron deficiency anemia, foods high in potassium may prevent hypokalemia with diuretic therapy, and salty foods along with water help to prevent problems associated with excessive perspiration. For people unable to eat, intravenous fluids and electrolytes are usually given. Generally, oral food intake or tube feeding is preferable to intravenous therapy.
3. Treat underlying disorders that contribute to mineral–electrolyte deficiency or excess. Thus, measures to relieve anorexia, nausea, vomiting, diarrhea, pain and other symptoms help to increase intake or decrease output of certain minerals. Measures to increase urine output such as forcing fluids help to increase output of some minerals in the urine and therefore prevent excess states from developing.
4. Mineral supplements are recommended only for current or potential deficiencies. They provide no beneficial effects in the absence of deficiency, and all are toxic if taken in excessive amounts. When deficiencies are identified, treat with foods when possible. Next, use oral mineral supplements. Finally, use parenteral supplements only for clear-cut indications, since they are potentially the most hazardous.
5. For clients who have nasogastric tubes to suction, irrigate the tubes with isotonic sodium chloride solution. The use of tap water is contraindicated because it is hypotonic and would ''pull'' electrolytes into the stomach. Then, electrolytes are lost in the aspirated and discarded stomach contents. For the same reason, only 2 to 3 teaspoons of ice chips or water are allowed per hour. Clients often request ice chips or water frequently and in larger amounts than desirable. The nurse must explain the reason for the restrictions.
6. If tap water enemas are ordered to be given until clear of feces, give no more than three. Isotonic sodium chloride is preferred to tap water. Still, no more than three enemas should be given consecutively.

DIET SUPPLEMENTS

Some people take mineral preparations as dietary supplements in an effort to promote health and prevent deficiencies. They are rarely needed for this purpose by people who are able to eat a balanced and varied diet, who have no increased needs for nutrients such as growth or pregnancy, and who have no abnormal losses of nutrients such as those caused by gastrointestinal diseases. In fact, dietary supplements in a person who eats adequately could exceed nutrient needs by more than 100%. No known benefit to health results from ingesting more mineral nutrients than the body needs, and harm may result because all minerals are toxic at high doses. If, despite these precautions, mineral supplements are taken, they should include only those minerals known to be essential for human nutrition. Additional ingredients such as liver, wheat germ, choline, and bioflavonoids apparently serve no nutritional advantage.

PREVENTION OF EXCESS STATE

When a mineral is given to correct a deficiency state, there is a risk of producing an excess state. Since both deficiency and excess states may be harmful, the amount of mineral supplement should be titrated as closely as possible to the amount needed by the body. Larger doses are needed to treat deficiency states than are needed to prevent deficiencies from developing. In addition to producing potential toxicity, large doses of one mineral may cause a relative deficiency of another mineral or nutrient.

DRUG SELECTION

Oral drug preparations are preferred, when feasible, for preventing or treating mineral disorders. They are generally safer, less likely to produce toxicity, convenient to administer, and less expensive.

PRINCIPLES OF TREATING SODIUM DISORDERS

Hyponatremia

Treatment of hyponatremia is aimed toward restoring normal levels of serum sodium. This can be done with isotonic sodium chloride solution when hyponatremia is caused by sodium depletion and with restriction of water when hyponatremia is caused by overhydration or water intoxication. Occasionally, in severe, symptomatic hyponatremia, a hypertonic sodium chloride solution (3%) is given. Such treatment is potentially hazardous and may result in circulatory overload and life-threatening pulmonary edema. It is rarely indicated.

Hypernatremia

Treatment of hypernatremia requires administration of sodium-free fluids, either orally or intravenously, until serum sodium levels return to normal. Milder states usually respond to increased water intake through the gastrointestinal tract; more severe hypernatremia is likely to require intravenous administration of 5% dextrose in water.

PRINCIPLES OF TREATING POTASSIUM DISORDERS

Hypokalemia

1. Assess for conditions contributing to hypokalemia, and attempt to eliminate them or reduce their impact. Such conditions are generally inadequate intake, excessive loss or some combination of the two.
2. Assess the extent or severity of the hypokalemia. This is probably best done on the basis of serum potassium levels and clinical manifestations. Serum potassium levels alone are not adequate because they may not accurately reflect depletion of body potassium.
3. Potassium supplements are indicated in the following circumstances:
   a. When serum potassium level is below 3 mEq/liter on repeated measurements, even if the client is asymptomatic
   b. When serum potassium is 3 to 3.5 mEq/liter and clear-cut symptoms or electrocardiographic changes indicate hypokalemia. Some clinicians advocate treatment in the absence of symptoms.
   c. In clients receiving digitalis preparations, if necessary to maintain serum potassium levels above 3.5 mEq/liter. Such usage is indicated because hypokalemia increases digitalis toxicity.
4. Although opinions differ, potassium supplements are probably not indicated for prevention of hypokalemia except in clients with hypokalemic periodic paralysis, a rare disorder. Thus, use of potassium supplements with diuretic therapy is not indicated unless hypokalemia develops or digitalis preparations are being given.
5. When potassium supplements are necessary, oral administration is preferred. Oral preparations are usually effective and less likely to cause hyperkalemia than intravenous preparations.
6. Potassium chloride is the drug of choice in most instances because it replaces both potassium and chloride. Liquids, powders, and effervescent tablets for oral use must be diluted in at least 4 ounces of water or juice to improve taste and decrease gastric irritation. Potassium gluconate and some other potassium preparations are reportedly more palatable and better tolerated than KCl. Liquid preparations of potassium have been recommended because tablets have caused intestinal ulcerations. Tablets of KCl in a wax matrix are now available and are apparently both safe and effective.
7. Intravenous KCl is indicated when a client is unable to take an oral preparation or has severe hypokalemia. Serum potassium level should be measured, estimates of total body deficit made, and adequate urine output established before intravenous potassium therapy.
   a. Intravenous KCl must be well diluted to prevent sudden hyperkalemia and cardiotoxic effects as well as pain and phlebitis at the venipuncture site. The usual dilution is KCl 20 to 60 mEq/1000 ml of intravenous fluid.
   b. Dosage must be individualized. Clients receiving intravenous fluids only are usually given 40 to 60 mEq of KCl daily. This can be given quite safely with 20 mEq KCl/liter of fluids and a flow rate of 100 to 125 ml/hour. In severe deficits, a higher concentration and a higher flow rate may be necessary. In these situations, an infusion pump to accurately control flow rate and continuous cardiac monitoring for detection of hyperkalemia are necessary. Also, serum potassium levels must be checked frequently and dosage adjusted if indicated. No more than 100 to 200 mEq KCl should be given within 24 hours, even if several days are required to replace the estimated deficit.
   c. Do not administer potassium-containing intravenous solutions into a central venous catheter. There is a risk of hyperkalemia and cardiac arrhythmias or arrest because there is limited time for the solution to be diluted in the blood returning to the heart.
   d. In critical situations, KCl should usually be given in sodium chloride solutions rather than dextrose solutions. Administering dextrose solutions may increase hypokalemia by causing

some potassium to leave the serum and enter cells.

Hyperkalemia

1. Eliminate any exogenous sources of potassium such as potassium supplements, penicillin G potassium, salt substitutes, and blood transfusion with old blood.
2. Treat acidosis, if present, because potassium leaves cells and enters the serum with acidosis.
3. Use measures that antagonize the effects of potassium, that cause potassium to leave the serum and reenter cells, and that remove potassium from the body. Which measures are appropriate is determined mainly by serum potassium levels and electrocardiographic (ECG) changes. Continuous cardiac monitoring is required.

   Severe hyperkalemia (serum potassium above 7 mEq/liter and ECG changes indicating hyperkalemia) requires urgent treatment. Immediate intravenous administration of sodium bicarbonate 45 mEq, over a 5-minute period, causes rapid movement of potassium into cells. This can be repeated in a few minutes if ECG changes persist.

   Calcium gluconate 10%, 5 to 10 ml intravenously, is also given early in treatment. It acts to decrease the cardiotoxic effects of hyperkalemia. It is contraindicated if the client is receiving digitalis, and it cannot be added to fluids containing sodium bicarbonate because insoluble precipitates are formed.

   The next step is intravenous infusion of glucose and insulin. This also causes potassium to move into cells, although not as quickly as sodium bicarbonate.
4. When hyperkalemia is less severe or when it has been reduced by the above measures, sodium polystyrene sulfonate, a cation exchange resin, can be given orally or rectally to remove potassium from the body. Each gram of the resin combines with 1 mEq potassium, and both are excreted in feces.

   The resin is usually mixed with water and sorbitol, a poorly absorbed, osmotically active alcohol that has a laxative effect. The sorbitol offsets the constipating effect of the resin and aids its expulsion. Oral administration is preferred, and several doses daily may be given until serum potassium is normal. When given as an enema, the solution must be retained from 1 to several hours, or repeated enemas must be given for therapeutic effect.
5. If the above measures fail to reduce hyperkalemia, peritoneal dialysis or hemodialysis may be used.

PRINCIPLES OF TREATING MAGNESIUM DISORDERS

Hypomagnesemia

1. Prevent, when possible, by giving parenteral fluids with magnesium when the fluids are the only source of nutrients. Multiple electrolyte intravenous solutions contain magnesium chloride or acetate and magnesium can be added to solutions for total parenteral nutrition.
2. Magnesium sulfate, intravenously or intramuscularly, can be given daily as long as hypomagnesemia persists or continuing losses occur. Initial dosage may be larger, but the usual maintenance dose is about 8 mEq daily. A 10% solution is available in 10-ml vials that contain 8 mEq of magnesium sulfate for adding to intravenous solutions. A 50% solution is available in 2-ml vials (8 mEq) for intramuscular administration.
3. Check serum magnesium levels daily.

Hypermagnesemia

1. Stop any source of exogenous magnesium such as magnesium sulfate or magnesium-containing antacids, cathartics, or enemas.
2. Have calcium gluconate available for intravenous administration. It is an antidote for the sedative effects of magnesium excess.
3. Increase urine output by increasing fluid intake, if feasible. This increases removal of magnesium from the body in urine.
4. People with chronic renal failure, who are most likely to develop hypermagnesemia in the first place, are likely to require peritoneal dialysis or hemodialysis to lower serum magnesium levels.

PRINCIPLES OF TREATING IRON DEFICIENCY AND EXCESS

Iron deficiency anemia

1. Anemia is a symptom, not a disease. Therefore, the underlying cause must be identified and eliminated, if possible.
2. Assess the client's intake of and attitude toward foods with high iron content. Encourage increased dietary intake of these foods.
3. Use oral iron preparations when possible. They are generally safe, effective, convenient to administer, and relatively inexpensive. Ferrous preparations (sulfate, gluconate, fumarate) are better absorbed than ferric preparations. Other iron salts do not

differ significantly from ferrous sulfate. Ferrous sulfate is usually the drug of choice for oral iron therapy. Slow-release or enteric-coated products tend to decrease absorption of iron. Adding acid such as ascorbic acid to iron products tends to increase both absorption and adverse reactions.

4. Dosage calculations are done in terms of elemental iron. Iron preparations vary greatly in the amount of elemental iron they contain. Ferrous sulfate, for example, contains 20% iron. Thus, each 300-mg tablet furnishes about 60 mg of elemental iron. With the usual regimen of one tablet three times daily, a daily dose of 180 mg of elemental iron is given. For most clients, probably half that amount (30 mg three times daily) would correct the deficiency. However, tablets are not manufactured in sizes to allow this regimen, and liquid preparations are not very popular with clients. Thus, relatively large doses are usually given, but smaller doses may be just as effective, especially if gastrointestinal symptoms become a problem with higher dosages. Whatever the dose, apparently only about 10% to 15% of the iron is absorbed. Most of the remainder is excreted in feces, which turn dark green or black.
5. Oral iron preparations are better absorbed if taken on an empty stomach. However, since gastric irritation is a common adverse reaction, they are more often given with or immediately after meals.
6. Although normal hemoglobin levels return after about 2 months of oral iron therapy, an additional 6-month period of drug therapy is recommended to replenish the body's iron stores.
7. Reasons for failure to respond to iron therapy include continued blood loss, failure to take the drug as prescribed, or defective iron absorption. These factors must be reevaluated if no therapeutic response is evident within 3 to 4 weeks after drug therapy is begun.
8. Parenteral iron is indicated when oral preparations may further irritate a diseased gastrointestinal tract, when the client is unable or unwilling to take the oral drugs, or when the anemia must be corrected relatively rapidly.
9. For severe iron deficiency anemia, blood transfusions may be most effective.

Iron excess

1. Acute iron overdosage requires treatment as soon as possible, even if overdosage is only suspected and the amount taken is unknown. It is not necessary to wait until serum iron level is measured.

   If treatment is begun shortly after oral ingestion of iron, induced vomiting or aspiration of stomach contents by nasogastric tube is helpful. This can be followed by lavage with 1% sodium bicarbonate solution to form insoluble iron carbonate compounds. The next step is to instill in the stomach 5 to 8 g of deferoxamine dissolved in 50 ml of distilled water to bind the iron remaining in the gastrointestinal tract and prevent its absorption. Finally, deferoxamine is given intramuscularly or intravenously to bind with iron in tissues and allow its excretion in the urine. Throughout the treatment period, supportive measures may be needed for gastrointestinal hemorrhage, acidosis, and shock.
2. For chronic iron overload or hemochromatosis, the first step in treatment is to stop the source of iron, if possible. Phlebotomy may be the treatment of choice for most clients because withdrawal of 500 ml of blood removes about 250 mg of iron. Phlebotomy may be needed as often as weekly and for as long as 2 to 3 years. For clients resistant to or intolerant of phlebotomy, deferoxamine can be given. About 10 to 50 mg of iron is excreted daily in the urine with deferoxamine administration.

PRINCIPLES OF TREATING ACID-BASE DISORDERS

Metabolic acidosis

1. Assess the extent and severity of acidosis. Suspected acidosis can be confirmed or rejected by measurement of arterial blood gases. Results reflecting acidosis are decreased *p*H (less than 7.35) and decreased bicarbonate (less than 22 mEq/liter).
2. Assess and treat the underlying condition, such as diabetic ketoacidosis.
3. If this does not relieve acidosis, or if acidosis is severe (arterial blood *p*H less than 7.2), sodium bicarbonate is given parenterally to alkalinize the blood. It can be given by direct injection into a vein or as a continuous intravenous infusion. Ampules and prefilled syringes are available in 8.4% solution (50 ml contains 50 mEq) or 7.5% solution (50 ml contains 44.6 mEq). Intravenous solutions of 5% and 1.4% sodium bicarbonate are also available in 500-ml bottles.
4. Monitor arterial blood gases and serum potassium levels frequently. Overtreatment of acidosis with sodium bicarbonate will produce alkalosis. Serum potassium levels may change from high to normal levels initially (because acidosis causes potassium to be drawn into the bloodstream) to severely low levels as potassium reenters cells with treatment of acidosis. Thus, potassium replacement is likely to be needed during treatment of acidosis.

5. When the acidosis accompanying cardiac arrest is being treated, administration of sodium bicarbonate is stopped when the pulse returns.
6. During cardiac arrest or severe acidosis from other causes, effective ventilation measures are needed along with sodium bicarbonate to remove carbon dioxide from the blood.
7. In lactic acidosis, much larger doses of sodium bicarbonate may be required than in other types of acidosis. This is because of continued production of large amounts of lactic acid by body metabolism.
8. Chronic metabolic acidosis may occur with chronic renal failure. Sodium bicarbonate or citrate (which is converted to bicarbonate in the body) can be given orally in a dose sufficient to maintain a normal serum bicarbonate level.

Metabolic alkalosis

1. Assess the severity of the alkalosis. Suspected alkalosis can be confirmed with arterial blood gas reports showing increased *p*H (above 7.45) and increased bicarbonate (above 26 mEq/liter).
2. Assess and treat the underlying condition. Often, volume depletion and hypochloremia are present and can be corrected with isotonic 0.9% sodium chloride solution. If hypokalemia and hypochloremia are present, potassium chloride will likely replace both deficits.
3. In severe alkalosis that does not respond to the above therapy, ammonium chloride can be given. It must be given very cautiously to avoid inducing acidosis.

NURSING ACTIONS: MINERAL–ELECTROLYTE PREPARATIONS

Nursing Actions	*Rationale/Explanation*
1. Administer accurately	
a. Give oral mineral–electrolyte preparations with food or immediately after meals.	To decrease gastric irritation. Iron and possibly some other agents are better absorbed when taken on an empty stomach. However, they are better tolerated when taken with food.
b. Give intravenous preparations slowly, as a general rule.	The primary danger of rapid intravenous injection or infusion is a transient excess in serum, which may cause cardiac arrhythmias or other serious problems.
c. Do not mix minerals and electrolytes with any other drug in a syringe.	High risk of physical incompatibility and precipitation of drugs
d. For intravenous infusion, most minerals and electrolytes are compatible with solutions of dextrose or sodium chloride. Do not mix with other solutions until compatibility is determined.	To avoid physical incompatibility and precipitation of contents.
e. For intravenous NaCl solutions	
(1) Give fluids at the prescribed flow rate.	Flow rates depend largely on reasons for use. For example, if a client is receiving no oral fluids (NPO) or only small amounts, the flow rate is often 100 to 125 ml/hour or 2400–3000 ml/24 hours. If used as a vehicle for intravenous antibiotics, the rate is often 50 ml/hour or keep open rate (KOR). If the client is dehydrated, 150 to 200 ml/hour may be given for a few hours or until a certain amount has been given. (Restrictions in time or amount are necessary to avoid circulatory overload or pulmonary edema.)
(2) Give hypertonic saline solutions (3% or 5% sodium chloride injection) slowly. Also, give no more than 200 to 400 ml at one time.	To avoid circulatory overload and sclerosing the veins
f. For potassium supplements	
(1) Mix liquids, powders, and effervescent tablets in at least 4 oz of juice, water, or carbonated beverage.	To dilute, disguise the unpleasant taste and decrease gastric irritation

Nursing Actions	**Rationale/Explanation**
(2) Give oral preparations with or after meals.	To decrease gastric irritation
(3) Never give undiluted potassium chloride (KCl) intravenously.	A transient hyperkalemia may cause life-threatening cardiotoxicity. Severe pain and vein sclerosis may also result.
(4) Dilute intravenous KCl 20–60 mEq in 1000 ml of intravenous solution such as dextrose in water. Be sure that KCl is mixed well with the intravenous solution.	Dilution decreases risks of hyperkalemia and cardiotoxicity. It also prevents or decreases pain at the infusion site.
(5) Give potassium-containing intravenous solutions at a rate that administers no more than 10 mEq/h.	This is the safest amount and rate of potassium administration. It is also usually effective.
(6) If severe hypokalemia is present, higher concentrations or faster flow rates of potassium-containing fluids may be used. In such situations, attach a cardiac monitor to the client.	Risks of hyperkalemia and life-threatening cardiotoxicity are greatly increased with high concentrations or rapid flow rates. Constant monitoring of the electrocardiogram is the best way to detect hyperkalemia.
g. For magnesium sulfate ($MgSO_4$)	
(1) Read the drug label very carefully to be sure of having the correct preparation for the intended use.	Magnesium sulfate is available in concentrations of 10%, 25%, and 50% and in sizes of 2-, 10-, and 20-ml ampules as well as a 30-ml multidose vial.
(2) For intramuscular administration, small amounts of 50% solution are usually used (1 g $MgSO_4$ = 2 ml of 50% solution)	
(3) For intravenous use, a 5% or 10% solution is used for direct injection, intermittent infusion, or continuous infusion. Whatever concentration is used, administer no more than 150 mg/minute (1.5 ml/minute of 10% solution; 3 ml/minute of 5% solution).	
h. For sodium bicarbonate ($NaHCO_3$)	
(1) Read the label carefully to be sure of having the correct solution.	Sodium bicarbonate is available in several concentrations and sizes such as 50-ml ampules or prefilled syringes with 50 mEq drug (8.4% solution) or 44.6 mEq drug (7.5% solution), 500-ml bottles with 297.7 mEq drug (5% solution) or 83 mEq drug (1.4% solution).
(2) Inject directly into the vein or into the tubing of a flowing intravenous solution in emergencies such as cardiac arrest.	
(3) In nonemergency situations, titrate flow rate of infusions according to arterial blood gases.	To avoid iatrogenic alkalosis
(4) Do not add any other medications to an intravenous infusion containing $NaHCO_3$.	$NaHCO_3$ is highly alkaline and may cause precipitation of other drugs.
(5) Monitor arterial blood gases for increased *p*H after each 50 to 100 mEq of $NaHCO_3$.	To avoid overtreatment and metabolic alkalosis
i. For iron preparations	
(1) Dilute liquid iron preparations, give with a straw, and have the client rinse his or her mouth afterward.	To prevent temporary staining of teeth
(2) To give iron dextran intramuscularly, use a 2- to 3-inch needle and Z-track technique to inject the drug into the upper outer quadrant of the buttock.	To prevent discomfort and staining of subcutaneous tissue and skin
(3) To give iron dextran intravenously (either directly or diluted in dextrose or sodium chloride solution and given over several hours), do not use the multidose vial.	The multidose vial contains phenol as a preservative and is not suitable for intravenous use. Ampules of 2 ml or 5 ml are available without preservative.
j. Refer to the individual drugs or package literature for instructions regarding administration of ammonium chloride, deferoxamine, penicillamine, tromethamine, and multiple electrolyte solutions.	

Nursing Actions	**Rationale/Explanation**
2. Observe for therapeutic effects	
a. With NaCl, observe for decreased symptoms of hyponatremia and increased serum sodium level.	Therapeutic effects should be evident within a few hours.
b. With KCl or other potassium preparations, observe for decreased signs of hypokalemia and increased serum potassium levels.	
c. With $MgSO_4$, observe for decreased signs of hypomagnesemia, increased serum magnesium levels, or control of convulsions.	
d. With zinc sulfate ($ZnSO_4$), observe for improved wound healing.	
e. With sodium bicarbonate ($NaHCO_3$), observe for decreased manifestations of acidosis and a rise in blood *p*H and bicarbonate levels.	
f. With iron preparations, observe for (1) Increased vigor and feeling of well being (2) Improved appetite (3) Less fatigue (4) Increased RBC, hemoglobin (hgb), and hematocrit (hct), on CBC (5) With parenteral iron, observe for an average increase in hemoglobin of 1 g/week.	Therapeutic effects are usually evident within a month unless other problems are also present (*e.g.,* vitamin deficiency, achlorhydria, infection, malabsorption).
3. Observe for adverse effects	
a. Mineral–electrolyte excess states	These are likely to occur with excessive dosages of supplements. They can usually be prevented by using relatively low doses in nonemergency situations and by frequent monitoring of serum levels of electrolytes and iron.
(1) With sodium chloride injection, observe for hypernatremia and circulatory overload.	These are most likely to occur with rapid infusion of large amounts or with heart or kidney disease, which decreases water excretion and urine output. They may also occur with hypertonic solutions (*e.g.,* 3% NaCl), but these are infrequently used.
(2) With potassium preparations, observe for hyperkalemia.	This is most likely to occur with rapid intravenous administration or high dosages or concentrations or in the presence of renal insufficiency and decreased urine output.
(3) With magnesium preparations, observe for hypermagnesemia.	See potassium preparations, above.
(4) With sodium bicarbonate, observe for metabolic alkalosis.	This is most likely to occur when large amounts of $NaHCO_3$ are given intravenously in the treatment of cardiac arrest.
b. Gastrointestinal symptoms—anorexia, nausea, vomiting, diarrhea, and abdominal discomfort from gastric irritation	Most oral preparations of minerals and electrolytes are likely to cause gastric irritation. Taking the drugs with food or 8 oz of fluid may decrease symptoms.
c. Cardiovascular symptoms	
(1) Cardiac arrhythmias	Potentially fatal arrhythmias may occur with hyperkalemia or hypermagnesemia.
(2) Hypotension, tachycardia, and other symptoms of shock	These may occur with deferoxamine and iron dextran injections.
(3) Circulatory overload and possible pulmonary edema	Most likely to occur with large amounts of NaCl or $NaHCO_3$.
d. With Kayexelate, observe for hypokalemia, hypocalcemia, hypomagnesemia, and edema.	Although this drug is used to treat hyperkalemia, it removes calcium and magnesium ions as well as potassium ions. Since

Nursing Actions	Rationale/Explanation
	it acts by trading sodium for potassium, the sodium retention may lead to edema.
4. Observe for drug interactions	
a. Drugs that *increase* effects of minerals and electrolytes and related drugs	
(1) Acidifying agents (ammonium chloride): effects are increased by sodium chloride, potassium chloride, and ascorbic acid.	Systemic acidification by increased serum chloride; also increased urine acidity
(2) Alkalinizing agents (sodium bicarbonate): effects are increased by antacids such as magnesium hydroxide, calcium carbonate, and aluminum hydroxide.	Small amounts of antacids may be absorbed to produce additive effects.
(3) Cation exchange resin (Kayexelate): diuretics increase potassium loss; other sources of sodium increase the likelihood of edema.	Additive effects
(4) Iron salts	
(a) Allopurinol (Zyloprim)	This drug may increase the concentration of iron in the liver. It should not be given concurrently with any iron preparation.
(b) Ascorbic acid (vitamin C)	In large doses of 1 g or more, ascorbic acid increases absorption of iron by acidifying gastrointestinal secretions.
(5) Potassium salts	
(a) Spironolactone, triamterene, and amiloride	These drugs are potassium-saving diuretics. They should *not* be given with a potassium supplement because of additive risks of producing life-threatening hyperkalemia.
(b) Salt substitutes (*e.g.,* Neo-Curtasol)	These contain potassium rather than sodium and may cause hyperkalemia if given with potassium supplements.
(c) Penicillin G potassium	This potassium salt of penicillin contains 1.7 mEq of potassium per 1 million units. It may produce hyperkalemia if given in combination with potassium supplements.
b. Drugs that *decrease* effects of minerals and electrolytes and related drugs	
(1) Acidifying agents: effects are decreased by alkalinizing agents.	Alkalinizing agents neutralize the effects of acidifying agents.
(2) Alkalinizing agents: effects are decreased by acidifying drugs.	Acidifying drugs neutralize effects of alkalinizing agents.
(3) Oral iron salts	
(a) Antacids containing carbonate	The antacids decrease iron absorption by forming an insoluble, nonabsorbable compound of iron carbonate.
(b) Magnesium trisilicate	This antacid decreases absorption of iron.
(c) Pancreatic extracts	These inhibit iron absorption by increasing alkalinity of gastrointestinal fluids.
(4) Potassium salts	
(a) Calcium gluconate	Decreases cardiotoxic effects of hyperkalemia and is therefore useful in the treatment of hyperkalemia.
(b) Sodium polystyrene sulfonate (Kayexelate)	Used in treatment of hyperkalemia because it removes potassium from the body.
5. Teach clients	
a. The best source of minerals is a well-balanced diet with a variety of foods.	A well-balanced diet contains all the minerals needed for health in most people. An exception is iron, which is often needed as a dietary supplement in women and children.
b. The safest course of action is to take mineral supplements only on a physician's advice, in the amounts, and for the length of time prescribed.	All minerals are toxic when taken in excess. Also, there is no benefit from taking more minerals than the body needs.

Nursing Actions	Rationale/Explanation
c. Keep all mineral supplements out of reach of children.	To prevent accidental overdosage. Acute iron intoxication is a relatively common problem among small children.
d. With iron preparations, teach	
(1) To take with or after meals, at least initially	To decrease gastric irritation. If no anorexia, nausea, vomiting, or other problems occur, the drug can be tried before meals because it is better absorbed from an empty stomach.
(2) To dilute and take liquid iron preparations through a straw	To avoid staining the teeth
(3) That the drug causes stools to be dark green or black	
e. Potassium preparations *must* be taken as directed.	The unpleasant taste of oral solutions apparently reduces compliance with physician's orders.
(1) Mix oral solutions or effervescent tablets with at least 4 oz of water or juice.	To improve the taste
(2) Take after meals.	To further dilute the drug and decrease gastric irritation
(3) Do *not* stop taking the drug without notifying the physician who prescribed it, especially if also taking digitalis or diuretics.	Serious problems may develop from low levels of potassium in the blood.

Selected References

American Medical Association (AMA) Division of Drugs: AMA Drug Evaluations, 5th ed. New York, John Wiley & Sons, 1983

Antoniou L: Zinc in clinical medicine. Drug Ther 14:92–102, August 1984

Ball M, Phillips LJ: Nutritional disorders. In Wiener MB, Pepper GA: Clinical Pharmacology and Therapeutics in Nursing, 2d ed, pp 353–388. New York, McGraw-Hill, 1985

Groer MW, Shekleton ME: Basic Pathophysiology: A Conceptual Approach, 2d ed. St. Louis, CV Mosby, 1983

Hansten PD: Drug Interactions: Clinical Significance of Drug–Drug Interactions, 5th ed. Philadelphia, Lea & Febiger, 1985

Hayter J: Trace elements: Implications for nursing. J Adv Nurs 5:91–101, January 1980

Hillman RS: Vitamin B_{12}, folic acid, and the treatment of megaloblastic anemias. In Gilman AG, Goodman LS, Rall TW, Murad F (eds): The Pharmacological Basis of Therapeutics, 7th ed, pp 1323–1337. New York, Macmillan, 1985

Hillman RS, Finch CA: Drugs effective in iron-deficiency and other hypochromic anemias. In Gilman AG, Goodman LS, Rall TW, Murad F (eds): The Pharmacological Basis of Therapeutics, 7th ed, pp 1308–1322. New York, Macmillan, 1985

Kopyt N, Narins RG: How should hypokalemia by treated? Drug Ther 15:93–113, May 1985

Mudge GH: Agents affecting volume and composition of body fluids. In Gilman AG, Goodman LS, Rall TW, Murad F (eds): The Pharmacological Basis of Therapeutics, 7th ed, pp 846–878. New York, Macmillan, 1985

Rodman MJ, Karch AM, Boyd EH, Smith DW: Pharmacology and Drug Therapy in Nursing, 3rd ed. Philadelphia, J B Lippincott, 1985

VI

DRUGS USED TO TREAT AND PREVENT INFECTIONS

33

GENERAL CHARACTERISTICS OF ANTI-INFECTIVE DRUGS

Anti-infective drugs are used to prevent or treat infections caused by pathogenic (disease-producing) microorganisms. People are surrounded by microorganisms, few of which cause disease in normal circumstances. Infections are usually prevented by the body's defense mechanisms, which keep pathogenic microorganisms from entering infectable tissues. If infections do occur, these mechanisms help eliminate them. Conditions that impair the defense mechanisms increase the incidence and severity of infections. The type, number, and virulence of the infective microorganism are also influential factors. To participate effectively in antimicrobial drug therapy, the nurse must be knowledgable about the host and the microorganism as well as about antimicrobial drugs.

Host defense mechanisms

The major defense mechanisms of the human body are intact skin and mucous membranes, various anti-infective secretions, mechanical movements, phagocytic cells, and the immune and inflammatory processes. The skin prevents penetration of foreign particles, and its secretions and indigenous bacterial flora inhibit growth of pathogenic microorganisms. Secretions of the gastrointestinal, respiratory, and genitourinary tracts (*e.g.*, gastric acid, mucus) kill, trap, or inhibit growth of microorganisms. Coughing, swallowing, and peristalsis help to remove foreign particles and pathogens trapped in mucus, as does the movement of cilia. Phagocytic cells in various organs and tissues engulf and digest pathogens and cellular debris. The immune system produces lymphocytes and antibodies. The inflammatory process is the body's response to injury by microorganisms, foreign particles, chemical agents, or physical irritation of tissues. Inflammation localizes, destroys, neutralizes, and dilutes or removes the injurious agent so that tissue healing can occur.

Many factors impair host defense mechanisms and predispose to infection by disease-producing microorganisms. These include the following:

1. Breaks in the skin and mucous membranes related to trauma, inflammation, open lesions, or insertion of prosthetic devices, tubes, and catheters for diagnostic or therapeutic purposes
2. Impaired blood supply
3. Neutropenia and other blood disorders
4. Malnutrition
5. Poor personal hygiene
6. Suppression of indigenous bacterial flora by antimicrobial drugs
7. Suppression of the immune system and the inflammatory response by immunosuppressive drugs, cytotoxic antineoplastic drugs, and adrenal corticosteroids
8. Diabetes mellitus and other chronic diseases
9. Advanced age

Microorganisms and infections

Microorganisms are everywhere in the environment, including air, food, water, and soil. They are also present in the human body, especially on the skin and in the mouth, upper respiratory tract, genitals, and colon. These microorganisms (bacteria, viruses, fungi, and others) usually live in a state of balance with the human host and do not cause disease. Infection results when the balance is upset by decreased host resistance or increased numbers and virulence of microorganisms. In an infection, microorganisms invade tissues, multiply, and produce injurious effects.

1. Microorganisms are classified according to groups or species.
   a. Bacterial species are subclassified according to whether they are aerobic (require oxygen) or anaerobic (cannot live in the presence of oxygen), their reaction to Gram stains (gram positive or gram negative), and their shape (cocci [oval], bacilli [rod shaped], spirilla [spiral]). In addition, various strains develop as an organism adapts to its environment. Many bacteria can survive in living (humans, animals) or nonliving (objects, air, food, soil, water) environments.
   b. Viruses are intracellular parasites that survive only in living tissues. They are classified in several different ways according to host, origin, and other characteristics. Like bacteria, viruses produce many strains.
   c. Fungi are plantlike organisms that live as parasites on living tissue or as saprophytes on decaying organic matter. About 50 species are pathogenic in humans.
2. The human body normally has areas that are sterile and areas that contain microorganisms.
   a. Sterile areas are the lower respiratory tract (trachea, bronchi, lungs), much of the gastrointestinal and genitourinary tracts, the musculoskeletal system, and the body cavities. Body fluids are also sterile.
   b. Indigenous skin flora includes staphylococci, streptococci, diphtheroids, and transient environmental organisms. The upper respiratory tract contains staphylococci, streptococci, pneumococci, diphtheroids, and *Hemophilus influenzae.* The external genitalia contain skin organisms; the vagina contains lactobacilli, *Candida,* and *Bacteroides.* The colon contains *Escherichia coli, Klebsiella, Enterobacter, Proteus, Pseudomonas, Bacteroides, Clostridia,* lactobacilli, streptococci, and staphylococci. Microorganisms that are part of the indigenous flora and are nonpathogenic in one area of the body may become pathogenic in other parts of the body. For example, *E. coli* often cause urinary tract infections.
3. Common human pathogens are viruses, gram-positive streptococci and staphylococci, and gram-negative intestinal organisms (*E. coli, Bacteroides, Klebsiella, Proteus, Pseudomonas* species, and others) (Table 33-1). These microorganisms are usually spread by air, direct contact with an infected person, or contaminated hands, food, water, and objects. Some may also be spread by a carrier (a person who transmits a pathogenic organism but does not have an active infection). For example, some people "carry" pathogenic strains of staphylococci in their upper respiratory tracts (*e.g.,* anterior nares).
4. "Opportunistic" microorganisms may be part of the indigenous flora and are usually nonpathogenic. They become pathogens, however, in hosts whose defense mechanisms are impaired. Opportunistic infections are likely to occur in people with severe burns, cancer, prolonged intravenous fluid therapy, in-dwelling urinary catheters, and antibiotic or corticosteroid drug therapy.
   a. Opportunistic bacterial infections may involve drug-resistant gram-negative microorganisms. These infections are serious and may be life threatening.
   b. Fungi of the *Candida* genus, especially *Candida albicans,* may cause life-threatening bloodstream or deep tissue infections such as brain abscesses.
   c. Viral infections may cause fatal pneumonia in renal, cardiac, and bone marrow transplant recipients.
5. Microorganisms may develop resistance to antimicrobial drugs by producing enzymes that destroy or inactivate the drug, by reducing their permeability to the drug, and by changing their structures or metabolic pathways. Resistant organisms can grow and multiply when indigenous flora is changed by certain antimicrobial drugs.
6. Infections are sometimes categorized as community acquired or hospital acquired (nosocomial). Nosocomial infections are often difficult to manage because they are likely to be caused by drug-resistant microorganisms and to occur in people whose resistance to disease is impaired. Drug-resistant strains of staphylococci, *Pseudomonas,* and *Proteus* are common causes of nosocomial infections.

TABLE 33-1. COMMON BACTERIAL PATHOGENS

Gram-positive bacteria	
Staphylococci	Some species of staphylococci are pathogenic. They may produce endotoxins that destroy tissue cells. Some produce enterotoxins and cause a common type of food poisoning. *Staphylococcus aureus,* one of the most widespread human pathogens, is commonly present on skin and mucous membrane of the nose and mouth. It is spread by direct and indirect contact with people who are carriers, people with staphylococcal infections, animals, and nonliving environments such as mop water and the cooling coils of air-conditioning systems. *S. aureus* causes boils, carbuncles, surgical wound infections, and internal abscesses. Staphylococcal infections are characterized by formation of yellow pus.
Streptococci	*Streptococcus viridans, Streptococcus pneumoniae,* and *Streptococcus pyogenes* are three strains that are pathogenic to humans. *S. viridans* (alpha-hemolytic streptococcus) is part of the indigenous bacterial flora of the upper respiratory tract. It does not cause disease unless the mucosal barrier is damaged by trauma, previous infection, or surgical manipulation. Such damage allows the organisms to enter the bloodstream and gain access to other parts of the body. For example, the organisms may cause subacute bacterial endocarditis if they reach damaged heart valves. *S. pneumoniae* causes about three fourths of all bacterial pneumonias. *S. pyogenes* (beta-hemolytic streptococcus) causes severe pharyngitis ("strep throat"), scarlet fever, rheumatic fever, and acute bacterial endocarditis. These infections are usually spread by inhalation of droplets from the upper respiratory tracts of carriers or people with infections. The organism also grows in milk.
Gram-negative bacteria	
Bacteroides	*Bacteroides* are anaerobic bacteria normally found in the digestive, respiratory, and genital tracts. They may also be found in the bloodstream and necrotic tissue. The most common bacteria in the colon, they greatly outnumber *Escherichia coli. Bacteroides fragilis* is the species most often seen.
Escherichia coli	*E. coli* inhabits the intestinal tract of humans and animals and is normally nonpathogenic in the intestinal tract. The organism may be beneficial by synthesizing vitamins and by competitively discouraging growth of possible pathogens. It may cause infection when allowed access to other parts of the body. For example, *E. coli* causes most urinary tract infections. The presence of *E. coli* in milk or water indicates fecal contamination.
Klebsiella	*Klebsiella* organisms are often associated with respiratory infections and may also infect the urinary tract, bloodstream, and meninges. *Klebsiella pneumoniae* is a relatively common cause of pneumonia, especially in people with bronchitis or other pulmonary disease.
Proteus	Proteus organisms are normally found in the intestinal tract and in decaying matter. They most often cause urinary tract and wound infections but may infect any tissue. Infection usually occurs with antibiotic therapy, which decreases drug-sensitive bacteria and allows drug-resistant bacteria to proliferate.
Pseudomonas	These organisms are found in water, soil, and normal skin and intestines. *Pseudomonas aeruginosa* is the species most often associated with human disease. It can cause infections of wounds, burns, eyes, and ears as well as pneumonia. Infection is more likely to occur in hosts who are very young or very old or who have decreased resistance.
Serratia	*Serratia marcescens* is found in infected people, water, soil, milk, and feces. Formerly believed nonpathogenic to humans, the organism is now known to cause septicemia and infections of the urinary tract, respiratory tract, skin, and burn wounds. It may also cause hospital epidemics and produce drug-resistant strains.
Salmonella	About 1400 species of *Salmonella* have been identified; several are pathogenic to humans. The organisms cause gastroenteritis, typhoid fever, septicemia, and a severe, sometimes fatal type of food poisoning.
Shigella	*Shigella* contains several species that cause gastrointestinal problems ranging from mild diarrhea to severe and often fatal dysentery.

Characteristics of anti-infective drugs

TERMINOLOGY

Several terms are used to describe these drugs, including *antimicrobial, antibacterial,* and *antibiotic,* as well as *anti-infective.* Antibiotic is probably the most frequently used term. Other terms include *broad spectrum,* for drugs effective against several groups of microorganisms, and *narrow spectrum,* for drugs effective against only one or two groups. The action of an anti-infective drug is usually described as *bactericidal* (kills the microorganism) or *bacteriostatic* (inhibits growth of the microorganism). Whether a particular drug is bactericidal or bacteriostatic depends on its concentration at the infection site and the susceptibility of the microorganism to the drug.

MECHANISMS OF ACTION

Anti-infectives act against microorganisms by several mechanisms, including the following:

1. Inhibition of bacterial cell wall synthesis or activation of enzymes that disrupt bacterial cell walls (*e.g.*, penicillins, cephalosporins, cycloserine, vancomycin, bacitracin).
2. Inhibition of protein synthesis by bacteria or production of abnormal bacterial proteins (*e.g.*, chloramphenicol, tetracyclines, erythromycin, clindamycin, aminoglycosides)
3. Disruption of bacterial cell membranes (*e.g.*, polymyxins, colistimethate)
4. Inhibition of bacterial reproduction by interfering with nucleic acid synthesis (*e.g.*, rifampin)
5. Inhibition of cell metabolism and growth (*e.g.*, sulfonamides, trimethoprim)

INDICATIONS

The clinical indications for use of anti-infectives are prevention and treatment of infections. Generally accepted prophylactic uses include the following:

1. Penicillin in group A streptococcal infections to prevent rheumatic fever, rheumatic heart disease, and glomerulonephritis
2. Antibiotics to prevent bacterial endocarditis in clients with cardiac valvular disease
3. Isoniazid to prevent tuberculosis in selected situations (see Chap. 41)
4. Antibiotics during the perioperative period for selected high-risk clients (those whose resistance to infection is lowered owing to age, poor nutrition, disease, or drugs) and for selected high-risk surgical procedures (cardiac surgery, gastrointestinal surgery, certain orthopedic procedures)
5. Antibiotics (usually penicillin) to prevent gonorrhea and syphilis after exposure has occurred

Principles of therapy: anti-infective drugs

ASSESSMENT GUIDELINES

Assess for current or potential infection:

1. General signs and symptoms of infection are the same as those of inflammation, although the terms are not synonymous. Inflammation is the normal response to any injury; infection requires the presence of a microorganism. The two often occur together. Inflammation may weaken tissue, allowing microorganisms to invade and cause infection. Infection (tissue injury by microorganisms) arouses inflammation. Local signs include redness, heat, edema, and pain; systemic signs include fever and leukocytosis. Specific manifestations depend on the site of infection. Common sites are the respiratory tract, surgical or other wounds, and the genitourinary tract. Check urinalysis and culture reports of urine, sputum, and wound drainage when available.
2. Assess each client for the presence of factors that increase risks of infection (see "Host defense mechanisms," above).

NURSING INTERVENTIONS

1. Use measures to control spread of infection.
   a. Wash hands thoroughly and often. This is probably the single most effective method of preventing infections.
   b. Prevent spread of viral and bacterial infections of the respiratory tract by the following means:
      (1) Wash hands after coughing, sneezing, or contact with infected persons.
      (2) Cover mouth and nose with tissues when sneezing or coughing and dispose of tissues by placing in a paper bag and burning.
      (3) Expectorate sputum (swallowing may cause reinfection).
      (4) Avoid crowds.
      (5) Recommend annual influenza vaccine to high-risk populations: people with chronic diseases such as diabetes, heart, lung, or renal problems, the elderly, and health care personnel who are often exposed.
   c. Wear a scrub gown in critical care or isolation areas of health care agencies.
   d. Handle *all* body secretions carefully. Always wash hands after handling and use gloves freely.
   e. Use sterile technique in changing any dressing. If a wound is not infected, sterile technique helps prevent infection; if the wound is already infected, sterile technique avoids introducing new bacteria. For all but the smallest of dressings without drainage, remove the dressing with clean gloves, discard it in a plas-

tic or foil-lined moistureproof bag, and wash hands before putting on sterile gloves to apply the new dressing.

f. To minimize spread of staphylococcal infections, infected personnel with skin lesions should not work until lesions are healed; infected patients should be isolated. Personnel with skin lesions probably spread more staphylococci than clients because personnel are more mobile.

2. Support natural defense mechanisms to prevent infection or, if it occurs, to promote rapid recovery.
   a. Promote general health measures—nutrition, fluid and electrolyte balance, rest, and exercise. Specific measures must be based on a thorough assessment of each client.
   b. In respiratory infections, assist the client with pulmonary hygiene measures to remove secretions because secretions furnish good culture media for bacterial growth. These measures include ambulation, turning, coughing and deep breathing exercises, and incentive spirometry.
   c. Keep the client's skin clean and dry, especially the hands, underarms, groin, and perineum, since these areas harbor large numbers of microorganisms. Also, take care to prevent trauma to the skin and mucous membrane.

LIMITATIONS ON USE OF ANTIBACTERIAL DRUGS

Antibacterial drugs are indicated only when a significant bacterial infection is diagnosed or strongly suspected or when there is an established indication for prophylaxis. These drugs should not be used for viral or trivial infections. They are not effective in viral infections; they may allow the growth of drug-resistant organisms in trivial infections.

COLLECTION OF SPECIMENS

Collect specimens for culture and Gram stain before giving the first dose of an anti-infective. For best results, specimens must be collected accurately and taken directly to the laboratory. If delayed, contaminants may overgrow pathogenic microorganisms.

DRUG SELECTION

The choice of an anti-infective for treating an infection should generally be based on culture and susceptibility studies. Culture identifies the causative organism; susceptibility tests determine which drugs are likely to be effective against the organism. Culture and susceptibility studies are especially important with suspected gram-negative infections because of the high incidence of drug-resistant microorganisms. Because these tests require 48 to 72 hours, the physician usually prescribes for immediate administration a drug that is likely to be effective.

ROUTE OF ADMINISTRATION

Route of administration depends largely on the severity of the infection. In serious infections, the intravenous route is usually preferred. Oral administration is preferred for initial therapy only in relatively mild infections.

DURATION OF THERAPY

Duration of therapy varies from a single dose to years, depending on the reason for use. For most acute infections, the average duration is approximately 7 to 10 days or until the recipient has been afebrile and asymptomatic for 48 to 72 hours.

PERIOPERATIVE USE

When used to prevent infections associated with surgery, anti-infective drugs are often given 1 hour preoperatively. This provides effective tissue concentration during the procedure, when contamination is highest. The choice of drug depends on the pathogen most likely to enter the operative area. A single dose is often adequate. If surgery is delayed or prolonged, a second dose may be given. Postoperative anti-infectives are probably indicated only with dirty, traumatic wounds or ruptured viscera.

USE IN RENAL INSUFFICIENCY

In renal insufficiency or failure, anti-infective drug therapy requires extreme caution. Many drugs are excreted primarily by the kidneys. Some drugs are nephrotoxic and may further damage the kidneys. In the presence of renal failure, they are likely to accumulate and produce toxic effects. Thus, dosage reductions are necessary for some drugs. Methods of calculating dosage are usually based on rates of creatinine clearance. Dosage may be reduced by giving smaller individual doses, by increasing the time interval between doses, or both. Anti-infective drugs can be categorized as follows in relation to renal disease:

1. Drugs that should never be given in the presence of renal disease (*i.e.*, creatinine clearance of less than 30 ml/minute). These drugs include all tetracyclines except doxycycline (Vibramycin).
2. Drugs that are not used in renal disease unless the infection is caused by organisms resistant to safer drugs. If used, dosage must be carefully adjusted, renal function must be closely monitored, and the recipient must be closely observed for adverse effects. These drugs include all the aminoglycosides, carbenicillin, cephalexin, colistin, amphotericin B, ethambutol, and flucytosine. Serum drug levels are recommended for monitoring aminoglycoside antibiotics.
3. Drugs that require dosage adjustment in severe renal failure. These include penicillin G, ampicillin, methicillin, oxacillin, trimethoprim-sulfamethoxazole, and most cephalosporins.
4. Drugs that require little or no dosage adjustment. These include cloxacillin, dicloxacillin, nafcillin, erythromycin, doxycycline, clindamycin, chloramphenicol, rifampin, and isoniazid.

An additional factor is important in clients with chronic renal failure who are receiving hemodialysis or peritoneal dialysis: some drugs are removed by dialysis, and an extra dose may be needed during or after dialysis.

USE IN LIVER DISEASE

In severe liver disease, anti-infective drugs that are excreted by the liver must be reduced in dosage. These include erythromycin, clindamycin, and chloramphenicol. The antitubercular drugs rifampin and isoniazid have longer half-lives in clients with cirrhosis. Dosing in liver disease is not well defined.

USE IN PREGNANCY AND LACTATION

During pregnancy and lactation, anti-infective drug therapy requires caution, primarily because of potential adverse effects on the fetus or infant. Many drugs have not been evaluated for safety during these periods. Although insufficient data are available regarding several anti-infective agents, it is probably safer to assume that most of the drugs reach the fetus by placental transfer and the nursing infant by excretion in breast milk. Even with this basic assumption, it is not generally known whether most drugs reach significant levels in the fetus or infant. Despite these limitations, some guidelines for use of anti-infective drugs include the following:

1. Penicillins cross the placenta and enter breast milk but apparently produce no adverse effects on the fetus. They are generally considered safe to use.
2. All tetracyclines are contraindicated during pregnancy and lactation. In the pregnant woman, there is a risk of fatal hepatic necrosis. In the fetus or nursing infant, dental and bone abnormalities may occur.
3. Cephalosporins have not been established as safe during pregnancy, and insufficient data are available regarding excretion in breast milk.
4. Aminoglycosides cross the placenta and may cause nephrotoxicity and ototoxicity in the fetus. Therefore, they should be used only when no alternative is available. During lactation, it is thought unlikely that significant amounts reach the infant. However, excretion in breast milk and potential for toxicity are unknown.
5. Chloramphenicol is contraindicated in late pregnancy because of the possible occurrence of "gray baby syndrome." This is the name given to a type of severe toxicity observed in both premature and full-term infants who required chloramphenicol for severe infections. The infants often became cyanotic and ash-gray. Diarrhea, respiratory problems, and collapse of peripheral blood vessels are other characteristics of this often fatal reaction. Chloramphenicol is contraindicated during lactation because levels in breast milk are about half the mother's serum level. Thus, adverse effects may occur, but levels are probably too low to cause gray baby syndrome.
6. Sulfonamides should not be used during the last 2 weeks of pregnancy because they displace bilirubin from albumin-binding sites and may cause kernicterus in the neonate.
7. Nitrofurantoin should not be used during late pregnancy. Hemolytic anemia may occur in the neonate, related to immature drug-metabolizing systems.

GERIATRIC CONSIDERATIONS

In geriatric anti-infective drug therapy, penicillins, cephalosporins, and erythromycin are generally safe. With impaired renal function, nitrofurantoin, tetracyclines, and aminoglycosides are contraindicated if less toxic drugs are effective against causative organisms. If these drugs are used, extreme caution must be exercised.

GENERAL NURSING ACTIONS: ANTI-INFECTIVE DRUGS

Nursing Actions	*Rationale/Explanation*
1. Administer accurately	
a. Schedule at evenly spaced intervals around the clock.	To maintain therapeutic blood levels
b. Give most oral anti-infective drugs on an empty stomach (1 hour before or 2 hours after meals). Notable exceptions are amoxicillin and bacampicillin, which can be scheduled without regard to meals.	To prevent drug inactivation by gastric acid and to promote absorption.
c. For oral and parenteral solutions from powder forms, follow label instructions for mixing and storing. Also, check expiration dates.	Several antimicrobial drugs are marketed in powder forms because they are unstable in solution. When mixed, measured amounts of diluent must be added for drug dissolution and the appropriate concentration, usually expressed in milligrams per milliliter (mg/ml). Parenteral solutions are often prepared in the pharmacy. Most solutions require refrigeration for longer periods of stability. None of the solutions should be used after the expiration date because drug decomposition is likely.
d. Give parenteral anti-infective solutions *alone;* do not mix with any other drug in a syringe or intravenous solution.	To avoid chemical and physical incompatibilities that may cause drug precipitation or inactivation
e. Give intramuscular anti-infective drugs deeply into large muscle masses (preferably gluteal muscles) and rotate injection sites.	Most parenteral solutions are irritating to tissues. Intramuscular injection is not the preferred route for most anti-infective drugs.
f. For intravenous administration, use dilute solutions and give slowly.	Most anti-infective drugs that are given intravenously can be given by intermittent infusion. Although instructions vary with specific drugs, most reconstituted drugs can be further diluted with 50 to 100 ml of intravenous fluid (D_5W, NS, $D_5-\frac{1}{4}\%$ or $D_5-\frac{1}{2}\%$ NaCl) and infused over 20 to 60 minutes. This method causes less vein irritation and thrombophlebitis, avoids drug deactivation, and provides therapeutic serum levels.
2. Observe for therapeutic effects **a.** With local infections, observe for decreased redness, edema, heat, and pain	Signs and symptoms of inflammation and infection usually subside within about 48 hours after anti-infective therapy is begun. Although systemic manifestations of infection are similar regardless of the cause, specific manifestations vary with the type or location of the infection.
b. With systemic infections, observe for decreased fever and white blood cell count, increased appetite, and reports of feeling better	
c. With wound infections, observe for decreased signs of local inflammation and decreased drainage. Drainage may also change from purulent to serous.	
d. With respiratory infections, observe for decreased dyspnea, coughing, and secretions. Secretions may change from thick and colored to thin and white.	
e. With urinary tract infections, observe for decreased urgency, frequency, and dysuria. If urinalysis is done, check the laboratory report for decreased bacteria and white blood cells.	
3. Observe for adverse effects	
a. Hypersensitivity	Hypersensitivity may occur with most anti-infectives but is more common with penicillins.

Nursing Actions	Rationale/Explanation
(1) Anaphylaxis—hypotension, respiratory distress, urticaria, angioedema, vomiting, diarrhea	Anaphylaxis usually occurs within minutes after taking the drug. Hypotension results from vasodilation and circulatory collapse. Respiratory distress results from bronchospasm or laryngeal edema.
(2) Serum sickness—fever, vasculitis, generalized lymphadenopathy, edema of joints, bronchospasm, and urticaria	This is a delayed allergic reaction, occurring a week or more after the drug is started. Signs and symptoms are caused by inflammation.
b. Superinfection	Superinfection is a new or secondary infection that occurs during anti-infective therapy of a primary infection. Superinfections are relatively common and potentially serious because responsible microorganisms are often drug-resistant staphylococci, gram-negative organisms (*Proteus* or *Pseudomonas*) or fungi (*Candida*). Infections with these organisms are often difficult to treat.
(1) Stomatitis—sore mouth, white patches on oral mucosa, black furry tongue (2) Diarrhea (3) Monilial vaginitis—rash in perineal area, itching, vaginal discharge (4) New localized signs and symptoms—redness, heat, edema, pain, drainage, cough (5) Recurrence of systemic signs and symptoms—fever, malaise	
c. Phlebitis at venipuncture sites; pain at intramuscular injection sites	Parenteral solutions of many anti-infective drugs are irritating to tissues.
d. Gastrointestinal symptoms—nausea, vomiting, diarrhea	These are common with oral anti-infective agents and probably result from irritation of gastrointestinal mucosa and changes in gastrointestinal flora.
4. Observe for drug interactions	See following chapters. The most significant interactions are those that alter anti-infective effectiveness or increase drug toxicity.
5. Teach clients	
a. Take all of prescribed anti-infectives—do not stop when symptoms subside.	To prevent recurrence of infection and emergence of drug-resistant microorganisms
b. Do not take anti-infectives left over from a previous illness or prescribed for someone else.	Even if infection is present and anti-infective treatment appears needed, the likelihood of having the appropriate drug on hand, and in adequate amounts, is extremely small. Thus, taking drugs not prescribed for the particular illness tends to maximize risks and minimize benefits. Also, if the infection is viral, most anti-infectives are not effective.
c. Take oral anti-infectives on an empty stomach, 1 hour before or 2 hours after a meal unless instructed otherwise.	Food decreases absorption of most oral anti-infectives. If the drug causes intolerable nausea or vomiting, a few bites of food (*e.g.,* crackers) may be taken
d. Report any other drugs being taken or allergies to the prescribing physician.	Drug interactions may occur, and changes in drug therapy may be indicated.
e. The importance of hand washing, maintaining nutrition and fluid balance, obtaining adequate rest, and handling secretions correctly	These measures help the body to fight the infection, prevent further infection, and enhance the effectiveness of anti-infective drugs.
f. Report nausea, vomiting, diarrhea, skin rash, recurrence of symptoms for which the anti-infective drug was prescribed, or signs of new infection (*e.g.,* fever, cough, sore mouth, drainage).	These problems may indicate adverse effects of the drug, lack of therapeutic response to the drug, or a superinfection. Any of these requires evaluation and may indicate changes in drug therapy.

Selected References

American Medical Association (AMA) Division of Drugs: AMA Drug Evaluations, 5th ed. New York, John Wiley & Sons, 1983

Antimicrobial prophylaxis for surgery. Med Lett Drugs Ther 25:113–116, December 1983

Burnakis TG: Surgical antimicrobial prophylaxis: Principles and guidelines. Pharmacotherapy 4:248–271, September–October 1984

Charles D, Larsen B: Placental transfer of antibiotics. In Ristuccia AM, Cunha BA (eds): Antimicrobial Therapy, pp 519–533. New York, Raven Press, 1984

Davies J: Microbial resistance to antimicrobial agents. In Ristuccia AM, Cunha BA (eds): Antimicrobial Therapy, pp 11–21. New York, Raven Press, 1984

Garner JS, Simmons BP: CDC guidelines, for the prevention and control of nosocomial infections: Guidelines for isolation precautions in hospitals. Am J Infect Control 12:103, April 1984

Gibbs RS, Weinstein AJ: Antibiotic Therapy in Obstetrics and Gynecology. New York, John Wiley & Sons, 1981

Ginsberg M, Tager I: Practical Guide to Antimicrobial Agents. Baltimore, Williams & Wilkins, 1980

Hansten PD: Drug Interactions: Clinical Significance of Drug-Drug Interactions, 5th ed. Philadelphia, Lea & Febiger, 1985

Leff RD, Roberts RJ: Host factors influencing the response to antimicrobial agents. Pediatr Clin North Am 30:93–102, February 1983

Lefkowitz S, Jones S, Johnson C: Infectious disorders. I. General principles of antimicrobial therapy and acute bacterial infections. In Wiener MB, Pepper GA (eds): Clinical Pharmacology and Therapeutics in Nursing, 2d ed, pp 443–496. New York, McGraw-Hill, 1985

May C: Antibiotic therapy at home. Am J Nurs, 84:348–349, March 1984

Medical Letter on Drugs and Therapeutics: Handbook of Antimicrobial Therapy, rev ed. New Rochelle, NY, 1984

Neuman M (ed): Useful and Harmful Interactions of Antibiotics. Boca Raton, FL, CRC Press, 1985

Orr ML: Drugs and renal diseases. Am J Nurs 81:969–971, May, 1981

Ristuccia AM, Cunha BA (eds): Antimicrobial Therapy. New York, Raven Press, 1984

Root RK, Sande MA (eds): New Dimensions in Antimicrobial Therapy. New York, Churchill Livingstone, 1984

Sager DP, Bomar SK: Intravenous Medications: A Guide to Preparation, Administration and Nursing Management. Philadelphia, J B Lippincott, 1980

Sande MA, Mandell GL: Antimicrobial agents: General considerations. In Gilman AG, Goodman LS, Rall TW, Murad F (eds): The Pharmacological Basis of Therapeutics, 7th ed, pp 1066–1094. New York, Macmillan, 1985

Smith IM: Infections in elderly patients: Practice guidelines for treatment. Drug Ther 8:33–45, July 1983

Smith LG: Factors in antibiotic selection. In Ristuccia AM, Cunha BA (eds): Antimicrobial Therapy, pp 1–9. New York, Raven Press, 1984

Snavely SR, Hodges GR: The neurotoxicity of antibacterial agents. Ann Intern Med 101:92–104, July 1984

Weinstein AJ, Alanis A: Antibiotic side effects. In Ristuccia AM, Cunha BA (eds): Antimicrobial Therapy, pp 339–363. New York, Raven Press, 1984

34 PENICILLINS

Description and uses

The penicillins are effective, safe, and widely used antimicrobial agents. The group includes natural extracts from the *Penicillium* mold and several semisynthetic derivatives. When penicillin G, the prototype, was introduced, it was effective against streptococci, staphylococci, gonococci, meningococci, *Treponema pallidum,* and other organisms. It had to be given parenterally because it was destroyed by gastric acid and intramuscular injections were very painful. With extensive use, strains of drug-resistant staphylococci appeared. Later penicillins were developed to increase gastric acid stability, beta-lactamase stability, and antimicrobial spectrum of activity, especially against gram-negative microorganisms.

The basic chemical structure of penicillin is 6-aminopenicillanic acid, which contains a beta-lactam ring and side chains. The beta-lactam ring is essential for antibacterial activity, and penicillins are frequently called beta-lactam antibiotics. Most penicillins are susceptible to destruction by beta-lactamases, which are a group of enzymes produced by some bacteria that open the beta-lactam ring and inactivate the drug. Penicillinase is a beta-lactamase enzyme that acts specifically on penicillins. This is a major mechanism by which microorganisms develop resistance to beta-lactam antibiotics (penicillins and cephalosporins). Semisynthetic derivatives are formed by adding side chains to the penicillin nucleus.

Penicillins kill bacteria by inhibiting synthesis of the bacterial cell wall. The probable mechanism of their antibacterial action involves binding of drug molecules to protein molecules (called penicillin-binding proteins or PBPs) in bacterial cell membranes. This binding produces a defective cell wall that allows intracellular contents to leak out, destroying the microorganism. In subbactericidal concentrations, penicillins may inhibit growth, decrease viability, and alter the shape and structure of organisms. The latter characteristic may help to explain the development of mutant strains of microorganisms exposed to the drugs. Penicillins are most effective when bacterial cells are dividing.

After absorption, penicillins are widely distributed and achieve therapeutic concentrations in most body fluids, including joint, pleural, and pericardial fluids and bile. Therapeutic levels are not usually obtained in intraocular and cerebrospinal fluids unless inflammation is present because normal cell membranes act as barriers to drug penetration. Penicillins are rapidly excreted by the kidneys and produce high drug concentrations in the urine. An exception is nafcillin, which is excreted by the liver.

Clinical indications for use of penicillins include bacterial infections caused by susceptible microorganisms. They are the drugs of choice for treatment of streptococcal pharyngitis, pneumococcal pneumonia, gonorrhea, and syphilis and for prevention of bacterial endocarditis in clients with valvular heart disease who must undergo dental or surgical procedures. They are often useful in respiratory infections, cholecystitis, and cellulitis. Contraindications include hypersensitivity or allergic reactions to any penicillin preparation.

INDIVIDUAL PENICILLINS

Penicillin subgroups are discussed in the following paragraphs. Individual penicillins are listed, with routes of administration and dosage ranges, in Table 34-1.

Penicillins G and V

Penicillin G, the prototype of the penicillins, is widely used. Because of its effectiveness and minimal toxicity, it is recommended for treatment of infections caused by susceptible microorganisms. Although most staphylococci and some gonococci have developed resistance to penicillin G, the drug is still effective in most streptococcal infections. Thus it is the drug of choice for the treatment of streptococcal pharyngitis and for prevention of rheumatic fever, a complication of streptococcal pharyngitis.

Numerous preparations of penicillin G are available for various purposes and routes of administration. They cannot be used interchangeably. Only aqueous preparations can be given intravenously. Preparations containing benzathine or procaine can only be given intramuscularly. Long-acting repository forms have additives that decrease their solubility in tissue fluids and delay their absorption. When penicillin G is given orally, large doses must be given to offset the portion destroyed by gastric acid.

Penicillin V is derived from penicillin G and has the same antibacterial spectrum. It is not destroyed by gastric acid and is given only by the oral route. It is better absorbed and produces higher blood levels than penicillin G. The potassium salt is preferred because it is better absorbed than plain penicillin V.

Penicillinase-resistant (antistaphylococcal) penicillins

This group includes five drugs (**cloxacillin, dicloxacillin, methicillin, nafcillin,** and **oxacillin**) that are effective in infections caused by staphylococci resistant to penicillin G. They are specifically formulated to resist the action of beta-lactamase (penicillinase) enzymes that inactivate other penicillins. These drugs are recommended for use only in known or suspected staphylococcal infections. They are not effective against gram-negative bacteria.

Ampicillins

Ampicillin is a broad-spectrum, semisynthetic penicillin that is bactericidal for several types of gram-positive and gram-negative bacteria. It has been effective against *Proteus mirabilis, Salmonella, Shigella,* and most strains of *Escherichia coli.* However, many resistant forms of *Shigella* and *E. coli* are being encountered. Ampicillin is not used against gram-positive cocci because penicillin G or V is less expensive and more effective. It is ineffective against penicillinase-producing staphylococci and gonococci. It is excreted mainly by the kidneys; thus it may be useful in urinary tract infections. Some is excreted in bile; thus it may be useful in biliary tract infections not caused by biliary obstruction. It is widely used in treatment of respiratory infections such as bronchitis and sinusitis and of otitis media.

Amoxicillin is similar to ampicillin but is reportedly better absorbed and produces more rapid and higher blood levels. It may also cause less gastrointestinal distress. A new preparation, Augmentin, contains amoxicillin and potassium clavulanate, a salt of clavulanic acid. Clavulanic acid is a beta-lactam drug that lacks antibacterial activity of its own but inhibits beta-lactamase enzymes and thereby enhances antibacterial activity of the antibiotic component. Potassium clavulanate protects amoxicillin from degradation and increases its effectiveness, even in infections caused by bacteria that are normally resistant to amoxicillin and other beta-lactam antibiotics. Augmentin is available in 250-mg and 500-mg tablets, each of which contains 125-mg of potassium clavulanate. Thus, two 250-mg tablets are not equivalent to one 500-mg tablet.

Cyclacillin closely resembles ampicillin; **hetacillin** and **bacampicillin** are "pro-drugs" that are converted to ampicillin in the body. Bacampicillin has a longer duration of action and can be given twice daily. Dosage of these drugs should be reduced in the presence of renal insufficiency.

Extended-spectrum (antipseudomonal) penicillins

This group is comprised of five drugs (**carbenicillin, ticarcillin, azlocillin, mezlocillin,** and **piperacillin**) that have a broad spectrum of antimicrobial activity. They are especially effective against gram-negative organisms such as *Pseudomonas, Proteus,* and *E. coli.* They are drugs of choice for pseudomonal infections and are usually given concomitantly with aminoglycoside antibiotics. Carbenicillin, the first of this group to be developed, may be given parenterally for systemic infections. Carbenicillin indanyl sodium, an ester of carbenicillin, is acid stable and can therefore be given orally. Relatively low plasma levels are obtained with the oral drug, but therapeutic levels are obtained in urine. Consequently, oral carbenicillin is used only for

(Text continues on p. 350.)

TABLE 34-1. PENICILLINS

	Generic name	Trade name	Routes and dosage ranges: Adults	Routes and dosage ranges: Children
Penicillins G and V	Penicillin G sodium Penicillin G potassium	Pfizerpen, Pentids, others	PO 600,000–3 million units daily IM 300,000–8 million units daily IV 6–20 million units daily by continuous or intermittent infusion q2–4h. Up to 60 million units daily have been given in certain serious infections	PO 25,000–90,000 units/kg/day in divided doses q6–8h IM, IV 50,000–250,000 units/kg/day in divided doses q4h
	Penicillin G benzathine	Bicillin	PO 400,000–600,000 units q4–6h IM 1.2–2.4 million units in a single dose Prophylaxis of rheumatic fever, IM 1.2 million units monthly or 600,000 units every 2 weeks Treatment of syphilis, IM 2.4 million units (1.2 million units in each buttock) in a single dose	PO 25,000–90,000 units/kg/day in 3–6 divided doses IM 50,000 units/kg in one dose Prophylaxis of rheumatic fever, IM 1.2 million units monthly or 600,000 units every 1–2 weeks
	Penicillin G procaine	Wycillin, others	IM 600,000–1.2 million units daily in 1–2 doses Prevention or treatment of uncomplicated gonorrhea, IM 4.8 million units in a single dose, divided into two or more injections and given at different sites. Probenecid 1 g is given 30 minutes before the penicillin	IM 25,000–50,000 units/kg/day in divided doses q12h
	Penicillin V	V-Cillin K, PenVee K, others	PO 125–500 mg 4–6 times daily	Same as adults Infants: PO 15–50 mg/kg/day in 3–6 divided doses
Penicillinase-resistant (antistaphylococcal) penicillins	Cloxacillin	Tegopen	PO 250–500 mg q6H	Weight 20 kg or more: Same as adults Weight under 20 kg: PO 50–100 mg/kg/day in 4 divided doses q6h
	Dicloxacillin	Dynapen	PO, IM 125–250 mg q6h	Weight 40 kg or more: Same as adults Weight under 40 kg: 12.5–25 mg/kg/day in 4 divided doses q6h
	Methicillin	Staphcillin	IM 1 g q4–6h IV 1–2 g in 50 ml sodium chloride injection, infused at 10 ml/minute q4–6h	IM 100–200 mg/kg/day in 4 divided doses q6h
	Nafcillin	Unipen	IM 500 mg q4–6h IV 500 mg–2 g in 15–30 ml sodium chloride injection, infused over 5–10 minutes, q4h; maximal daily dose, 12 g for serious infections	IM, IV 50–100 mg/kg/day in 4–6 divided doses q4–6h
	Oxacillin	Prostaphlin	PO, IM, IV 500 mg–1 g q4–6h. For direct intra-	Weight over 40 kg: Same as adults

TABLE 34-1. PENICILLINS (*Continued*)

	Generic name	Trade name	Routes and dosage ranges: Adults	Routes and dosage ranges: Children
			venous injection, the dose should be well diluted and given over 10–15 minutes.	Weight 40 kg or less: PO, IM, IV 50–100 mg/kg/day in 4 divided doses q6h
Ampicillins	Ampicillin	Omnipen, Penbriten, others	PO, IM, IV 250–500 mg q6h. In severe infections, doses up to 2 g q4h may be given IV	Weight over 20 kg: Same as adults Weight 20 kg or less: PO, IM, IV 50–100 mg/kg/day in divided doses q6h
	Amoxicillin	Amoxil, Larotid, others	PO 250–500 mg q8h	Weight over 20 kg: Same as adults Weight 20 kg or less: 20–40 mg/kg/day in divided doses q8h
	Amoxicillin and potassium clavulanate	Augmentin	PO 250–500 mg q8h	Weight under 40 kg: 20–40 mg/kg/day in divided doses q8h
	Bacampicillin	Spectrobid	PO 400–800 mg q12h	Weight over 25 kg: Same as adults
	Cyclacillin	Cyclapen	PO 250–500 mg q6h	PO 50–100 mg/kg/day in divided doses q6h
	Hetacillin	Versapen	PO 225–450 mg 4 times daily	Weight over 40 kg: Same as adults Weight under 40 kg: PO 22.5–45 mg/kg/day in divided doses
Extended-spectrum (antipseudomonal) penicillins	Carbenicillin disodium	Geopen	Urinary tract infections, IM, IV 1–2 g q6h Septicemia and severe systemic, respiratory or soft-tissue infections, IV 25–30 g daily in divided doses q4h	Urinary tract infections, IM, IV 50–200 mg/kg/day in divided doses Serious infections, IV 400–600 mg/kg/day in 4–6 divided doses; Maximal daily dose, 40 g
	Carbenicillin indanyl sodium	Geocillin	PO 1–2 tablets (382 mg carbenicillin/tablet) 4 times daily	PO 30–50 mg/kg/day in divided doses q8h
	Ticarcillin	Ticar	IM, IV 1–3 g q6h. IM injections should not exceed 2 g/injection	Weight under 40 kg: 100–300 mg/kg/day q6–8h
	Ticarcillin/clavulanate	Timentin	IV 3.1 g q4–6h	Weight under 60 kg: 200–300 mg/kg/day in divided doses q4–6h
	Azlocillin	Azlin	IV 200–350 mg/kg/day in 4–6 divided doses. Usual adult dosage, 3 g q4h; maximal dose, 24 g daily	Acute pulmonary exacerbation of cystic fibrosis, 450 mg/kg/day; maximum daily dose, 24 g
	Mezlocillin	Mezlin	IM, IV 200–300 mg/kg/day in 4–6 divided doses. Usual adult dose 3 g q4h or 4 g q6h	Age 1 month–12 years: 300 mg/kg/day in 6 divided doses, q4h
	Piperacillin	Pipracil	IV, IM 200–300 mg/kg/day in divided doses q4–6h. Usual adult dose 3–4 g q4–6h; maximal daily dose, 24 g	Age under 12 years: Dosage not established
Amidinopenicillin	Amdinocillin	Coactin	IV, IM 40–60 mg/kg/day in divided doses q4–6h	

treating urinary tract infections caused by susceptible pathogens. Carbenicillin delivers a relatively high amount of sodium to recipients. Ticarcillin is very similar to carbenicillin except that it is more potent on a weight basis and delivers less sodium because the dosage is lower. Ticarcillin/clavulanate (Timentin) recently became available. Clavulanate is a beta-lactamase enzyme inhibitor. (See amoxicillin/clavulanate, above.) The other drugs in this group deliver even less sodium and may be more effective against *Pseudomonas* organisms. The newer drugs may be preferred in clients with cardiovascular or other disorders in which sodium intake should be limited. Dosage of these drugs should be reduced in renal failure.

Amidinopenicillins

This is a new group of penicillins currently represented by only one drug, **amdinocillin** (Coactin). Amdinocillin differs from other penicillins in chemical structure, protein-binding pattern, gastric acid stability, and beta-lactamase stability. It has a 6-beta-amidinopenicillanic nucleus and attaches to PBP 2. Beta-lactam antibiotics that bind to PBP 2 are apparently resistant to beta-lactamase enzymes. Other penicillins reportedly bind to PBPs 1 and 3.

Amdinocillin is approved for treatment of urinary tract infections caused by susceptible strains of *E. coli, Klebsiella pneumoniae,* or *Enterobacter* and bacteremia caused by *E. coli.* Although its mechanism of action is mainly bacteriostatic, high drug levels produce bactericidal effects in the urinary tract. It acts synergistically with other beta-lactam antibiotics, and, if given concomitantly, dosage of amdinocillin should be reduced. It is given parenterally only. When given intravenously piggyback, the primary infusion should be temporarily discontinued.

Principles of therapy: penicillins

GUIDELINES RELATED TO HYPERSENSITIVITY TO PENICILLINS

1. Before giving the initial dose of any penicillin preparation, ask the client specifically if he or she has ever taken penicillin and, if so, whether an allergic reaction occurred. Penicillin is the most common cause of drug-induced hypersensitivity, and a person known to be hypersensitive should generally be given another type of antibiotic.
2. In the relatively rare instance in which penicillin is considered essential, a skin test may be helpful in assessing hypersensitivity. Benzylpenicilloylpolylysine (Pre-Pen) or a dilute solution of the penicillin to be administered (10,000 units/ml) may be applied topically to a skin scratch made with a sterile needle. If the scratch test is negative (no urticaria, erythema, or pruritus), the preparation may be injected intradermally. Allergic reactions, including fatal anaphylactic shock, have occurred with skin tests and following negative skin tests.
3. Anaphylactic shock may occur with administration of the penicillins, especially by parenteral routes. Therefore, emergency drugs and equipment must be readily available. Treatment may require parenteral epinephrine, oxygen, and insertion of an endotracheal or tracheostomy tube if laryngeal edema occurs.

DRUG SELECTION, ROUTE, AND DOSAGE

1. Choice of penicillin preparation depends primarily on the organism causing the infection. In many infections penicillin G is the drug of choice. In many gram-negative infections ampicillin is useful. In most *Pseudomonas* and *Proteus* infections, an antipseudomonal penicillin is preferred. Most staphylococcal infections are caused by organisms that produce penicillinase, an enzyme that inactivates the above drugs. Thus, in those infections, penicillinase-resistant penicillins are required. Nafcillin is the intravenous agent of choice, and dicloxacillin is the oral agent of choice.
2. Choice of route and dosage depends largely on the seriousness of the infection being treated. For serious infections, penicillins are given intravenously in large doses. Most penicillins must be given every 4 to 6 hours to maintain therapeutic blood levels. The intramuscular route is infrequently used in hospitalized clients but is used more often in ambulatory settings. The oral route is often used, especially for less serious infections and for long-term prophylaxis of rheumatic fever.

USE IN SPECIFIC SITUATIONS

Streptococcal infections

When used for streptococcal infections, pencillins should be given for the full prescribed course to prevent complications such as rheumatic fever, endocarditis, and glomerulonephritis.

Sexually transmitted diseases

When used for sexually transmitted diseases, it is advisable to refer to the guidelines established by the

Centers for Disease Control. Recommendations vary according to patterns of bacterial resistance. For example, penicillin-resistant strains of *Neisseria gonorrhoeae* are being encountered with increasing frequency.

With an aminoglycoside

A penicillin is often given concomitantly with an aminoglycoside antibiotic for some serious infections, such as those caused by *Pseudomonas aeruginosa.* In this instance, the drugs should not be mixed in a syringe or an intravenous solution because that inactivates the aminoglycoside.

With probenecid

Probenecid (Benemid) can be given concurrently with penicillins to increase serum drug levels. Probenecid acts by blocking renal excretion of the penicillins. This action may be useful when high serum levels are needed with oral penicillin preparations or when a single large dose is given for prevention or treatment of gonorrhea or syphilis.

USE IN PREGNANCY AND LACTATION

During pregnancy and lactation, penicillins are considered safer than other antibiotics, although they should still be used only if necessary. Teratogenesis has not been reported with penicillins. The drugs are excreted in breast milk and may cause diarrhea or candidiasis in nursing infants.

PEDIATRIC CONSIDERATIONS

In pediatrics, penicillins are considered safe and effective. Amdinocillin (Coactin), a newer drug, has not been established as safe and effective in children under 12 years of age. In neonates, penicillins are eliminated more slowly because of immature renal function.

GERIATRIC CONSIDERATIONS

In geriatric drug therapy, penicillins are safer than other antibiotics. Dosage of some drugs must be reduced with impaired renal function, a condition often present in the elderly adult.

POTENTIAL ELECTROLYTE DISTURBANCES

Excessive amounts of potassium or sodium may be ingested during penicillin therapy. Potassium excess may occur with large intravenous doses of penicillin G potassium, which contains 1.7 mEq of potassium per 1 million units. Hyperkalemia is unlikely with normal renal function but may occur with impaired renal function. Sodium excess is likely to occur when carbenicillin (5.6 mEq sodium/g) or ticarcillin (5.6 mEq sodium/g) is given to clients with renal impairment or congestive heart failure. Hypokalemic metabolic acidosis may occur with carbenicillin or ticarcillin in clients whose renal function is impaired. This occurs because potassium loss is enhanced by high sodium intake.

NURSING ACTIONS: PENICILLINS

Nursing Actions	*Rationale/Explanation*
1. Administer accurately	
a. Give most oral penicillins on an empty stomach, about 1 hour before or 2 hours after a meal. Penicillin V, amoxicillin, and bacampicillin may be given without regard to meals.	To decrease binding to foods and inactivation by gastric acid. The latter three drugs are not significantly affected by food.
b. Give intramuscular penicillins deeply into a large muscle mass.	To decrease tissue irritation
c. For intravenous administration, generally dilute reconstituted penicillins in 50 to 100 ml of 5% dextrose or 0.9% sodium chloride injection and infuse over 30 to 60 minutes.	To minimize vascular irritation and phlebitis. Amounts and types of intravenous solutions may vary. Check manufacturers' literature for specific drugs to ensure compatibility and safety.
d. Prepare crystalline penicillin G for intravenous use just before giving.	The drug in crystalline (powder) form is stable for a long time. When diluent is added to form a solution, the drug loses activity rapidly.

Nursing Actions	***Rationale/Explanation***
e. Give reconstituted ampicillin intravenously or intramuscularly within 1 hour.	The drug is stable for a limited time in solution.
f. Do not give methicillin as a continuous intravenous infusion.	Methicillin is unstable at acid *p*H, and most solutions used for intravenous infusions are acidic enough to start breakdown of methicillin in about 20 minutes.
2. Observe for therapeutic effects	Depend on type of infection. See Chapter 33.
a. Decreased signs and symptoms of infection for which given	
b. Absence of signs and symptoms of infection when given prophylactically	
3. Observe for adverse effects:	
a. Hypersensitivity—anaphylaxis, serum sickness	Hypersensitivity is more likely to occur with penicillins than with other anti-infectives. Anaphylaxis may occur within 5 to 30 minutes of penicillin administration. See "Nursing Actions," Chapter 33 for signs and symptoms of hypersensitivity.
b. Superinfection	See Chapter 33 for signs and symptoms.
c. Nausea, vomiting, diarrhea	These gastrointestinal disturbances are more likely to occur with high doses of oral drugs and are probably caused by local irritation of mucosa and changes in gastrointestinal flora.
d. Thrombophlebitis at venipuncture sites and pain at intramuscular injection sites.	
e. With carbenicillin and ticarcillin, observe for congestive heart failure (dyspnea, edema, fatigue) and bleeding.	These drugs contain relatively large amounts of sodium. Congestive heart failure is more likely to occur in clients with heart or kidney disease. Bleeding tendencies result from decreased platelet aggregation.
4. Observe for drug interactions	
a. Drugs that *increase* effects of penicillins	
(1) Gentamicin	Synergistic activity against *Pseudomonas* organisms when given concomitantly with extended-spectrum (antipseudomonal) penicillins Synergistic activity against enterococci that cause subacute bacterial endocarditis, brain abscess, meningitis, or urinary tract infection Synergisic activity against *Staphylococcus aureus* when used with nafcillin or methicillin
(2) Probenecid (Benemid)	Decreases renal excretion of penicillins, thus elevates and prolongs penicillin blood levels
b. Drugs that *decrease* effects of penicillins	
(1) Acidifying agents (ammonium chloride, ascorbic acid, cranberry juice, methenamine, methionine, orange juice)	Most oral penicillins are destroyed by acids, including gastric acid. Ampicillin, penicillin V, and phenethicillin are acid stable.
(2) Erythromycin	Erythromycin inhibits the bactericidal activity of penicillins against most organisms but potentiates activity against resistant strains of *S. aureus*.
(3) Tetracyclines	These bacteriostatic antibiotics slow multiplication of bacteria and thereby inhibit the penicillins, which act against rapidly multiplying bacteria.
5. Teach clients	See Chapter 33.

Selected References

American Medical Association (AMA) Division of Drugs: AMA Drug Evaluations, 5th ed. New York, John Wiley & Sons, 1983

Amoxicillin clavulanic acid (Augmentin). Med Lett Drugs Ther 26:99–100, November 1984

Anderson PD: Basic Human Anatomy and Physiology: Clinical Implications for the Health Professions. Monterey, CA, Wadsworth, 1984

Brooks GF, Barriere SL: Clinical use of the new beta-lactam antimicrobial drugs. Ann Intern Med 98:530–535, April 1983

Eichenwald HF: Using the newer penicillins in pediatric practice. Drug Ther 13:239–253, October 1983

Facts and Comparisons. St. Louis, J B Lippincott (Updated monthly)

Hansten PD: Drug Interactions: Clinical Significance of Drug–Drug Interactions, 5th ed. Philadelphia, Lea & Febiger, 1985

Mandell GL, Sande MA: Penicillins, cephalosporins, and other beta-lactam antibiotics. In Gilman AG, Goodman LS, Rall TW, Murad F (eds): The Pharmacological Basis of Therapeutics, 7th ed, pp 1115–1149. New York, Macmillan, 1985

Molavi A, Le Frock JL: Antistaphylococcal penicillins. In Ristuccia AM, Cunha BA (eds): Antimicrobial Therapy, pp 183–195. New York, Raven Press, 1984

Parry MF, Pancoast SJ: Antipseudomonal penicillins. In Ristuccia AM, Cunha BA (eds): Antimicrobial Therapy, pp 197–207. New York, Raven Press, 1984

Prince AS, Neu HC: New penicillins and their use in pediatrics. Pediatr Clin North Am 30:3–16, February 1983

Rodman MJ, Karch AM, Boyd EH, Smith DW: Pharmacology and Drug Therapy in Nursing, 3rd ed. Philadelphia, J B Lippincott, 1985

Ticarcillin-clavulanic acid (Timentin). Med Lett Drugs Ther 27:69–70, August 1985

35 CEPHALOSPORINS

Description and uses

Cephalosporins are a widely used group of antimicrobial drugs that are derived from a fungus. Although technically cefoxitin (a cephamycin derived from a different fungus) and moxalactam (a synthetic drug) are not cephalosporins, they are categorized with the cephalosporins because of their similarities to the group. Cephalosporins are also called beta-lactam antibiotics because their chemical structure contains a beta-lactam ring (like the penicillins). They have the same mechanism of action as the penicillins; that is, they inhibit formation of bacterial cell walls. They are broad-spectrum antimicrobial agents with a wide range of activity against both gram-positive and gram-negative bacteria. Compared to penicillins, they are generally less active against gram-positive organisms but more active against gram-negative organisms. Most cephalosporins are given parenterally; only four are available for oral administration. Once absorbed, they are widely distributed into most body fluids and tissues with maximum concentrations in the liver and kidneys. Most cephalosporins do not reach therapeutic levels in cerebrospinal fluid. Exceptions are cefurozime, a second-generation drug, and the third-generation agents. These drugs reach therapeutic levels when meninges are inflamed. Cephalosporins are excreted through the kidneys except for cefoperazone, which is excreted in bile.

Early cephalosporins (now called first-generation cephalosporins) have essentially the same spectrum of antimicrobial activity and can be described as a group with cephalothin (Keflin) as the prototype. They are effective against streptococci (except *Streptococcus faecalis*), staphylococci (except methicillin-resistant *Staphylococcus aureus*), *Neiserria, Salmonella, Shigella, Escherichia, Klebsiella, Bacillus, Corynebacterium diphtheriae, Proteus mirabilis,* and *Bacteroides* (except *Bacteroides fragilis*). They are not effective against *Enterobacter, Pseudomonas,* and *Serratia.*

Second-generation cephalosporins differ from first-generation drugs but are similar to each other. They are more active against some gram-negative organisms than older drugs. Thus, they may be effective in infections resistant to other antibiotics, including infections caused by *Hemophilus influenzae, Enterobacter, Klebsiella, Escherichia coli,* and some strains of *Proteus.* Since each of these drugs has somewhat different antimicrobial spectra, susceptibility tests must be performed for each drug rather than for the entire group, as was feasible with first-generation drugs. Cefoxitin (Mefoxin), for example, is active against *B. fragilis,* an organism resistant to most drugs.

Third-generation cephalosporins further extend the spectrum of activity against gram-negative organisms. In addition to activity against usual enteric pathogens (*e.g., E. coli, Proteus, Klebsiella*), they are also active against several strains resistant to other antibiotics and to first- and second-generation cephalosporins. Thus, they may be useful in infections caused by unusual strains of enteric organisms such as *Citrobacter, Serratia, Providencia,* and *Enterobacter.* Another difference is that third-generation cephalosporins penetrate inflamed meninges to reach therapeutic concentrations in cerebrospinal fluid. Thus, they may be useful in meningeal infections caused by many common pathogens, including *H. influenzae, Neisseria meningitidis,* and *Streptococcus pneumoniae.* Although the drugs are active against *Pseudomonas* organisms, drug-resistant strains emerge when a cephalosporin is used alone for treatment of pseudomonal infection.

Overall, cephalosporins gain gram-negative activity and lose gram-positive activity as they move from the first to the third generation. The second- and third-generation drugs are more active against gram-negative organisms because they are more resistant to the beta-lactamase enzymes (cephalosporinases) produced by some bacteria to inactivate cephalosporins.

Clinical indications include surgical prophylaxis and treatment of infections of the respiratory tract, skin and soft tissues, bones and joints, urinary tract, and bloodstream (septicemia). Although a cephalosporin is the initial drug of choice only in infections caused by *K. pneumoniae,* these drugs are often used as alternative drugs in infections caused by organisms resistant to other drugs. Cephalosporins are most important clinically for gram-negative infections. In most infections with streptococci and staphylococci, penicillins are more effective and less expensive. In infections caused by methicillin-resistant *S. aureus,* cephalosporins are not clinically effective even if testing indicates susceptibility.

A major contraindication to the use of cephalosporins is a previous anaphylactoid reaction to penicillin. The chemical structure of cephalosporins is similar to that of penicillins (both groups are beta-lactam antibiotics), and there is some risk of cross sensitivity between the two groups. However, incidence of cross sensitivity is considered to be low, especially in clients who have had delayed reactions (*e.g.,* skin rash) to penicillins. Another contraindication is cephalosporin allergy. Immediate allergic reactions with anaphylaxis, bronchospasm, and urticaria occur less often than delayed reactions with skin rash, drug fever, and eosinophilia.

Individual cephalosporins are listed in Table 35-1.

Principles of therapy: cephalosporins

ASSESSMENT GUIDELINES

Before giving the initial dose of a cephalosporin, ask the client about any previous penicillin therapy. If the client ever had a sudden, severe reaction to penicillin, do not give the cephalosporin. Clients who are hypersensitive to penicillin may have an allergic reaction to a cephalosporin (cross allergenicity).

DRUG SELECTION

Choice of cephalosporin depends primarily on causative organisms, severity of infection, and other factors. Guidelines include the following:

1. In choosing an antimicrobial agent, a cephalosporin may be a good choice when it can be used alone for prophylaxis or treatment. If the cephalosporin must be combined with another antimicrobial agent, a noncephalosporin is preferred. For example, cephalosporins cannot be used alone in the treatment of *Pseudomonas* infections because first- and second-generation drugs are not effective and third-generation drugs allow emergence of drug-resistant organisms. A cephalosporin could be given concomitantly with an aminoglycoside, but an antipseudomonal penicillin is preferred. Penicillins are less nephrotoxic and less expensive than third-generation cephalosporins.
2. First-generation cephalosporins are frequently used for surgical prophylaxis, especially with prosthetic implants, since most postimplant infections are caused by gram-positive organisms such as staphylococci. They may also be used alone for treatment of infections caused by any susceptible organisms in body sites where drug penetration and host defenses are not a problem. Cefazolin (Kefzol) and cephapirin (Cefadyl) are frequently used parenteral agents. Cefazolin reportedly reaches a higher serum concentration, is more protein bound, and has a slower rate of elimination than other first-generation drugs. These factors prolong serum half-life, so that cefazolin can be given in smaller doses or less frequently. Cefazolin is also preferred for intramuscular administration because it is less irritating to body tissues.
3. Second-generation cephalosporins are also frequently used for surgical prophylaxis, especially for gynecologic and colorectal surgery. They are also used for treatment of intra-abdominal infections such as pelvic inflammatory disease, diverticulitis, penetrating wounds of the abdomen, and other infections caused by organisms inhabiting pelvic and colorectal areas. Newer drugs in this group, cefonicid and ceforanide, are similar in effectiveness to the older drugs and have the advantage of once- or twice-daily administration.
4. Third-generation cephalosporins are recommended for serious infections caused by susceptible organisms that are resistant to first- and second-generation cephalosporins. They are often used in the treatment of infections caused by *E. coli, Proteus, Klebsiella, Serratia,* and other Enterobacteriaceae, especially when the infections occur in body sites not readily reached by other drugs (*e.g.,* cerebrospinal fluid, bone) and in clients with im-

(Text continues on p. 358.)

TABLE 35-1. CEPHALOSPORINS

	Generic name	Trade name	Characteristics	Routes and dosage ranges: Adults	Routes and dosage ranges: Children
First generation	Cephalothin	Keflin	1. Prototype of first-generation cephalosporins 2. Active against streptococci, staphylococci, *Neisseria, Salmonella, Shigella, Escherichia, Klebsiella, Listeria, Bacillus, Hemophilus influenzae, Corynebacterium diphtheriae, Proteus mirabilis,* and *Bacteroides* except *Bacteroides fragilis* 3. Inactive against enterococci, *Enterobacter, Pseudomonas,* and *Serratia*	IV, IM 1–2 g q4–6h, depending on severity of infection	IV, IM 75–160 mg/kg/day in divided doses q4–6h
	Cefaclor	Ceclor	May be more active against *H. influenza, E. coli* than cephalothin	PO 250–500 mg q8h	PO 20–40 mg/kg/day in 3 divided doses q8h
	Cefadroxil	Duricef	A derivative of cephalexin with no apparent advantage over the parent drug	PO 1–2 g twice daily	30 mg/kg/day in 2 doses q12h
	Cefazolin	Kefzol, Ancef	More active against *E. coli* and *Klebsiella* species than cephalothin	IM, IV 250 mg–1 g q6–8h	IM, IV 50–100 mg/kg/day in 3–4 divided doses
	Cephalexin	Keflex	1. Somewhat less active against penicillinase-producing staphylococci than cephalothin 2. First oral cephalosporin, still used extensively	PO 250–500 mg q6h, increased to 4 g q6h if necessary in severe infections	PO 25–50 mg/kg/day in divided doses q6h
	Cephapirin	Cefadyl	No significant differences from cephalothin	IV, IM 500 mg–1 g q4–6h, up to 12 g daily, IV, in serious infections	IV, IM 40–80 mg/kg/day in 4 divided doses (q6h)
	Cephradine	Anspor, Velosef	Essentially the same as cephalexin except it can also be given parenterally	PO 250–500 mg q6h, up to 4 g daily in severe infections IV, IM 500 mg–1 g 2–4 times daily, depending on severity of infection	PO 25–50 mg/kg/day in divided doses q6h. In severe infections, up to 100 mg/kg/day may be given. IV, IM 75–125 mg/kg/day in divided doses q6h
Second generation	Cefamandole	Mandol	1. More active against some gram-negative organisms than cephalothin and other first-generation cephalosporins, especially *H. influenzae, Enterobacter* and *Klebsiella* species, indole-positive strains of *Proteus,* and *E. coli* 2. Major clinical usefulness is treatment of gram-negative infections caused by organisms resistant to other cephalosporins.	IV, IM 0.5–2 g q4–6h, up to 12 g daily in life-threatening infections	IV, IM 50–150 mg/kg/day in 4–6 divided doses q4–6h
	Cefonocid	Monocid	1. Antimicrobial spectrum similar to other second-generation cephalosporins 2. Has a long half-life and can therefore be given once daily	IV, IM 1 g daily (q24h) Surgical prophylaxis, IV, IM 1 g 1 hour before the procedure	

TABLE 35-1. CEPHALOSPORINS (*Continued*)

	Generic name	Trade name	Characteristics	Routes and dosage ranges — Adults	Routes and dosage ranges — Children
			3. Not approved for use in children		
	Ceforanide	Precef	1. Similar to other second-generation cephalosporins 2. Has a relatively long half-live and can therefore be given twice daily	IV, IM 0.5–1 g q12h Surgical prophylaxis, IV, IM 0.5–1 g 1 hour before the procedure	20–40 mg/kg/day in divided doses q12h
	Cefoxitin	Mefoxin	1. The first cephamycin (derived from a different fungus than cephalosporins) 2. Compared to cephalothin, cefoxitin is more active against gram-negative bacteria and less active against gram-positive bacteria. 3. Compared to cefamandole, cefoxitin is more active against indole-positive *Proteus* and *Serratia* but less active against gram-positive bacteria and gram-negative *Enterobacter* and *H. influenzae.* 4. A major clinical use may stem from increased activity against *B. fragilis,* an organism resistant to most other antimicrobial drugs.	IV, IM 1–2 g q4–6h	IV, IM 80–160 mg/kg/day in divided doses q4–6h. Do not exceed 12 g/day.
	Cefuroxime	Zinacef	1. Similar to other second-generation cephalosporins 2. Penetrates cerebrospinal fluid in presence of inflamed meninges	IV, IM 750 mg–1.5 g q8h Surgical prophylaxis, IV 1.5 g 30–60 minutes before initial skin incision, then 750 mg IV or IM q8h if procedure is prolonged	Over 3 months of age: IV, IM 50–100 mg/kg/day in divided doses q6–8h Bacterial meningitis, IV 200–240 mg/kg/day in divided doses q6–8h, reduced to 100 mg/kg/day upon clinical improvement
Third generation	Cefotaxime	Claforan	1. Antibacterial activity against most gram-positive and gram-negative bacteria, including several strains resistant to other antibiotics. It has activity against some strains of *Pseudomonas aeruginosa* resistant to both first- and second-generation cephalosporins. 2. Cefotaxime is recommended for serious infections caused by susceptible microorganisms.	IV, IM 1 g q6–8h; maximum dose, 12 g/24 hours	
	Ceftazidime	Fortaz	1. Active against gram-positive and gram-negative organisms 2. Especially effective against gram-negative organisms, including *Pseudomonas aeruginosa* and other bacterial strains re-	IV, IM 1 g q8–12h	1 month to 12 years: IV 30 to 50 mg/kg q8h, not to exceed 6 g/day Under 1 month of age: IV 30 mg/kg q12h

TABLE 35-1. CEPHALOSPORINS (*Continued*)

Generic name	Trade name	Characteristics	Routes and dosage ranges: Adults	Routes and dosage ranges: Children
		sistant to aminoglycosides 3. Indicated for serious infections caused by susceptible organisms		
Ceftizoxime	Cefizox	1. Broader gram-negative and anaerobic activity, especially against *B. fragilis* 2. More active against gram-positive organisms than moxalactam and more active against *Enterobacteriaceae* than cefoperazone 3. Dosage must be reduced with even mild renal insufficiency (creatinine clearance <80 ml/minute)	IV, IM 1–2 g q8–12h Gonorrhea, uncomplicated, IM 1 g as a single dose	Over 6 months of age: IV, IM 50 mg/kg q6–8h, increased to a total daily dose of 200 mg/kg if necessary
Ceftriaxone	Rocephin	1. First third-generation cephalosporin approved for once-daily dosing	IV, IM 1–2 g once daily (q24h) Surgical prophylaxis, IV, IM 1 g ½–2 hours before the procedure	IV, IM 50–75 mg/kg day, not to exceed 2 g daily, in divided doses q12h Meningitis, IV, IM 100 mg/kg/day, not to exceed 4 g daily, in divided doses, q12h
Cefoperazone	Cefobid	1. Active against gram-negative and gram-positive organisms, including gram-negative organisms resistant to earlier cephalosporins 2. Has increased activity against *Pseudomonas* organisms but cannot be used for single-agent treatment of systemic pseudomonal infections 3. Excreted primarily in bile; half-life prolonged in hepatic failure	IV, IM 2–4 g/day in divided doses q8–12h	
Moxalactam	Moxam	Antibacterial spectrum is similar to that of cefotaxime, but moxalactam has better activity against anaerobic bacteria and better penetration into cerebrospinal fluid.	IM, IV 1–2 g q8h	

munosuppression. Although these drugs are effective against 50% to 75% of *Pseudomonas* strains, they should not be used alone in treating pseudomonal infections because drug resistance develops.

5. Individual drugs of choice and guidelines for rational usage are still being developed for this group of drugs, since they are new and clinical use is limited. Moxalactam, one of the more extensively used drugs, has caused concern because of its association with bleeding problems, especially in the presence of renal or hepatic disease. Although the reasons are not clear, possible causes include drug-induced deficiency in vitamin K–dependent clotting factors and impaired platelet aggregation. It is now recommended that clients at high risk of bleeding be given 10 mg of vitamin K before receiving moxalactam. Included are clients who are elderly or malnourished, those with chronic liver disease or obstructive biliary tract disorders, those with preexisting coagulation disorders, and those with severe renal impairment (creatinine clearance <20 ml/minute). Administration of vitamin K will not restore normal platelet function or normal bacterial flora in the intestine.

ADMINISTRATION AND DOSAGE

Route of administration and dosage also depend on several factors. Only a few cephalosporins are sufficiently well absorbed for oral administration. These are most often used in mild infections and urinary tract infections. Although some cephalosporins can be given intramuscularly, the injections cause considerable pain and induration. Cefazolin is preferred for intramuscular administration because it is less irritating to tissues. The intravenous route is often used, especially with severe infections. Dosages are higher with severe infections and lower with renal failure (except with cefoperazone, which is excreted through the biliary tract).

PERIOPERATIVE USE

Most of the cephalosporins are used in surgical prophylaxis. The particular drug depends largely on the type of organism likely to be encountered in the operative area. First-generation drugs are often used for procedures associated with gram-positive postoperative infections, such as prosthetic implant surgery. Second-generation cephalosporins are often used for abdominal procedures, especially gynecologic and colorectal surgery, in which enteric gram-negative infections may occur postoperatively. Thus far, third-generation drugs seem to have little, if any, advantage over older drugs.

When used perioperatively, a cephalosporin should be given about 30 to 60 minutes before the first skin incision is made. To be effective, the drug must be present in therapeutic serum and tissue concentrations at the time of surgery. A single dose of a long-acting or several doses of a shorter-acting agent may be given. In most cases, "coverage" for about 24 hours is adequate; in prosthetic implants such as arthroplasty and open-heart surgery, the drug may be continued for 3 to 5 days.

MONITORING SERUM DRUG LEVELS

Although serum drug levels are not routinely required with cephalosporins, they may be indicated in some circumstances, as follows:

1. When tests indicate organism susceptibility to a cephalosporin but clinical effectiveness is lacking
2. When renal function is changing, to determine whether dosage reductions are needed
3. When toxicity may be present
4. When oral agents are used to treat serious infections (*e.g.*, osteomyelitis) in which therapeutic serum concentrations should be confirmed

USE IN PREGNANCY

During pregnancy, cephalosporins cross the placenta, and, although they seem to be safe, they have not been studied extensively in pregnancy. They apparently have shorter half-lives, lower serum concentrations, and a faster rate of elimination during pregnancy.

USE IN LACTATION

During lactation, the drugs are excreted in breast milk in small amounts and may alter the infant's bowel flora.

PEDIATRIC CONSIDERATIONS

In pediatric drug therapy, cephalosporins have not been extensively studied, although they are frequently used. A longer half-life and drug accumulation have been reported in neonates, probably due to immature renal function.

GERIATRIC CONSIDERATIONS

In geriatric drug therapy, there is apparently no contraindication to using cephalosporins. However, dosage may need to be reduced if renal function is impaired.

USE IN RENAL FAILURE OR IMPAIRMENT

In renal failure (creatinine clearance <20 to 30 ml/minute), dosage of all cephalosporins except cefoperazone should be reduced by 50%. Cefoperazone is excreted primarily through the bile and therefore does not accumulate with renal failure. Dosage of moxalactam and ceftizoxime should be reduced even with moderate renal impairment (creatinine clearance <80 ml/minute).

POTENTIAL ELECTROLYTE DISTURBANCES

In clients with severe renal disease or congestive heart failure, the sodium content of parenteral cephalosporins may need to be considered. Cephradine contains 6.0 mEq/g; cefamandole contains 3.3 mEq/g; cephalothin, cefazolin, cephapirin, and cefoxitin contain 2 to 3 mEq/g.

EFFECT ON URINE GLUCOSE TESTS

In clients receiving cephalosporins, testing urine for glucose with copper sulfate reagents (*e.g.*, Clinitest tablets) may produce black–brown colors that can be erroneously interpreted as positive for glucose. Clinistix and Tes-Tape (glucose oxidase reagents) should be used instead.

NURSING ACTIONS: CEPHALOSPORINS

Nursing Actions	*Rationale/Explanation*
1. Administer accurately	
a. Give oral cephalosporins 1 hour before or 2 hours after meals. Give with food if nausea occurs.	Food delays absorption but does not affect amount of drug absorbed
b. Give intramuscular cephalosporins deeply into a large muscle mass.	These drugs are irritating to tissues and cause pain, induration, and possibly sterile abscess. The intramuscular route is infrequently used except for cefazolin.
c. For intravenous administration, dilute cephalosporins in 50 to 100 ml of 5% dextrose or 0.9% sodium chloride injection and infuse over 20 to 30 minutes.	These drugs are irritating to veins and cause phlebitis. This problem can be minimized by adequate dilution of the drug and relatively slow injection rates. Also, changing venipuncture sites helps avoid prolonged irritation of the same vein. Thrombophlebitis is more likely to occur with doses of more than 6 grams/day for longer than 3 days.
2. Observe for therapeutic effects	See Chapter 33.
a. Decreased signs of local and systemic inflammation	
b. Decreased signs of infection for which given	
3. Observe for adverse effects	
a. Hypersensitivity—anaphylaxis, serum sickness	Hypersensitivity reactions are similar to those with penicillins but are uncommon.
b. Superinfection	See Chapter 33 for signs and symptoms
c. Thrombophlebitis at venipuncture sites and pain at intramuscular injection sites.	See 1b and c, above.
d. Nephrotoxicity—increased BUN and serum creatinine, and casts in urine	Renal toxicity is not common with cephalosporins but may occur. Cephaloridine, the most nephrotoxic cephalosporin, has largely been replaced by other cephalosporins.
e. Nausea, vomiting, and diarrhea	These gastrointestinal disturbances may occur with cephalosporins.
4. Observe for drug interactions	
a. Drugs that *increase* effects of cephalosporins	
(1) Loop diuretics (furosemide, ethacrynic acid)	Increased renal toxicity
(2) Gentamicin and other aminoglycoside antibiotics	Additive renal toxicity, especially in older clients, those with renal impairment, those receiving high dosages, and those receiving probenecid.
(3) Probenecid	Increases blood levels by decreasing renal excretion of the cephalosporins. This may be a desirable interaction to increase blood levels and therapeutic effectiveness or allow smaller doses.
b. Drugs that *decrease* effects of cephalosporins	
Tetracyclines	Tetracyclines are bacteriostatic and slow the rate of bacterial reproduction. Cephalosporins are bactericidal and are most effective against rapidly multiplying bacteria. Thus, tetracyclines should not be given concurrently with cephalosporins.
5. Teach clients	See Chapter 33.

Selected References

American Medical Association (AMA) Division of Drugs: AMA Drug Evaluations, 5th ed. New York, John Wiley & Sons, 1983

Bertino JS Jr, Speck WT: The cephalosporin antibiotics. Pediatr Clin North Am 30:17–26, February 1983

Brooks GF, Barriere SL: Clinical use of the new beta-lactam antimicrobial drugs. Ann Intern Med 98:530–535, April 1983

Cefonocid sodium (Monocid). Med Lett Drugs Ther 26:71–72, August 1984

Ceforanide (Precef). Med Lett Drugs Ther 26:91–92, October 1984

Ceftriazone sodium (Rocephin): Med Lett Drugs Ther 27:37–39, April 1985

Eichenwald HF: Using cephalosporins in children. Drug Ther 13:221–231, January 1983.

Facts and Comparisons. St. Louis, J B Lippincott (Updated monthly)

Malseed RT: Pharmacology: Drug Therapy and Nursing Considerations, 2d ed. Philadelphia, J B Lippincott, 1985

Mandell GL, Sande MA: Penicillins, cephalosporins, and other beta-lactam antibiotics. In Gilman AG, Goodman LS, Rall TW, Murad F (eds): The Pharmacological Basis of Therapeutics, 7th ed, pp 1115–1149. New York, Macmillan, 1985

Quintiliana R, Nightingale CH, Rossi JG, et al: Cephalosporins: An overview. In Ristuccia AM, Cunha BA (eds): Antimicrobial Therapy, pp 289–303. New York, Raven Press, 1984

36 AMINOGLYCOSIDES

Description and uses

The aminoglycoside antibiotics, derived from fungi, are effective against a broad spectrum of organisms. They are used clinically to treat infections caused by gram-negative microorganisms such as *Pseudomonas, Proteus, Escherichia coli,* and *Klebsiella–Enterobacter–Serratia* species. They kill bacteria by interfering with protein synthesis and preventing cell reproduction.

The clinical importance of the aminoglycosides lies in the increasing incidence of gram-negative infections. The majority of hospital-acquired infections are caused by gram-negative organisms. These infections have become more common with control of other types of infections, widespread use of antimicrobial drugs, and treatment measures that lower host resistance (*e.g.,* radical surgery and antineoplastic and immunosuppressive drug therapy). The infections occur in the respiratory and genitourinary tracts, skin, wounds, bowel, and bloodstream. Any infection with gram-negative organisms is serious and potentially life threatening. Management is difficult because the organisms are generally less susceptible to antibacterial drugs, and drug-resistant strains develop rapidly. Few drugs are effective against them, and those that are available are relatively toxic.

Most aminoglycosides are given parenterally to prevent or treat systemic infections. They reach therapeutic levels in blood, urine, bone, inflamed joints, and pleural and ascitic fluids. They are poorly distributed to the central nervous system (CNS) and intraocular fluids; small amounts reach the biliary tract. They are excreted unchanged by the kidney and therefore accumulate in the presence of renal failure if dosage is not reduced. The major clinical indication for parenteral aminoglycoside antibiotics is serious infection unlikely to respond to less toxic drugs. Adverse effects, including nephrotoxicity and ototoxicity, limit the usefulness of these agents. Dosage of aminoglycosides must be reduced in the presence of renal failure according to results of renal function tests (*e.g.,* creatinine clearance).

Some aminoglycosides are given orally to suppress intestinal bacteria. Neomycin and kanamycin may be given before colonoscopy or bowel surgery and to treat hepatic coma. In hepatic coma, intestinal bacteria produce ammonia, which enters the bloodstream and causes encephalopathy. Drug therapy to suppress intestinal bacteria decreases ammonia production. Paromomycin is used only in the treatment of intestinal amebiasis. Oral aminoglycosides are poorly absorbed from the gastrointestinal tract and are excreted in the feces. Systemic absorption and adverse effects are unlikely with normal renal function but may occur with impaired renal function. A few aminoglycosides are administered topically to the eye or to the skin. These are discussed in Chapters 65 and 66, respectively.

Individual aminoglycosides

Amikacin (Amikin) is a semisynthetic derivative of kanamycin. It has a broader spectrum of antibacterial activity than other aminoglycosides because it resists degradation by most enzymes that inactivate gentamicin, kanamycin, and tobramycin. Consequently, its major clinical use is in infections caused by organisms resistant to other aminoglycosides (*e.g., Pseudomonas, Proteus, E. coli, Klebsiella–Enterobacter–Serratia*), whether community or hospital acquired.

Routes and dosage ranges

Adults: IM, IV 15 mg/kg/day in 2–3 divided doses, q8–12h; maximal daily dose, 1.5 g
Children and older infants: IM, IV, same as adults
Neonates: IM, IV 10 mg/kg initially, then 7.5 mg/kg q12h

Gentamicin (Garamycin) is a frequently prescribed aminoglycoside. Although effective against several gram-positive organisms, including penicillin-resistant staphylococci, gentamicin is not the drug of choice in infections caused by these organisms. Penicillins and cephalosporins are effective and less toxic. Similarly, although effective against a number of gram-negative organisms, gentamicin is primarily used to treat *Pseudomonas* and *Proteus* infections, which are often resistant to other antibiotics. As a result of widespread use, gentamicin-resistant organisms are emerging. This development might, in the future, limit the usefulness of the drug. Gentamicin acts synergistically with carbenicillin or ticarcillin against *Pseudomonas* infections. The combination also inhibits the emergence of resistant organisms that may occur when either drug is used alone.

Routes and dosage ranges

Adults: IV, IM 3–5 mg/kg/day in 3 divided doses, q8h (dosage adjusted according to renal function)
Children: IV, IM 6–7.5 mg/kg/day in 3 divided doses, q8h
Infants and neonates: IV, IM 7.5 mg/kg/day in 3 divided doses, q8h
Premature infants and neonates less than 1 week of age: IV, IM 5 mg/kg/day in 2 divided doses, q12h

Kanamycin (Kantrex), because of its toxicity and lack of activity against *Pseudomonas* organisms, has largely been replaced by newer aminoglycosides in treating systemic gram-negative infections. It is sometimes used, however, to decrease bowel bacteria before diagnostic procedures (*e.g.,* colonoscopy) or surgery and in hepatic coma.

Routes and dosage ranges

Adults: IM 15 mg/kg/day in 2–3 divided doses, q8–12h; maximal daily dose, 1.5 g
Hepatic coma, PO 8–12 g daily in divided doses
Bowel sterilization, PO 1 g q1h for 4 hours followed by 1 g q6h for 36–72 hours
Children: PO 50 mg/kg/day in 4 divided doses, q6h
IM up to 15 mg/kg/day in 2–4 divided doses, q6–12h
Infants and neonates: IV, IM 5–15 mg/kg/day in 2–4 divided doses, q6–12h

Neomycin (Mycifradin, Otobiotic) is the most toxic aminoglycoside and is recommended for oral or topical use only. It is given orally to decrease bacterial flora in the colon before colonoscopy or bowel surgery and in hepatic coma. Although the drug is poorly absorbed from the gastrointestinal tract, toxic amounts may be absorbed when renal disease is present. It is used topically, often in combination with other drugs, for infections of the eye, ear, and skin (burns, wounds, ulcers, dermatoses). When it is used for wound or bladder irrigations, systemic absorption may occur if the area is large or if drug concentration exceeds 0.1%.

Routes and dosage ranges

Adults: Before bowel surgery, PO 4–8 g daily in 4 divided doses for 1–3 days
Hepatic coma, PO 4–8 g daily in 4 divided doses for 5–6 days
Infectious diarrhea, PO 50 mg/kg/day in 4 divided doses
External otitis, topically to ear 2 drops of otic solution 3–4 times daily
Skin lesions, topically to skin, application of topical ointment or cream 2–4 times daily
Continuous bladder irrigation, 1 ml Neosporin GU irrigant (neomycin 40 mg and polymyxin B 200,000 units/ml) in 1000 ml 0.9% sodium chloride irrigating solution over 24 hours
Infants and children: Infectious diarrhea, PO 50–100 mg/kg/day in 4 divided doses
External otitis and skin lesions, same as for adults
Neonates and premature infants: Infectious diarrhea, PO 10–50 mg/kg/day in 4 divided doses

Netilmicin (Netromycin), the most recently approved aminoglycoside, is similar to gentamicin in its antimicrobial spectrum but is reportedly less active against *Pseudomonas aeruginosa.* It may also be less nephrotoxic and ototoxic than other aminoglycosides.

Routes and dosage ranges

Adults: IM, IV 4–6.5 mg/kg/day in 2–3 divided doses, q8–12h
Infants and children (6 weeks to 12 years): 5.5–8 mg/kg/day in 2–3 doses, q8–12h
Neonates (under 6 weeks): 4–6.5 mg/kg/day, in divided doses, q12h

Streptomycin was the first aminoglycoside to be developed and is usually considered the prototype. It is active against a variety of microorganisms but is used clinically in only a few infections. It is used with penicillin in enterococcal endocarditis, with tetracyclines in brucellosis, plague, and tularemia, and occasionally with other drugs in tuberculosis. The major disadvantages of streptomycin are toxicity to the eighth cranial (acoustic) nerve and rapid development of drug-resistant microorganisms. Streptomycin-resistant organisms may develop within 48 hours if the drug is used alone. In most infections requiring aminoglycoside antibiotics, gentamicin and others are preferred over streptomycin.

Routes and dosage ranges

Adults: IM 1 g daily
Children: IM 20–40 mg/kg/day in 2 divided doses, q12h

Tobramycin (Nebcin) is very similar to gentamicin in its antibacterial spectrum, although it may be more active against *Pseudomonas* organisms, especially when ticarcillin is given concurrently. Tobramycin may also be indicated in serious staphylococcal infections when penicillins or other less toxic drugs are contraindicated or ineffective. When first introduced, tobramycin was recommended in infections caused by gentamicin-resistant organisms. Currently, use of tobramycin is increasing because some studies suggest it is less toxic than gentamicin. It is often used with other antibiotics for septicemia and infections of burn wounds, other soft tissues, bone, the urinary tract, and the CNS. Dosage must be reduced with impaired renal function.

Routes and dosage ranges

Adults: IM, IV 3–5 mg/kg/day in 3–4 divided doses, q6–8h
Children: IM, IV same as adults
Neonates (1 week or less): IM, IV up to 4 mg/kg/day in 2 divided doses, q12h

Principles of therapy: aminoglycosides

LIMITATIONS ON USE

Because of a high incidence of toxicity, aminoglycoside antibiotics should be used only in serious infections caused by susceptible microorganisms and for which less toxic drugs are not available.

ASSESSMENT GUIDELINES

1. Before starting aminoglycoside antibiotics, renal and eighth cranial nerve functions should be assessed. Renal function may be assessed to some extent by checking laboratory reports of urinalysis, blood urea nitrogen (BUN), and serum creatinine or creatinine clearance. Eighth cranial nerve function can be assessed by audiometry.
2. During aminoglycoside therapy, serum drug levels should be assessed as well as renal and eighth cranial nerve function. These measures are needed to prevent or minimize nephrotoxicity and ototoxicity.

NURSING INTERVENTIONS

Keeping recipients of aminoglycosides well hydrated helps to decrease damage to the renal tubules. If signs of kidney damage do occur, fluid intake should be increased.

DOSAGE AND DURATION OF THERAPY

1. Dosage of aminoglycosides must be carefully regulated because therapeutic doses are close to toxic doses. Some guidelines include the following:
   a. An initial loading dose is given to achieve therapeutic serum levels rapidly. The amount is based on weight and desired peak serum level. If the client is obese, ideal body weight should be used because aminoglycosides are not significantly distributed in body fat. For gentamicin, tobramycin, and netilmicin, the recommended loading dose is 1.5 to 2 mg/kg of body weight; for amikacin the loading dose is 5 to 7.5 mg/kg.
   b. Maintenance doses should be based on serum drug levels. Peak serum levels occur 30 to 60 minutes after drug administration (5 to 8 μg/ml for gentamicin and tobramycin, 20 to 30 μg/ml for amikacin, and 4 to 12 μg/ml for netilmicin). Measurement of both peak and trough levels is needed to establish and maintain therapeutic serum levels without excessive toxicity. For gentamicin and tobramycin, peak levels above 10 to 12 μg/ml and trough levels above 2 μg/ml for prolonged periods have been associated with nephrotoxicity. For accuracy, blood samples must be drawn at the correct times.
   c. The above guidelines relate to clients with normal renal function. If renal function is impaired, the dosage of aminoglycoside antibiotics must be reduced. Various methods may be used. Measuring serum drug levels is probably the best method. Another method is to lengthen the time interval between doses according to creatinine clearance levels. For spe-

cific instructions, consult the manufacturer's literature on gentamicin, tobramycin, amikacin, and netilmicin.

d. In urinary tract infections, smaller doses can be used than in systemic infections because the aminoglycosides reach high concentrations in the urine. Also, alkalinizing the urine increases the effectiveness of drug therapy. The drugs are much more active in an alkaline environment than in an acid one.

2. Duration of aminoglycoside therapy is preferably no longer than 10 days.

USE IN PREGNANCY AND LACTATION

Aminoglycosides should not be used during pregnancy unless necessary. These drugs cross the placenta, and fetal serum levels may reach 15% to 50% of maternal serum levels. Small amounts of streptomycin and netilmicin are excreted in breast milk.

PEDIATRIC CONSIDERATIONS

In pediatric drug therapy, there is greater risk of toxicity in premature infants and neonates because of immature renal function and impaired excretion. Neomycin is not recommended for use in infants or children.

GERIATRIC CONSIDERATIONS

In geriatric drug therapy, there is greater risk of toxicity than for younger adults because renal function is frequently impaired.

NURSING ACTIONS: AMINOGLYCOSIDES

Nursing Actions	*Rationale/Explanation*
1. Administer accurately	
a. For intravenous administration, dilute gentamicin, tobramycin, amikacin, or netilmicin in 50 to 100 ml of 5% dextrose or 0.9% sodium chloride injection and infuse over 30 to 60 minutes. Concentration of gentamicin should not exceed 1 mg/ml.	To achieve therapeutic blood levels.
b. Give intramuscular aminoglycosides in a large muscle mass and rotate sites.	To avoid local tissue irritation. This is less likely to occur with aminoglycosides than with most other antibiotics.
2. Observe for therapeutic effects	
a. Decreased local and systemic signs of infection	See Chapter 33.
b. Decreased signs and symptoms of the specific infection for which the drug is being given	
3. Observe for adverse effects	Adverse effects are more likely to occur with parenteral administration of large doses for prolonged periods. However, they may occur with oral administration in the presence of renal impairment and with usual therapeutic doses.
a. Nephrotoxicity—casts, albumin, red or white blood cells in urine, decreased creatinine clearance, increased serum creatinine, increased BUN	Renal damage is most likely to occur in clients who are elderly, who receive high doses or prolonged therapy, who have prior renal damage, or who receive other nephrotoxic drugs. This is the most serious adverse reaction. Risks of kidney damage can be minimized by using the drugs appropriately and detecting early signs of renal impairment.
b. Ototoxicity—deafness or decreased hearing, tinnitus, dizziness, ataxia	This results from damage to the eighth cranial nerve. Incidence of ototoxicity is increased in older clients, those with previous auditory damage, high doses or prolonged duration, and concurrent use of other ototoxic drugs.
c. Neurotoxicity—respiratory paralysis and apnea	This is caused by neuromuscular blockade and is more likely to occur after rapid intravenous injection, administration to a

Nursing Actions	Rationale/Explanation
	client with myasthenia gravis, or concomitant administration of general anesthetics or neuromuscular blocking agents (*e.g.,* succinylcholine, tubocurarine). This effect may also occur if an aminoglycoside is administered shortly after surgery, owing to the residual effects of anesthetics or neuromuscular blockers. Neostigmine or calcium may be given to counteract apnea.
d. Hypersensitivity—skin rash, urticaria	This an uncommon reaction except with topical neomycin, which may cause sensitization in as many as 10% of recipients.
e. Nausea, vomiting, diarrhea, peripheral neuritis, paresthesias	Uncommon with parenteral aminoglycosides. Diarrhea often occurs with oral administration.
4. Observe for drug interactions	
a. Drugs that *increase* effects of aminoglycosides	Except for the antipseudomonal penicillins, the listed drugs increase toxicity.
(1) Carbenicillin, ticarcillin, mezlocillin, azlocillin, piperacillin	The combination is synergistic in treating infections caused by *P. aeruginosa.* However, the drugs are chemically and physically incompatible. Therefore, do not mix them in a syringe or an intravenous fluid because the aminoglycoside will be deactivated.
(2) Loop diuretics (furosemide, ethacrynic acid, bumetanide)	Increased nephrotoxicity apparently caused by increased drug concentration in serum and tissues when the client is relatively "dehydrated" by potent diuretics
(3) Methoxyflurane (Penthrane) and nephrotoxic antimicrobial agents (amphotericin B, cephalosporins, colistimethate, polymyxin)	Increased nephrotoxicity
(4) Drugs with neuromuscular blocking activity (methoxyflurane, procainamide, promethazine, quinidine, sodium citrate, succinylcholine, tubocurarine)	Increased neuromuscular blockade with possible paralysis of respiratory muscles and apnea. This is most likely to occur with succinylcholine and tubocurarine (see 3[c] above).
5. Teach clients	
a. Report ringing in the ears, loss of hearing, dizziness or unsteady gait.	These are symptoms of ototoxicity.
b. Drink 2000 to 3000 ml of fluid/day if not contraindicated or received by intravenous infusion.	To reduce damage to the kidneys
c. Wash hands thoroughly and often, especially after contact with any secretions or urine.	To help prevent spread of infection and development of drug-resistant organisms

Selected References

American Medical Association (AMA) Division of Drugs: AMA Drug Evaluations, 5th ed. New York, John Wiley & Sons, 1983

Blumer JL, Reed MD: Clinical pharmacology of aminoglycoside antibiotics in pediatrics. Pediatr Clin North Am 30:195–208, February 1983

Facts and Comparisons. St. Louis, J B Lippincott (Updated monthly)

Hansten PD: Drug Interactions: Clinical Significance of Drug–Drug Interactions, 5th ed. Philadelphia, Lea & Febiger, 1985

Malseed RT: Pharmacology: Drug Therapy and Nursing Considerations, 2d ed. Philadelphia, J B Lippincott, 1985

Ristuccia AM: Aminoglycosides. In Ristuccia AM, Cunha BA (eds): Antimicrobial Therapy, pp 305–328. New York, Raven Press, 1984

Rodman MJ, Karch AM, Boyd EH, Smith DW: Pharmacology and Drug Therapy in Nursing, 3rd ed. Philadelphia, J B Lippincott, 1985

Sande MA, Mandell GL: The aminoglycosides. In Gilman AG, Goodman LS, Rall TW, Murad F (eds): The Pharmacological Basis of Therapeutics, 7th ed, pp 1150–1169. New York, Macmillan, 1985

37
TETRACYCLINES

Description and uses

The tetracyclines are broad-spectrum, bacteriostatic antimicrobial drugs that are similar in chemical structure, pharmacologic properties, and antimicrobial activity. They act by inhibiting intracellular protein synthesis. They are effective against a wide range of gram-positive and gram-negative organisms as well as rickettsiae, mycoplasmas, some protozoa, spirochetes, and others. They can be given orally or parenterally and are widely distributed into most body tissues and fluids. They are excreted in urine and feces. The older tetracyclines are excreted mainly in urine, the newer ones (doxycycline and minocycline) mainly in feces. All tetracyclines are excreted in bile, enter the intestine, and are partially reabsorbed (enterohepatic recirculation).

Despite a broad spectrum of antimicrobial activity, a tetracycline is the first drug of choice in only a few, relatively uncommon infections (cholera, granuloma inguinale, chancroid, Rocky Mountain spotted fever, psittacosis, typhus, trachoma). Other drugs (*e.g.*, penicillin) are usually preferred in gram-positive infections, and most gram-negative organisms are resistant to tetracyclines. However, a tetracycline may be used if bacterial susceptibility is confirmed. Specific clinical indications for tetracyclines include the following:

1. Treatment of uncomplicated urethral, endocervical, or rectal infections caused by *Chlamydia* organisms.
2. Adjunctive treatment, with other antimicrobials, in the treatment of pelvic inflammatory disease and sexually transmitted diseases.
3. Long-term treatment of acne. They interfere with the production of free fatty acids and decrease *Corynebacterium* in sebum. These actions decrease the inflammatory, pustular lesions associated with severe acne.
4. They can sometimes be substituted for penicillin in penicillin-allergic clients. They are effective in treating gonorrhea and syphilis when penicillin cannot be given. They should not be substituted for penicillin in treating streptococcal pharyngitis because microbial resistance is common, and tetracyclines do not prevent rheumatic fever. In addition, they should not be substituted for penicillin in any serious staphylococcal infection because microbial resistance commonly occurs.
5. Treatment of pericardial and pleural effusions caused by malignant tumors and other conditions. Intravenous tetracycline is instilled into the chest cavity, where it causes sclerosis and adherence of serosal surfaces.
6. Doxycycline may be used to prevent traveler's diarrhea due to enterotoxic strains of *Escherichia coli.*
7. Demeclocycline may be used to inhibit antidiuretic hormone in the management of chronic inappropriate antidiuretic hormone secretion.

Tetracyclines decrease effectiveness of penicillins and cephalosporins and should not be given concurrently with them. Tetracyclines are bacteriostatic and slow the rate of bacterial multiplication; penicillins and cephalosporins are bactericidal agents that are most effective against rapidly multiplying bacteria.

The major contraindication to the use of tetracy-

TABLE 37-1. TETRACYCLINES

Generic name	Trade name	Characteristics	Routes and dosage ranges: Adults	Routes and dosage ranges: Children
Tetracycline	Achromycin, others	1. Prototype drug 2. Marketed under generic and numerous trade names 3. Probably the most frequently used tetracycline	PO 250–500 mg q6h IM 250–500 mg daily in 2 divided doses, depending on severity of infection IV 250–500 mg q12h (do not exceed 2 g daily)	PO 22–44 mg/kg/day in 4 divided doses IM same as adults for children weighing more than 40 kg. For those weighing less than 40 kg, 15–25 mg/kg/day in 2–3 divided doses
Demeclocycline	Declomycin	1. Has a longer half-life than tetracycline, and smaller doses produce therapeutic serum levels 2. The tetracycline most likely to cause photosensitivity 3. May be used to promote diuresis when fluid retention is caused by inappropriate secretion of antidiuretic hormone	PO 150 mg q6h or 300 mg q12h Gonorrhea in penicillin-sensitive clients, PO 600 mg initially, followed by 300 mg q12h for 4 days	Age over 8 years, PO 3–6 mg/kg/day in 2–4 divided doses
Doxycycline	Vibramycin	1. A newer tetracycline that is better absorbed from the gastrointestinal tract than older preparations. Oral administration yields serum drug levels equivalent to those obtained by parenteral administration 2. Can be given in smaller doses and less frequently than other tetracyclines because of long serum half-life (about 18 hours) 3. Excreted by kidneys to a lesser extent than other tetracyclines and is the only tetracycline considered safe for clients with impaired renal function	PO 100 mg q12h for 2 doses, then once daily or in divided doses. Severe infections, 100 mg q12h IV 200 mg the first day, then 100–200 mg daily in 1–2 doses	PO, IV same as adults for children weighing at least 45 kg Those weighing less than 45 kg: PO 4.4 mg/kg (2 mg/lb) q12h for 2 doses, then 1 mg/kg/day in a single dose. Severe infections, 2 mg/kg q12h IV 4.4 mg/kg/day in 1–2 doses, then 1–2 mg/kg/day, depending on severity of infection
Methacycline	Rondomycin	A semisynthetic tetracycline that is similar to the parent drug	PO 600 mg daily in 2–4 divided doses q6–12h	PO 10 mg/kg/day in 3 divided doses q8h
Minocycline	Minocin	1. A relatively new tetracycline that is well absorbed after oral administration 2. Metabolized more than other tetracyclines, and smaller amounts are excreted in urine and feces	PO, IV 200 mg initially, then 100 mg q12h	Over 12 years old, PO, IV same as adults Under 12 years old, PO, IV 4 mg/kg initially, then 2 mg/kg q12h
Oxytetracycline	Terramycin	One of the first tetracyclines to be developed	PO 250–500 mg q6h, up to 4 g daily in severe infections IM 250 mg daily in a single dose or 200–400 mg daily in 2–3 divided doses IV 500 mg–1 g daily in 2 doses; maximal daily dose, 2 g	PO 22–44 mg/kg q6h IM 15–25 mg/kg/day in 2–3 divided doses IV 10–20 mg/kg/day in 2 divided doses

clines is renal failure. Tetracyclines inhibit protein synthesis in body cells. This antianabolic effect increases tissue breakdown (catabolism) and the amount of waste products to be excreted by the kidneys. The increased "workload" can be handled by normally functioning kidneys, but waste products are retained when renal function is impaired. This leads to azotemia, increased blood urea nitrogen (BUN), hyperphosphatemia, hyperkalemia, and acidosis. If a tetracycline is necessary because of an organism's sensitivity or the host's inability to take other antimicrobial drugs, the only one that can be given safely in renally impaired clients is doxycycline.

Nephrotoxicity has occurred from the use of outdated tetracyclines. Expiration dates should be monitored, and outdated drugs discarded.

Tetracyclines are also contraindicated in pregnant women and in children up to 8 years of age. During pregnancy, tetracyclines may cause fatal hepatic necrosis in the mother. In the fetus and young child, tetracyclines are deposited in bones and teeth along with calcium. If given during active mineralization of these tissues, tetracyclines can cause permanent brown coloring (mottling) of tooth enamel and depress bone growth. Tetracyclines should not be used in children unless other drugs are not effective or are contraindicated.

Individual tetracyclines are listed in Table 37-1.

Principles of therapy: tetracyclines

1. Culture and sensitivity studies are needed before tetracycline therapy because many strains of organisms are either resistant or vary greatly in drug susceptibility. Cross sensitivity and cross resistance among tetracyclines is usually the rule.
2. The oral route of administration is usually effective and preferred. Parenteral therapy is used when oral administration is contraindicated or for initial treatment of severe infections. Intramuscular injections cause pain, and intravenous infusions cause thrombophlebitis.
3. Tetracycline is almost insoluble in water above *p*H 3. Consequently, injectable tetracycline hydrochloride preparations are usually buffered with about three times their weight of ascorbic acid to produce a low *p*H.
4. Parenteral tetracycline preparations may cause a false-positive urine glucose with Clinitest tablets. Clinistix or Tes-Tape may be used instead.
5. Tetracyclines decompose with age, exposure to light, and extreme heat and humidity. Because the breakdown products may be toxic, it is very important to store these drugs correctly. Also, the manufacturer's expiration dates on containers should be noted and outdated drugs discarded.

NURSING ACTIONS: TETRACYCLINES

Nursing Actions	*Rationale/Explanation*
1. Administer accurately	
a. Give oral tetracycline preparations 1 hour before or 2 hours after meals.	Food interferes with absorption.
b. Give oral tetracyclines at least 1 hour before or 2 hours after antacids or milk products.	Substances containing aluminum, magnesium, or calcium combine with the drug to form poorly absorbed compounds.
c. If an oral tetracycline and an iron preparation are ordered, give them as far apart as possible (*e.g.*, tetracycline 3 hours before or 2 hours after the iron supplement).	Iron combines with tetracyclines as do other metallic ions to inhibit absorption. Tetracyclines reach only 10% to 50% of expected serum levels if given with iron.
d. Give intramuscular tetracyclines deep into a large muscle mass.	The drug is very irritating to tissues, and deep injection helps to minimize pain, induration and tissue damage. The intramuscular route is infrequently used.
e. After dissolving an intravenous preparation of tetracycline, dilute further in at least 100 ml of 5% dextrose or 0.9% sodium chloride injection. Administer over 60 min-	These preparations are highly irritating to tissues. Dilution decreases irritation and phlebitis. Rapid intravenous administration or high dosage (above 750 mg) has been associated with

Nursing Actions	***Rationale/Explanation***
utes. The drug may also be diluted in 500 to 1000 ml of intravenous solution and given over 6 to 12 hours. Avoid rapid administration.	a high incidence of nausea, vomiting, chills, fever, and hypotension.
f. Give the reconstituted drug within 12 hours.	The drug is stable in solution for 12 hours.
2. Observe for therapeutic effects	
a. Decreased local and systemic signs of infection	See Chapter 33.
b. Decreased signs and symptoms of the specific infection for which the drug is being given.	
3. Observe for adverse effects	
a. Nausea, vomiting, diarrhea	These are the most common adverse reactions and are probably caused by local irritation of gastrointestinal mucosa. After several days of tetracycline therapy, diarrhea may be caused by superinfection.
b. Superinfection—sore mouth, white patches on oral mucosa, black, furry tongue, diarrhea, skin rash and itching in the perineal area	These signs usually indicate monilial infection. Meticulous oral and perineal hygiene helps prevent these problems. A potentially serious but less common superinfection is colitis, caused by tetracycline-resistant staphylococci. Superinfection is more likely to occur with tetracyclines than with other antibiotics.
c. Photosensitivity	This may occur with any tetracycline, but it occurs most often with demeclocycline. It may be prevented by avoiding exposure to sunlight or other sources of ultraviolet light, wearing protective clothing, and using sunscreen lotions.
d. Pain and induration with intramuscular injections	This can be minimized by injecting the drug deep into a large muscle mass (*e.g.,* gluteal) and rotating injection sites.
e. Thrombophlebitis at the venipuncture site	These drugs are irritating to tissues and cause phlebitis if injected into the same vein for more than 48 to 72 hours.
f. Increased BUN and serum creatinine in clients with renal impairment	
g. Hepatotoxicity—elevated serum glutamic-oxaloacetic transaminase and other enzymes	Liver toxicity is most likely to occur when renal insufficiency allows accumulation of drug in the blood. It may also occur in pregnant women.
h. Blood disorders (neutropenia, thrombocytopenia, anemia) and allergic reactions (skin rash, urticaria, angioedema, anaphylaxis)	These effects rarely occur.
4. Observe for drug interactions	
a. Drugs that *increase* effects of tetracycline	
(1) Methoxyflurane (Penthrane)	This anesthetic plus parenteral tetracycline may cause severe nephrotoxicity and death.
(2) Sulfonamides	The combination is synergistic in certain infections such as *Nocardia* in brain abscesses, pulmonary or other lesions, lymphogranuloma venereum, and trachoma.
b. Drugs that *decrease* effects of tetracycline	
(1) Aluminum, calcium, iron or magnesium preparaions (*e.g.,* antacids, ferrous sulfate)	These metals combine with oral tetracyclines to produce insoluble, nonabsorbable compounds that are excreted in feces.
(2) Cathartics	Decrease absorption
(3) Sodium bicarbonate	Decreases absorption of tetracyclines about 50%

Nursing Actions	Rationale/Explanation
(4) Enzyme inducers (*e.g.*, barbiturates, other sedative–hypnotics, phenytoin, carbamazepine)	May increase metabolism of doxycycline
5. Teach clients	
a. Store tetracyclines in a cool, dry, dark place.	The drugs decompose with age and exposure to light, heat, and humidity.
b. Take oral tetracyclines on an empty stomach 1 hour before or 2 hours after meals.	Food decreases drug absorption.
c. If antacids, iron supplements, or vitamin preparations containing iron must be taken while tetracyclines are also taken, take them as far apart from the tetracyclines as possible (*e.g.*, 3 hours before or 2 hours after the tetracycline).	These drugs combine with tetracyclines with the result that little tetracycline is absorbed.
d. Do not take milk or milk products with tetracyclines.	Calcium in milk products combines with oral tetracyclines to produce nonabsorbable compounds.
e. Report severe nausea, vomiting, diarrhea, skin rash, or perineal itching to the physician.	These symptoms may indicate a need for changing or discontinuing tetracycline drug therapy.
f. Avoid intense or prolonged exposure to sunlight or to artificial ultraviolet light. If exposure is unavoidable, wear protective clothing and use a sunscreen lotion.	Tetracyclines, especially demeclocycline, may cause a sunburn or rash reaction.
g. If the entire prescription of oral tetracycline is not taken, discard the remaining amount.	To avoid having anyone take decomposed tetracyclines, which may have serious results

Selected References

American Medical Association (AMA) Division of Drugs: AMA Drug Evaluations, 5th ed. New York, John Wiley & Sons, 1983

Berkowitz RL, Coustan DR, Mochizuki TK: Handbook for Prescribing Medications During Pregnancy. Boston, Little, Brown & Co, 1981

Facts and Comparisons. St. Louis, J B Lippincott (Updated monthly)

Gibbs RS, Weinstein AJ: Antibiotic Therapy in Obstetrics and Gynecology. New York, John Wiley & Sons, 1981

Hansten PD: Drug Interactions: Clinical Significance of Drug–Drug Interactions, 5th ed. Philadelphia, Lea & Febiger, 1985

Malseed RT: Pharmacology: Drug Therapy and Nursing Considerations, 2d ed. Philadelphia, J B Lippincott, 1985

Rodman MJ, Karch AM, Boyd EH, Smith DW: Pharmacology and Drug Therapy in Nursing, 3rd ed. Philadelphia, J B Lippincott, 1985

Sande MA, Mandell GL: Tetracyclines, chloramphenicol, erythromycin, and miscellaneous antibacterial agents. In Gilman AG, Goodman LS, Rall TW, Murad F (eds): The Pharmacological Basis of Therapeutics, 7th ed., pp 1170–1198. New York, Macmillan, 1985

38

MACROLIDES AND LINCOSAMIDES

Description and uses

The macrolide antibiotics include erythromycin and troleandomycin. Erythromycin is commonly used; troleandomycin is rarely used. The lincosamides include lincomycin and clindamycin. Lincomycin is obsolete because clindamycin is more effective and produces fewer adverse reactions. Consequently, this chapter focuses on erythromycin and clindamycin.

Erythromycin and clindamycin have different chemical structures but similar pharmacologic and therapeutic characteristics. Their mechanisms of action and antimicrobial spectra are nearly identical, and bacteria resistant to erythromycin are usually resistant to clindamycin. They are bacteriostatic rather than bactericidal, except at high doses, and they act by inhibiting protein synthesis within the bacterial cell. They are effective against gram-positive cocci, including group A streptococci, pneumococci, and most staphylococci. They are also effective against species of *Corynebacterium, Treponema, Neisseria,* and *Mycoplasma* and against some anaerobic organisms such as *Bacteroides* and *Clostridia.* Gram-negative organisms such as *Proteus, Pseudomonas, Escherichia coli, Klebsiella,* and *Enterobacter* are usually resistant.

Erythromycin and clindamycin are widely distributed in body tissues and fluids, with the exception of cerebrospinal fluid. They are metabolized primarily in the liver and excreted in bile, with some reabsorption from the gastrointestinal tract. About 20% is excreted in urine.

Erythromycin is considered one of the safest antibiotics available. It is often used as a penicillin substitute in clients who are allergic to penicillin. Specific clinical indications include the following:

1. Suppression of intestinal bacteria before colonoscopy or bowel surgery. It is used with neomycin for this purpose.
2. Legionnaire's disease. Erythromycin is the drug of choice for this pneumonialike disease caused by a gram-negative bacillus (*Legionella pneumophila*).
3. Infections caused by *Mycoplasma pneumoniae.*
4. Prevention of whooping cough in household contacts.
5. Elimination of the diphtheria carrier state as an adjunct to diphtheria antitoxin.
6. Substitution for penicillin in prophylaxis of rheumatic fever, gonorrhea, and syphilis and in treatment of pneumococcal pneumonia, streptococcal pharyngitis, and syphilis.

Clindamycin may be useful as a penicillin substitute in clients who are allergic to penicillin and who have streptococcal, staphylococcal, or pneumococcal infections in which the causative organism is sensitive to clindamycin. It is the drug of choice in infections caused by *Bacteroides fragilis.* Since these bacteria are usually mixed with gram-negative organisms from the gynecologic or gastrointestinal tracts, clindamycin is usually given with another drug, such as gentamicin, to treat mixed infections adequately. Because of a high incidence of diarrhea and risk of pseudomembranous colitis, clindamycin is indicated only in infections in which it is clearly superior to other drugs.

Individual macrolides and lincosamides

Erythromycin is available in numerous preparations, none of which is more effective than erythromycin base or erythromycin stearate. Oral forms except the estolate salt are coated or buffered to prevent destruction by gastric acid. The estolate salt is stable in gastric acid. Topical and ophthalmic preparations are discussed in other chapters. For trade names, routes of administration, and dosage ranges, see Table 38-1.

Troleandomycin (Tao) is a macrolide antibiotic with an antibacterial spectrum similar to erythromycin. It is less active and offers no advantage over erythromycin. Thus, it is used only when infecting microorganisms are not susceptible to more effective agents.

Route and dosage ranges

Adults: PO 250–500 mg 4 times daily
Children: PO 7–12 mg/kg q6h

Clindamycin (Cleocin) is most useful in treating infections caused by anaerobic microorganisms, particularly *B. fragilis,* which are often resistant to other drugs. A major limitation to use is the occurrence of diarrhea and pseudomembranous colitis. Although these effects may occur with other antibiotics, they are more common with oral clindamycin. Clindamycin may also enhance neuromuscular blocking agents.

Routes and dosage ranges

Clindamycin hydrochloride

Adults: PO 150–300 mg q6h, up to 450 mg q6h for severe infections

TABLE 38-1. ERYTHROMYCIN PREPARATIONS

Generic name	Trade name	Usual routes and dosage ranges: Adults	Usual routes and dosage ranges: Children	Remarks
Erythromycin (base)	E-mycin, Ilotycin	PO 250–500 mg q6h. Severe infections, up to 4 g or more daily in divided doses.	PO 30–50 mg/kg/day in divided doses q6–12h. Severe infections, 100 mg/kg/day in divided doses	
Erythromycin estolate	Ilosone	PO 250 mg q6h; maximal daily dose, 4 g	Weight over 25 kg, PO same as adults Weight 10–25 kg, PO 30–50 mg/kg/day in divided doses Weight under 10 kg, PO 10 mg/kg/day in divided doses q6–12h Dosages may be doubled in severe infections.	This preparation may cause cholestatic jaundice and hepatotoxicity. It should not be used with known or suspected hepatic insufficiency.
Erythromycin ethylsuccinate	E.E.S., Pediamycin	PO 400 mg 4 times daily. Severe infections, up to 4 g or more daily in divided doses	PO 30–50 mg/kg/day in 4 divided doses q6h. Severe infections, 60–100 mg/kg/day in divided doses.	
Erythromycin gluceptate	Ilotycin gluceptate	IV 15–20 mg/kg/day, in divided doses up to 4 g daily	IV same as adults	IV administration painful, causes phlebitis, infrequently used
Erythromycin lactobionate	Erythrocin lactobionate	IV 15–20 mg/kg/day in divided doses. Severe infections, up to 4 g daily	IV same as adults	
Erythromycin stearate	Erythrocin stearate	PO 250 mg q6h or 500 mg q12h. Severe infections, up to 4 g daily	PO 30–50 mg/kg/day in 4 divided doses q6h. Severe infections, 60–100 mg/kg/day	

Children: PO 8–16 mg/kg/day in 3–4 divided doses, q6–8h, up to 20 mg/kg/day in severe infections

Clindamycin phosphate

Adults: IM 600 mg–2.7 g daily in 2–4 divided doses, q6–8h
IV 600 mg–2.7 g daily in 2–4 divided doses, up to 4.8 g daily in life-threatening infections

Children: IM, IV 15–40 mg/kg/day in 3–4 divided doses, q6–8h, up to 40 mg/kg/day in severe infections

Clindamycin palmitate hydrochloride (Cleocin Pediatric—75 mg/ml)

Children: PO 8–12 mg/kg/day in 3–4 divided doses, up to 25 mg/kg/day in very severe infections. For children weighing 10 kg or less, the minimum dose is 37.5 mg, 3 times daily.

Principles of therapy: erythromycin and clindamycin

1. Specimens for culture and sensitivity studies should be obtained before the first drug dose. This is necessary because these drugs have a narrow spectrum of antibacterial activity. They are mainly effective against gram-positive organisms, and a number of organisms are resistant. Drug therapy is often started before results are available, especially with serious infections.
2. When erythromycin is used for preoperative bowel preparation, erythromycin base, rather than estolate or stearate, is routinely used. Neomycin and erythromycin base is a useful combination because it suppresses the entire bacterial flora of the colon. However, antibiotic bowel preparation is adjunctive to mechanical bowel cleansing (*e.g.*, liquid diet, laxatives, enemas).
3. If a client receiving clindamycin develops diarrhea, stools should be checked for white blood cells, blood, and mucus, and a proctoscopy should be done to determine whether the client has pseudomembranous colitis, a potentially fatal adverse reaction. If lesions are seen on proctoscopy, the drug should be stopped immediately.
4. In renal failure, the dosage of erythromycin and clindamycin does not need reduction because the drugs are excreted primarily by extrarenal routes.
5. In moderate to severe liver disease, other drugs should be substituted or dosage reduced to prevent accumulation and toxic effects.

USE IN PREGNANCY AND LACTATION

Erythromycin is considered safe during pregnancy. Although a portion reaches the fetus, no fetal abnormalities have been reported. Clindamycin has not been established as safe during pregnancy and should be given only when infection with *B. fragilis* is suspected. Clindamycin is excreted in breast milk.

NURSING ACTIONS: ERYTHROMYCIN AND CLINDAMYCIN

Nursing Actions	*Rationale/Explanation*
1. Administer accurately	
a. With erythromycin	
(1) Give oral preparations on an empty stomach.	To aid absorption and maintenance of therapeutic serum drug levels
(2) Give intramuscular injections deeply into a large muscle mass and rotate sites.	The drug is very irritating to tissues and may cause pain, myositis, abscess, or necrosis. This route is infrequently used. Tissue irritation can be minimized by switching to an oral preparation as soon as feasible.
(3) For intravenous administration, consult the manufacturer's instructions for dissolving, diluting, and administering the drug.	The gluceptate and lactobionate salts used for intravenous injection are stable in a limited number of solutions and for a limited time. Instructions must be carefully followed to maintain drug stability and achieve therapeutic effects. Instructions differ according to the preparation and method of administration (intermittent or continuous infusion). Intravenous erythromycin is the treatment of choice for Legionnaire's disease. Otherwise, it is infrequently used.

Nursing Actions	***Rationale/Explanation***
b. With clindamycin	
(1) Give capsules with a full glass of water.	To avoid esophageal irritation
(2) Do not refrigerate reconstituted oral solution.	Refrigeration may thicken the solution and make it difficult to pour.
(3) Give intramuscular injections deeply and rotate sites. Do not give more than 600 mg in a single injection.	To decrease pain, induration, and abscess formation
(4) For intravenous administration, dilute 300 mg in at least 50 ml of any fluid and give over 10 minutes, *or* dilute 600 mg in 100 ml and give over 20 minutes. *Do not* give clindamycin undiluted or by direct injection.	Dilution decreases risks of phlebitis. Cardiac arrest has been reported with bolus injections of undiluted clindamycin.
2. Observe for therapeutic effects	
a. Decreased local and systemic signs of infection	See Chapter 33.
b. Decreased signs and symptoms of the specific infection for which the drug is being given	
3. Observe for adverse effects	
a. Nausea, vomiting, diarrhea	These are the most frequent adverse reactions and are usually rather minor with erythromycin. With clindamycin, though, they may be severe enough to require stopping the drug. Diarrhea may indicate pseudomembranous colitis, a serious adverse reaction.
b. Pain and induration at intramuscular injection sites	May be minimized by injecting deeply into a large muscle mass and rotating sites. With erythromycin, changing to oral administration as soon as feasible will also be helpful.
c. Phlebitis—heat, redness, edema, pain—at intravenous injection sites	May be decreased by diluting the drugs well, administering rather slowly, and not using the same vein more than 48 to 72 hours, if possible
d. Hepatotoxicity—nausea, vomiting, abdominal cramps, fever, leukocytosis, abnormal liver function, and possibly jaundice	Reported only with the estolate formulation of erythromycin
e. Pseudomembranous colitis—severe diarrhea, fever, stools containing neutrophils and shreds of mucous membrane	Although this problem may occur with other antibiotics, it is most common with oral clindamycin. It is attributed to superinfection caused by *Clostridium difficile*. The organism produces a toxin that kills mucosal cells and produces superficial ulcerations that are visible with sigmoidoscopy. Discontinuing the drug and giving oral vancomycin are curative measures.
f. Skin rash or urticaria	Occasionally occurs
g. Anaphylaxis	Rarely occurs
4. Observe for drug interactions	
a. Drugs that *increase* effects of erythromycin	
(1) Chloramphenicol (Chloromycetin)	The combination is effective against some strains of resistant *Staphylococcus aureus*.
(2) Streptomycin	The combination is effective against the enterococcus in bacteremia, brain abscess, endocarditis, meningitis, and urinary tract infections.
b. Drugs that significantly decrease effects of erythromycin or alter effects of clindamycin have not been reported.	

Nursing Actions	*Rationale/Explanation*
5. Teach clients	See Chapter 33.
a. Take oral erythromycin with water and minimize food intake just before or after taking the drug.	To increase drug absorption and therapeutic benefits
b. Report severe nausea, vomiting, diarrhea, skin rash, or "hives."	These are adverse reactions, and their occurrence may require discontinuation of the drug, decrease in dosage, or other alterations in therapy.

Selected References

American Medical Association (AMA) Division of Drugs: AMA Drug Evaluations, 5th ed. New York, John Wiley & Sons, 1983

Facts and Comparisons. St. Louis, J B Lippincott (Updated monthly)

Gibbs RS, Weinstein AJ: Antibiotic Therapy in Obstetrics and Gynecology. New York, John Wiley & Sons, 1981

Ginsberg M, Tager I: Practical Guide to Antimicrobial Agents. Baltimore, Williams & Wilkins, 1980

Hansten PD: Drug Interactions: Clinical Significance of Drug–Drug Interactions, 5th ed. Philadelphia, Lea & Febiger, 1985

Oral erythromycins. Med Lett Drugs Ther 27:1–3, January 4, 1985

Rodman MJ, Karch AM, Boyd EH, Smith DW: Pharmacology and Drug Therapy in Nursing, 3rd ed. Philadelphia, J B Lippincott, 1985

Sande MA, Mandell GL: Tetracyclines, chloramphenicol, erythromycin, and miscellaneous antibacterial agents. In Gilman AG, Goodman LS, Rall TW, Murad F (eds): The Pharmacological Basis of Therapeutics, 7th ed, pp 1170–1198. New York, Macmillan, 1985

Sasso SC: Erythromycin for eye prophylaxis. Maternal–Child Nursing 9:417, November–December 1984

39

MISCELLANEOUS ANTI-INFECTIVES

The drugs included in this chapter have limited clinical usefulness. In most infections other drugs are effective and less toxic. In certain circumstances, however, these drugs may be life saving. Since they have varied characteristics and indications for use, they are discussed individually.

Individual drugs

Chloramphenicol (Chloromycetin) is a broad-spectrum, bacteriostatic antibiotic that is active against most gram-positive bacteria, most gram-negative bacteria, rickettsiae, chlamydiae, and treponemes. Chloramphenicol acts by interfering with bacterial protein synthesis. It is well absorbed and diffuses well into body tissues and fluids, including cerebrospinal fluid. Low drug levels are obtained in urine, however. It is metabolized in the liver and excreted in the urine.

Chloramphenicol is rarely used in infections caused by gram-positive organisms because of the effectiveness and low toxicity of penicillins, cephalosporins, and erythromycin. However, it may be the drug of choice in several gram-negative infections. Generally, chloramphenicol should be used for serious infections for which no adequate substitute drug is available. Specific infections for which chloramphenicol may be used include the following:

1. Meningococcal, pneumococcal, or hemophilus meningitis in penicillin-allergic persons
2. Serious ampicillin-resistant infection with *Hemophilus influenzae* organisms
3. Typhoid fever
4. *Bacteroides fragilis* infections
5. Anaerobic brain abscess
6. Rickettsial infections (*e.g.,* typhus, Rocky Mountain spotted fever) when tetracyclines are contraindicated owing to hypersensitivity, reduced renal function, or pregnancy
7. Brucellosis, when tetracyclines are contraindicated
8. Acute pyelonephritis when no other effective and safer drug is available
9. Infections caused by *Klebsiella pneumoniae* that are resistant to cephalosporins and aminoglycosides

Chloramphenicol is contraindicated during late pregnancy because of placental transfer and possible adverse effects on the fetus. It is contraindicated during lactation because concentration in breast milk reaches about half the mother's serum concentration and may produce adverse effects in the infant.

Routes and dosage ranges

Adults: PO, IV 50–100 mg/kg/day, in 4 divided doses, q6h

Children and full-term infants over 2 weeks: PO 50 mg/kg/day, in 3–4 divided doses, q6–8h

Premature infants: PO 25 mg/kg/day, in 2 divided doses, q12h

Full-term infants under 2 weeks: PO 25 mg/kg/day in 4–6 divided doses, q4–6h

Nitrofurazone (Furacin) is a topical anti-infective agent that is effective against a broad spectrum of gram-positive and gram-negative organisms. Some strains of *Pseudomonas* and *Proteus* are resistant. The drug is recommended for adjunctive use to prevent bacterial infections in second- and third-degree burn wounds and skin-graft sites. The drug is available as a cream, as a gauze dressing impregnated with cream (Furacin soluble dressing), and as a powder.

Route and dosage range

Adults: Topically to burn wounds or graft sites once daily or every few days when dressings are changed

The polymyxins, **polymyxin B** (Aerosporin) and **colistin** (Coly-Mycin S), and **colistimethate** (Coly-Mycin M) are older, rarely used drugs that are bactericidal against *Pseudomonas* and other gram-negative microorganisms except *Proteus.* They act by changing permeability of the bacterial cell membrane and allowing leakage of intracellular content. They penetrate poorly into tissues. Their clinical usefulness is limited by their toxicity and the availability of effective, safer drugs (*e.g.,* aminoglycosides, carbenicillin, ticarcillin, and third-generation cephalosporins). The polymyxins are used mainly in infections caused by gram-negative bacteria, especially *Pseudomonas,* which are resistant to penicillins and aminoglycosides. These include severe urinary tract infections, infections of skin, mucous membrane, eye, and ear, and bacterial diarrhea caused by *Shigella* or other gram-negative organisms.

Polymyxins are given parenterally in systemic infections. When given orally, they act within the bowel lumen because they are poorly absorbed from the gastrointestinal tract. They are used topically, usually combined with one or two other antibacterial agents such as neomycin or bacitracin. A commonly used topical combination preparation is Neosporin. Little systemic absorption occurs with topical use.

When given parenterally, these drugs are nephrotoxic and neurotoxic. Extreme caution is indicated if the drugs are used in persons with impaired renal function.

Routes and dosage ranges

Colistimethate

Adults with normal renal function: IM, IV 2.5–5 mg/kg/day in 2–4 divided doses q6–12h; maximal daily dose, 300 mg

Children: IM, IV same as adults

Colistin sulfate

Adults: PO 5–15 mg/kg/day in 3 divided doses
Otic suspension, 3–4 drops into ear canal 3–4 times daily

Children: PO 3–5 mg/kg/day in 3 divided doses q8h

Polymyxin B sulfate

Adults: IV 15,000–25,000 units/kg/day in 1–2 infusions, each given over a 60- to 90-minute period
IM 25,000–30,000 units/kg/day in divided doses q4–6h
Intrathecal 50,000 units once daily for 3–4 days, then 50,000 units every other day
Otic solution, 3–4 drops, 3–4 times daily

Children: IV same as adults. Infants may receive up to 40,000 units/kg/day.
Intrathecal, same as adults for children over 2 years. Under 2 years, 20,000 units once daily for 3–4 days or 25,000 units once every other day. Continue with a dosage of 25,000 units once every other day.

Bacitracin (Baciguent) is effective against gram-positive organisms. Because of its high toxicity, the drug is usually administered only by the topical route. Preparations are available for dermatologic and ophthalmic use. When used in skin infections, the ointment is applied to lesions once or twice daily. For ophthalmic use, see Chapter 65.

Spectinomycin (Trobicin) is used for treatment of gonococcal infections in people who are allergic to penicillin or whose infection is caused by penicillin-resistant organisms. Safety for use in pregnancy, lactation, and for children has not been established.

Route and dosage range

Adults: IM 2 g in a single dose, or 4 g divided into 2 equal parts and administered in 2 gluteal injection sites.

Vancomycin (Vancocin) is active only against gram-positive microorganisms. It acts by inhibiting cell-wall synthesis. It is not absorbed from the gastrointestinal tract after oral administration and is usually given intravenously in systemic infections. Intramuscular injections cause pain and necrosis. When given orally, it acts within the bowel lumen. Vancomycin is mainly used in severe infections caused by penicillin-resistant staphylococci. It is also used in pseudomembranous colitis induced by antibiotics, for reduction of bacterial flora in the bowel, and in staphylococcal enterocolitis. Vancomycin is nephrotoxic and ototoxic.

Routes and dosage ranges

Adults: PO 500 mg q6h or 1 g q12h; maximal daily dose, 4 g
IV 2 g daily in 2–4 divided doses, q6–12h
Children: PO, IV 40 mg/kg/day in divided doses

Principles of therapy: chloramphenicol, polymyxins, bacitracin, spectinomycin, and vancomycin

1. Owing to their activity against a limited number of microorganisms and their relatively high incidence of toxicity, these drugs should be used only when specifically indicated by clinical and bacteriologic data.
2. Clients receiving chloramphenicol need a complete blood count, platelet count, reticulocyte count, and serum iron every 3 days. These tests are necessary for monitoring drug toxicity, since chloramphenicol may cause bone marrow depression and blood disorders.
3. Dosage of chloramphenicol must be reduced in clients with impaired liver function, in premature infants, and in full-term infants less than 2 weeks of age. In these circumstances, impaired metabolism leads to accumulation and adverse effects. If available, frequent measurements of serum drug levels are probably the most reliable guides for dosage. Therapeutic serum levels are 10 to 20 μg/ml.
4. Parenteral polymyxin B should be given only to hospitalized clients. Dosage must be reduced in the presence of renal insufficiency. The drug should be discontinued if signs and symptoms of nephrotoxicity occur.
5. Dosage of vancomycin must be reduced with impaired renal function, and serum levels should be monitored. Therapeutic serum levels are 10 to 25 μg/ml.

NURSING ACTIONS: CHLORAMPHENICOL, POLYMYXINS, BACITRACIN, SPECTINOMYCIN, VANCOMYCIN

Nursing Actions	*Rationale/Explanation*
1. Administer accurately	
a. Mix intravenous chloramphenicol in 50 to 100 ml of 5% dextrose in water and infuse over 15 to 30 minutes.	
b. Give intravenous polymyxin B in 300 to 500 ml of 5% dextrose in water as a continuous infusion.	
c. Dilute intravenous vancomycin in at least 200 ml of glucose or saline solution and rotate venipuncture sites.	To decrease pain and phlebitis at injection sites
2. Observe for therapeutic effects	See Chapter 33.
a. Decreased local and systemic signs of infection	
b. Decreased signs of the specific infection for which the drug is being given	
3. Observe for adverse effects	
a. Blood dyscrasias with chloramphenicol (1) Anemia, leukopenia, thrombocytopenia (2) Clinical signs of infection, bleeding	This is the major and most serious adverse reaction to chloramphenicol. It is caused by bone marrow depression.
b. Nephrotoxicity with polymyxin and vancomycin (1) Oliguria (2) Increased blood urea nitrogen and serum creatinine levels (3) Cells, casts, and protein in urine	

Nursing Actions	Rationale/Explanation
c. Neurotoxicity with polymyxin, vancomycin, and chloramphenicol	
(1) Ototoxicity with impaired hearing	
(2) Neuromuscular blockade with respiratory depression or apnea	The likelihood of respiratory muscle paralysis is increased when these drugs are given with others causing neuromuscular blockade (see *Observe for Drug Interactions,* below).
(3) Paresthesias, ataxia, vertigo, optic and peripheral neuritis	
4. Observe for drug interactions	
a. Drugs that *increase* effects of polymyxins	
(1) Aminoglycoside antibiotics, anesthetics, anticholinesterases, skeletal muscle relaxants	Additive neuromuscular blockade resulting in respiratory depression and apnea
(2) Cephalosporin antibiotics	Additive nephrotoxicity
(3) Sulfonamides	The combination of colistin and a sulfonammide has synergistic activity against *Pseudomonas* and *Proteus* species.
5. Teach clients	
Report bleeding (in skin, urine, stool), fever, sore throat, decreased urine output, dizziness	These reactions may indicate that the drug should be discontinued or reduced in dosage.

Selected References

American Medical Association (AMA) Division of Drugs: AMA Drug Evaluations, 5th ed. New York, John Wiley & Sons, 1983

Facts and Comparisons. St. Louis, J B Lippincott (Updated monthly)

Malseed RT: Pharmacology: Drug Therapy and Nursing Considerations, 2d ed. Philadelphia, J B Lippincott, 1985

Rodman MJ, Karch AM, Boyd EH, Smith DW: Pharmacology and Drug Therapy in Nursing, 3rd ed. Philadelphia, J B Lippincott, 1985

Sande MA, Mandell GL: Tetracyclines, chloramphenicol, erythromycin, and miscellaneous antibacterial agents. In Gilman AG, Goodman LS, Rall TW, Murad F (eds): The Pharmacological Basis of Therapeutics, 7th ed, pp 1170–1198. New York, Macmillan, 1985

40

SULFONAMIDES AND URINARY ANTISEPTICS

Description and uses

Sulfonamides were the first synthetic antibacterial agents to be developed. They are bacteriostatic against a wide range of bacteria, including pneumococci, *Neisseria, Escherichia coli, Klebsiella, Proteus, Enterobacter,* and *Hemophilus influenzae.* They act as antimetabolites of para-aminobenzoic acid (PABA), which microorganisms require to produce folic acid; folic acid, in turn, is required for the production of bacterial intracellular proteins. Sulfonamides enter into the reaction instead of PABA, compete for the enzyme involved, and cause formation of nonfunctional derivatives of folic acid. Thus, sulfonamides halt multiplication of new bacteria but do not kill mature, fully formed bacteria. With the exception of the topical sulfonamides used in burn therapy, the presence of pus, serum, or necrotic tissue interferes with sulfonamide action because these materials contain PABA. Some bacteria are able to change their metabolic pathways to use precursors or other forms of folic acid and thereby develop resistance to the antibacterial action of sulfonamides. Once resistance to one sulfonamide develops, cross resistance to others is common.

Individual sulfonamide drugs vary in extent of systemic absorption and clinical indications. Some are well absorbed and can be used in systemic infections; others are poorly absorbed and exert more local effects. In systemic infections, sulfonamides have largely been replaced by newer, more effective antibacterial agents. A major clinical indication for use is urinary tract infection caused by *E. coli* strains or by *Proteus* or *Klebsiella* species. These drugs are most useful in the treatment of acute and chronic cystitis. They are also used in asymptomatic bacteriuria. In acute pyelonephritis, other agents are usually preferred. Additional uses include ulcerative colitis and uncommon infections such as chancroid, lymphogranuloma venereum, nocardiosis, toxoplasmosis, and trachoma. Topical sulfonamides are used in prevention of burn wound infections and in treatment of ocular, vaginal, and other soft-tissue infections. For specific clinical indications of individual drugs, see Table 40-1.

Sulfonamides are contraindicated during late pregnancy and lactation and in premature and newborn infants. If an infant receives a sulfonamide by placental transfer, in breast milk, or by direct administration, kernicterus may occur because the drug displaces bilirubin from binding sites on albumin. These

(Text continues on p. 384.)

TABLE 40-1. SULFONAMIDE PREPARATIONS

Generic name	Trade name	Characteristics	Clinical indications	Usual routes and dosage ranges: Adults	Usual routes and dosage ranges: Children
Single agents					
Sulfacytine	Renoquid	A short-acting agent that is rapidly absorbed and rapidly excreted	Urinary tract infection	PO 500 mg initially, then 250 mg 4 times daily	
Sulfadiazine	Microsulfon	1. A short-acting, rapidly absorbed, rapidly excreted agent for systemic infections 2. Low solubility 3. Therapeutic blood levels are 10–15 mg/100 ml	1. Urinary tract infection 2. Prophylaxis of rheumatic fever in clients who are allergic to penicillin 3. Nocardiosis 4. Meningococcal meningitis	PO 2–4 g initially, then 2–4 g daily in 3–6 divided doses	Over 2 months of age: PO 75 mg/kg initially, then 150 mg/kg/day in 4–6 divided doses; maximal daily dose, 6 g Prophylaxis of rheumatic fever, PO 500 mg once daily for children weighing less than 30 kg, 1 g daily for children weighing over 30 kg
Sulfamethoxazole	Gantanol	1. Similar to sulfisoxazole in therapeutic effects but absorbed and excreted more slowly. More likely to produce excessive blood levels and crystalluria than sulfisoxazole. 2. An ingredient in mixtures with trimethoprim and phenazopyridine (see Combination Agents, below).	1. Systemic infections 2. Urinary tract infections	PO 2 g initially, then 1–2 g 2–3 times daily	Over 2 months of age: PO 50–60 mg/kg initially, then 30 mg/kg q12h; maximal daily dose, 75 mg/kg
Sulfamethizole	Thiosulfil	A highly soluble, rapidly absorbed, and rapidly excreted agent that is similar to sulfisoxazole in actions and uses	Urinary tract infections	PO 500 mg–1 g 3–4 times daily	Over 2 months of age: PO 30–45 mg/kg/day in 4 divided doses
Sulfasalazine	Azulfidine	1. Poorly absorbed, acts within the bowel lumen 2. Does not alter normal bacterial flora in the intestine. Effectiveness in ulcerative colitis may be due to antibacterial (sulfapyridine) and anti-inflammatory (aminosalicylic acid) metabolites.	1. Ulcerative colitis 2. Regional enteritis (Crohn's disease)	PO 3–4 g daily in divided doses initially; 2 g daily in 4 doses for maintenance; maximal daily dose, 8 g	PO 40–60 mg/kg/day in 3–6 divided doses initially, followed by 30 mg/kg/day in 4 divided doses
Sulfisoxazole	Gantrisin	1. A rapidly absorbed, rapidly excreted sulfonamide that is widely used 2. Highly soluble and less likely to cause crystalluria than most other sulfonamides 3. Available in tablets, parenteral solution, oral suspension and syrup, vaginal cream, and ophthalmic solution and ointment	1. Urinary tract infections 2. Systemic infections 3. Vaginitis 4. Ocular infections 5. Nocardiosis	PO, IV, SC 2–4 g initially, then 4–8 g daily in 3–6 divided doses Intravaginally, 2.5–5 g of vaginal cream (10%) twice daily	Over 2 months of age: PO 75 mg/kg of body weight initially, then 150 mg/kg/day in 4–6 divided doses; maximal daily dose, 6 g
Combination agents					
Sulfamethoxazole–trimethoprim	Bactrim, Septra	1. Synergistic effectiveness against many gram-positive and gram-negative organisms, including streptococci (*Strep-*	1. Acute and chronic urinary tract infections 2. Acute exacer-	Urinary tract infections, trimethoprim 160 mg and	Urinary tract infections, otitis media, and shigellosis, PO 8

TABLE 40-1. SULFONAMIDE PREPARATIONS (*Continued*)

Generic name	Trade name	Characteristics	Clinical indications	Usual routes and dosage ranges: Adults	Usual routes and dosage ranges: Children
		tococcus pneumoniae, Streptococcus viridans, Streptococcus faecalis); staphylococci (*Staphylococcus epidermidis, Staphylococcus aureus*); *E. coli; Proteus; Enterobacter; Salmonella; Shigella; Serratia; Klebsiella; Nocardia* and others. Most strains of *Pseudomonas* are resistant. 2. The two drugs have additive antibacterial effects because they interfere with different steps in bacterial synthesis and activation of folic acid, an essential nutrient. 3. The combination is less likely to produce resistant bacteria than either agent alone. 4. Oral preparations contain different amounts of the two drugs, as follows: a. "Regular" tablets contain trimethoprim 80 mg and sulfamethoxazole 400 mg. b. Double-strength tablets (*e.g.*, Bactrim D.S., Septra D.S.) contain trimethoprim 160 mg and sulfamethoxazole 800 mg. c. The oral suspension contains trimethoprim 40 mg and sulfamethoxazole 200 mg in each 5 ml. 5. An intravenous preparation contains trimethoprim 80 mg and sulfamethoxazole 400 mg in 5 ml. 6. Dosage must be reduced in renal insufficiency. 7. The preparation is contraindicated if creatinine clearance is less than 15 ml/minute	bations of chronic bronchitis 3. Acute otitis media (in children) and acute maxillary sinusitis (in adults) caused by susceptible strains of *H. influenzae* and *S. pneumoniae* 4. Shigellosis 5. Typhoid fever 6. Salmonella infections 7. Infection by *Pneumocystis carinii* (prevention and treatment) 8. Acute gonococcal urethritis 9. Intravenous preparation indicated for *P. carinii* pneumonia, severe urinary tract infections, and shigellosis	sulfamethoxazole 800 mg PO q12h for 10–14 days Shigellosis, same dose as above for 5 days Severe urinary tract infections, PO 8–10 mg (trimethoprim component)/kg/day in 2–4 divided doses, up to 14 days *P. carinii* pneumonia, 15–20 mg (trimethoprim component)/kg/day in 3–4 divided doses, q6–8h, up to 14 days	mg/kg trimethoprim and 40 mg/kg sulfamethoxazole in 2 divided doses q12h for 10 days Severe urinary tract infections, IV 8–10 mg (trimethoprim component)/kg in 2–4 divided doses q6–8h or q12h up to 14 days *P. carinii* pneumonia, IV 15–20 mg (trimethoprim component)/kg/day in 3–4 divided doses q6–8h up to 14 days
Sulfamethoxazole–phenazopyridine	Azo-Gantanol	No added benefit beyond that of the drugs given separately.	Urinary tract infection with dysuria, frequency, and urgency	PO 4 tablets initially, then 2 tablets twice daily for 2–3 days	
Sulfisoxazole–phenazopyridine	Azo-Gantrisin	Same as sulfamethoxazole–phenazopyridine	Same as sulfamethazole–phenazopyridine	PO 4–6 tablets initially, then 2 tablets 4 times daily for 2–3 days	
Topical sulfonamides					
Mafenide	Sulfamylon	1. Effective against most gram-negative and gram-positive organisms, especially *Pseudomonas*. 2. Application causes pain and burning. 3. Mafenide is absorbed systemically and may produce metabolic acidosis.	Prevention of bacterial colonization and infection of severe burn wounds	Topical application to burned area, once or twice daily, in a thin layer	Same as adults

TABLE 40-1. SULFONAMIDE PREPARATIONS (*Continued*)

Generic name	Trade name	Characteristics	Clinical indications	Usual routes and dosage ranges: Adults	Usual routes and dosage ranges: Children
Silver sulfadiazine	Silvadene	1. Effective against most *Pseudomonas* species, the most common pathogen in severe burn sepsis, *E. coli, Klebsiella, Proteus,* staphylococci, and streptococci 2. Application is painless. 3. Does not cause electrolyte or acid–base imbalances 4. Significant amounts may be absorbed systemically with large burned areas and prolonged use.	Same as mafenide. Usually the preferred drug.	Same as mafenide	Same as mafenide

drugs are also contraindicated in clients who are allergic to them.

Urinary antiseptics are drugs used only to prevent or treat urinary tract infections. They are not used in systemic infections because they do not attain therapeutic plasma levels. They are potentially bactericidal for sensitive organisms in the kidneys and bladder because the drugs are concentrated in renal tubules and produce high levels in urine.

Individual drugs

Sulfonamides are listed in Table 40-1.

URINARY ANTISEPTICS

Cinoxacin (Cinobac) is a synthetic antibacterial agent used for treatment of initial and recurrent urinary tract infections in adults. It is effective against most gram-negative bacteria that commonly cause urinary tract infections (*E. coli* and *Klebsiella, Enterobacter,* and *Proteus* species). It exerts bactericidal effects by inhibiting bacterial replication of deoxyribonucleic acid. Thus far, the incidence of bacterial resistance to the drug has been low.

Route and dosage range

Adults: PO 1 g daily, in 2–4 divided doses, for 7–14 days

Methenamine mandelate (Mandelamine) and **methenamine hippurate** (Hiprex) are salts of methenamine that have antibacterial activity only when urine *p*H is acidic. At a urine *p*H below 5.5, the drugs are degraded to form formaldehyde, which is the antibacterial component. Acidification of urine is a prerequisite to methenamine effectiveness. Supplemental drug therapy with ascorbic acid or other urinary acidifiers is usually needed. Formaldehyde is active against several gram-positive and gram-negative organisms, including *E. coli.* It is most useful for long-term suppression of bacteria in chronic, recurrent infections. It should generally not be used in acute infections because other anti-infective drugs are more effective. It should also not be used to prevent urinary tract infections in clients with in-dwelling urinary catheters. Several hours are required for methenamine to be hydrolyzed into formaldehyde and become bacteriostatic. Because catheters continuously empty the bladder, methenamine hydrolyzes in the urine drainage bag rather than the bladder. Methenamine is contraindicated in renal failure.

Route and dosage range

Methenamine mandelate

Adults: PO 1 g 4 times daily

Children: PO 500 mg 4 times daily for ages 6–12 years; 50 mg/kg/day, in 3 divided doses, for ages under 6 years

Methenamine hippurate

Adults: PO 1 g twice daily

Children: PO 500 mg–1 g twice daily

Nalidixic acid (NegGram) is effective against most gram-negative organisms that cause urinary tract infections, including *E. coli* and *Proteus, Klebsiella,* and *Enterobacter* species. Bacterial resistance to this drug may develop rapidly (within 48 to 72 hours).

Route and dosage ranges

Adults: PO 4 g daily in 4 divided doses for 1–2 weeks, then 2 g daily if long-term treatment is required
Children: PO 55 mg/kg/day in 4 divided doses, reduced to 33 mg/kg/day for long-term use in children under 12 years of age. Contraindicated in infants under 3 months of age

Nitrofurantoin (Furadantin, Macrodantin) has a wide spectrum of antibacterial activity against most gram-positive and gram-negative organisms, including *E. coli*, streptococci, staphylococci, and *Klebsiella, Enterobacter, Salmonella, Shigella,* and some *Proteus* species. It is ineffective against *Pseudomonas* and *Proteus mirabilis.* Despite its broad spectrum, nitrofurantoin is generally not used in systemic infections. It is used primarily for short-term treatment of urinary tract infections or long-term suppression of bacteria in chronic, recurrent urinary tract infections. An advantage of nitrofurantoin is that bacterial resistance develops slowly and to a limited degree. In contrast to most anti-infective drugs, nitrofurantoin's effectiveness is increased when given with or just after food intake. Macrodantin, a macrocrystalline form of the drug, reportedly causes fewer gastrointestinal adverse effects than Furadantin, a microcrystalline form. Nitrofurantoin is contraindicated in severe renal disease.

Route and dosage ranges

Adults: PO 50–100 mg 4 times daily
Prophylaxis of recurrent urinary tract infection in women, 50–100 mg at bedtime
Children: 5–7 mg/kg/day, in 4 divided doses, to children over 3 months of age

OTHER DRUGS USED IN URINARY TRACT INFECTIONS

Phenazopyridine (Pyridium) is an azo dye that acts as a urinary tract analgesic. It relieves symptoms of dysuria, burning, and frequency and urgency of urination, which occur with cystitis or urethritis. It has no anti-infective action. It turns urine orange-red, which may be mistaken for blood. It is contraindicated in renal insufficiency and severe hepatitis. It is available alone or in fixed-dose combinations with sulfamethoxazole and sulfisoxazole. When indicated, phenazopyridine is better given alone. It can usually be discontinued after 2 to 3 days, whereas the sulfonamide component usually must be given longer.

Route and dosage range

Adults: PO 200 mg 3 times daily after meals
Children 6–12 years of age: PO 12 mg/kg/day, in 3 divided doses

Trimethoprim (Proloprim, Trimpex) is a folate antagonist drug with antibacterial effects. For some time, it was marketed only in fixed-dose combination with sulfamethoxazole (see Table 40-1). It is now available as a single agent for treatment of urinary tract infections caused by susceptible strains of *E. coli, Proteus, Klebsiella,* and *Enterobacter.* It is contraindicated in clients with hypersensitivity to trimethoprim or with megaloblastic anemia due to folate deficiency. Rash and pruritus are the most common adverse effects. Nausea, vomiting, glossitis, thrombocytopenia, leukopenia, anemia, and methemoglobinemia occasionally occur.

Route and dosage range

Adults: PO 100 mg q12h for 10 days

Principles of therapy: sulfonamides and urinary antiseptics

1. With systemically absorbed sulfonamides, an initial loading dose may be given to produce therapeutic blood levels (12 to 15 mg/100 ml) more rapidly. The amount is usually twice that of the maintenance dose.
2. Urine *p*H is important in drug therapy with sulfonamides and urinary antiseptics.
   a. With sulfonamide therapy, alkaline urine increases drug solubility and helps prevent crystalluria. It also increases the rate of sulfonamide excretion and the concentration of sulfonamide in the urine. The urine can be alkalinized by giving sodium bicarbonate. Alkalinization is less likely to be needed with sulfisoxazole, since the drug is highly soluble, with the sulfonamides used to treat intestinal infections, since they are not absorbed systemically to any significant extent, or with topical agents used for burn wounds, since there is little systemic absorption.
   b. With mandelamine therapy, urine *p*H must be acidic (*p*H below 5.5) for the drug to be effective. At higher *p*H, mandelamine does not hydrolyze to formaldehyde, the antibacterial component. Urine can be acidified by concomitant administration of ascorbic acid.

3. Urine cultures and sensitivity tests are indicated in suspected urinary tract infection because of the great variability in possible pathogens and in their susceptibility to antibacterial drugs, even within the same species or organism. Best results are obtained by using drug therapy indicated by the microorganisms isolated from each client.

NURSING INTERVENTIONS

1. During sulfonamide therapy, sufficient fluids should be taken to produce a urine output of at least 1200 to 1500 ml daily. A high fluid intake decreases the risk of crystalluria (precipitation of crystals in the urine).
2. Use measures to prevent urinary tract infections.
   a. Teach women to cleanse themselves from the urethral area toward the rectum after voiding or defecating to avoid contamination of the urethral area with bacteria from the vagina and rectum. Also, voiding after sexual intercourse probably helps cleanse the lower urethra and prevent urinary tract infection.
   b. Avoid urinary catheterization when possible. If catheterization is necessary, use sterile technique. The urinary tract is normally sterile except for the lower one third of the urethra. Introduction of any bacteria into the bladder may cause infection.
      (1) A single catheterization has about a 6% chance of introducing infection. With in-dwelling catheters, bacteria colonize the bladder and produce infection within 2 to 3 weeks, even with meticulous care.
      (2) When in-dwelling catheters must be used, measures to decrease incidence and severity of urinary tract infection include the following: using a closed drainage system; keeping the perineal area clean; forcing fluids, if not contraindicated, to maintain a dilute urine; and removing the catheter as soon as possible, since infection occurs if the catheter is in place more than a few days. In addition, do not disconnect the system and irrigate the catheter unless obstruction is suspected. *Never* raise the urinary drainage bag above bladder level.
3. Force fluids in anyone with urinary tract infection unless contraindicated. Bacteria do not multiply as rapidly in dilute urine. In addition, emptying the bladder frequently allows it to refill with uninfected urine. This decreases the bacterial population of the bladder.

NURSING ACTIONS: SULFONAMIDES AND URINARY ANTISEPTICS

Nursing Actions	*Rationale/Explanation*
1. Administer accurately	
a. Give oral sulfonamide preparations before or after meals.	Food in the stomach may delay but does not prevent drug absorption. Giving the drugs before meals probably improves absorption. However, giving with food decreases gastric irritation, anorexia, nausea, and vomiting. Therefore, time of administration in relation to meals can be altered according to the client's tolerance.
b. Consult the manufacturer's instructions before giving any sulfonamide parenterally, including intravenous trimethoprim–sulfamethoxazole.	Parenteral use is infrequent, and available parenteral preparations require specific administration techniques.
c. Give nitrofurantoin with or after meals.	Food decreases nausea, vomiting, and diarrhea.
d. Apply a thin layer of topical sulfonamides to burn wounds with a sterile gloved hand after the surface has been cleansed of previously applied medication.	Burn wounds can be cleansed in several ways, including immersion in Hubbard tank or whirlpool, shower or tub bath, and spot cleansing with sterile saline, 4 × 4 gauze pads, and gloves.
2. Observe for therapeutic effects	
a. Decreased symptoms of urinary tract infection—less burning on urination, decreased frequency and urgency of voiding, less fever, sterile urinalysis report	

Nursing Actions	Rationale/Explanation
b. Less diarrhea with ulcerative colitis or bacillary dysentery	
c. Lack of fever, wound drainage in burn wounds, evidence of wound healing	Topical sulfonamides for burn therapy are used to prevent rather than treat infection.
3. Observe for adverse effects	
a. Anorexia, nausea, and vomiting	These gastrointestinal symptoms commonly occur with sulfonamides and urinary tract antiseptics, owing to gastric irritation or stimulation of the vomiting center in the medulla.
b. Hypersensitivity—skin rash, fever, urticaria, pruritus, serum sickness, and occasional anaphylaxis	This is more likely to occur with sulfonamides than urinary tract antiseptics. Sensitization may occur with exposure to a sulfonamide drug or to sulfonamide derivatives such as thiazide diuretics and oral antidiabetic drugs. The drug should be discontinued if a skin rash appears.
c. Nephrotoxicity—oliguria, crystalluria, hematuria	This occurred more often with older, less soluble sulfonamides when drug crystals would form and damage tissues in the urinary tract. Most sulfonamides currently used are relatively soluble. However, adequate fluid intake to produce at least 1200 to 1500 ml of urine daily may prevent crystalluria. Also, alkalinizing urine increases drug solubility and prevents crystals from forming. Nephrotoxicity with urinary antiseptics is uncommon.
d. Blood dyscrasias—hemolytic anemia, agranulocytosis, aplastic anemia, and others	These are uncommon but potentially life threatening.
e. Central nervous system effects—headache, dizziness, lethargy, and mental depression	These may occur with sulfonamides.
4. Observe for drug interactions	
a. Drugs that *increase* effects of sulfonamides	
(1) Alkalinizing agents (*e.g.,* sodium bicarbonate)	Increase rate of urinary excretion, thereby raising levels of sulfonamides in the urinary tract and increasing effectiveness in urinary tract infections.
(2) Methenamine compounds, urinary acidifiers, paraldehyde	These drugs increase the risk of nephrotoxicity. They should *not* be used with sulfonamides. They may cause precipitation of sulfonamide with resultant blockage of renal tubules.
(3) Tetracyclines	The combination of a tetracycline plus a sulfonamide is preferred treatment of *Nocardia* in brain abscess and lesions of the lungs and other organs, against organisms causing lymphogranuloma venereum, and against organisms causing trachoma. These infections are rather rare.
(4) Salicylates (*e.g.,* aspirin), nonsteroidal anti-inflammatory agents (*e.g.,* ibuprofen, indomethacin), oral anticoagulants, phenytoin, methotrexate	Increase toxicity of sulfonamides by displacing sulfonamides from plasma protein-binding sites, thereby increasing plasma levels of free drug
b. Drugs that *decrease* effects of sulfonamides	
(1) Alkalinizing agents (*e.g.,* sodium bicarbonate)	Alkalinizing agents decrease gastrointestinal absorption of sulfonamides. This results in decreased therapeutic effectiveness in systemic illness. The agents also decrease crystalluria, an adverse effect, by alkalinizing the urine and increasing sulfonamide solubility.
(2) Local anesthetics containing PABA (*e.g.,* procaine, benzocaine)	Increasing the concentration of PABA decreases activity of sulfonamides.
c. Drugs that alter effects of nitrofurantoin	
(1) Antacids, alkalinizing agents	May reduce the effectiveness of nitrofurantoin; antacids may impair gastrointestinal absorption of nitrofurantoin

Nursing Actions	Rationale/Explanation
(2) Acidifying agents	Increase antibacterial activity of nitrofurantoin by decreasing renal excretion. Nitrofurantoin is most active against organisms causing urinary tract infection when urine *p*H is 5.5 or less.
(3) Probenecid	Decreases renal clearance of nitrofurantoin and may thereby increase its toxicity
d. Drugs that alter effects of methenamine	
(1) Acetazolamide (Diamox)	Decreases effect by making urine alkaline. Methenamine requires an acidic *p*H (5.5 or less) for releasing formaldehyde, the antibacterial product of methenamine breakdown.
(2) Acidifying agents	Increase effects by increasing the rate of liberation of formaldehyde.
(3) Alkalinizing agents	Decrease effect by decreasing conversion to formaldehyde
(4) Sulfonamides	See 4a(2), above.
5. Teach clients	
a. Take medication for the full time prescribed.	Sulfonamides and urinary antiseptics are bacteriostatic, and bacterial resistance develops rather readily. Therefore, to be most effective and decrease resistance, these drugs should not be stopped when symptoms subside.
b. Take medications before meals; if nausea and vomiting occur, take them with meals.	Absorption from the gastrointestinal tract is probably better if the drugs are taken on an empty stomach. However, symptoms of gastrointestinal distress often occur and can be prevented or minimized by taking the medications with food.
c. Drink at least 3 quarts of fluid daily, if not contraindicated.	With sulfonamides, an adequate fluid intake and a urine output of at least 1500 ml/day reduce or prevent crystals from forming and damaging the urinary tract. With urinary tract infections, fluids decrease the bacterial population of the urinary tract.
d. Report skin rash, fever, sore throat, abnormal bleeding (blood in urine, nose bleed, bruises).	These symptoms may indicate adverse drug effects and the need to discontinue or reduce dosage of the drugs.
e. With phenazopyridine, inform the client that the drug turns urine orange-red.	To prevent the client from mistaking the discolored urine for blood from the urinary tract
f. Use measures to prevent urinary tract infection (especially in women).	Urinary tract infection is much more common in women. Incidence can be reduced by keeping the perineal area clean, cleansing from the urethra toward the rectum, and urinating after sexual intercourse.

Selected References

American Medical Association (AMA) Division of Drugs: AMA Drug Evaluations, 5th ed. New York, John Wiley & Sons, 1983

Facts and Comparisons. St Louis, J B Lippincott (Updated monthly)

Hansten PD: Drug Interactions: Clinical Significance of Drug–Drug Interactions, 5th ed. Philadelphia, Lea & Febiger, 1985

Hughes WT: Trimethoprim–sulfamethoxazole. Pediatr Clin North Am 30:27–30, February 1983

Malseed RT: Pharmacology: Drug Therapy and Nursing Considerations, 2d ed. Philadelphia. J B Lippincott, 1985

Mandell GL, Sande MA: Sulfonamides, trimethoprim–sulfamethoxazole, and agents for urinary tract infections. In Gilman AG, Goodman LS, Rall TW, Murad F (eds): The Pharmacological Basis of Therapeutics, 7th ed, pp 1095–1114. New York, Macmillan, 1985

41

ANTITUBERCULAR DRUGS

Description and uses

Tuberculosis is an infectious disease that usually affects the respiratory system but may involve the kidneys, meninges, bone, adrenal glands, and gastrointestinal tract. It is caused by *Mycobacterium tuberculosis,* the tubercle bacillus. These organisms have unique characteristics that influence the disease process and drug therapy. They multiply slowly, they may lie dormant within the body for many years, encapsulated in calcified tubercles, they resist phagocytosis and survive within phagocytic cells, and they rapidly develop resistance to single-drug therapies.

The only effective treatment for tuberculosis is drug therapy. Antitubercular drugs are bacteriostatic, with the exceptions of isoniazid and rifampin. Drug therapy is long term (9 to 36 months), and multiple drugs are required to inhibit emergence of drug-resistant bacteria. These factors may contribute to lack of client compliance with prescribed medication regimens.

Two developments may promote increased compliance. One of these is being called short-course chemotherapy (SCC) and involves administration of isoniazid and rifampin for 9 months in selected clients. The other development involves twice-weekly drug administration for a minimum of 12 months for clients who are unable or unwilling to administer their own medications on a daily basis.

Antitubercular drugs are subdivided into primary and secondary drugs. Primary drugs are used in initial treatment of tuberculosis; secondary drugs are used when organisms develop resistance to primary drugs. Compared to primary drugs, secondary drugs are less effective or more toxic or both.

Individual antitubercular drugs

PRIMARY DRUGS

Isoniazid (INH) (Laniazid, Nydrazid) is the single most important antitubercular drug. It is thought to act by inhibiting intracellular protein synthesis in the tubercle bacillus. It is well absorbed from the gastrointestinal tract and widely distributed in body tissues and fluids, including cerebrospinal fluid.

Isoniazid is acetylated in the liver to acetylisoniazid, which is more efficiently excreted by the kidneys. Metabolism of INH is genetically determined; some people are "slow acetylators" and others are "rapid acetylators." The rate of acetylation in a person may be significant in determining response to INH. Slow acetylators have less N-acetyl transferase, the acetylating enzyme, in their livers. In these clients, INH is more likely to accumulate to toxic concentrations, and the development of peripheral neuropathy is more likely. However, there is no significant difference in the clinical effectiveness of isoniazid. Rapid acetylators may require unusually high doses of isoniazid. They may also be more susceptible to serious liver injury related to the formation of hepatotoxic metabolites.

Isoniazid is used for both prevention and treatment of tuberculosis. Chemoprophylaxis is indicated in household contacts and other close contacts of clients with recently diagnosed tuberculosis. It is also indicated in clients who are recent converters from negative to positive skin tests; in those who have leukemia, lymphoma, or silicosis; or in those who are receiving corticosteroids or other immunosuppressive drugs. Chemoprophylaxis with INH is contraindicated in clients with hepatic disease, in those who have had reactions to the drug, and in pregnant women. Isoniazid is given alone for chemoprophylaxis, usually 3 months for contacts with negative skin tests and 12 months for people with positive skin tests.

In chemotherapy of active tuberculosis, INH should be part of any drug regimen. It is always used in conjunction with one or two other primary antitubercular drugs to inhibit emergence of drug-resistant organisms.

Routes and dosage ranges

Adults: Treatment of active disease, PO, IM 4–5 mg/kg, up to 300 mg total, daily in a single dose
Chemoprophylaxis, PO, IM 300 mg/day in a single dose for 3–12 months
SCC, PO, IM 300 mg/day for 9 months; or 300 mg/day for 1 month, followed by 900 mg twice weekly for 8 months
Disseminated tuberculosis or pulmonary disease resulting from atypical mycobacteria, PO, IM 10–20 mg/kg/day

Children: Treatment of active disease, PO, IM 10–20 mg/kg/day, up to 300–500 mg total daily dose
Chemoprophylaxis, 10 mg/kg/day in a single dose, up to 300 mg total daily dose, for 3–12 months
SCC, 10 mg/kg/day (maximal daily dose, 300 mg) for 9 months

Ethambutol (Myambutol) is a tuberculostatic drug that has largely replaced para-aminosalicylic acid (PAS) as a primary agent because it produces fewer adverse effects. Ethambutol inhibits synthesis of ribonucleic acid and thus interferes with mycobacterial protein metabolism. It is well absorbed from the gastrointestinal tract, even when given with food. The extent of tissue distribution is not clear except that diffusion into cerebrospinal fluid is limited. It is excreted primarily by the kidneys, either unchanged or as metabolites. Mycobacterial resistance to ethambutol develops slowly.

Dosage is determined by body weight because no practical method of measuring serum drug levels is available. Also, dosage is changed during treatment if significant changes in body weight occur. Dosage must be reduced with impaired renal function. To obtain therapeutic serum levels, the total daily dose is given at one time.

Route and dosage ranges

Adults: Initial treatment, PO 15 mg/kg/day in a single dose
Retreatment, 25 mg/kg/day for 2 months, then 15 mg/kg/day

Children: PO same as adult dosage if over 13 years of age; not recommended for children under 13

Rifampin (Rifadin) is a semisynthetic antibacterial drug that inhibits growth of many gram-positive and gram-negative bacteria, including *Escherichia coli, Pseudomonas, Proteus, Klebsiella, Staphylococcal aureus,* and meningococci, as well as mycobacteria causing tuberculosis. It acts by causing defective, nonfunctional proteins to be produced by the bacterial cell. It is also able to penetrate intact cells and kill intracellular bacteria. This unique ability contributes to its effectiveness in treating tuberculosis because mycobacteria are harbored within host cells. Despite rifampin's effectiveness against other microorganisms, its use is largely limited to treatment of tuberculosis. This limitation is caused by the ability of many bacteria to become rifampin resistant. Rifampin is well absorbed following oral administration and diffuses well into body tissues and fluids, with highest concentrations being obtained in the liver, lungs, gallbladder, and kidneys. It is metabolized in the liver and excreted primarily in bile; a small amount is excreted in urine. The drug discolors various body secretions red-orange including urine, tears, saliva, sputum, perspiration, and feces.

Rifampin is always used with other drugs to prevent the occurrence of drug-resistant organisms. Rifampin and INH in combination eliminate tuberculosis bacilli from sputum and produce clinical improvement faster than any other drug regimen. However, some authorities recommend that rifampin be reserved for use in drug-resistant or life-threatening tuberculosis. Rifampin is currently the drug of choice to treat INH-resistant tuberculosis, since it is both bactericidal and less toxic than other available drugs. Rifampin is more expensive than other antitubercular drugs.

Rifampin is a drug of choice for prophylaxis of meningitis in close contacts of clients with meningitis. It is being investigated for use in other infections as well, including those caused by some staphylococci, atypical mycobacteria, viruses, and fungi.

Route and dosage ranges

Adults: Treatment of active disease, PO 600 mg or 10–20 mg/kg/day, in a single dose
SCC, PO 600 mg daily for 9 months; or 600 mg daily for 1 month followed by 600 mg twice weekly for 8 months
Children: Treatment of active disease, PO 10–20 mg/kg once daily; maximal daily dose, 600 mg
SCC, 10–20 mg/kg/day, up to 600 mg daily

Streptomycin is an aminoglycoside antibacterial drug that is effective against a variety of gram-positive and gram-negative organisms as well as the tubercle bacillus. It is widely distributed in body tissues, including tubercular cavities and caseous granulomas. Like other aminoglycosides, streptomycin may cause damage to the kidneys and the eighth cranial nerve. Because of its toxicity and the development of effective oral antitubercular drugs, streptomycin is used less often than formerly for treatment of tuberculosis. When used for this purpose, it is always combined with other drugs to inhibit emergence of drug-resistant tubercle bacilli.

Route and dosage range

Adults: IM 1 g daily for 2 months, then 1–2 g 3 times weekly

SECONDARY DRUGS

Para-aminosalicylic acid (PAS), capreomycin (Capastat), **cycloserine** (Seromycin), **ethionamide** (Trecator-SC), **kanamycin** (Kantrex), and **pyrazinamide** are diverse drugs that share tuberculostatic properties. These secondary antitubercular drugs are generally less effective or more toxic than primary drugs. They are indicated for use only when other agents are contraindicated or in disease caused by drug-resistant organisms. They must be given concurrently with other tuberculostatic drugs to inhibit emergence of resistant mycobacteria.

Routes and dosage ranges

Para-aminosalicylic acid, sodium aminosalicylate

Adults: PO 14–16 g daily in 2–3 divided doses
Children: PO 275–420 mg/kg/day in 3–4 divided doses

Capreomycin

Adults: IM (deep) 20 mg/kg (about 1 g) daily for 2–4 weeks, then 1 g 2–3 times weekly for 6–12 months or longer
Children: No dosage established

Cycloserine

Adults: PO 10 mg/kg/day in 2 divided doses
Children: No dosage established

Ethionamide

Adults: PO 0.5–1 g/day in 3 divided doses
Children: PO 12–15 mg/kg/day, in 3 divided doses; maximal daily dose, 750 mg

Kanamycin

Adults: IM (deep), 15 mg/kg (maximal dose, 1 g) 3–5 times weekly
Children: Same as for adults

Pyrazinamide

Adults: PO 20–35 mg/kg/day in 3–4 doses; maximal daily dose, 3 g
Children: No dosage established

Principles of therapy: antitubercular drugs

ASSESSMENT GUIDELINES

Assess for current or potential tuberculosis.

1. For current disease, clinical manifestations include fatigue, weight loss, anorexia, malaise, fever, and a productive cough. In early phases, however, there may be no symptoms. If available, check diagnostic test reports for indications of tuberculosis (chest x-ray, tuberculin skin test, sputum smear and culture).
2. For potential tuberculosis, identify high-risk clients. These include the following: those who are close contacts of someone with active tuberculosis; those who are elderly or undernourished; those who have diabetes mellitus, silicosis, Hodgkin's disease, or leukemia; those who are alcoholics; and those who are receiving immunosuppressive drugs. Most new cases of tuberculosis develop in people previously infected.

HOSPITALIZATION AND ISOLATION GUIDELINES

1. To prevent the spread of tuberculosis, people with newly diagnosed or active disease should be hospitalized initially. During hospitalization, diagnostic tests can be done, drug therapy can be closely monitored, and client education about the disease and self-care measures can be implemented. In addition, the client can be isolated until drug therapy

renders him or her noninfectious, usually within 2 or 3 weeks.

2. Hospital policies vary regarding isolation techniques. The client may be taught to cover the mouth and nose when coughing, to expectorate into tissues, to dispose of tissues properly, and to wear a mask when outside the room. Personnel may need to wear masks only if clients are unable to handle secretions correctly. Frequent and thorough handwashing is necessary for both clients and personnel.

DRUG REGIMENS

Drug therapy for tuberculosis differs in several respects from drug therapy for other bacterial infections. Some guidelines include the following:

1. Sputum culture and susceptibility reports require 3 to 6 weeks because the tubercle bacillus multiplies slowly. Consequently, initial drug therapy is based on other factors, such as the extent of disease and whether the client has previously received antitubercular drugs.
2. Multiple drugs are required to inhibit emergence of drug-resistant organisms. Isoniazid and one or two other primary drugs are drugs of choice. The most intensive treatment is given during the first 6 to 12 weeks to decrease the bacterial population rapidly.
3. Duration of drug therapy varies with extent of disease and clinical response but averaged about 18 to 36 months until 1980. At that time, the American Thoracic Society and the Centers for Disease Control recommended SCC for selected persons, which involves at least 9 months of treatment with INH and rifampin, the two most effective antitubercular drugs and the only ones that are bactericidal rather than bacteriostatic. In one regimen, INH and rifampin are given daily for 9 months. In another, the drugs are given daily for 1 month, then twice weekly for 12 months. The latter regimen may be used if the client is unreliable in self-administration of drugs. However, SCC is not recommended in clients with extrapulmonary tuberculosis, drug-resistant disease, or immunosuppressive diseases.
4. Whatever the drug therapy regimen, close supervision is needed during treatment to monitor response and compliance and during the year after completion of drug therapy, since most relapses occur during that time.

EFFECTS OF DRUGS ON URINE GLUCOSE TESTS

Streptomycin, INH, and aminosalicylic acid may produce false-positive tests for glycosuria when urine is tested with copper-containing reagents such as Clinitest tablets. Urine can be tested accurately with glucose oxidase reagents such as Tes-tape or Clinistix.

NURSING ACTIONS: ANTITUBERCULAR DRUGS

Nursing Actions	*Rationale/Explanation*
1. Administer accurately	
a. Give INH, ethambutol, and rifampin in a single dose, once daily.	A single dose with the resulting higher blood levels is more effective. Also, fewer doses may increase client compliance with drug therapy.
b. Give PAS and ethionamide with food.	To minimize nausea, vomiting, and diarrhea
c. Give rifampin 1 hour before or 2 hours after a meal.	Food delays absorption.
d. Give capreomycin, kanamycin, streptomycin, and parenteral INH by deep intramuscular injection into a large muscle mass, and rotate injection sites.	To decrease local pain and tissue irritation
2. Observe for therapeutic effects	Therapeutic effects are usually apparent within the first 2 or 3 weeks of drug therapy.
a. Clinical improvement (1) Decreased cough, sputum, fever, night sweats, and fatigue	

Nursing Actions	Rationale/Explanation
(2) Increased appetite, weight, and feeling of well being	
b. Negative sputum smear and culture	
c. Improvement in chest x-ray studies	
3. Observe for adverse effects	
a. Nausea, vomiting, diarrhea	These symptoms are likely to occur with any of the oral antitubercular drugs and are usually most severe with PAS.
b. Neurotoxicity	
(1) Eighth cranial nerve damage—vertigo, tinnitus, hearing loss	A major adverse reaction to streptomycin and kanamycin
(2) Optic nerve damage—decreased vision and color discrimination	The major adverse reaction to ethambutol
(3) Peripheral neuritis—tingling, numbness, paresthesias	Often occurs with INH but can be prevented by administering pyridoxine (vitamin B_6). Also may occur with ethambutol.
(4) Central nervous system changes—confusion, convulsions, depression	More often associated with INH but similar changes may occur with ethambutol
c. Hepatotoxicity—increased serum glutamic-oxaloacetic transaminase (SGOT), serum glutamic-pyruvic transaminase (SGPT), and serum bilirubin; jaundice; and other symptoms of hepatitis	May occur with INH, especially if the client is also receiving rifampin or already has liver damage
d. Nephrotoxicity—increased blood urea nitrogen and serum creatinine; cells in urine; oliguria	A major adverse reaction to streptomycin or kanamycin
e. Hypersensitivity—fever, tachycardia, anorexia, and malaise are early symptoms. If the drug is not discontinued, exfoliative dermatitis, hepatitis, renal abnormalities, and blood dyscrasias may occur.	Hypersensitivity reactions are more likely to occur between the third and eighth weeks of drug therapy. Early detection and drug discontinuance are necessary to prevent progressive worsening of the client's condition. Severe reactions can be fatal.
4. Observe for drug interactions	
a. Drugs that *increase* effects of antitubercular drugs Other antitubercular drugs	Potentiate antitubercular effects. These drugs are always used in combination of two or more for treatment of tuberculosis. For chemoprophylaxis, INH is used alone.
b. Drugs that alter the effects of INH	
(1) Alcohol and oral antacids *decrease* effects	Alcohol induces hepatic enzymes, which accelerate the rate of isoniazid metabolism and may increase the likelihood of toxicity. Oral antacids may decrease absorption of oral INH.
(2) Disulfiram	May cause behavioral changes and impairments in coordination
(3) Pyridoxine (vitamin B_6)	Pyridoxine decreases peripheral neuritis, a common adverse effect of INH, and is usually combined with INH for this purpose.
(4) Sympathomimetics	May result in increased blood pressure owing to the monoamine oxidase–inhibitory activity of INH.
c. Drugs that alter effects of rifampin Halothane and INH *increase* effects	Additive risk of hepatotoxicity
d. Drugs that alter effects of streptomycin	See Chapter 36.
5. Teach clients	
a. About the disease process and the necessity for long-term treatment and follow up	This is extremely important for both the person and the community, since lack of knowledge and failure to comply with the

Nursing Actions	***Rationale/Explanation***
	therapeutic regimen lead to disease progression and spread. Many helpful pamphlets, written for the general public, may be obtained from the local chapter of the American Lung Association and given to clients and their families. These should not be substituted for personal contact, however.
b. Measures to prevent spread of tuberculosis	
(1) Cover mouth and nose when coughing or sneezing.	This prevents the expulsion of droplet nuclei containing the tubercle bacillus into the surrounding air, where it can be inhaled by and infect others.
(2) Cough and expectorate sputum into at least two layers of tissue, place used tissues in a waterproof bag, and dispose of the bag, preferably by burning.	
(3) Wash hands after coughing or sneezing.	
c. Report adverse reactions to drug therapy	
(1) Severe gastrointestinal problems	
(2) Yellowing of sclera, dark urine, clay-colored stools	Characteristics of jaundice and possible liver damage
(3) Any changes in vision or hearing	May indicate need to change dosage or discontinue drugs
(4) Numbness or tingling of hands or feet	May indicate peripheral neuritis, which can usually be controlled by taking an additional medication, that is, pyridoxine (vitamin B_6)
(5) Any other changes in usual patterns, such as drowsiness, dizziness, decreased urine output, skin rash, or fever	These may indicate adverse reactions to drugs but must be evaluated by the physician, since they may be caused by other conditions as well.
d. If taking PAS, discard any tablets that turn brownish or purplish.	PAS deteriorates rapidly in contact with water, heat, and sunlight. Deterioration is manifested by discoloration of the tablets.
e. If taking rifampin, urine, tears, saliva, and other body secretions become red. Discoloration of secretions is harmless, except that contact lenses may be permanently stained.	

Selected References

American Medical Association (AMA) Division of Drugs: AMA Drug Evaluations, 5th ed. New York, John Wiley & Sons, 1983

Coleman DA: TB: The disease that's not dead yet. RN 47:48–57, September 1984

Facts and Comparisons. St. Louis, J B Lippincott (Updated monthly)

Mandell GL, Sande MA: Drugs used in the chemotherapy of tuberculosis and leprosy. In Gilman AG, Goodman LS, Rall TW, Murad F (eds): The Pharmacological Basis of Therapeutics, 7th ed, pp 1199–1218. New York, Macmillan, 1985

Reed MD, Blumer JL: Clinical pharmacology of antitubercular drugs. Pediatr Clin North Am 30:177–193, February 1983

Rodman MJ, Karch AM, Boyd EH, Smith DW: Pharmacology and Drug Therapy in Nursing, 3rd ed. Philadelphia, J B Lippincott, 1985

Snider DE, Cohn DE, Davidson PT, et al: Standard therapy for tuberculosis 1985. Chest 87(Suppl):117S–124S, February 1985

42

ANTIVIRAL DRUGS

Description and uses

The incidence of viral infections in human beings is high, and many potentially pathogenic viral strains exist. For example, more than 150 distinct viruses infect the human respiratory tract, including about 100 types of rhinovirus that cause the common cold. Viral infections vary from mild, localized disease with few symptoms to severe systemic illness and death. Severe infections are more common when host defense mechanisms are impaired by disease or by drugs or other treatment measures (*e.g.,* organ transplants). Viral infections are more often primary infections, although viruses may be opportunists as well, particularly the herpes group. Additional characteristics of viruses and viral infections include the following:

1. Viruses can live and reproduce only while inside other living cells.
2. Viruses are spread by secretions from infected persons. For example, influenza and cold viruses spread when infected droplet nuclei are expelled into the air with a cough or sneeze and inhaled into the respiratory tract of an uninfected person. Hepatitis and poliomyelitis viruses are spread by ingestion of contaminated food or water. Less common viral infections such as rabies and mosquito-borne encephalitis can be transmitted through breaks in skin or mucous membrane. This allows the viruses direct access to the bloodstream.
3. Viruses can cause infection either by coming into direct contact with target cells (cold, influenza) or by gaining access to the bloodstream and then being transported to the target cells. Target cells must have specific receptors for the particular viruses, much as a key fits into a lock, before the virus can pass into the human cell and start reproducing itself. The viruses causing hepatitis, for example, apparently have target cells in the liver.
4. Viruses induce antibodies and immunity. Antibodies are proteins that defend against microbial or viral invasion. They are very specific; that is, an antibody will protect only against a specific virus or other antigen. For instance, a person who has had measles develops antibody protection (immunity) against future infection by the measles virus but does not develop immunity against other viral infections, such as chickenpox or hepatitis.
5. It is apparently the protein coat of the virus that allows the immune system of the host to recognize the virus as a "foreign invader" and to produce antibodies against it. This system works efficiently for most viruses but does not work for the influenza A virus. Apparently, the influenza A virus is able to alter its protein covering so much and so often that the immune system does not recognize it as foreign to the body. Thus, last year's antibody cannot recognize and neutralize this year's virus. This characteristic of the virus is the major obstacle to vaccine development.
6. Antibodies against infecting viruses can function to prevent their reaching the bloodstream, or, if they have reached the bloodstream, prevent their invasion of host cells. Once the virus has pene-

trated the cell, it is protected from antibody action, and the host depends on cell-mediated immunity (lymphocytes and macrophages) to eradicate the virus along with the cell harboring it.

7. Viral infection may occur without signs and symptoms of illness. If illness does occur, the clinical course is usually short and self-limited. Recovery occurs as the virus is eliminated from the body. Some viruses, however, are apparently able to survive in host cells for a long time and can cause chronic infection. Also, autoimmune diseases may be caused by viral alteration of host cells so that lymphocytes are fooled into thinking the host's own tissues are foreign.
8. Symptoms usually associated with acute viral infections include fever, headache, cough, malaise, muscle pain, nausea and vomiting, diarrhea, insomnia, and photophobia. White blood cell count is usually normal.

Drug therapy for viral infections is very limited and primarily geared toward relieving symptoms rather than the infection itself. Development of effective antiviral drugs is extremely difficult owing to the relationship between viruses and their host cells. Viruses depend on the enzymatic, genetic, and nutritional systems of the host cells for all their own vital functions. Consequently, the search for drugs that will suppress multiplication or transmission of viruses without being excessively toxic to host tissues has been rather unsuccessful.

Currently available antiviral drugs are expensive, relatively toxic, and effective in only a few specific infections. They are of potential use in treating established infection if given promptly and in chemoprophylaxis if given before, or as soon as possible after, exposure. Protection conferred by chemoprophylaxis is immediate but lasts only while the drug is being taken.

Individual antiviral drugs

Acyclovir (Zovirax) is a synthetic antiviral agent that is effective against herpes simplex virus types 1 and 2, varicella-zoster virus, Epstein-Barr virus, and cytomegalovirus. The drug penetrates human host cells, interferes with production of deoxyribonucleic acid, and thereby prevents viral reproduction. Acyclovir is indicated in the treatment of mucosal and cutaneous infections caused by herpes simplex virus. The major use is for genital herpes, an infectious viral disease transmitted primarily by sexual contact or contact with lesions. The disease is characterized by blisterlike lesions, pruritus, and pain. It occurs in an exacerbation–remission pattern and is infectious when lesions are present. Acyclovir decreases viral shedding and the duration of skin lesions and pain. The drug does not eliminate inactive virus in the body and thus does not prevent transmission or recurrence of the disease unless oral drug therapy is continued. Acyclovir is also indicated for treatment of herpes labialis ("cold sores" or "fever blisters") or other herpes simplex infections in immunocompromised clients. Prolonged or repeated courses of acyclovir therapy may result in the emergence of acyclovir-resistant viral strains. This is most likely to occur in immunocompromised clients.

Initially available only as an ointment for topical application to lesions, acyclovir is now available for intravenous and oral administration. Intravenous use is recommended only for severe genital herpes in nonimmunocompromised clients and any herpes infections in immunocompromised clients. The drug is excreted through the kidneys, and dosage must be reduced in the presence of renal failure. Safety and effectiveness of acyclovir during pregnancy and lactation have not been established. Oral acyclovir has not been approved for use in children.

Routes and dosage ranges

Adults: IV 5 mg/kg q8h for 5–7 days
PO 1000 mg daily, in divided doses, for 10 days in initial herpes genitalis, for 5 days in recurrent herpes genitalis, for up to 6 months to suppress recurrent episodes
Topically to lesions q3h or at least 6 times daily for 7 days
Children under 12 years: IV 250 mg/m^2 q8h for 7 days

Amantadine (Symmetrel) is a synthetic antiviral agent that prevents viral penetration into human host cells. It is most effective in preventing infections caused by the influenza A virus. It may be given to clients having contact with active influenza cases. In confirmed epidemics of influenza A infections, amantadine is recommended for clients at high risk who have not been vaccinated. The high-risk population includes those who are elderly, who have chronic lung disease, or who have immunodeficiency disorders. Amantadine may be given daily throughout the epidemic (5 to 6 weeks) or, if the client is vaccinated at the beginning of amantadine therapy, for 10 to 14 days. The drug may also be useful in treatment of influenza A infections if started as early as possible after onset and continued for 5 to 7 days.

Amantadine is excreted in the urine unchanged; it accumulates in the body when renal function is impaired. Dosage should be reduced with renal impairment. The drug is contraindicated during pregnancy and must be used cautiously in clients with cerebral atherosclerosis, psychiatric disorders, or a history of epilepsy.

Route and dosage ranges

Adults: PO 200 mg daily in 1–2 doses
Children: PO 200 mg daily in 1–2 doses for children over 9 years; 4.4–8.8 mg/kg daily for children 1–9 years (maximal daily dose, 150 mg)

Idoxuridine (Stoxil) is most effective when used topically to treat corneal ulcer caused by the herpes simplex virus (herpetic keratitis). It is not effective in treating systemic herpes infections, and results have been disappointing when it has been used to treat herpetic ulcers of the skin and the genital mucous membranes. Viral resistance may develop, but this has presented no difficulty with topical use. It is available as an ophthalmic solution and an ophthalmic ointment.

Route and dosage range

Adults: Topical instillation in the eye, 0.1% solution, 1 drop in the conjunctival sac q1h daytime and q2h nighttime until improvement apparent, then 1 drop q2h daytime and q4h during the night; 0.5% ointment, apply q4h during the day and at bedtime. The drug is continued for 5 days after healing is complete

Trifluridine (Viroptic) is used for topical treatment of keratoconjunctivitis and recurrent epithelial keratitis due to herpes simplex virus. Trifluridine may promote more rapid healing of corneal ulcers than other drugs. There is little systemic absorption, and no systemic adverse effects have been reported. Local burning, stinging, or eyelid edema may occur. The drug should not be used longer than 21 days because of possible ocular toxicity.

Route and dosage range

Adults: Topical instillation in the eye, 1% ophthalmic solution, 1 drop q2h while awake (maximum 9 drops daily) until reepithelialization of corneal ulcer occurs; then 1 drop q4h (maximum, 5 drops daily) for 7 days

Vidarabine (Vira-A) is an antiviral agent that is active against vaccinia, herpes simplex, and varicella-zoster viruses and some strains of cytomegalovirus. It is used most often in encephalitis or keratoconjunctivitis caused by the herpes simplex virus. Vidarabine is given parenterally for encephalitis. Dosage must be reduced with impaired renal function. It is applied topically to the eye for keratoconjunctivitis. It is as effective as idoxuridine for this purpose and causes less tissue irritation. Vidarabine is also used in herpes zoster infections in clients whose immune systems are impaired. It is not recommended for treatment of herpes zoster in unimpaired hosts. It has mutagenic and teratogenic properties.

Routes and dosage ranges

Adults: IV 15 mg/kg/day, dissolved in 2500 ml of fluid and given over 12–24 hours daily for 10 days
Topical instillation in the eye, 3% ophthalmic ointment, applied q3h until reepithelialization has occurred, then twice daily for 7 days

Interferon is a naturally occurring antiviral agent produced by body cells in response to viral infection that prevents growth of viruses within the infected cells. It also enters surrounding tissues and the bloodstream to protect uninfected cells from viral invasion. In contrast to antibody production by the immune system, interferon is immediately available and exerts antiviral activity against all viruses, not specific ones. However, only human interferon is effective in human viral infections. Commercial interferon production has been hampered by a number of difficulties. Thus far, relatively small amounts have been available (most produced from human leukocytes) for investigational purposes.

Principles of therapy: antiviral drugs

1. Drug therapy has a limited place in treating viral infections. Management mainly involves preventive measures such as vaccination, handwashing, teaching infected clients to cover the mouth and nose when coughing or sneezing, treatment of symptoms, and recognition and treatment of complications.
2. Viral vaccines are used for active immunization of clients before exposure or to control epidemics of viral disease in a community. Vaccines for prevention of poliomyelitis, measles, rubella, mumps, smallpox, and yellow fever and for protection against influenza and rabies are available (see Chap. 45).
3. Live attenuated viral vaccines are generally quite safe and nontoxic. However, they probably should not be used in clients who are pregnant, who are immunodeficient, or who are receiving corticosteroids, antineoplastic or immunosuppressive drugs, or irradiation.

4. Influenza vaccines prevent infection in most clients. If infection does occur, less virus is shed in respiratory secretions. Thus, vaccination reduces transmission of influenza by decreasing the number of susceptible people and by decreasing transmission by immunized people who still become infected.
5. The multiplicity of rhinoviruses (common cold), enteroviruses, and respiratory viruses precludes imminent development of practical vaccines for these common clinical diseases.
6. Antiviral drugs are available to prevent or treat a few specific virus infections. They should not be used unless the etiologic diagnosis is certain.
7. Antibacterial drugs should not be used in viral infections in the hope of preventing complications. They do have a role, however, in treating bacterial complications of viral infections.

NURSING ACTIONS: ANTIVIRAL DRUGS

Nursing Actions	Rationale/Explanation
1. Administer accurately	
a. With intravenous acyclovir, dissolve contents in 10 ml of sterile water for injection, add to 50 to 100 ml of an appropriate intravenous solution, and infuse over at least 1 hour.	A concentration of 7 mg/ml or lower is recommended and infusion over at least 1 hour helps prevent precipitation of drug in the renal tubules and the possible renal damage that may occur with a bolus or rapid administration. Renal damage is also less likely to occur if the client is well hydrated.
With topical acyclovir, wear a glove to apply.	To prevent spread of infection, since lesions contain herpes virus
b. Give amantadine in two divided doses.	To reduce adverse reactions, which are more likely if the full daily dose is given at one time
c. Give the second daily dose of amantadine at least 6 hours before bedtime.	To decrease the insomnia that may occur during amantadine therapy
2. Observe for therapeutic effects	
a. With acyclovir, observe for healing of lesions and decreased pain and itching.	
b. When amantadine is given for influenza A prophylaxis, absence of symptoms indicates therapeutic benefit.	
c. When amantadine is given in active influenza A infection, observe for decreased fever, cough, muscle aches, and malaise.	
d. With idoxuridine and ophthalmic vidarabine, observe for decreased signs of eye infection.	
e. With parenteral vidarabine, observe for decreased fever and headache and increased mental alertness.	Vidarabine is not effective in clients with herpes simplex encephalitis who are comatose when drug therapy is initiated.
3. Observe for adverse effects	
a. With acyclovir, observe for nausea, vomiting, diarrhea, headache, dizziness, skin rash, itching and burning, and increased serum creatinine. Rare but potentially serious encephalopathy may be manifested by lethargy, confusion, tremors, seizures, or coma.	Adverse effects are usually infrequent and mild. Gastrointestinal effects and headache are most common; CNS effects are most likely to occur with intravenous administration.

Nursing Actions	Rationale/Explanation
b. Central nervous system (CNS) effects with amantadine—insomnia, hyperexcitability, ataxia, dizziness, slurred speech, mental confusion	Symptoms may be similar to those caused by atropine and amphetamines. Adverse reactions are more likely to occur in the elderly and those with renal impairment.
c. Pain, itching, edema, or inflammation of eyelids with ophthalmic antiviral preparations	These symptoms are more likely to occur with idoxuridine than vidarabine. They result from tissue irritation or hypersensitivity reactions.
4. Observe for drug interactions	
a. With acyclovir, probenecid increases effects	Prolongs half-life and slows renal excretion of acyclovir
b. Drugs that alter effects of amantadine	
(1) Anticholinergics (*e.g.,* atropine)	Increased anticholinergic effects, such as blurred vision, mouth dryness, urine retention, constipation
(2) CNS stimulants and psychotropic drugs	Amantadine has CNS and psychic effects ranging from stimulation (insomnia, nervousness, hyperexcitability) to depression (decreased ability to concentrate, confusion, mental depression). Therefore, other drugs with these effects potentiate amantadine.
c. Drugs that alter effects of idoxuridine	
(1) Boric acid	Boric acid and idoxuridine ophthalmic solutions should not be administered at the same time or close together, since the combination may irritate tissues
(2) Corticosteroids	These drugs may accelerate the spread of a viral infection such as herpes simplex keratitis. Therefore, they should not be used with idoxuridine unless absolutely necessary.
(3) Other medications	To ensure stability, do not mix idoxuridine ophthalmic solution with other ophthalmic drugs.
5. Teach clients	
a. With acyclovir,	
(1) Avoid sexual intercourse when visible lesions are present	
(2) Always wash hands after touching any lesion	
(3) Start oral acyclovir for recurrent genital herpes as soon as signs and symptoms begin	
(4) Use gloves to apply ointment to lesions	
b. With amantadine, do not operate machinery of any kind if feeling dizzy or drowsy.	Amantadine causes CNS changes that may impair physical and mental responses, and thus safety may be impaired.
c. Report insomnia, ataxia, and other adverse effects with amantadine.	
d. Correct administration of eye medications (*e.g.,* washing hands before and after instilling eye drops or ointments, not touching the tip of the medication container to the eye or any other surface)	To avoid spreading infection and contaminating medications

Selected References

American Medical Association (AMA) Division of Drugs: AMA Drug Evaluations, 5th ed. New York, John Wiley & Sons, 1983

Cesario TC: The clinical implications of interferon. Med Clin North Am 67:1147–1162, September 1983

Corey L, Holmes KK: Genital herpes simplex virus infections:

Current concepts in diagnosis, treatment and prevention. Ann Intern Med 98:973–983, June 1983
Douglas RG: Antiviral drugs. Med Clin North Am 67:1163–1172, September 1983
Facts and Comparisons. St. Louis, J B Lippincott (Updated monthly)
Hirsch MS, Schooley MN: Treatment of herpesvirus infections. N Engl J Med 309:963–970, October 1983
Intravenous acyclovir (Zovirax). Med Lett Drugs Ther 25:34–36, April 1983
Oral acyclovir for genital herpes simplex infection. Med Lett Drugs Ther 27:41–43, May 1985
Rodman MJ, Karch AM, Boyd EH, Smith DW: Pharmacology and Drug Therapy in Nursing, 3rd ed. Philadelphia, J B Lippincott, 1985
Sande MA, Mandell GL: Antifungal and antiviral agents. In Gilman AG, Goodman LS, Rall TW, Murad F (eds): The Pharmacological Basis of Therapeutics, 7th ed, pp 1219–1239. New York, Macmillan, 1985
Schinazi RF, Prusoff WH: Antiviral agents. Pediatr Clin North Am 30:77–92, February 1983
Scott TM, Parish LC, Witkowski JA: Herpes simplex virus infections. II. Diagnosis and treatment. Drug Ther 15:135–143, October 1985

43

ANTIFUNGAL DRUGS

Description and uses

Fungi are plantlike, parasitic microorganisms of which about 50 species cause human disease. Humans are often unavoidably exposed to pathogenic fungi; conditions in which exposure is followed by infection are not fully known. Mechanisms of infection include inhalation of airborne spores, oral ingestion, and implantation of the fungus under the skin as a result of an injury. Fungal infections (mycoses) range from mild, superficial infections to life-threatening systemic infections. Additional characteristics of fungi and fungal infections include the following:

1. Fungi that cause superficial infections of the skin, hair, and nails are called *dermatophytes.* These fungi are often present on the body without causing infection. They obtain nourishment from keratin, a protein in skin, hair, and nails. Dermatophytic infections include tinea pedis (athlete's foot) and tinea capitis (ringworm of the scalp) (see also Chap. 66).
2. *Candida albicans* is usually part of the indigenous microbial flora of the skin, mouth, intestine, and vagina. It causes infection in certain circumstances. Vaginal candidiasis is common during pregnancy, in women with diabetes mellitus, and in women who take oral contraceptives. Oral candidiasis (thrush) is common in newborns. Oral, intestinal, vaginal, and systemic candidiasis can occur with antibiotic, antineoplastic, and corticosteroid drug therapy. Systemic candidiasis also occurs in clients receiving parenteral nutrition and in those with burn wounds. *Candida* may cause endocarditis after insertion of a prosthetic heart valve.
3. Fungi that cause other serious infections are not part of the indigenous microbial flora. These fungi grow independently in soil and decaying organic matter. Fungal infections such as histoplasmosis, coccidioidomycosis, and blastomycosis usually occur as pulmonary disease but may be systemic. Severity of disease increases with intensity of exposure.
   (a) Histoplasmosis is endemic in many parts of the world. It usually occurs as an acute, self-limiting respiratory tract infection. It occasionally occurs as a rapidly fatal infection involving the liver, spleen, and other organs. Healed lung lesions may calcify and be confused with the lesions of tuberculosis. The fungus causing histoplasmosis is found in soil and organic debris, especially around chicken houses, bird roosts, and caves inhabited by bats.
   (b) Coccidioidomycosis usually occurs as an acute, self-limiting respiratory infection but may occur as a chronic, diffuse disease involving almost any body part.
   (c) Blastomycosis most often causes respiratory infection that resembles pneumonia or tuberculosis. Other organs may be involved, how-

TABLE 43-1. SELECTED ANTIFUNGAL DRUGS

Generic name	Trade name	Clinical indications	Routes and dosage ranges: Adults	Routes and dosage ranges: Children
Acrisorcin	Akrinol	Tinea versicolor	Topically to skin lesions, twice daily for at least 6 weeks	
Amphotericin B	Fungizone	Systemic mycoses (*e.g.,* candidiasis, histoplasmosis, blastomycosis, and others) Cutaneous candidiasis	Intravenous individualized according to disease severity and client tolerance. Average dose, 0.25–0.5 mg/kg/day Topically to skin lesions, 2–4 times daily for 1–4 weeks	Same as for adults
Ciclopirox	Loprox	Tinea infections, cutaneous candidiasis	Topically to skin lesions, twice daily for 2–4 weeks	
Clotrimazole	Lotrimin, Mycelex	Cutaneous dermatophytosis; oral, cutaneous, and vaginal candidiasis	Orally 1 troche dissolved in mouth 5 times daily Topically to skin twice daily Intravaginally once daily	Same as for adults Dosage not established
Econazole	Spectazole	Tinea infections, cutaneous candidiasis	Topically to skin lesions once or twice daily for 2–4 weeks	
Flucytosine	Ancobon	Systemic mycoses due to *Candida* species or *Cryptococcus neoformans*	PO 50–150 mg/kg/day in divided doses q6h. Dosage must be decreased with impaired liver function	Same as for adults
Griseofulvin	Fulvicin	Dermatophytosis (skin, hair, and nails)	Microsize, PO 500 mg–1 g daily in divided doses q6h Ultramicrosize, PO 250–500 mg daily	Microsize, PO 10 mg/kg in divided doses q6h Ultramicrosize, 5–7 mg/kg/day
Haloprogin	Halotex	Dermatophytosis, mainly tinea pedis (athlete's foot), cutaneous candidiasis	Topically to skin, 1% cream or solution twice daily for 2–4 weeks	Dosage not established
Ketoconazole	Nizoral	Candidiasis, histoplasmosis, coccidioidomycosis, paracoccidioidomycosis	PO 200 mg once daily, increased to 400 mg once daily if necessary in severe infections	Weight above 40 kg: PO 200 mg once daily Weight 20–40 kg: PO 100 mg (½ tablet) once daily Weight under 20 kg: 50 mg (¼ tablet) once daily
Miconazole	Monistat	Systemic mycoses Dermatophytosis, cutaneous and vulvovaginal candidiasis	IV 600 mg–1 g q8h Topically to skin, once or twice daily for 4 weeks Intravaginally, once daily for 2 weeks	20–40 mg/kg/day in divided infusions
Natamycin	Natacyn	Fungal infections of the eye	Topically to eye, 1 drop q1–2h for 3–4 days, then 1 drop 6–8 times daily for 14–24 days	
Nystatin	Mycostatin	Candidiasis of skin, mucous membrane, and intestinal tract	Oral or intestinal infection, PO 400,000–600,000 units 4 times daily	Oral infection, PO 100,000 units 3–4 times daily

TABLE 43-1. SELECTED ANTIFUNGAL DRUGS (*Continued*)

Generic name	Trade name	Clinical indications	Routes and dosage ranges	
			Adults	*Children*
			Topically to skin lesions, 2–3 times daily, continued for 1 week after cure Intravaginally, 1 vaginal tablet once daily for 14 days	
Tolnaftate	Tinactin	Cutaneous mycoses (dermatophytosis)	Topically to skin lesions, twice daily for 2–6 weeks	Same as for adults
Triacetin	Enzactin	Dermatophytosis (*e.g.*, athlete's foot), cutaneous candidiasis	Topically to skin lesions, twice daily until 1 week after symptoms are relieved	Same as for adults
Zinc undecylenate	Desenex	Dermatophytosis	Topically to skin twice daily for 2 to 4 weeks	Same as for adults

ever, especially the skin. Skin pustules, ulcerations, and abscesses may occur.

4. Systemic mycoses are confirmed by recovery of organisms from specimens of body tissues or fluids.

Individual antifungal drugs are listed in Table 43-1.

Principles of therapy: antifungal drugs

ASSESSMENT GUIDELINES

Assess for fungal infections. Specific signs and symptoms vary with location and type of infection.

1. Superficial lesions of skin, hair, and nails are usually characterized by pain, burning, and itching. Some lesions are moist; others are dry and scaling. They may also appear inflamed or discolored.
2. Candidiasis occurs in warm, moist areas of the body. Skin lesions are likely to occur in perineal and intertriginous areas. They are usually moist, inflamed, pruritic areas with vesicles and pustules. Oral lesions are white patches that adhere to the buccal mucosa. Vaginal infection causes a cheesy vaginal discharge, burning, and itching. Intestinal infection causes diarrhea.
3. Histoplasmosis, coccidioidomycosis, and blastomycosis often simulate tuberculosis or pneumonia, with cough, fever, malaise, and other manifestations.

NURSING INTERVENTIONS

Use measures to prevent spread of fungal infections. Superficial infections (*e.g.*, ringworm or tinea) are highly contagious and can be spread by sharing towels and hairbrushes. Systemic mycoses are not contagious.

DIAGNOSTIC AND THERAPEUTIC FACTORS

1. An etiologic diagnosis should be made before an antifungal drug is used. Local infections can be caused by bacteria or fungi or a combination. Most antifungal drugs are not effective in bacterial infections. Antifungal drugs effective in candidiasis are not usually effective in dermatophytic infections, and vice versa.
2. Candidal infections of blood or urine often respond to the removal of predisposing factors, such as antibiotics, corticosteroids, immunosuppressive drugs, and in-dwelling intravenous or bladder catheters. Candidal endocarditis, which may occur after prosthetic heart valve replacement, is best treated by surgical removal of the infected prosthesis and administration of amphotericin B.
3. Most antifungal drug therapy is long term (several weeks to months).

NURSING ACTIONS: ANTIFUNGAL DRUGS

Nursing Actions	Rationale/Explanation
1. Administer accurately	
a. Check the package insert for complete instructions before giving intravenous amphotericin B. Some major points of administration include the following:	
(1) Use sterile water without a bacteriostatic agent for initial dissolution of the powdered drug; use 5% dextrose in water for further dilution to a 0.1 to 0.2 mg/ml concentration.	Use of any other solution causes precipitation of amphotericin B.
(2) Use a large vein and a scalp vein needle to administer.	To decrease phlebitis and pain at the venipuncture site. In addition, heparin and hydrocortisone may be added to the infusion solution to prevent local reactions.
(3) Administer each day's dose over a 6-hour period.	To decrease adverse reactions
b. For intravenous miconazole, dilute in at least 200 ml of 0.9% saline or 5% dextrose and infuse over 60 minutes or longer.	To prevent cardiorespiratory toxicity during infusion
c. For ketoconazole, do not give antacids, anticholinergics, or cimetidine within 2 hours of administration of ketoconazole. For clients with achlorhydria, dissolve ketoconazole tablets in 4 ml aqueous solution of 0.2 N hydrochloric acid and have them drink the mixture through a straw and then drink 8 oz of tap water.	The drug is dissolved and absorbed only in an acid environment.
d. For nystatin, the suspension should be swished in the mouth for a few minutes before swallowing.	To increase contact with oral lesions
2. Observe for therapeutic effects	
a. Decreased fever and malaise, with systemic mycoses	
b. Healing of lesions on skin and mucous membranes	
c. Diminished diarrhea with intestinal candidiasis	
d. Decreased vaginal discharge and discomfort with vaginal candidiasis	
3. Observe for adverse effects	
a. With amphotericin B, observe for fever, chills, anorexia, nausea, vomiting, renal damage (elevated blood urea nitrogen and serum creatinine, hypokalemia, hypomagnesemia, headache, stupor, coma, convulsions), anemia from bone marrow depression, phlebitis at venipuncture sites, anaphylaxis.	Amphotericin B is a highly toxic drug, and most recipients develop some adverse reactions, including some degree of renal damage. Antipyretic and antiemetic drugs may be given to help minimize adverse reactions and promote patient comfort. Adequate hydration may decrease renal damage.
b. With flucytosine, observe for nausea, vomiting, and diarrhea.	These are common effects. Hepatic, renal, and hematologic functions may also be affected. Drug resistance often develops when flucytosine is used alone.
c. With intravenous miconazole, observe for nausea, phlebitis, anemia, thrombocytopenia, and pruritus.	
d. With ketoconazole, observe for nausea, vomiting, pruritus, and abdominal pain.	Adverse effects are mild and transient.
e. With griseofulvin, observe for gastrointestinal symptoms, hypersensitivity (urticaria, photosensitivity, skin	Incidence of serious reactions is very low.

Nursing Actions	Rationale/Explanation
rashes, angioedema), headache, mental confusion, fatigue, dizziness, peripheral neuritis, and blood dyscrasias (leukopenia, neutropenia, granunlocytopenia)	
f. With topical drugs, observe for skin rash and irritation	Adverse reactions are usually minimal with topical drugs, although hypersensitivity may occur.
4. Observe for drug interactions	
a. Drugs that alter effects of amphotericin B	
(1) Antibiotics, especially nephrotoxic ones such as aminoglycosides	Additive nephrotoxicity, since each drug alone is nephrotoxic
(2) Antineoplastic drugs	Increased bone marrow depression and blood dyscrasias. However, clients receiving antineoplastic drugs are highly susceptible to systemic fungal infections, and amphotericin B may be required concomitantly. The combination is indicated only if the illness is more life threatening than the drug toxicity.
(3) Corticosteroids	Systemic mycoses sometimes develop in clients receiving corticosteroids because corticosteroids depress the immune system. They should not be given with amphotericin B unless absolutely necessary to control reactions to the drug or to treat the underlying disease.
(4) Potassium-losing diuretics, corticosteroids	Additive hypokalemia
(5) Minocycline, rifampin, flucytosine	Potentiate antifungal activity of amphotericin B
b. Drugs that alter effects of griseofulvin	
Barbiturates, glutethimide, and other sedative–hypnotics that induce liver enzymes	Enzyme inducers inhibit effects of griseofulvin by increasing its rate of metabolism.
c. Drugs that alter effects of ketoconazole	
Antacids, anticholinergics, and cimetidine	These drugs decrease dissolution and absorption of ketoconazole by decreasing gastric acidity.
5. Teach clients	
a. Take drugs as prescribed.	To avoid recurrence of the infection. Drugs must often be taken several weeks after symptoms subside.
b. Report severe adverse effects.	Drug administration may need to be altered or discontinued.
c. With skin lesions, wash hands often; do not share towels, hair brushes, or other personal items.	To avoid spreading infection
d. With histoplasmosis and other potentially serious fungal infections, avoid or minimize future exposure to chicken, pigeon, and bat excreta.	To prevent recurrence of serious, often fatal, systemic fungal infections

Selected References

Comer JB: Amphotericin B: Ten common questions. Am J Nurs 81:1166–1167, June 1981

Drugs for treatment of systemic fungal infections. Med Lett Drugs Ther 26:36–38, March 1984

Facts and Comparisons. St. Louis, J B Lippincott (Updated monthly)

Harvey SC: Antiseptics and disinfectants; fungicides; ectoparasiticides. In Gilman AG, Goodman LS, Rall TW, Murad F (eds): The Pharmacological Basis of Therapeutics, 7th ed, pp 959–979. New York, Macmillan, 1985

Koldin MH, Medoff G: Antifungal chemotherapy. Pediatr Clin North Am 30:49–61, February 1983

New topical antifungal drugs. Med Lett Drugs Ther 25:98–100, October 1983

Rees PL, Dixon DM: Opportunistic mycoses. Am J Nurs 81:1160–1165, June 1981

Sande MA, Mandell GL: Antifungal and antiviral agents. In Gilman AG, Goodman LS, Rall TW, Murad F (eds): The Pharmacological Basis of Therapeutics, 7th ed, pp 1219–1239. New York, Macmillan, 1985

44 ANTIPARASITICS

A parasite is a living organism that survives at the expense of another organism, called the host. Parasitic infestations are among the most common human ailments worldwide. The effects of parasitic diseases on human hosts vary from minor and annoying to major and life threatening. Parasitic diseases in this chapter are those caused by protozoa, helminths (worms), the itch mite, and pediculi (lice). Protozoa and helminths can infect the digestive tract and other body tissues. The itch mite and pediculi affect the skin.

Protozoal infections

AMEBIASIS

Amebiasis is a common disease seen most often in tropical regions, but it can occur in any geographic area with poor sanitary conditions. In the United States it is most likely to occur in institutions for mentally retarded children and elderly adults.

Amebiasis is caused by the pathogenic protozoan *Entamoeba histolytica,* which exists in two forms. The cystic form is inactive, resistant to drugs, heat, cold, and drying, and able to live outside the body for long periods. Amebiasis is acquired by ingesting food or water contaminated with human feces containing amebic cysts. Once ingested, some cysts break open in the ileum to release amebae, which produce trophozoites. Other cysts remain intact to be expelled in feces and continue the chain of infection. Trophozoites are active amebae that feed, multiply, move about, and produce clinical manifestations of amebiasis. Trophozoites produce an enzyme that allows them to invade body tissues. They may form erosions and ulcerations in the intestinal wall and cause diarrhea (this form of the disease is called *intestinal amebiasis* or *amebic dysentery*), or they may penetrate blood vessels and be carried to other organs, where they form abscesses. These abscesses are usually found in the liver (hepatic amebiasis), but they may also occur in the lungs or brain.

Drugs used for treatment of amebiasis (amebicides) are classified according to their site of action. Some drugs (*e.g.,* iodoquinol, paromomycin) are called *intestinal amebicides* because they act within the lumen of the bowel. Other drugs (*e.g.,* chloroquine, emetine) are called *tissue* or *extraintestinal amebicides* because they act in the bowel wall, liver, and other tissues. Metronidazole (Flagyl) is effective in both intestinal and extraintestinal amebiasis. No currently available amebicides are recommended for prophylaxis of amebiasis.

Dehydroemetine and diloxanide furoate (Furamide) are amebicides available to physicians from the Parasitic Diseases Division, Centers for Disease Control (CDC), Atlanta, Georgia. These drugs are not discussed individually, since clinical information is dispensed with them.

MALARIA

Malaria is a common cause of morbidity and mortality in many parts of the world, especially in tropical regions. In the United States, malaria is rare and almost always imported by travelers or immigrants from malarious areas.

Malaria is caused by four species of protozoa of the genus *Plasmodium*. The human being is the only natural reservoir of these parasites. All types of malaria are transmitted only by *Anopheles* mosquitoes. *Plasmodium vivax, Plasmodium malariae,* and *Plasmodium ovale* cause recurrent malaria by forming reservoirs in the human host. In these types of malaria, signs and symptoms may occur months or years after the initial attack. *Plasmodium falciparum* causes the most life-threatening type of malaria but does not form a reservoir. This type of malaria may be cured and prevented from recurring.

Plasmodia have a life cycle in which one stage of development occurs within the human body. When a mosquito bites a person with malaria, it ingests blood that contains gametocytes (male and female forms of the protozoan parasite). From these forms, sporozoites are produced and transported to the mosquito's salivary glands. When the mosquito bites the next person, the sporozoites are injected into that person's bloodstream. From the bloodstream, the organisms lodge in the liver and other tissues, where they reproduce asexually and form merozoites. The liver cells containing the parasite eventually rupture and release the merozoites into the bloodstream, where they invade red blood cells. After a period of growth and asexual reproduction, merozoites rupture red blood cells, invade other erythrocytes, form gametocytes, and continue the cycle. After several cycles, clinical manifestations of malaria occur because of the large numbers of parasites. The characteristic cycles of chills and fever correspond to the release of merozoites from erythrocytes.

Antimalarial drugs act at different stages in the life cycle of plasmodial parasites. Some drugs (*e.g.,* chloroquine) are effective against erythrocytic forms and are therefore useful in preventing or treating acute attacks of malaria. These drugs do not prevent infection with the parasite, but they do prevent clinical manifestations. Other drugs (*e.g.,* primaquine) act against exoerythrocytic or tissue forms of the parasite to prevent initial infection and recurrent attacks or to cure some types of malaria. Combination drug therapy, administered concomitantly or consecutively, is common with antimalarial drugs.

TRICHOMONIASIS

The most common form of trichomoniasis is a vaginal infection caused by the protozoan *Trichomonas vaginalis.* The disease is usually spread by sexual intercourse. Antitrichomonal drugs may be administered systemically (*i.e.,* metronidazole) or applied locally as douche solutions or vaginal creams.

MISCELLANEOUS PROTOZOAL INFECTIONS

Giardiasis is a protozoal infection caused by *Giardia lamblia.* This disease is similar to amebiasis in that it is spread by food or water contaminated with human feces containing encysted forms of the organism. This disease is uncommon in the United States but may occur in people who camp or hike in wilderness areas or who drink untreated well water in areas where sanitation is poor.

Pneumocystosis is an acute pneumonialike lung infection caused by the parasitic protozoa *Pneumocystis carinii.* Pneumocystosis occurs primarily in immunosuppressed persons (*i.e.,* those receiving corticosteroids, antineoplastic or other immunosuppressive drugs, or radiation therapy).

Helminthiasis

Helminthiasis, an infestation with parasitic worms, is a major disease in many parts of the world. Helminths are most often found in the gastrointestinal tract. However, several types of parasitic worms penetrate body tissues or produce larvae, which migrate to the blood, lymph channels, lungs, liver, and other body tissues. Specific types of helminthiasis include the following:

1. Hookworm infections are caused by *Necator americanus,* a species found in the United States, and *Ancylostoma duodenale,* a species found in Europe, the Middle East, and North Africa. Hookworm is spread by ova-containing feces from infected persons. Ova develop into larvae when deposited on the soil. Larvae burrow through the skin (*e.g.,* if the person walks on the soil with bare feet), enter blood vessels, and migrate through the lungs to the pharynx, where they are swallowed. Larvae develop into adult hookworms in the small intestine and attach themselves to the intestinal mucosa.
2. Pinworm infections (enterobiasis), caused by *Enterobius vermicularis,* are the most common parasitic worm infections in the United States. Pinworm infections are highly communicable; they often involve schoolchildren and household contacts. Infection occurs from contact with ova in food or water or on bed linens. The female pinworm migrates from the bowel to the perianal area to deposit eggs, especially at night. Touching or scratching the perianal area deposits ova on hands

and any objects touched by the contaminated hands.

3. Roundworm infections (ascariasis), caused by *Ascaris lumbricoides*, are the most common parasitic worm infections in the world. They occur most often in tropical regions but may occur wherever sanitation is poor. The infection is transmitted by ingesting food or water contaminated with feces from infected persons. Ova are swallowed and hatch into larvae in the intestine. Like the hookworm larvae, roundworm larvae penetrate blood vessels and migrate through the lungs before returning to the intestines, where they develop into adult worms.
4. Tapeworms attach themselves to the intestinal wall and may attain lengths of several yards. Segments called proglottids, which contain tapeworm eggs, are expelled in feces. Tapeworms are transmitted by ingestion of contaminated, raw, or improperly cooked beef, pork, or fish. Beef and fish tapeworm infections are not usually considered serious illnesses. Pork tapeworm, which is uncommon in the United States, is more serious because it produces larvae that enter the bloodstream and migrate to other body tissues (*i.e.*, muscles, liver, lungs, and brain).
5. Threadworm infections (strongyloidiasis), caused by *Strongyloides stercoralis*, are potentially serious infections. This parasitic worm burrows into the mucosa of the small intestine, where the female lays eggs. The eggs hatch into larvae that are capable of penetrating all body tissues.
6. Trichinosis, a parasitic worm infection caused by *Trichinella spiralis*, occurs worldwide, with a relatively high incidence in Europe and the United States. It is caused by inadequately cooked meat, especially pork. Encysted larvae are ingested in infected pork. In the intestine, the larvae excyst, mature, and produce eggs that hatch into new larvae. The larvae enter blood and lymphatic vessels and are transported throughout the body. They penetrate various body tissues (*e.g.*, muscles and brain) and evoke inflammatory reactions. Eventually, the larvae are reencysted or walled off in the tissues and may remain for 10 years or longer.
7. Whipworm infections (trichuriasis) are caused by *Trichuris trichiura*. Whipworms attach themselves to the wall of the colon.

Drugs used for treatment of helminthiasis are called *anthelmintics*. Most anthelmintics act locally to kill or cause expulsion of parasitic worms from the intestines; some anthelmintics act systemically against parasites that have penetrated various body tissues. The goal of anthelmintic therapy may be to eradicate the parasite completely or to decrease the magnitude of infestation ("worm burden").

Scabies and pediculosis

Scabies and pediculosis are parasitic infestations of the skin. Scabies is caused by the itch mite (*Sarcoptes scabiei*), which burrows into the skin and lays eggs that hatch in 4 to 8 days. The burrows may produce visible skin lesions, most often between the fingers and on the wrists, but other parts of the body may be affected as well. Pediculosis is caused by three types of lice, which are blood-sucking insects. Pediculosis capitus (head lice) is the most common type of pediculosis in the United States. It is diagnosed by finding louse eggs (nits) attached to hair shafts close to the scalp. Pediculosis corporis (body lice) is diagnosed by finding lice in clothing, especially in seams. Body lice can transmit typhus and other diseases. Pediculosis pubis (pubic or crab lice) is diagnosed by finding lice in the pubic and genital areas. Occasionally, these lice infest the axillae, mustache, or eyelashes.

Although scabies and pediculosis are caused by different parasites, the conditions have several characteristics in common. These are listed as follows:

1. Scabies and pediculosis are more likely to occur in areas of poverty, overcrowding, and poor sanitation. However, they may occur in any geographic area and socioeconomic group.
2. Scabies and pediculosis are highly communicable. The diseases are transmitted by direct contact with an infected person or the person's personal effects (*e.g.*, clothing, combs and hair brushes, bed linens).
3. Pruritus is usually the major symptom of scabies and pediculosis. It results from an allergic reaction to parasite secretions and excrement. In addition to the intense discomfort associated with pruritus, scratching is likely to cause skin excoriation with secondary bacterial infection and formation of vesicles, pustules, and crusts.
4. Some of the same medications, applied topically, are used in both scabies and pediculosis.

Individual antiparasitic drugs

AMEBICIDES

Chloroquine (Aralen) is a drug used primarily for antimalarial effects. When used as an amebicide, the drug is effective in extraintestinal amebiasis (*i.e.*, hepatic amebiasis) but generally ineffective in intestinal amebiasis. The phosphate salt is given orally. When the oral route is contraindicated, when severe nausea and vomiting occur, or when the infection is severe, the hydrochloride salt can be given intramuscularly. Treatment is usually combined with an intestinal amebicide.

Routes and dosage ranges

Chloroquine phosphate

Adults: PO 1 g daily for 2 days, then 500 mg daily for 2–3 weeks
Children: PO 20 mg/kg/day, in 2 divided doses, for 2 days, then 10 mg/kg/day for 2–3 weeks

Chloroquine hydrochloride

Adults: IM 200–250 mg daily for 10–12 days
Children: IM 15 mg/kg/day for 2 days, then 7.5 mg/kg/day for 2–3 weeks

Emetine hydrochloride is an effective but highly toxic tissue amebicide. It acts against amebae in the intestinal wall and extraintestinal sites such as the liver and lungs. It is more effective against active amebae (trophozoites) than against the cystic form. Emetine is used with other drugs for treatment of severe amebic dysentery and amebic hepatitis. Adverse effects occur in approximately 50% to 75% of emetine recipients. During emetine therapy, clients are hospitalized and maintained on bed rest. Emetine accumulates in the body, and the risk of serious adverse reactions increases with repeated courses of therapy. Therefore, a course of therapy should be followed by an interval of at least 6 weeks before starting a second course. Emetine is generally contraindicated in pregnancy, cardiac or renal disease, and elderly or debilitated clients.

Routes and dosage ranges

Adults: IM, SC 1 mg/kg/day, for up to 5 days (10 days in hepatitis); maximal daily dose, 60 mg
Children: IM, SC 1 mg/kg/day, for up to 5 days; maximal daily dose, 10 mg for children under 8 years and 20 mg for children over 8 years

Iodoquinol or diiodohydroxyquin (Yodoxin) is an iodine compound that acts against active amebae (trophozoites) in the intestinal lumen. Iodoquinol may be used alone in asymptomatic intestinal amebiasis to decrease the number of amebic cysts passed in the feces. When given for symptomatic intestinal amebiasis (*e.g.*, amebic dysentery), iodoquinol is usually given with other amebicides in concurrent or alternating courses. Iodoquinol is ineffective in amebic hepatitis and abscess formation. Its use is contraindicated with iodine allergy and liver disease. A related drug, *clioquinol* or iodochlorhydroxyquin (Vioform), is also an effective ambecide. Clioquinol tablets for oral administration are not marketed in the United States. Both iodoquinol and clioquinol are ingredients in various dermatologic and vaginal preparations for topical application.

Route and dosage ranges

Adults: Asymptomatic carriers, PO 650 mg daily
Symptomatic intestinal amebiasis, PO 650 mg 3 times daily, after meals, for 20 days. If necessary, the 20-day course of therapy may be repeated after a drug-free interval of 2–3 weeks
Children: PO 30–40 mg/kg/day in 2–3 divided doses, for 20 days (maximal daily dose, 2 g). Repeat after 2–3 weeks if necessary

Metronidazole (Flagyl) is effective against protozoa that cause amebiasis, giardiasis, and trichomoniasis and against gram-negative bacilli such as *Bacteroides, Clostridia,* and *Gardnerella* vaginalis. In amebiasis, metronidazole is amebicidal at both intestinal and extraintestinal sites of infection. It is probably the drug of choice for all forms of amebiasis except asymptomatic intestinal amebiasis (in which amebic cysts are expelled in the feces). In trichomoniasis, metronidazole is the only systemic trichomonacide available, and it is more effective than any locally active agent.

Because trichomoniasis is transmitted by sexual intercourse, some authorities recommend simultaneous treatment of both partners to prevent reinfection. Metronidazole is given orally for protozoal infections and intravenously for anaerobic bacterial infections. It is generally contraindicated during the first trimester of pregnancy and must be used with caution in clients with central nervous system (CNS) or blood disorders. The drug is carcinogenic in rodents and mutagenic in bacteria. Therefore, it should be used only when necessary.

Routes and dosage ranges

Adults: Amebiasis, PO 500–750 mg 3 times daily for 5–10 days
Trichomoniasis, PO 250 mg 3 times daily for 7 days, 1 g twice daily for 1 day, or 2 g in a single dose. If necessary, the course of treatment may be repeated after 4–6 weeks.
Gardnerella vaginalis vaginitis, PO 500 mg twice daily for 7 days
Anaerobic bacterial infection, IV 15 mg/kg as a loading dose, infused over 1 hour, followed by 7.5 mg/kg q6h as a maintenance dose, infused over 1 hour; maximal dose, 4 g/24 hours
Children: Amebiasis, PO 35–50 mg/kg/day in 3 divided doses, for 10 days

Paromomycin sulfate (Humatin) is an aminoglycoside antibiotic (see Chap. 36) that acts against amebae in the intestinal lumen. It may be used alone or in combination with other drugs in intestinal amebiasis, but it is ineffective for extraintestinal sites of amebic infection. Paromomycin has antibacterial effects on pathogenic bacteria in the colon. Thus, superinfection may occur. Paromomycin is poorly absorbed from the gastrointestinal tract and is therefore unlikely to cause the ototoxicity and nephrotoxicity associated with aminoglycoside antibiotics. However, systemic absorption may be increased in the presence of inflammatory or ulcerative bowel disease.

Route and dosage ranges

Adults: PO 25–35 mg/kg/day, in 3 divided doses, with meals, for 5–10 days. The course of therapy may be repeated after 2 weeks, if necessary.
Children: PO same as adults

Tetracycline (Achromycin), and **oxytetracycline** (Terramycin) are broad-spectrum antibiotics (see Chap. 37) that act against amebae in the intestinal lumen. These drugs are not directly amebicidal; instead, they exert their effects by altering the bacterial flora required for amebic viability. One of these drugs may be used with other amebicides in the treatment of all forms of amebiasis except asymptomatic intestinal amebiasis.

Route and dosage ranges

Adults: PO 250–500 mg q6h, up to 14 days
Children: PO 25–50 mg/kg/day, in 4 divided doses, for 7–10 days

ANTIMALARIAL AGENTS

Chloroquine (Aralen) is one of the most widely used antimalarial agents. Chloroquine acts against erythrocytic forms of plasmodial parasites to prevent or treat malarial attacks. When used for prophylaxis, chloroquine is given before, during, and after travel or residence in endemic areas. When used for treatment of malaria caused by *P. vivax, P. malariae,* or *P. ovale,* chloroquine relieves symptoms of the acute attack. However, chloroquine does not prevent recurrence of malarial attacks because the drug does not act against the tissue (exoerythrocytic) forms of the parasite. When used for treatment of malaria caused by *P. falciparum,* chloroquine relieves symptoms of the acute attack and, since *P. falciparum* does not have tissue reservoirs, eliminates the parasite from the body. However, chloroquine-resistant strains of *P. falciparum* have developed in some geographic areas.

Chloroquine is also used in protozoal infections other than malaria. These include extraintestinal amebiasis and giardiasis. Chloroquine is occasionally used for its anti-inflammatory effects in rheumatoid arthritis and discoid lupus erythematosus. Chloroquine should be used with caution in clients with hepatic disease or severe neurologic, gastrointestinal, or blood disorders.

Hydroxychloroquine sulfate (Plaquenil) is a derivative of chloroquine with essentially the same actions, uses, and adverse effects as chloroquine.

Routes and dosage ranges

Chloroquine phosphate

Adults: Prophylaxis of malaria, PO 5 mg/kg (base) weekly (maximum of 300 mg of chloroquine base weekly), starting 2 weeks before entering a malarious area and continuing for 8 weeks after return
Treatment of an acute attack of malaria, PO 1 g (600 mg of base) initially, then 500 mg (300 mg of base) after 6–8 hours, then 500 mg daily for 2 days (total of 2.5 g in 4 doses)
Children: Treatment of an acute attack of malaria, PO 10 mg/kg of chloroquine base initially, then 5 mg/kg after 6 hours, then 5 mg/kg/day for 2 days (total of 4 doses)

Chloroquine hydrochloride

Adults: Treatment of malarial attacks, IM 250 mg (equivalent to 200 mg of chloroquine base) initially, repeated q6h if necessary, to a maximal dose of 800 mg of chloroquine base in 24 hours
Children: Treatment of malarial attacks, IM 5 mg/kg chloroquine base initially, repeated after 6 hours if necessary; maximal dose, 10 mg/kg/24 hours

Hydroxychloroquine sulfate

Adults: Prophylaxis, PO 5 mg/kg, not to exceed 310 mg (of hydroxychloroquine base) once weekly for 2 weeks before entry to and 8 weeks after return from malarious areas
Treatment of acute malarial attacks, PO 620 mg initially, then 310 mg 6 hours later, and 310 mg daily for 2 days (total of 4 doses)
Children: Prophylaxis, PO 5 mg/kg (of hydroxychloroquine base) once weekly for 2 weeks before entry to and 8 weeks after return from malarious areas
Treatment of acute malarial attacks, PO 10 mg/kg initially, then 5 mg/kg 6 hours later, and 5 mg/kg/day for 2 doses (total of 4 doses)

Chloroquine phosphate (Aralen) with **primaquine phosphate** is a mixture that is available in tablets containing chloroquine phosphate 500 mg (equivalent to 300 mg of chloroquine base) and primaquine phosphate 79 mg (equivalent to 45 mg of primaquine base).

This combination is effective for prophylaxis of malaria and may be more acceptable to clients. It may also be more convenient for use in children, since there is no pediatric formulation of primaquine available.

Route and dosage ranges

Adults: Prophylaxis of malaria, PO 1 tablet weekly on the same day each week for 2 weeks before entering and 8 weeks after leaving malarious areas

Children: PO same as adults, for children weighing over 45 kg; one half tablet for children weighing 25–45 kg. For younger children, a suspension is prepared, using the tablets and chocolate syrup or fruit juice. The usual concentration is 40 mg of chloroquine base and 6 mg of primaquine base in 5 ml of suspension. Dosages are then 2.5 ml for children weighing 5–7 kg; 5 ml for 8–11 kg; 7.5 ml for 12–15 kg; 10 ml for 16–20 kg; 12.5 ml for 21–24 kg. These dosages are administered weekly, on the same day of the week, for 2 weeks before entering and 8 weeks after leaving malarious areas.

Primaquine phosphate is an antimalarial agent that is used to prevent the initial occurrence of malaria, to prevent recurrent attacks of malaria caused by *P. vivax, P. malariae,* and *P. ovale,* and to achieve "radical cure" of these three types of malaria. (Radical cure involves eradicating the exoerythrocytic forms of the plasmodium and also preventing the survival of the blood forms.) Clinical usefulness of primaquine stems primarily from the drug's ability to destroy tissue (exoerythrocytic) forms of the malarial parasite. Primaquine is especially effective in vivax malaria. Thus far, plasmodial strains causing the three relapsing types of malaria have not developed resistance to primaquine. When used to prevent initial occurrence of malaria (causal prophylaxis), primaquine is given concurrently with a suppressive agent (*e.g.,* chloroquine, amodiaquine, or hydroxychloroquine) after the client has returned from a malarious area. Primaquine is not effective for treatment of acute attacks of malaria.

Route and dosage ranges

Adults: Prophylaxis, PO 26.3 mg (equivalent of 15 mg of primaquine base) daily for 14 days, beginning immediately after leaving a malarious area, or 79 mg (45 mg of base) once a week for 8 weeks. To prevent relapse (*i.e.,* acute malarial attacks), the same dose is given with chloroquine or a related drug daily for 14 days.

Children: Prophylaxis of both the disease and relapse, PO 0.3 mg(base)/kg/day for 14 days, according to the schedule outlined above, or 0.9 mg(base)/kg/week for 8 weeks

Pyrimethamine (Daraprim) is a folic acid antagonist that is used to prevent malaria caused by susceptible strains of plasmodial parasites. Pyrimethamine is sometimes used with a sulfonamide and quinine to treat chloroquine-resistant strains of *P. falciparum.* Folic acid antagonists and sulfonamides act synergistically against plasmodial parasites because they block different steps in the synthesis of folinic acid, a nutrient required by the parasites.

Route and dosage ranges

Adults: Prophylaxis, PO 25 mg once *weekly,* starting 2 weeks before entering and continuing for 8 weeks after returning from malarious areas

Children: Prophylaxis, PO 25 mg once weekly, as above, for ages over 10 years; 6.25 mg–12.5 mg once weekly for ages under 10 years

Quinine sulfate (Quinamm) is a naturally occurring alkaloid derived from the bark of the cinchona tree. Quinine was the primary antimalarial drug for many years. Currently, quinine has been largely replaced by synthetic agents that cause fewer adverse reactions. However, it may still be used in the treatment of chloroquine-resistant falciparum malaria, usually in conjunction with pyrimethamine and a sulfonamide. Quinine also relaxes skeletal muscles and is used for prevention and treatment of nocturnal leg cramps.

Route and dosage range

Adults: Treatment of malaria, PO 650 mg q8h for 10–14 days
Leg cramps, PO 260–300 mg at bedtime

Children: Treatment of malaria, PO 25 mg/kg/day in divided doses q8h for 10–14 days

ANTITRICHOMONAL AGENTS

Metronidazole (Flagyl) see amebicides, above.

Povidone-iodine (Betadine) is an antiseptic (see Chap. 66) that is available in a douche solution for treatment of vaginal infections in general, possibly including trichomoniasis.

Route and dosage range

Adults: Topically to vagina, as a vaginal douche each morning for 10–15 days. Treatment should be continued through menstruation if it occurs.

Several mixtures containing aminacrine hydrochloride (an antiseptic), allantoin (a "debriding" agent), and sulfanilamide (an antimicrobial) are marketed for treatment of vaginal infections, including trichomoniasis. The effectiveness of these agents has not been clearly demonstrated, and topical sulfonamides may cause sensitization, which prevents future administration of systemic sulfonamides. Most of the mixtures are available in vaginal creams and suppositories. These products include AVC and Vagitrol.

ANTI-*PNEUMOCYSTIS CARINII* AGENT

Pentamidine isethionate (Pentam 300) is an antiprotozoal agent approved only for the treatment of *Pneumocystis carinii* pneumonia. This severe, often fatal form of pneumonia rarely occurs in the general population but is not uncommon in people whose immune systems are impaired. One particular group at risk includes victims of acquired immune deficiency syndrome (AIDS). Pentamidine apparently interferes with production of ribonucleic acid and deoxyribonucleic acid by the protozoa. The drug may cause several serious adverse effects, including leukopenia, thrombocytopenia, hypoglycemia, hypocalcemia, hypotension, acute renal failure, Stevens–Johnson syndrome, and ventricular tachycardia. Appropriate tests should be performed before and during pentamidine therapy to detect adverse effects (*e.g.*, complete blood count, platelet count, blood urea nitrogen, serum creatinine, blood glucose, serum calcium, electrocardiogram). Adverse effects are usually reversible. Pentamidine is excreted by the kidneys and accumulates in the presence of renal failure. Dosage should be reduced with renal failure.

Routes and dosage ranges

Adults: IM, IV 4 mg/kg once daily for 14 days
Children: Same as adults

ANTHELMINTICS

Mebendazole (Vermox) is a broad-spectrum anthelmintic drug that is effective in the treatment of parasitic infestations by hookworms, pinworms, roundworms, and whipworms. It is also useful but somewhat less effective in tapeworm infection. Mebendazole kills helminths by preventing uptake of the glucose necessary for parasitic metabolism. The helminths become immobilized and die slowly, so they may be expelled from the gastrointestinal tract up to 3 days after drug therapy is completed. Mebendazole acts locally within the gastrointestinal tract, and less than 10% of the drug is absorbed systemically.

Mebendazole is usually the drug of choice for single or mixed infections caused by the above parasitic worms. The drug is contraindicated during pregnancy because of teratogenic effects in rats; it is relatively contraindicated in children under 2 years of age because it has not been extensively investigated for use in this age group.

Route and dosage ranges

Adults: Most infections, PO 100 mg morning and evening for 3 consecutive days. For pinworms, a single 100-mg dose may be sufficient. A second course of therapy may be administered in 3 weeks, if necessary.
Children: Same as adults

Niclosamide (Niclocide) is an anthelmintic that is effective against beef, fish, and dwarf tapeworm infestations of the intestine. Clients are not considered cured until the stool has been negative for a minimum of 3 months.

Route and dosage ranges

Adults: Beef and fish tapeworm, PO 2g (4 tablets) as a single dose
Dwarf tapeworm, PO 2 g as a single daily dose for 7 days
Children over 34 kg (75 lb): Beef and fish tapeworm, PO 1.5 g as a single dose
Dwarf tapeworm, PO 1.5 g the first day, then 1 g daily for 6 days
Children 11 to 34 kg (25 to 75 lb): Beef and fish tapeworm, PO 1 g as a single dose
Dwarf tapeworm, PO 1 g the first day, then 0.5 g daily for 6 days

Piperazine citrate (Antepar) is an anthelmintic agent that is highly effective against roundworm and pinworm infestations. The drug is not parasiticidal; it causes expulsion of the parasitic worms. Roundworms are alive but paralyzed when expelled by peristalsis. Pinworms are alive and active and may cause reinfection if not disposed of properly. Good personal and environmental hygienic practices are necessary to prevent reinfection.

Piperazine citrate forms piperazine hexahydrate in solution, and it is the hexahydrate salt that exerts anthelmintic action. The drug is well absorbed after oral administration; a portion is metabolized in the liver, and the remainder is excreted in the urine. Piperazine is contraindicated in people with liver, kidney, or convulsive disorders.

Route and dosage ranges

Adults: Roundworms, PO 3.5 g/day for 2 days
Pinworms, PO 65 mg/kg/day for 7 days (maxi-

mal daily dose, 2.5 g of hexahydrate equivalent) In severe roundworm or pinworm infestations, the course of therapy may be repeated after 1 week

Children: Roundworms, PO 75 mg/kg/day for 2 days (maximal daily dose, 3.5 g of hexahydrate equivalent)
Pinworms, same as adults

Pyrantel pamoate (Antiminth) is effective in parasitic infestation of roundworms, pinworms, and hookworms. The drug acts locally to paralyze worms in the intestinal tract. Pyrantel is poorly absorbed from the gastrointestinal tract, and most of an administered dose may be recovered in feces. Pyrantel is contraindicated in pregnancy and is not recommended for children under 1 year of age.

Route and dosage ranges

Adults: Roundworms and pinworms, PO 11 mg/kg (maximal dose, 1 g) as a single dose; for hookworms, the same dose is given daily for 3 consecutive days. The course of therapy may be repeated in 1 month, if necessary.

Children: Same as adults

Pyrvinium pamoate (Povan) is a type of dye that is effective for treatment of pinworm infestations. The drug kills the worms by preventing absorption of the glucose required for metabolism. Pyrvinium acts locally within the intestinal tract; little drug is absorbed systemically. Because the drug is a dye, it colors vomitus, feces, or clothing a bright red. The tablets should be swallowed immediately, without chewing, to avoid staining of teeth.

Route and dosage range

Adults: Pinworms, PO 5 mg/kg in a single dose (maximal dose, 350 mg of pyrvinium base), repeated after 2–3 weeks to eliminate worms that have developed after the first dose.

Children: Same as adults

Thiabendazole (Mintezol) is an anthelmintic agent that is most effective against threadworms and pinworms. It is useful but somewhat less effective against hookworms, roundworms, and whipworms. Because of the broad spectrum of anthelmintic activity, thiabendazole may be especially useful in mixed parasitic infestations. In trichinosis, thiabendazole decreases symptoms and eosinophilia but apparently does not eliminate larvae from muscle tissues. The mechanism of anthelmintic action is uncertain but probably involves interference with parasitic metabolism. The drug is relatively toxic compared to other anthelmintic agents.

Thiabendazole is a first drug of choice for threadworm infestations. For other types of helminthiasis, it is usually considered an alternative drug. Thiabendazole is rapidly absorbed after oral administration. Most of the drug is excreted in urine within 24 hours. Thiabendazole should be used with caution in clients with liver or kidney disease.

Route and dosage ranges

Adults: PO 22 mg/kg (maximal single dose, 3 g) twice daily after meals; 1 day for pinworms, repeated after 1–2 weeks; 2 days for other infections, except trichinosis, which requires about 5 days.

Children: Same as adults

SCABICIDES AND PEDICULICIDES

Gamma benzene hexachloride or **lindane** (Kwell, Gamene) is probably the most frequently prescribed drug in both scabies and pediculosis. It is applied topically, and substantial amounts are absorbed through intact skin. CNS toxicity has been reported with excessive use especially in infants and children. The drug is available in a 1% concentration in a cream, lotion, and shampoo. A single application is usually sufficient to kill parasites and ova.

Route and dosage range

Adults: Scabies, topically to skin, applied to entire skin except the face, neck, and scalp, left in place for 24 hours then removed by shower bath. For pediculosis, use the cream or lotion (rub into the affected area, leave in place for 12 hours, then wash thoroughly) or shampoo (rub into the affected area for 4 minutes before rinsing thoroughly).

Children: Same as adults

Malathion (Prioderm) is a pediculicide used in the treatment of head lice. It is sprinkled on the hair and rubbed in until the hair is thoroughly moistened. The hair is allowed to dry naturally and uncovered. The drug is flammable and should not be used near open flames, nor should a hair dryer be used. In addition, recipients should not smoke while applying the drug or while the hair is wet. After 8 to 12 hours, the hair should be shampooed, rinsed, and combed with a fine-toothed comb to remove dead lice and eggs. If necessary, treatment can be repeated in 7 to 9 days.

Benzyl benzoate is used as a 25% lotion in the treatment of scabies and pediculosis. **Crotamiton** (Eurax) is used as a 10% cream or lotion for scabies. **Pyrethin** preparations (*e.g.,* A-200-Pyrinate, Barc) are available as gels, shampoos, and liquid suspensions for treatment of pediculosis. **Sulfur** solutions and ointments (*e.g.,* Sulfurated Lime Topical Solution, U.S.P., and Sulfur Ointment, U.S.P.) may be used for treatment of both scabies and pediculosis. All these topical agents are applied in the same manner as gamma benzene hexachloride, above.

Principles of therapy: antiparasitics

ASSESSMENT GUIDELINES

Assess for conditions in which antiparasitic drugs are used.

1. Assess for exposure to parasites. Although exposure is influenced by many variables (*e.g.,* geographic location, personal hygiene, environmental sanitation), some useful questions may include the following:
   a. Does the person reside in an institution, an area of poor sanitation, an underdeveloped country, a tropical region, or an area of overcrowded housing? All these conditions predispose to parasitic infestations with lice, the itch mite, protozoa, and worms.
   b. Are parasitic diseases present in the person's environment? For example, head lice, scabies, and pinworm infestations often affect several schoolchildren or family members.
   c. Has the person recently traveled (within the previous 1 to 3 weeks) in malarious regions? If so, were prophylactic measures used appropriately?
   d. With vaginal trichomoniasis, assess in relation to sexual activity. The disease is spread by sexual intercourse, and men may need treatment to prevent reinfection of women.
   e. With pubic (crab) lice, assess sexual activity. Lice may be transmitted by sexual and other close contact and by contact with infested bed linens.
2. Assess for signs and symptoms. These vary greatly, depending on the extent of parasitic infestation.
   a. With amebiasis, the person may be asymptomatic, have nausea, vomiting, diarrhea, abdominal cramping, and weakness or experience symptoms from ulcerations of the colon or abscesses of the liver (amebic hepatitis) if the disease is severe, prolonged, and untreated. Amebiasis is diagnosed by identifying cysts or trophozoites of *E. histolytica* in stool specimens.
   b. With malaria, initial symptoms may resemble those produced by influenza (*e.g.,* headache, myalgia). Characteristic paroxysms of chills, fever, and copious perspiration may not be present in early malaria. During acute malarial attacks, the cycles occur every 36 to 72 hours. Additional symptoms include nausea and vomiting, splenomegaly, hepatomegaly, anemia, leukopenia, thrombocytopenia, and hyperbilirubinemia. Malaria is diagnosed by identifying the plasmodial parasite in peripheral blood smears (by microscopic examination).
   c. With trichomoniasis, females usually have vaginal burning, itching, and yellowish discharge; males are usually asymptomatic. The condition is diagnosed by finding *T. vaginalis* organisms in a wet smear of vaginal exudate, semen, prostatic fluid, or urinary sediment (microscopic examination). Cultures may be necessary.
   d. With helminthiasis, light infestations may be asymptomatic. Heavy infestations produce symptoms according to the particular parasitic worm. Hookworm, roundworm, and threadworm larvae migrate through the lungs and may cause symptoms of pulmonary congestion. The hookworm may cause anemia by sucking blood from the intestinal mucosa; the fish tapeworm may cause megaloblastic or pernicious anemia by absorbing folic acid and vitamin B_{12}. Large masses of roundworms or tapeworms have caused intestinal obstruction. The major symptom usually associated with pinworms is intense itching in the perianal area (pruritus ani). Helminthiasis is diagnosed by microscopic identification of parasites or ova in stool specimens. Pinworm infestation is diagnosed by identifying ova on anal swabs, obtained by touching the adherent side of cellophane tape to the anal area. (Early morning swabs are best because the female pinworm deposits eggs during sleeping hours.)
   e. With scabies and pediculosis, pruritus is usually the primary symptom. Secondary symptoms result from scratching and often include skin excoriation and infection (*i.e.,* vesicles, pustules, and crusts). Pediculosis is diagnosed by visual identification of lice or ova (nits) on the client's body or clothing.

PREVENTION OF PARASITIC DISEASE

Use measures to avoid exposure to or prevent transmission of parasitic diseases.

1. Environmental health measures often attempt to interrupt the life cycle of parasites. Specific measures include the following:
   a. Sanitary sewers to prevent deposition of feces on surface soil and the resultant exposure to helminths
   b. Monitoring of community water supplies, food handling establishments, and food handling personnel
   c. Follow-up examination and possibly treatment of household and other close contacts of persons with helminthiasis, amebiasis, trichomoniasis, scabies, and pediculosis.
   d. Mosquito control in malarious areas and prophylactic drug therapy for travelers to malarious areas. The CDC publishes an annual report that identifies areas where there is risk of malarial infection.
2. Personal and other health measures include the following:
   a. Personal hygiene (*i.e.,* regular bathing and shampooing, handwashing before eating or handling food and after defecation or urination).
   b. Avoiding raw fish and undercooked pork products. Smoking, pickling, or other processing of pork does not prevent trichinosis.
   c. Avoiding contamination of streams or other water sources with feces.
   d. Controlling flies and avoiding foods exposed to flies (*e.g.,* raw fruits and vegetables, cooked foods).
   e. With scabies and pediculosis infestations, drug therapy must be accompanied by adjunctive measures to avoid reinfection or transmission to others. For example, clothes, bed linens, and towels should be washed and dried on hot cycles. Clothes that cannot be washed should be dry cleaned. With head lice, combs and brushes should be cleaned and disinfected; carpets and upholstered furniture should be vacuumed.
   f. With pinworms, clothing, bed linens, and towels should be washed daily on hot cycles. Toilet seats should be disinfected daily.
   g. Cooperating with follow-up measures such as stool specimens, vaginal examinations, anal swabs, smears, and cultures
   h. With vaginal infections, avoid sexual intercourse or have the male partner use a condom.

NURSING ACTIONS: ANTIPARASITICS

Nursing Actions	*Rationale/Explanation*
1. Administer accurately	
a. Give chloroquine and related drugs, iodoquinol, oral metronidazole, and paromomycin with or after meals.	To decrease gastrointestinal irritation
b. Check manufacturer's instructions before giving intravenous metronidazole.	The drug requires specific techniques for preparation and administration.
c. With pentamidine:	
(1) For IM administration, dissolve the drug in 3 ml of sterile water for injection and inject deeply in a large muscle mass.	Intramuscular administraion is painful and may cause sterile abscesses.
(2) For intravenous administration, dissolve the calculated dose in 3 to 5 ml of sterile water or 5% dextrose in water. Dilute further with 50 to 250 ml of 5% dextrose solution and infuse over 60 minutes.	
d. Give anthelmintics without regard to mealtimes or food ingestion. Mebendazole tablets may be chewed, swallowed, or crushed and mixed with food. Niclosamide tablets should be chewed or crushed.	Food in the gastrointestinal tract does not decrease effectiveness of most anthelmintics.

Nursing Actions	Rationale/Explanation
e. For scabicides, use the following sequence: (1) Have the client bathe. (2) Wearing gown and gloves, apply scabicide thinly to all skin surfaces except the face, neck, and scalp. (3) Have the client don clean clothing; remove soiled clothing for laundering. (4) Leave the medication in place for 12 to 24 hours; have the client bathe and again don clean clothing. (5) Wear gloves if direct contact is required while the medication is in place.	Because scabies is highly infectious, most of these procedures are aimed toward preventing reinfection of the client (*i.e.,* wearing clean clothes, laundering soiled clothing) or infection of the nurse (*i.e.,* wearing gloves with direct contact). Isolation is unnecessary. Gloves are unnecessary after 24 hours.
f. For pediculicides, rub cream or lotion into the affected area, leave in place for 12 hours, then wash thoroughly; rub shampoo into the scalp for 4 minutes, then rinse thoroughly.	These methods of administration are used for treatment of head and pubic lice. Skin treatment is not necessary with body lice because the parasites live in the clothing, especially in undergarments and seams.
2. Observe for therapeutic effects	
a. With chloroquine for acute malaria, observe for relief of symptoms and negative blood smears.	Fever and chills usually subside within 24 to 48 hours, and blood smears are negative for plasmodia within 48 to 72 hours.
b. With amebicides, observe for relief of symptoms and negative stool examinations.	Relief of symptoms does not indicate cure of amebiasis; laboratory evidence is required. Stool specimens should be examined for amebic cysts and trophozoites periodically for about 6 months.
c. With anthelmintics, observe for relief of symptoms, absence of the parasite in blood or stool for three consecutive examinations, or a reduction in the number of parasitic ova in the feces.	The goal of anthelmintic drug therapy may be complete eradication of the parasite or reduction of the "worm burden."
d. With pediculicides, inspect affected areas daily for lice or nits for 1 to 2 weeks.	For most clients, one treatment is effective. For others, a second treatment may be necessary about 1 week after the first (to eliminate newly hatched lice).
3. Observe for adverse effects	
a. With amebicides, observe for anorexia, nausea, vomiting, epigastric burning, diarrhea.	Gastrointestinal effects may occur with all amebicides.
(1) With iodoquinol, observe for agitation, amnesia, peripheral neuropathy, and optic neuropathy.	These effects are most likely to occur with large doses or long-term drug administration.
(2) With emetine, observe for cardiovascular effects (*e.g.,* hypotension, chest pain, dyspnea, tachycardia, electrocardiographic abnormalities) and local tissue reactions at injection sites (*e.g.,* pain, tenderness, weakness).	Emetine is a highly toxic drug. Adverse effects may be minimized by close observation during emetine therapy. The client is hospitalized and maintained on bed rest.
b. With antimalarial agents, observe for nausea, vomiting, diarrhea, pruritus, skin rash, headache, CNS stimulation.	These effects may occur with most antimalarial agents. However, adverse effects are usually mild because small doses are used for clinical prophylaxis, and the larger doses required for treatment of acute malarial attacks are only given for short periods. When chloroquine and related drugs are used for long-term treatment of rheumatoid arthritis or lupus erythematosus, adverse effects increase (*e.g.,* blood dyscrasias, retinal damage).
(1) With pyrimethamine, observe for anemia, thrombocytopenia, and leukopenia.	This drug interferes with folic acid metabolism.
(2) With quinine, observe for signs of cinchonism (headache, tinnitus, decreased auditory acuity, blurred vision).	These effects occur with usual therapeutic doses of quinine. They do not usually necessitate discontinuance of quinine therapy.

Nursing Actions	***Rationale/Explanation***
c. With metronidazole, observe for convulsions, peripheral paresthesias, nausea, diarrhea, unpleasant taste, vertigo, headache, and vaginal and urethral burning sensation.	CNS effects are most serious; gastrointestinal effects are most common.
d. With topical antitrichomonal agents, observe for hypersensitivity reactions (*e.g.,* rash, inflammation), burning, and pruritus.	Hypersensitivity reactions are the major adverse effects. Other effects are minor and rarely require that drug therapy be discontinued.
e. With scabicides and pediculicides, observe for irritation and allergic reactions (*e.g.,* rash, inflammation). In addition, gamma benzene hexachloride may cause CNS stimulation (nervousness, tremors, insomnia, convulsions).	Hypersensitivity reactions necessitate discontinuance of the drug. Inflammation should be allowed to subside before other topical scabicides and pediculicides are applied CNS stimulation may occur with gamma benzene hexachloride because the drug is absorbed systemically through intact skin. Adverse effects are uncommon if the drug is used correctly. They are more likely to occur with excessive application (*i.e.,* increased amounts, leaving in place longer than prescribed, or applying more frequently than prescribed).
4. Observe for drug interactions	Few clinically significant drug interactions occur, since many antiparasitic agents are administered for local effects in the gastrointestinal tract or on the skin. The drugs are also given for short periods.
a. Drugs that alter effects of chloroquine	
(1) Acidifying agents (*e.g.,* ascorbic acid)	Inhibit chloroquine by increasing the rate of urinary excretion
(2) Alkalinizing agents (*e.g.,* sodium bicarbonate)	Potentiate chloroquine by decreasing the rate of urinary excretion
(3) Monoamine oxidase (MAO) inhibitors	Increase risk of toxicity and retinal damage by inhibiting hepatic enzymes
b. Drugs that alter effects of metronidazole	
(1) Alcohol	Metronidazole may cause alcohol intolerance or a disulfiram-like reaction if alcohol is ingested. Metronidazole inhibits metabolism of alcohol to carbon dioxide and water. Instead, metronidazole promotes accumulation of acetaldehyde.
(2) Disulfiram (Antabuse)	Increased accumulation of acetaldehyde with possible psychosis. This combination should be avoided.
5. Teach clients	
a. Use antiparasitic drugs as prescribed	To achieve therapeutic effects without adverse effects
b. Measures to prevent parasitic infection or reinfection	

Selected References

Clore ER: Lice: Ancient pest with new resistance. Pediatr Nurs 9:347–350, October 1983

Drugs for parasitic infections. Med Lett Drugs Ther 26:27–34, March 1984

Harvey SC: Antiseptics and disinfectants; fungicides; ectoparasiticides. In Gilman AG, Goodman LS, Rall TW, Murad F (eds): The Pharmacological Basis of Therapeutics, 7th ed, pp 959–979. New York, Macmillan, 1985

McGowan K: How to find and treat amebiasis. Drug Ther 14:159–176, May 1984

Webster LT Jr: Drugs used in the chemotherapy of helminthiasis. In Gilman AG, Goodman LS, Rall TW, Murad F (eds): The Pharmacological Basis of Therapeutics, 7th ed, pp 1009–1028. New York, Macmillan, 1985

Webster LT Jr: Drugs used in the chemotherapy of protozoal infections. In Gilman AG, Goodman LS, Rall TW, Murad F (eds): The Pharmacological Basis of Therapeutics, 7th ed, pp 1029–1065. New York, Macmillan, 1985

45

IMMUNIZING AGENTS

Immune responses

Immunity indicates protection from or resistance to a disease. The process by which a person develops immunity is normally a powerful defense mechanism of the body. The immune response is essentially an antigen–antibody reaction. *Antigens,* substances that are foreign or perceived as foreign to the body's own tissues, are usually proteins or polysaccharides. *Antibodies* are proteins called immunoglobulins. An antibody opposes only the specific antigen that induced formation of the antibody.

Many antigens that activate the immune response are bacteria and viruses that cause infectious disease. In this instance, the immune response is a defense mechanism. In some instances, however, the immune response is initiated by ordinarily harmless substances (*e.g.,* foods, plant pollens) to produce allergic reactions in sensitized persons. In other instances, the immune response is activated by the body's own tissues and produces autoimmune diseases (*e.g.,* lupus erythematosus, rheumatoid arthritis).

In this chapter, the immune response is discussed in relation to infectious disease. The major elements of the immune response are humoral and cellular. These elements are described as follows:

1. Humoral immunity involves production of specific antibodies (*i.e.,* immunoglobulins) that combine with specific antigens. The antigens are thereby deactivated. Immunoglobulins are produced by B-lymphocytes. B-lymphocytes originate in lymphocytic stem cells in the bone marrow, differentiate into cells capable of forming antibodies, and migrate to lymphoid tissue. In lymphoid tissue, the cells may be dormant until exposed to an antigen. When exposed to an antigen, the cells enlarge, become plasma cells, multiply rapidly, and produce immunoglobulins. The immunoglobulins are secreted into lymph and transported to the bloodstream for circulation throughout the body. There are five classes of immunoglobulins.
   a. *Immunoglobulin G* (IgG) is the most abundant immunoglobulin in human serum (approximately 70% of antibodies). IgG opposes microorganisms by promoting phagocytosis and activating complement (a series of enzymatic proteins that break down antigen–antibody complexes). IgG also crosses the placenta to provide maternally acquired (passive) immunity to the infant.
   b. *Immunoglobulin A* (IgA) constitutes only 5% to 10% of serum antibodies but is concentrated in respiratory and gastrointestinal secretions, where it acts against pathogens entering those areas.
   c. *Immunoglobulin M* (IgM) constitutes about 10% of serum antibodies. IgM reacts with antigens in the bloodstream only because its large molecular size prevents transport through capillary walls. IgM activates complement to destroy microorganisms.
   d. *Immunoglobulin E* (IgE) is thought to be the immunoglobulin responsible for allergic reac-

tions, including anaphylaxis. Small amounts of IgE are present in the serum of nonallergic persons; larger amounts are produced by people with allergies.

e. *Immunoglobulin D* (IgD) is present in serum in trace amounts and probably functions in recognition of antigens.

2. Cellular immunity involves special cells, T-lymphocytes, which are able to oppose antigens. The T-lymphocytes originate in lymphocytic stem cells in the bone marrow, differentiate into cells capable of reacting with antigens in the thymus gland, enter the bloodstream, and migrate to lymphoid tissue, mainly lymph nodes and spleen. When exposed to an antigen, these specifically sensitized cells can produce large numbers of other cells by clonal growth. These cells enter the bloodstream to oppose the antigen.

   Cell-mediated immunity is involved in the development of delayed hypersensitivity, rejection of tissue transplants, and response to neoplasms and some infections.

Types of immunity

Natural immunity is present from birth and varies in persons, ethnic groups, and species. For example, one person may develop a disease while another does not, despite similar exposure to antigenic microorganisms. Similarly, whites have relatively high resistance to tuberculosis and little resistance to malaria, whereas the opposite reactions occur in blacks. Finally, many diseases occur in human beings that do not occur in most animals, and vice versa.

Acquired immunity is immunity that develops after birth. It may be active or passive. *Active immunity* occurs when the host develops antibodies against an antigen (*i.e.*, antibodies are formed endogenously). Exposure to the antigen and subsequent antibody formation may occur when the person has the disease produced by a specific antigen or when the antigen is artificially administered, usually by injection.

When an antigen is present for the first time, production of antibodies requires several days. As a result, the concentration of serum antibodies does not reach protective levels for about 1 week, and the host develops the disease. When the antigen is eliminated, the antibody titer gradually decreases over several weeks. Duration of active immunity may be relatively brief (*e.g.*, with the common cold and penumonia), or it may be long term (*i.e.*, years or even lifetime). Long-term active immunity has a unique characteristic called *memory*. When the host is reexposed to the antigen, production of antibodies is immediate and the host does not develop the disease. This characteristic allows "booster" doses of antigen to increase antibody levels and maintain active immunity against some diseases.

Passive immunity occurs when antibodies are formed exogenously and transferred to the host. The infant is normally protected for several months by antibodies received from the mother by placental transfer during gestation. In another instance, antibodies are formed in other people or animals and transferred to the host by an injection of immune serum. These preformed antibodies act against antigens immediately. Passive immunity is short term, lasting only a few weeks or months.

Immunization

Immunization or vaccination involves administration of an antigen to induce antibody formation (for active immunity) or serum from immune people or animals (for passive immunity). Preparations used for immunization are biologic products prepared by pharmaceutical companies and regulated by the Food and Drug Administration (FDA).

AGENTS FOR ACTIVE IMMUNITY

The biologic products used for active immunity are vaccines and toxoids. *Vaccines* are suspensions of microorganisms that have been killed or attenuated (weakened or reduced in virulence) so that they are able to induce antibody formation without causing the disease. *Toxoids* are bacterial toxins that have been modified to destroy toxicity while retaining antigenic properties (*i.e.*, ability to induce antibody formation).

Clinical indications for use of vaccines and toxoids include the following:

1. Routine immunization of all children against diphtheria, tetanus, pertussis (whooping cough), rubeola ("red" measles), rubella (German measles), mumps, and poliomyelitis
2. Immunization of adults against tetanus
3. Immunization of prepubertal girls or women of child-bearing age against rubella. Rubella during the first trimester of pregnancy is associated with a high incidence of birth defects in the newborn.
4. Immunization of people at high risk of serious morbidity or mortality from a particular disease. For example, influenza and pneumococcal vaccines are recommended for various groups of people (see Table 45-1).
5. Immunization of adults and children at high risk of exposure to a particular disease. For example, sev-

(Text continues on p. 427.)

TABLE 45-1. VACCINES AND TOXOIDS FOR ACTIVE IMMUNITY

Generic name	Trade name	Characteristics	Clinical indications	Routes and dosage ranges	
				Adults	*Children*
Cholera vaccine		1. Sterile suspension of killed cholera organisms. 2. Protects 60%–80% of recipients for 3–6 months. Does not prevent transmission of cholera. 3. Protection begins about 1 week after the initial dose.	1. Travel to endemic areas (Asia, Africa, Middle East). 2. Living in endemic areas.	IM, SC 0.5 ml initially, 0.5 ml 4 weeks later, then 0.5 ml every 6 months if indicated	Over age 10 years, same as adults Age 5–10 years, IM, SC 0.3 ml initially, 0.3 ml 4 weeks later, then 0.3 ml every 6 months if indicated Age 6 months–4 years, IM, SC 0.2 ml initially, 0.2 ml 4 weeks later, then 0.2 ml every 6 months if indicated
Hemophilus b polysaccharide vaccine	b-Capsa I	1. Adverse effects are usually mild and transitory (*e.g.,* fever, erythema and induration at injection sites) 2. It is not yet known whether revaccination is required	To prevent infection with Hib, which often occurs in the first 5 years of life and may cause bacterial meningitis and other serious conditions. It is recommended for all children 24 months to 6 years of age and children 18 to 24 months who are at high risk for Hib disease (*e.g.,* those attending day-care centers)		SC 0.5 ml (25 μg) of reconstituted vaccine in a single dose
Hepatitis B vaccine	Heptavax-B	1. A killed-virus vaccine prepared from particles of hepatitis B surface antigen (HB_sAg) obtained from the plasma of human HB_sAg carriers 2. Protection begins in 7–10 days and lasts a year or more 3. 90%–95% effective	Preexposure immunization of high-risk persons such as workers in blood centers and hemodialysis units, surgeons, dentists, drug addicts, male homosexuals, sexually promiscuous persons, clients with renal transplant or cancer, and those receiving hemodialysis or multiple blood transfusions or who are immunosuppressed	IM 1 ml initially, repeated in 1 month and 6 months Persons undergoing hemodialysis or who are immunosuppressed, IM 2 ml (in 2 divided doses, given at different sites) initially, repeated in 1 month and 6 months Booster may be needed every 5 years	Under age 10 years, IM 0.5 ml initially, repeated in 1 month and 6 months. Booster may be needed every 5 years
Influenza vaccine	Fluogen, others	1. Inactivated strains of A and B influenza viruses, usually reformulated annually to include current strains. 2. Protects 60%–75% of recipients for a	1. To reduce incidence and severity of influenza in high-risk people. 2. Recommended annually for people who are elderly; who are	SC 0.5 ml for 2 doses, 2 months apart initially, then 0.5 ml annually	Over age 3 months, same as adults

TABLE 45-1. VACCINES AND TOXOIDS FOR ACTIVE IMMUNITY (*Continued*)

Generic name	Trade name	Characteristics	Clinical indications	Routes and dosage ranges *Adults*	*Children*
		few months. Maximal antibody production occurs the second week after vaccination; the titer remains constant about 1 month, then gradually declines. 3. Grown in chick embryos, therefore contraindicated in clients who are highly allergic to eggs. 4. A disadvantage is that the vaccine may not contain currently active strains of influenza viruses.	nursing home patients; who have chronic pulmonary, cardiovascular or renal disease; who have diabetes mellitus; or who have adrenocortical insufficiency. 3. Not recommended for healthy adults or children.		
Measles vaccine	Attenuvax	1. Sterile preparation of live, attenuated measles (rubeola) virus. 2. Grown in chick embryos but allergic reactions have not been reported in people known to be allergic to egg protein. 3. Protects approximately 95% of recipients for several years or lifetime. 4. Usually given with mumps and rubella vaccines. A combination product containing all three antigens is available and preferred. 5. Measles vaccine should not be given for 3 months after administration of immune serum globulin, plasma, or whole blood. 6. Contraindicated during pregnancy, febrile illness, and upper respiratory infection and in clients with malignancy (*e.g.,* leukemia, lymphoma, generalized malignancy) or who are receiving immunosuppressive treatment (*e.g.,* corticosteroid or antineoplastic drugs or irradiation).	1. Routine immunization of children 1 year of age or older. 2. Immunization of adults not previously immunized.	SC 0.5 ml in a single dose.	SC, same as adults

TABLE 45-1. VACCINES AND TOXOIDS FOR ACTIVE IMMUNITY (*Continued*)

Generic name	Trade name	Characteristics	Clinical indications	Routes and dosage ranges	
				Adults	***Children***
Measles and rubella vaccine	M-R-Vax-II	A mixture of live attenuated rubeola virus (Attenuvax) and rubella (German measles) virus	Immunization of 15-month-old children against rubeola and rubella		SC, total volume of reconstituted vial
Measles, mumps, and rubella vaccine	M-M-R-II	1. A mixture of three vaccines (rubeola, rubella, mumps) 2. Usually preferred over single immunizing agents	Immunization from age 15 months to puberty		SC, total volume of reconstituted vial
Meningitis vaccine	Menomune A/C Menomune A/C/Y/W-135	A suspension prepared from groups A and C or A, C, Y, and W-135 of *Neisseria meningitides*	1. Immunization of persons at risk in epidemic or endemic areas 2. Type A only should be given to infants and children under 2 years of age	SC 0.5 ml	
Mumps vaccine	Mumpsvax	1. Sterile suspension of live, attenuated mumps virus. 2. Provides active immunity in about 97% of children and 93% of adults for at least 8 years. 3. Most often given in combination with measles and rubella vaccines. 4. Contraindicated in pregnancy, people who have dysgammaglobulinemia, people receiving immunosuppressive therapy (*i.e.*, corticosteroids, antineoplastic agents, irradiation), and people with acute infections.	Routine immunization of children (1 year and older) and adults.	SC 0.5 ml in a single dose of reconstituted vaccine. (Reconstituted vaccine retains potency for 8 hours if refrigerated. Discard if not used within 8 hours.)	Over 1 year, same as adults (vaccination not indicated in children under 1 year)
Pertussis vaccine		Usually given in combination with diphtheria and tetanus toxoids. Triogen is a formulation that contains the three components.	Routine immunization of infants and children up to 6 years of age.	Not recommended	Age 2 months–6 years, SC 0.5 ml every 4–6 weeks for 3 doses initially; 0.5 ml as booster dose 1 year after initial immunization and upon starting school
Plague vaccine		A sterile suspension of killed plague bacilli	Immunization of high-risk persons (*e.g.*, laboratory workers, people in disaster areas)	IM 1.0 ml initially, then 0.2 ml after 1–3 months and 3–6 months (total of 3 doses).	Age 5–10 years, $\frac{3}{5}$ adult dose Age 1–4 years, $\frac{2}{5}$ adult dose Age under 1 year, $\frac{1}{5}$ adult dose

TABLE 45-1. VACCINES AND TOXOIDS FOR ACTIVE IMMUNITY (*Continued*)

Generic name	Trade name	Characteristics	Clinical indications	Routes and dosage ranges: *Adults*	Routes and dosage ranges: *Children*
				Booster doses of 0.1–0.2 ml every 6 months during active exposure	
Pneumococcal vaccine, polyvalent	Pneumovax 23 Pnu-Imune 23	1. Consists of 23 strains of pneumococci, which cause approximately 85%–90% of the serious pneumococcal infections in the United States. 2. Protection begins about the third week after vaccination and lasts at least 3 years. 3. Not recommended for children under 2 years old because they may be unable to produce adequate antibody levels.	1. Adults with chronic cardiovascular or pulmonary diseases 2. Adults with chronic diseases associated with increased risk of pneumoccal infection (*e.g.,* splenic dysfunction, Hodgkin's disease, multiple myeloma, cirrhosis, alcohol dependence, renal failure, immunosuppression) 3. Adults 65 years or older who are otherwise healthy 4. Children 2 years or older with chronic diseases associated with increased risk of pneumococcal infection (*e.g.,* asplenia, nephrotic syndrome, immunosuppression)	SC, IM 0.5 ml as a single dose	Same as adults
Poliomyelitis vaccine, inactivated	IPV	A suspension of poliovirus types I, II, and III	Immunization in persons whose immune systems are suppressed or compromised by illness or immunosuppressant drugs	SC 1.0 ml every 4–6 weeks for a total of 3 doses, followed by a fourth dose after 6–12 months. Booster dose (1 ml) every 5 years	Same as adults
Poliovirus vaccine (Sabin, oral)	Orimune	1. Suspension of live, attenuated poliovirus types I, II, and III (trivalent preparation, which is most often used). 2. Provides rapid immunity of more than 90% of recipients. 3. Contraindicated in clients with impaired immunity due to leukemia, lymphoma, generalized malignancy, corticosteroids, antineoplastic drugs, or irradiation.	1. Routine immunization of all infants and children. 2. Immunization of high-risk adults (*e.g.,* hospital employees, people who live in or travel to epidemic or endemic areas).	Same as children and adolescents	Infants, PO 0.5 ml at 2, 4, and 6 months, followed by a fourth dose at approximately 15–18 months Children and adolescents, PO 0.5 ml for 2 doses, 6–8 weeks apart, followed by a third dose of 0.5 ml 8–12 months after the second

TABLE 45-1. VACCINES AND TOXOIDS FOR ACTIVE IMMUNITY (*Continued*)

Generic name	Trade name	Characteristics	Clinical indications	Routes and dosage ranges: Adults	Routes and dosage ranges: Children
					dose. All children who have received the series should be given a single booster dose at 4–6 years of age
Rabies vaccines		1. The rabies vaccine of choice for postexposure prophylaxis is human diploid cell cultures rabies vaccine (HDCV). This preparation is the rabies vaccine most recently approved for use in the United States. 2. Another vaccine (used for 14- or 21-day regimens) is inactivated viruses grown in rabbit brain tissue (Semple vaccine).	1. Preexposure immunization in persons at high-risk of exposure (veterinarians, animal handlers, laboratory personnel who work with rabies virus). 2. Postexposure prophylaxis in persons who have been bitten by potentially rabid animals or who have skin scratches or abrasions exposed to animal saliva (*e.g.,* animal licking of wound), urine, or blood.	HDCV: Preexposure prophylaxis, IM 1.0 ml for 3 doses. The second dose is given 1 week after the first; the third dose is given 4 weeks after the first. Thereafter, booster doses (1 ml) are given every 2 years in high-risk persons Postexposure, IM 1 ml for 5 doses. After the initial dose, remaining doses are given 3, 7, 14, and 28 days later. Rabies immune globulin is administered at the same time as the initial dose of HDVC vaccine	
Rubella vaccine	Meruvax II	1. Sterile suspension of live, attenuated rubella virus. 2. Grown in duck embryo 3. Protects approximately 95% of recipients for 8 years or longer. 4. Usually given with measles and mumps vaccines. A combination product containing all three antigens is available and preferred. 5. Rubella vaccine should not be given for 3 months after administration of immune serum globulin, plasma, or whole blood.	1. Routine immunization of children 1 year of age or older. 2. Initial or repeat immunization of adolescent girls or women of childbearing age *if* serum antibody levels are low.	SC 0.5 ml in a single dose	SC, same as adults

TABLE 45-1. VACCINES AND TOXOIDS FOR ACTIVE IMMUNITY (*Continued*)

Generic name	Trade name	Characteristics	Clinical indications	Routes and dosage ranges	
				Adults	*Children*
		6. Contraindicated during pregnancy, febrile illness, immunosuppressive therapy (*e.g.*, corticosteroid or antineoplastic drugs or irradiation), and malignancy (leukemia, lymphoma, generalized malignancy).			
Rubella and mumps vaccine	Biavax-II	1. A mixture of mumps and rubella virus strains 2. Less frequently used than measles, mumps, and rubella vaccine	Immunization of children		Age 1 year and older, SC, total volume of reconstituted vial
Smallpox vaccine		1. Preparation of live (cowpox) virus 2. Protection lasts 3–10 years, beginning 8 days after vaccination. 3. Not recommended for routine immunization because risks from vaccine are greater than risk of getting smallpox. 4. Available from Centers for Disease Control; no longer commercially manufactured in the United States	1. Foreign travel to Africa, Asia, Central America, and South America. 2. Health care personnel.	Intradermal, by multiple puncture technique, of one capillary tube	
Tuberculosis vaccine		1. Also called Bacillus Calmette-Guerin (BCG) vaccine. 2. Suspension of attenuated tubercle bacillus. 3. Converts negative tuberculin reactors to positive reactors. Therefore, precludes use of the tuberculin skin test for screening or early diagnosis of tuberculosis. 4. Contraindicated in clients who have not had a (negative) tuberculin skin test within the preceding 2 weeks; who are actually ill or suspected of having respiratory tract, skin, or other infection; who have dysgammaglobulinemia; and who have	Persons at high risk for exposure, including newborns of women with tuberculosis.	Intradermal, by multiple puncture technique, 0.1 ml	Newborns, intradermal, 0.05 ml Children, intradermal, 0.1 ml

TABLE 45-1. VACCINES AND TOXOIDS FOR ACTIVE IMMUNITY *(Continued)*

Generic name	Trade name	Characteristics	Clinical indications	Routes and dosage ranges: Adults	Routes and dosage ranges: Children
		a positive tuberculin skin test.			
Typhoid vaccine		1. Sterile suspension of killed typhoid bacilli. 2. Protects 70%–90% of recipients. 3. Not recommended for routine immunization.	High-risk persons (household contacts of typhoid carriers or people whose occupation or travel predisposes to exposure).	SC 0.5 ml for 2 doses at least 4 weeks apart, then a booster dose of 0.5 ml (or 0.1 ml intradermal) at least every 3 years for repeated or continued exposure	Age over 10 years, SC 0.5 ml for 2 doses at least 4 weeks apart, then a booster dose of 0.5 ml at least every 3 years for repeated or continued exposure Age 6 months–10 years, SC 0.25 ml for 2 doses, at least 4 weeks apart, then a booster dose of 0.25 ml (or 0.1 ml intradermal) every 3 years if indicated
Yellow fever vaccine	YF-Vax	1. Suspension of live, attenuated yellow fever virus. 2. Protects approximately 95% of recipients for 10 years or longer. 3. Contraindicated in clients who are allergic to eggs, who have febrile illnesses, who have dysgammaglobulinemia, or who are receiving corticosteroids, antineoplastic, or other immunosuppressive drugs.	1. Laboratory personnel at risk of exposure. 2. Travel to endemic areas (Africa, South America).	SC 0.5 ml; booster dose of 0.5 ml every 10 years if in endemic areas	Age over 6 months, SC same as adults
Diphtheria and tetanus toxoids and pertussis vaccine (DTP)	Tri-Immunol	Diphtheria component is a preparation of detoxified growth products of *Corynebacterium diphtheriae*	Routine immunization of infants and young children 6 years of age or younger		IM 0.5 ml for 3 doses at 4- to 6-week intervals, beginning at 2 months of age, followed by a reinforcing dose 7–12 months later and a booster dose when the child is 5–6 years of age
Diphtheria and tetanus toxoids adsorbed (pediatric type)		1. Also called DT 2. Contains a larger amount of diphtheria antigen than tetanus and diphtheria	Routine immunization of infants and children up to 6 years of age in whom pertussis vaccine is		Infants and children up to 6 years of age, IM 0.5 ml for 2 doses at

TABLE 45-1. VACCINES AND TOXOIDS FOR ACTIVE IMMUNITY (*Continued*)

Generic name	Trade name	Characteristics	Clinical indications	Routes and dosage ranges Adults	Children
		toxoids, adult type (Td)	contraindicated (*i.e.*, those who have adverse reactions to initial doses of DTP)		least 4 weeks apart, followed by a reinforcing dose 1 year later and at the time the child starts school
Tetanus toxoid, adsorbed		1. Preparation of detoxified growth products of *Clostridium tetani* 2. Protects approximately 100% of recipients for 10 years or more. 3. Usually given in combination with diphtheria toxoid and pertussis vaccine (DTP) or diphtheria toxoid (DT) for primary immunization of infants and children up to 6 years of age. 4. Usually given alone or combined with diphtheria toxoid (Td, adult type) for primary immunization of adults	1. Routine immunization of infants and young children. 2. Primary immunization of adults. 3. Prevention of tetanus in previously immunized persons who sustain a potentially contaminated wound.	Primary immunization in adults not previously immunized, IM 0.5 ml initially, followed by 0.5 ml in 4–6 weeks, followed by 0.5 ml 6–12 months later (total of 3 doses). Then, 0.5 ml booster dose every 10 years. Prophylaxis, IM, 0.5 ml if wound severely contaminated and no booster dose received for 5 years; 0.5 ml if wound clean and no booster dose received for 10 years	Primary immunization and prophylaxis, same as adults
Tetanus and diphtheria toxoids, adsorbed (adult type)		1. Also called Td 2. Contains a smaller amount of diphtheria antigen than diphtheria and tetanus toxoids, pediatric type (DT)	Primary immunization or booster doses in adults and children over 6 years of age	IM 0.5 ml for 2 doses, at least 4 weeks apart, followed by a reinforcing dose 6–12 months later and every 10 years thereafter	Age above 6 years, same as adults

eral diseases (*e.g.*, yellow fever, cholera) rarely occur in most parts of the world. Thus, immunization is recommended only for people who live in or travel to geographic areas where the disease can be contracted.

Vaccines and toxoids are generally contraindicated in people with febrile illnesses, impaired cellular immunity (*i.e.*, those receiving corticosteroid, antineoplastic, or immunosuppressive drugs or radiation therapy), leukemia, lymphoma or generalized malignancy, and dysgammaglobulinemia and during pregnancy.

AGENTS FOR PASSIVE IMMUNITY

The biologic products used for passive immunity are immune serums and antitoxins. These substances may be obtained from human or animal sources, and they may consist of whole serum or the immunoglobulin portion of serum in which the specific antibodies are concentrated. When possible, human serum is preferred to animal serum because risks of severe allergic reactions are reduced. Also, immunoglobulin fractions are preferred over whole serum because they are more likely to be effective. Human immune globulins are available for measles, hepatitis, rabies, mumps, pertussis, and tetanus. Mumps and pertussis immune globulins have not been proved effective.

To obtain antitoxins or animal immune serums, an animal such as a horse is injected with a purified toxin or toxoid. After antibodies have had time to develop, blood is withdrawn from the animal and prepared for clinical use. Antitoxins are available for rabies, botulism, diphtheria, gas gangrene, and tetanus. A major disadvantage of antitoxins is that a relatively high number of people are allergic to horse serum.

Immune serums and antitoxins are used to provide temporary immunity in persons exposed to or experiencing a particular disease. The goal of therapy is to prevent or modify the disease process (*i.e.*, decrease incidence and severity of symptoms). Antitoxins are contraindicated in clients who are allergic to horse serum.

Individual immunizing agents

Vaccines and toxoids are listed in Table 45-1; immune serums and antitoxins are shown in Table 45-2.

Principles of therapy: immunizing agents

ASSESSMENT GUIDELINES

Assess the client's immunization status by obtaining the following information:

1. Previous history of diseases for which immunizing agents are available (*e.g.*, measles, mumps, influenza)
2. Previous immunizations
   a. For which diseases were immunizations received?
   b. Which immunizing agent was received?
   c. Any adverse effects experienced? If so, what symptoms occurred and how long did they last?
   d. Any cuts or wounds for which tetanus toxoid was given?
   e. Any foreign travel that required immunizations?
3. Does the client have any conditions that contraindicate administration of immunizing agents (*e.g.*, malignancy, pregnancy, immunosuppressive drug therapy)?
4. For pregnant women not known to be immunized against rubella, serum antibody titer should be measured to determine resistance or susceptibility to the disease.
5. For clients with wounds, assess the type of wound and determine how, when, and where it was sustained. Such information may reveal whether tetanus immunization is needed.
6. For clients exposed to infectious diseases, try to determine the extent of exposure (*e.g.*, household or brief, casual contact) and when it occurred.

PREVENTION OF INFECTIOUS DISEASE

Use measures to prevent infectious diseases, and provide information about the availability of immunizing agents. General measures include those to promote health and resistance to disease (*e.g.*, nutrition, rest, and exercise). Additional measures include the following:

1. Education of the public, especially parents of young children, regarding the importance of immunizations to personal and public health. Include information about the diseases that can be prevented and where immunizations can be obtained. In addition, emphasize the importance of keeping accurate immunization records. This is a personal responsibility of all persons (or parents) because immunizations are often obtained at different places and over a period of years.
2. Prevention of disease transmission. The following are helpful measures:
   a. Handwashing, probably the most effective method
   b. Avoiding contact with people who have known or suspected infectious diseases, when possible
   c. Using isolation techniques when appropriate
   d. Using medical and surgical aseptic techniques
3. For someone exposed to rubeola, administration of measles vaccine within 48 hours is effective in preventing the disease.
4. For someone with a puncture wound or a dirty wound, administration of tetanus immune globulin may be needed to prevent tetanus, a life-threatening disease.
5. For someone with an animal bite, the wound should be washed immediately with large amounts of soap and water. Then, health care should be sought. Administration of rabies vaccine may be needed to prevent rabies, a life-threatening disease.

(Text continues on p. 432.)

TABLE 45-2. IMMUNE SERUMS AND ANTITOXINS FOR PASSIVE IMMUNITY

	Generic name	Trade name	Characteristics	Clinical indications	Routes and dosage ranges
Immune serums	Hepatitis B immune globulin, human	H-BIG, Hyper-Hep, Hep-B-Gammagee	A solution of immunoglobulins that contains antibodies to hepatitis B surface antigen	To prevent hepatitis after exposure	Adults and children: IM 0.06 ml/kg as soon as possible after exposure. Dose repeated in 1 month
	Immune serum globulin (human) (ISG)	Gammar	1. Commonly called gamma globulin. 2. Obtained from pooled plasma of normal donors. 3. Consists primarily of immunoglobulin G (IgG), which contains concentrated antibodies. 4. Produces adequate serum levels of IgG in 2–5 days	1. To decrease the severity of hepatitis, measles, and varicella after exposure 2. Replacement therapy for immunoglobulin deficiency states 3. Adjunct to antibiotics in severe bacterial infections and burns 4. To lessen possibility of fetal damage in pregnant women exposed to rubella virus (however, routine use in early pregnancy is not recommended)	Adults and children: Exposure to hepatitis A, IM 0.02–0.04 ml/kg Exposure to hepatitis B, IM 0.06 ml/kg, repeated in 1 month Exposure to measles, IM 0.22 ml/kg given within 6 days of exposure Exposure to varicella, IM 0.6–1.2 ml/kg Exposure to rubella (pregnant women only), IM 20 ml Immunoglobulin deficiency, IM 1.2 ml/kg initially, then 0.6 ml/kg every 3–4 weeks Bacterial infections, IM 0.5–3.5 ml/kg
	Immune serum globulin intravenous (IGIV)	Gamimune, Sandoglobulin	1. Given intravenously only 2. Provides immediate antibodies 3. Half-life about 3 weeks 4. Mechanism of Sandoglobulin's action in idiopathic thrombocytopenic purpura (ITP) unknown	1. Immunodeficiency syndrome 2. ITP (Sandoglobulin)	Gamimune: IV infusion, 100 mg/kg once a month. May be given more often or increased to 200 mg/kg if clinical response or serum level of immunoglobulin G (IgG) is insufficient Sandoglobulin: IV infusion, 200 mg/kg once a month. May be given more often or increased to 300 mg/kg if clinical response or level of IgG is inadequate. ITP IV infusion, 0.4 g/kg daily for 5 consecutive days
	Lymphocyte immune globulin	Atgam	1. Decreases number of T-lymphocytes (antilymphocytic action) 2. Contains antibodies against other formed elements of the blood 3. Alters both cell-mediated and humoral immunity	To prevent or treat rejection of transplanted organs	Adults: IV 10–30 mg/kg/day Children: IV 5–25 mg/kg/day

TABLE 45-2. IMMUNE SERUMS AND ANTITOXINS FOR PASSIVE IMMUNITY (*Continued*)

Generic name	Trade name	Characteristics	Clinical indications	Routes and dosage ranges
Rabies immune globulin (Human)	Hyperab	1. Gamma globulin obtained from plasma of people hyperimmunized with rabies vaccine. 2. Not useful in treatment of clinical rabies infection.	Postexposure prevention of rabies, in conjunction with rabies vaccine.	Adults and children: IM 20 units/kg (half the dose may be infiltrated around the wound) as soon as possible after possible exposure (*e.g.*, animal bite)
Rh_0 (D) immune globulin (human)	Gamulin Rh, HypRho-D, RhoGAM	1. Prepared from fractionated human plasma. 2. A sterile concentrated solution of specific immunoglobulin (IgG) containing anti-Rh_0(D). 3. For IM use only.	1. To prevent sensitization in a subsequent pregnancy to the Rh_0 (D) factor in an Rh-negative mother who has given birth to an Rh-positive infant by an Rh-positive father. 2. To prevent Rh_0(D) sensitization in Rh-negative clients accidentally transfused with Rh-positive blood. 3. Also available in microdose form (MICRhoGAM) for the prevention of maternal Rh immunization following abortion or miscarriage up to 12 weeks' gestation.	Obstetrical use: inject contents of 1 vial IM for every 15 ml fetal packed red cell volume within 72 hours following delivery, miscarriage, or abortion Transfusion accidents: inject contents of 1 vial IM for every 15 ml of Rh-positive packed red cell volume Consult package instructions for blood typing and drug administration procedures.
Tetanus immune globulin (human)	Hyper-Tet, others	1. Solution of globulins from plasma of people hyperimmunized with tetanus toxoid. 2. Tetanus toxoid should be given at the same time (in a different syringe and injection site) to initiate active immunization.	1. To prevent tetanus in clients with wounds possibly contaminated with *Clostridium tetani* and whose immunization history is uncertain or included less than 2 immunizing doses of tetanus toxoid. 2. Treatment of tetanus.	Adults and children: Prophylaxis, IM 250 units as a single dose Treatment of clinical disease, IM 3000–6000 units
Varicella-zoster immune globulin (human) (VZIG)	Varicella-zoster immune globulin	1. The globulin fraction of human plasma 2. Antibodies last 1 month or longer	To prevent or decrease severity of varicella infections (chickenpox, shingles) in children under 15 years of age who are immunodeficient because of illness (*e.g.*, leukemia, lymphoma), or drug therapy (*e.g.*, corticosteroids, antineoplastics) and who have had signifi-	IM 125 units/10 kg up to a maximum of 625 units as soon as possible after exposure, up to 96 hours after exposure. Minimal dose, 125 units

TABLE 45-2. IMMUNE SERUMS AND ANTITOXINS FOR PASSIVE IMMUNITY (*Continued*)

	Generic name	Trade name	Characteristics	Clinical indications	Routes and dosage ranges
				cant exposure to chickenpox or herpes zoster (*i.e.*, playmate, household or hospital contact) May be used in children under 15 and adults on an individualized basis	
Animal serums (antitoxins)	Antirabies serum, equine		A hyperimmune horse serum used only if human rabies immune globulin is not available.	To prevent rabies after severe exposure (*e.g.*, multiple, deep animal bites, especially around the head). Used in conjunction with rabies vaccine.	Adults and children: IM 55 units/kg (half the dose may be infiltrated around the wound) as soon as possible. A test for hypersensitivity to horse serum should precede administration.
	Botulism antitoxin		1. Obtained from blood of horses immunized against toxins of *Clostridium botulinus.* 2. The only specific agent available for treatment of botulism. Prompt use markedly decreases mortality. 3. May be obtained from the Centers for Disease Control.	For treatment of suspected botulism (a severe form of food poisoning that develops from raw or improperly preserved foods such as home canned vegetables). Botulism has a 20% to 35% mortality.	Adults and children: Consult the manufacturer's instructions regarding dosages and routes of administration. Testing for hypersensitivity to horse serum should precede administration of the antitoxin.
	Diphtheria antitoxin		1. Obtained from blood of horses hyperimmunized against diphtheria toxin. 2. Used in conjunction with antibiotics (*e.g.*, penicillin, tetracycline, erythromycin), which eliminate bacteria but do not eliminate bacterial toxins.	1. To prevent diphtheria in exposed, nonimmunized clients. 2. For treatment of diphtheria infection (based on clinical diagnosis, without waiting for bacteriologic confirmation of *Corynebacterium diphtheriae*).	Adults and children: Prophylaxis, IM 5000–10,000 units Treatment, IV 20,000–120,000 units
	Tetanus antitoxin		1. Obtained from the blood of horses hyperimmunized with tetanus toxin or toxoid. 2. Used only when tetanus immune globulin, human, is unavailable.	1. To prevent tetanus in nonimmunized clients with tetanus-prone wounds. 2. For treament of tetanus.	Adults and children: Prophylaxis, IM, SC 1500–5000 units within 24 hours after injury. If 48 hours have elapsed, 10,000–20,000 units. Treatment, IV IM 50,000–100,000 units Recommended to give a portion IV and the remainder IM

6. Contracting rubella or undergoing rubella immunization during pregnancy, especially during the first trimester, may cause severe birth defects in the infant. The goal of immunization is to prevent congenital rubella syndrome. Current recommendations are to immunize children against rubella at 12 to 15 months of age.

   It is recommended that previously unimmunized girls of ages 11 to 13 years be immunized. Further, nonpregnant women of child-bearing age should have rubella antibody tests. If antibody concentrations are low, the women should be immunized. Pregnancy should be avoided for 3 months after immunization.

IMMUNIZATION RECOMMENDATIONS

1. Recommendations regarding immunizations change periodically as additional information and new immunizing agents become available. Consequently, health care personnel should update their knowledge at least annually. The best sources of information regarding current recommendations are the local health department and the Centers for Disease Control (CDC), U.S. Public Health Service, Department of Health and Human Services, Atlanta, Georgia. Local health departments can be consulted on immunization requirements for foreign travel as well as routine immunizations.
2. Current recommendations for immunization of infants and children are listed as follows:
   a. Diphtheria, tetanus, and pertussis (DTP) and trivalent oral poliovirus vaccine (TOPV) at ages 2 months, 4 months, 6 months, 18 months, and 4 to 6 years.
   b. Measles, mumps, and rubella at 12 to 15 months of age, usually as a combined vaccine (*i.e.,* MMR). These vaccines are given later than DTP and TOPV because sufficient antibodies may not be produced until passive immunity acquired from the mother dissipates (at 12 to 15 months of age).
   c. Tetanus–diphtheria (Td, adult type) at 14 to 16 years of age and every 10 years thereafter.

   These recommendations apply only to children whose immunizations began in early infancy. Different schedules are recommended for children aged 1 to 5 years and for those over 6 years of age who are being immunized for the first time.

SELECTION OF PREPARATION

For routine immunizations, combined antigen preparations are preferred (*e.g.,* DTP and MMR). Single antigens are recommended only when other components are contraindicated. In addition, adsorbed DTP is preferred to fluid DTP becuse it is absorbed more slowly. Although the adsorbed preparation causes a more painful local reaction, it also stimulates antibody production for a longer time.

STORAGE OF VACCINES

To maintain effectiveness of vaccines and other biologic preparations, the products must be stored properly. Most products require refrigeration at 2°C to 8°C (35.6°F to 46.4°F); some require protection from light (*e.g.,* MMR). Follow the manufacturer's instructions for storage.

NURSING ACTIONS: IMMUNIZING AGENTS

Nursing Actions	*Rationale/Explanation*
1. Administer accurately	
a. Read the package insert and check the expiration date on all biologic products (*e.g.,* vaccines, toxoids, human immune serums, and antitoxins).	Concentration and dosage of biologic products may vary with manufacturers. Fresh products are preferred; avoid administration of expired products. In addition, reconstituted products are usually stable for only a few hours.
b. Give TOPV into the side of an infant's mouth with a dropper, by placing on a child's tongue or a sugar cube, or by mixing with milk, distilled water, or chlorine-free water.	Several methods of administration are effective and can be varied to meet the needs of individual infants or children. Avoid administering TOPV to a crying child because the dose may be lost or aspirated into the lungs.

Nursing Actions	***Rationale/Explanation***
c. Check the child's temperature before giving DTP.	If the temperature is elevated, do not give the vaccine.
d. Give DTP in the lateral thigh muscle of the infant.	The vastus lateralis is the largest skeletal muscle mass in the infant and the preferred site for all intramuscular injections.
e. With MMR vaccine, use only the diluent provided by the manufacturer, and administer the vaccine subcutaneously, within 8 hours after reconstitution.	The reconstituted preparation is stable for approximately 8 hours. If not used within 8 hours, discard the solution.
f. Give intramuscular human immune serum globulin with an 18- to 20-gauge needle, preferably in gluteal muscles. If the dose is 5 ml or more, divide it and inject it into 2 or more intramuscular sites. Follow manufacturer's instructions for preparation and administration of intravenous formulations.	To promote absorption and minimize tissue irritation and other adverse reactions
g. Test for sensitivity to horse serum before administering any antitoxin (*e.g.,* botulism, diphtheria, gas gangrene, tetanus). This test is preferably performed by the physician. If done by the nurse, a physician should be in close proximity. Also, a syringe with 1 ml of epinephrine 1:1000 should be prepared *before* testing. (1) For the intradermal test, inject 0.1 to 0.2 ml of a 1:1000 dilution of horse serum into the forearm. The test is positive (*i.e.,* indicates allergy to horse serum) if a wheal appears at the injection site within 30 minutes. (2) For the conjunctival test, 1 drop of a 1:10 dilution of horse serum in isotonic saline solution is instilled in one eye. The test is positive if lacrimation and conjunctivitis appear within 30 minutes.	Anaphylactic shock may occur. Epinephrine aqueous solution 1:1000 is used for emergency treatment of anaphylaxis. Epinephrine is injected subcutaneously in a dose of 0.5 ml for adults and 0.01 ml/kg for children. If sensitivity tests are positive and antitoxins are deemed necessary, special desensitization procedures may be performed. Follow the manufacturer's recommendations for desensitization.
h. Aspirate carefully before intramuscular or subcutaneous injection of any immunizing agent.	To avoid inadvertent intravenous administration and greatly increased risks of severe adverse effects
i. Have aqueous epinephrine 1:1000 readily available before administering any vaccine.	For immediate treatment of allergic reactions
j. After administration of an immunizing agent in a clinic or office setting, have the client stay in the area for at least 30 minutes.	To be observed for allergic reactions, which usually occur within 30 minutes
2. Observe for therapeutic effects	
a. Absence of diseases for which a person is immunized	
b. Decreased incidence and severity of symptoms when given to modify disease processes	
3. Observe for adverse effects	Immunizing agents may cause adverse, life-threatening reactions. The risk of serious adverse effects from immunization is usually much smaller than the risk of the disease immunized against. Adverse effects may be caused by the immunizing agent or by foreign protein incorporated with the immunizing agent (*e.g.,* egg protein in viral vaccines grown in chick embryos).
a. Pain, tenderness, redness at injection sites	Local tissue irritation may occur with any injected immunizing agent. It is especially likely to occur with adsorbed DTP or tetanus toxoid. With DTP, a nodule or lump may persist for months but eventually resolves.

Nursing Actions	***Rationale/Explanation***
b. Fever, malaise, myalgia	These adverse effects are relatively common with vaccines and toxoids. They rarely occur with human immune serums given for passive immunity.
c. Severe fever, shock, somnolence, convulsions, encephalopathy	These are rare adverse reactions to DTP. If they occur, they are thought to be caused by the pertussis antigen, and further administration of pertussis vaccine or DTP is contraindicated.
d. Paralysis (Guillain–Barré syndrome)	This is a rare reaction to oral poliovirus vaccine.
e. Anaphylaxis (cardiovascular collapse, shock, laryngeal edema, urticaria, angioneurotic edema, severe respiratory distress)	Anaphylaxis is most likely to occur with injections of antitoxins (horse serum) but may occasionally occur with other immunizing agents. Anaphylaxis is a medical emergency that requires immediate treatment with epinephrine (0.5 ml for adults; 0.01 ml/kg for children) administered subcutaneously. Anaphylaxis is most likely to occur within 30 minutes after immunizing agents are injected.
f. Serum sickness (urticaria, fever, arthralgia, enlarged lymph nodes)	Serum sickness is a delayed hypersensitivity reaction that occurs several days or weeks after an injection of serum. It is most likely to occur with antitoxins (horse serum). Treatment is symptomatic. Symptoms are usually relieved by aspirin, antihistamines, and corticosteroids.
4. Observe for drug interactions Drugs that alter effects of vaccines Immunosuppressant agents (*e.g.,* corticosteroids, antineoplastic drugs, phenytoin [Dilantin])	Vaccines are contraindicated in clients receiving immunosuppressive drugs. These persons are unable to produce sufficient amounts of antibodies for immunity and may develop the illness produced by the particular organism contained in the vaccine. The disease is most likely to occur with the live virus vaccines (measles, mumps, rubella). Similar effects occur when the client is receiving irradiation and phenytoin, an anticonvulsant drug that suppresses both cellular and humoral immune responses.
5. Teach clients **a.** Maintain immunization records for themselves and their children	This is important because immunizations are often obtained at different places and over a period of years. Memory is not reliable; written, accurate, up-to-date records help to prevent disease and unnecessary immunizations.
b. If a physician recommends immunization and it is uncertain whether the client has had a particular immunization or disease, it is probably safer to have the immunization than risk having the disease.	Immunization after a client has been previously immunized or has had the disease is generally not harmful.
c. Give aspirin or acetaminophen (Tylenol) every 4 to 6 hours to children who develop fever 24 to 48 hours after DTP injection.	For symptomatic relief and comfort
d. Report adverse reactions other than discomfort at the injection site, minor fever, malaise, and muscle aches.	This is especially important when vaccines are given in serial doses or booster doses. Subsequent doses may need to be reduced.
e. Women of child-bearing age who receive rubella vaccine must avoid becoming pregnant (*i.e.,* use effective contraceptive methods) for 3 months.	To avoid rubella-induced abnormalities in fetal development

Selected References

American Academy of Pediatrics: Recommendations for using pneumococcal vaccine in children. Pediatrics 75:1153–1158, June 1985

Anderson PD: Basic Human Anatomy and Physiology: Clinical Implications for the Health Professions. Monterey, CA, Wadsworth, 1984

Facts and Comparisons. St. Louis, J B Lippincott (Updated monthly)

Ferguson CK, Roll LJ: Human rabies. Am J Nurs 81:1174–1179, June 1981

Haemophilus Influenzae Type b vaccine. Med Lett Drugs Ther 27:61–62, July 1985

Immunizations and chemoprophylaxis for travelers. Med Lett Drugs Ther 27:33–36, April 1985

Kirkmann-Liff BL, Dandoy S: Hepatitis B: What price exposure? Am J Nurs 84:988–990, August 1984

Leibel RL: Pertussis vaccination: Benefits and risks. Drug Ther 14:103–108, October 1984

Magily JK, Tong TG, Bonk JR, et al: Community health care. In Wiener MB, Pepper GA (eds): Clinical Pharmacology and Therapeutics in Nursing, 2d ed., pp 1004–1044. New York, McGraw-Hill, 1985

Mayer TR: Optimum use of rubella immunization. Am Fam Physician 23:143–145, January 1981

Rodman MJ, Karch AM, Boyd EH, Smith DW: Pharmacology and Drug Therapy in Nursing, 3rd ed. Philadelphia, J B Lippincott, 1985

VII

DRUGS AFFECTING THE RESPIRATORY SYSTEM

46

PHYSIOLOGY OF THE RESPIRATORY SYSTEM

The respiratory system helps meet the basic human need for oxygen (O_2). Oxygen is necessary for the oxidation of foodstuffs, by which energy for cellular metabolism is produced. When the oxygen supply is inadequate, cell function is impaired; when oxygen is absent, cells die. Permanent brain damage occurs within 4 to 6 minutes of anoxia. In addition to providing oxygen to all body cells, the respiratory system also removes carbon dioxide (CO_2), a major waste product of cell metabolism. Excessive accumulation of CO_2 damages or kills body cells. The efficiency of the respiratory system depends on the quality and quantity of air inhaled, the patency of air passageways, the ability of the lungs to expand and contract, and the ability of O_2 and CO_2 to cross the alveolar–capillary membrane. In addition to the respiratory system itself, the circulatory, nervous, and musculoskeletal systems have important functions in respiration. Some characteristics of the respiratory system and the process of respiration include the following:

1. *Respiration* is the process of gas exchange by which O_2 is obtained and CO_2 eliminated. This gas exchange occurs between the lung and the blood across the alveolar–capillary membrane and between the blood and body cells. The first phase of respiration depends on the adequacy of air flow to and from alveoli in the lungs (ventilation). The second phase depends on the adequacy of the circulatory system.
2. The respiratory tract is a series of branching tubes with progressively smaller diameters. These tubes (nose, pharynx, larynx, trachea, bronchi, and bronchioles) function as air passageways and as air "conditioners" that filter, warm, and humidify incoming air. Most of the conditioning is done by the ciliated mucous membrane that lines the entire respiratory tract except the pharynx and alveoli. *Cilia* are tiny, hairlike projections that sweep mucus toward the pharynx to be expectorated or swallowed. The mucous membrane secretes mucus, which forms a protective blanket and traps foreign particles such as bacteria or dust.
   a. When air is inhaled through the nose, it is conditioned by the nasal mucosa. When the nasal passages are blocked, the mouth serves as an alternate airway. The oral mucosa may warm and humidify air but is unable to filter it.
   b. Air passes from the nasal cavities to the *pharynx* (throat). Its walls are composed of skeletal muscle, and its lining is composed of mucous membrane. The pharynx contains the palatine tonsils, which are large masses of lymphatic tissue. The pharynx is a passageway for food and fluids as well as for air. Food and fluids go

from the pharynx to the esophagus, and air passes from the pharynx into the trachea.

c. The *larynx* is composed of nine cartilages joined by ligaments and controlled by skeletal muscles. It contains the vocal cords and forms the upper end of the trachea. It closes on swallowing to prevent aspiration of food and fluids into the lungs.

d. The *trachea* is the passageway between the upper respiratory tract and the lungs. It divides into right and left primary or mainstem *bronchi,* which branch into secondary and smaller bronchi, then into bronchioles. *Bronchioles* are about the size of broomstraws. The walls of the bronchioles contain smooth muscle, which is controlled by the autonomic nervous system. Parasympathetic nerves cause constriction; sympathetic nerves cause relaxation or dilation. The bronchioles give rise to the *alveoli,* which are grapelike clusters of air sacs surrounded by capillaries.

e. Gas exchange occurs across the alveolar–capillary membrane by passive diffusion. O_2 enters the bloodstream to be transported to body cells; CO_2 enters the alveoli to be exhaled from the lungs.

3. Beginning with the bronchi, the respiratory structures are contained in the *lungs.*

   a. Each lung is divided into lobes. The right lung has three lobes, and the left has two. Each lobe is supplied by a secondary bronchus. The lobes are further subdivided into bronchopulmonary segments, supplied by smaller bronchi. The bronchopulmonary segments contain lobules, which are the functional units of the lung (the site where gas exchange takes place). Each lobule is supplied by a bronchiole and by an arteriole, a venule, and a lymphatic vessel.

   b. The lungs are encased in a membrane called the *pleura,* which is composed of two layers. The inner layer, which adheres to the surface of the lung, is called the *visceral pleura.* The outer layer, which lines the thoracic cavity, is called the *parietal pleura.* The potential space between the layers is called the pleural cavity. It contains fluid that allows the layers to glide over each other and minimizes friction.

   c. The lungs expand and relax in response to changes in pressure relationships (intrapulmonic and intrapleural pressures). Elastic tissue in the bronchioles and alveoli allows the lungs to stretch or expand to accommodate incoming air. This ability is called *compliance.* The lungs also recoil (like a stretched rubber band) to expel air. Some air remains in the lungs after expiration, which allows gas exchange to continue between respirations.

4. The nervous system regulates rate and depth of respiration by the respiratory center in the medulla oblongata, the pneumotaxic center in the pons, and the apneustic center in the reticular formation. The respiratory center is stimulated primarily by increased CO_2 in the fluids of the center. (However, excessive CO_2 will depress the respiratory center.) When the center is stimulated, rate and depth of breathing are increased and excessive CO_2 is exhaled. A lesser stimulus to the respiratory center is decreased oxygen in arterial blood.

   The nervous system also operates several reflexes important to respiration. The cough reflex is especially important because it helps protect the lungs from foreign particles, air pollutants, bacteria, and other potentially harmful substances. Cough occurs when nerve endings in the respiratory tract mucosa are stimulated by dryness, pressure, cold, irritant fumes, and excessive secretions.

5. The circulatory system transports O_2 and CO_2. After oxygen enters the bloodstream across the alveolar–capillary membrane, it combines with hemoglobin in red blood cells for transport to body cells, where it is released. CO_2 combines with hemoglobin at the cells for return to the lungs and elimination from the body.

6. The musculoskeletal system participates in chest expansion and contraction. Normally, the diaphragm and external intercostal muscles expand the chest cavity and are called muscles of inspiration. The abdominal and internal intercostal muscles are the muscles of expiration.

7. To summarize, normal respiration requires the following:

   a. Atmospheric air containing at least 21% O_2

   b. Adequate ventilation. Ventilation, in turn, requires patent airways, expansion and contraction of the chest, expansion and contraction of the lungs, and maintenance of a normal range of intrapulmonic and intrapleural pressures.

   c. Adequate diffusion of O_2 and CO_2 through the alveolar–capillary membrane. Factors influencing diffusion include the thickness and surface area of the membrane and pressure differences between gases on each side of the membrane.

   d. Adequate perfusion or circulation of blood and sufficient hemoglobin to carry needed O_2

8. Normal breathing occurs 16 to 20 times per minute and is quiet, rhythmic, and effortless. About 500 cc of air is inspired and expired with a normal breath (tidal volume); deep breaths or "sighs" occur 6 to 10 times per hour to ventilate more alveoli. Fever,

exercise, pain, and emotions such as anger tend to increase respirations. Sleep or rest and various medications such as tranquilizers, sedatives, and narcotic analgesics tend to slow respiration.

The respiratory system is subject to many disorders that interfere with respiration. Common disorders include respiratory tract infections, allergic disorders, inflammatory disorders, and conditions that obstruct air flow (*e.g.*, excessive respiratory tract secretions, emphysema, and other chronic obstructive pulmonary diseases). Common signs and symptoms of respiratory disorders include cough, increased secretions, mucosal congestion, and bronchospasm. As a general rule, drug therapy is more effective in relieving symptoms than in curing the underlying disorders that cause the symptoms. Major drug groups used to treat respiratory symptoms are bronchodilating and antiasthmatic agents (Chap. 47), antihistamines (Chap. 48), and nasal decongestants, antitussives, mucolytics, and cold remedies (Chap. 49).

Selected References

Anderson PD: Basic Human Anatomy and Physiology: Clinical Implications for the Health Professions. Monterey, CA, Wadsworth, 1984

Groer MW, Shekleton ME: Basic Pathophysiology: A Conceptual Aproach, 2d ed. St. Louis, C V Mosby 1983

Guyton AC: Textbook of Medical Physiology, 7th ed. Philadelphia, W B Saunders, 1986

Rodman MJ, Karch AM, Boyd EH, Smith DW: Pharmacology and Drug Therapy in Nursing, 3rd ed. Philadelphia, J B Lippincott, 1985

47

BRONCHODILATING AND ANTIASTHMATIC DRUGS

Description and uses

Bronchodilating and antiasthmatic agents are used in the treatment of bronchospasm and bronchial asthma. Bronchospasm is the spasmodic contraction of smooth muscles in the bronchioles. As a result, airways are narrowed, air flow to and from the lungs is decreased, and acute respiratory distress occurs. Bronchospasm occurs in bronchial asthma and may occur in bronchitis and emphysema. Bronchial asthma is a chronic pulmonary disorder characterized by intermittent attacks of acute bronchospasm, mucosal edema and inflammation, and excessive mucus production. Asthmatics are usually symptom free between attacks. Bronchial asthma may occur at any age but is especially common in childhood and early adulthood. Chronic bronchitis and emphysema are chronic obstructive pulmonary diseases characterized by progressive anatomic and physiologic changes in the lungs. The changes are irreversible and lead to increasing dyspnea over several years. These conditions usually affect middle-aged or elderly people.

In adults and children known to have asthma, acute bronchospasm may be precipitated by several factors including minor respiratory or other infections, odors, smoke, chemical fumes or air pollutants, cold air, exercise, emotional upsets, or tartrazine (a yellow dye found in many foods and drugs). In some asthmatics, nonsteroidal anti-inflammatory drugs (*e.g.*, aspirin, ibuprofen, indomethacin) may cause severe bronchoconstriction. When lung tissues are exposed to these factors, mast cells release substances that cause bronchoconstriction. Mast cells are found throughout the body in connective tissue, and they are abundant in tissues surrounding capillaries in the lungs. Bronchoconstrictive substances include histamine, serotonin, slow-reacting substance of anaphylaxis (SRS-A), prostaglandins, and acetylcholine. These substances are antagonized by the action of cyclic AMP (3′,5′-adenosine monophosphate). Cyclic AMP is an intracellular substance that initiates various intracellular activities, depending on the type of cell. In lung cells, cyclic AMP inhibits release of bronchoconstrictive substances and promotes bronchodilation.

Bronchodilating drugs produce therapeutic effects by increasing the amount of cyclic AMP in bronchial tissue. Sympathomimetic bronchodilators stimulate the enzyme adenyl cyclase to increase production of cyclic AMP; methylxanthine bronchodilators increase cyclic AMP by inhibiting the enzyme phosphodiesterase, which metabolizes cyclic AMP.

Adrenergic (sympathomimetic) drugs, of which epinephrine is the prototype, exert widespread effects on body tissues. These drugs are discussed more extensively in Chapter 18. When used to relieve bronchospasm, these drugs are given primarily for their ability to stimulate $beta_2$-adrenergic receptors in bronchial smooth muscle and produce bronchodilation. However, some drugs (*e.g.*, epinephrine, isoproterenol) also stimulate $beta_1$ receptors in the heart and produce cardiac stimulation. Cardiac effects are considered adverse reactions when the drugs are used in respiratory disorders. Newer sympathomimetic bronchodilators (*e.g.*, metaproterenol, albuterol, terbutaline) act more selectively on $beta_2$-adrenergic receptors and cause fewer cardiac effects. In addition, they are effective with oral administration and have a longer duration of action.

Methylxanthine bronchodilators are theophylline and its derivatives. Theophylline is related chemically to caffeine and theobromine (see Chap. 16) and exerts widespread effects on body tissues. In addition to producing bronchodilation, xanthines increase cardiac output, increase coronary artery blood flow and exert a mild diuretic effect, and stimulate the central nervous system (CNS). Effects on the heart and CNS are considered adverse reactions.

Other drugs used in the treatment of asthma include cromolyn and adrenal corticosteroids. Cromolyn is a unique agent used only to prevent acute attacks of asthma. Adrenal corticosteroids are potent therapeutic agents and are discussed in Chapter 24. They are used in acute bronchospasm and severe chronic asthma when bronchodilators do not relieve respiratory distress. Numerous corticosteroids are available for various purposes and routes of administration: three of these, beclomethasone (Vanceril), flunisolide (AeroBid), and triamcinolone (Azmacort), were developed for topical administration (by oral inhalation) in asthma and bronchospasm.

Individual bronchodilating and antiasthmatic drugs

ADRENERGIC BRONCHODILATORS

Epinephrine (Adrenalin, Bronkaid) is administered subcutaneously in an acute attack of bronchospasm. Therapeutic effects may occur within 5 minutes and last for 4 hours. Epinephrine is available in a pressurized aerosol form without a physician's prescription (*e.g.*, Primatene). When given by inhalation, epinephrine rapidly relieves bronchospasm associated with asthma, bronchitis, or emphysema. Almost all over-the-counter aerosol products promoted for use in asthma contain epinephrine. These products are frequently abused. Clients should be cautioned that excessive use may produce tolerance and hazardous adverse effects.

Routes and dosage ranges

Adults: Aqueous solution (epinephrine 1:1000), SC 0.2–0.5 ml. The dose may be repeated after 20 minutes if necessary.
Aqueous suspension (Sus-Phrine 1:200), SC 0.1–0.3 ml. The dose may be repeated after 4 hours if necessary.
Inhalation by inhaler, 1–2 inhalations 4–6 times daily
Inhalation by nebulizer, 0.25–0.5 ml of 2.25% racemic epinephrine in 2.5 ml normal saline

Children: Aqueous solution (epinephrine 1:1000), SC 0.01 ml/kg q4h as needed. A single dose should not exceed 0.5 ml.
Aqueous suspension (Sus-Phrine 1:200), SC 0.005 ml/kg q8–12h if necessary
Inhalation, same as adults for both inhaler and nebulizer

Albuterol (Proventil) is a relatively selective $beta_2$-adrenergic agent approved for use in treatment of bronchospasm. Although albuterol has less effect on the cardiovascular system than epinephrine or isoproterenol, the drug should be used with caution in clients with cardiac disorders.

Routes and dosage ranges

Adults: PO 2–4 mg 3 to 4 times daily
Inhalation, 1–2 inhalations (90 μg/puff) q4–6h

Children: Safety and effectiveness in children under 12 years of age have not been established.

Bitolterol (Tornalate) is a relatively selective $beta_2$-adrenergic receptor agonist used for prevention and treatment of asthma and bronchospasm. A prodrug, it must be metabolized to colterol, the active form.

Route and dosage ranges

Adults: Bronchospasm, 2 inhalations (0.37 mg/puff) at least 1–3 minutes apart, followed by a third if necessary
Prevention of bronchospasm, 2 inhalations q8h; maximal recommended dose, 3 inhalations q6h or 2 inhalations q4h

Children over 12 years: Same as adults

Ephedrine is an adrenergic drug used in long-term treatment of asthma. It has a long duration of action and is effective with oral administration. Ephedrine stimulates the CNS. Because the stimulant effects cause insomnia and nervousness, it is often given in combination with a barbiturate or an anti-anxiety agent. Such combinations are not recommended for use, although they are widely prescribed. Children may react to ephedrine with somnolence rather than CNS stimulation. Use of ephedrine in treatment of asthma is declining, since more selective beta$_2$-adrenergic agonists have become available.

Route and dosage range

Adults: PO 25–50 mg q3–4h. Sustained-release preparations, 30–60 mg q8–12h
Children: PO 3 mg/kg/day in 4–6 divided doses

Isoetharine (Bronkosol, Bronkometer) is available for use as a solution for nebulization or in a pressurized container for inhalation. Isoetharine is used for relief of acute attacks of asthma or bronchospasm. Although isoetharine acts more selectively on beta$_2$-adrenergic receptors than on beta$_1$ receptors, cardiac and CNS stimulation may occur with high doses. Isoetharine is relatively short acting (duration of 1–3 hours).

Route and dosage range

Adults: Inhalation by nebulizer, 0.25–0.5 ml of 1% isoetharine in 2.5 ml of normal saline
Inhalation by inhaler, 1–2 inhalations (0.34 mg/dose) 4 times daily
Children: Same as adults

Isoproterenol (Isuprel) is a potent bronchodilator and cardiac stimulant. When used for treatment of bronchospasm, isoproterenol is given by inhalation, alone or in combination with other agents. The drug is also available in sublingual tablets and oral solutions. These preparations are not recommended because sublingual tablets are erratically absorbed and oral solutions are inactivated in the gastrointestinal tract. Isoproterenol is a short-acting agent (approximate duration of 1–3 hours).

Route and dosage range

Adults: Inhalation by nebulizer, 0.25–0.5 ml of 1:200 Isuprel solution in 2.5 ml of saline
Inhalation by inhaler, 1–2 inhalations (0.075–0.125 mg/puff) 4 times daily; maximal dose, 3 inhalations per attack of bronchospasm
Children: Same as adults

Metaproterenol (Alupent), a relatively selective beta$_2$-adrenergic agonist, is an effective, long-acting bronchodilating agent. The drug may be given orally or by metered-dose inhaler. Metaproterenol is used to treat acute asthma attacks or bronchospasm and to prevent exercise-induced asthma. In high doses, metaproterenol loses some of its selectivity and may cause cardiac and CNS stimulation.

Routes and dosage ranges

Adults: Inhalation 1–3 puffs (0.65 mg/dose), 4 times daily; maximal dose, 12 inhalations/day
PO 10–20 mg q6–8h
Children: Inhalation, not recommended for use in children under 12 years of age
Under 9 years or weight under 27 kg, PO 10 mg q6–8h
Over 9 years or weight over 27 kg, PO 20 mg q6–8h

Terbutaline (Brethine, others) is a relatively selective beta$_2$-adrenergic agonist that is a long-acting bronchodilator. When given subcutaneously, terbutaline loses its selectivity and has little advantage over epinephrine. Muscle tremor is the most frequent side-effect with this agent.

Routes and dosage ranges

Adults: PO 2.5–5 mg q6–8h; maximal daily dose, 15 mg
SC 0.25 mg, repeated in 15–30 minutes if necessary, q4–6h
Inhalation, 2 inhalations (400 μg/dose) q4–6h
Children: PO 2.5 mg 3 times daily for children 12 years of age or older; maximal daily dose, 7.5 mg
SC dosage not established
Inhalation, same as adults for children 12 years and older

XANTHINE BRONCHODILATORS

Theophylline is widely used in the prevention and treatment of bronchospasm associated with asthma, bronchitis, and emphysema. It is often the first oral bronchodilator prescribed and may be the only drug required.

Numerous preparations of theophylline are available for clinical use. Dosage forms include tablets, capsules, long-acting or sustained-release tablets and capsules, elixirs, suspensions, enemas, and rectal suppositories. Most formulations contain anhydrous theophylline (100% theophylline) as the active ingredient; some formulations contain theophylline salts. For example, theophylline ethylenediamine (aminophylline) is a frequently used preparation that contains approximately 85% theophylline and is the only theophylline preparation that can be given intravenously. Oxtriphylline (Choledyl) is a choline salt of theophylline that contains 64% theophylline. In addition to the single-drug formulations, many combination products are available. These products contain other active ingredients, such as an adrenergic drug (*e.g.*, ephedrine), an expectorant (*e.g.*, guaifenesin, potassium iodide), or a sedative (*e.g.*, phenobarbital, hydroxyzine). Selected theophylline preparations are listed in Table 47-1.

ANTIASTHMATIC AGENTS

Cromolyn (Intal) has no bronchodilating or anti-inflammatory effects. It is a specific antiasthmatic drug that prevents acute asthma attacks by stabilizing sensitized mast cells. This action prevents the release of histamine and other bronchoconstrictive substances when mast cells are confronted with an allergen.

Cromolyn is approved as an adjunctive drug in the management of clients with severe perennial bronchial asthma. The drug is effective in allergic asthma and exercise-induced asthma. Utilization of cromolyn may allow reduction or elimination of corticosteroid drugs. Cromolyn is used prophylactically; it should not be used in acute bronchospasm or status asthmaticus.

Cromolyn is available in a capsule and a solution for inhalation. The capsule is placed in a special turboinhaler (Spinhaler), which punctures the capsule. When the client places the turboinhaler in the mouth and inhales, the capsule spins and vibrates, causing the

TABLE 47-1. THEOPHYLLINE PREPARATIONS

	Generic name	Trade name	Routes and dosage ranges	
			Adults	*Children*
Short-acting preparations	Theophylline anhydrous (100% theophylline)	Elixophyllin, Theolair, others	PO 100–250 mg q6h	PO 50–100 mg q6h
	Theophylline ethylenediamine (85% theophylline) (aminophylline)	Aminophyllline, others	PO 500 mg initially, then 200–300 mg q6–8h Rectal suppository 250–500 mg q8–12h Acute bronchospasm, IV 6 mg/kg over a 20- to 30-minute period, followed by a maintenance infusion of 0.1–1.2 mg/kg/hour. Dilute the dose in 5% dextrose injection or 0.9% sodium chloride injection to a concentration of 2 mg of aminophylline/ml of intravenous solution.	PO 7.5 mg/kg initially, then 5–6 mg/kg q6–8h Acute bronchospasm, IV 6 mg/kg over a 30-minute period as a loading dose, followed by a maintenance infusion of 0.6–0.9 mg/kg/hour
	Theophylline monothanolamine (75% theophylline)	Fleet Theophylline	Rectally, as a retention enema, 250–500 mg twice daily	Not recommended
	Theophylline sodium glycinate (49% theophylline)	Synophylate, Theofort	Tablets, elixir PO 330–660 mg q6–8h	Ages 6–12 years, PO 220–330 mg q6–8h Ages under 6 years, PO 6–12 mg/kg q6–8h
	Oxtriphylline (64% theophylline)	Choledyl	PO 200 mg 4 times daily	PO 15 mg/kg daily, in 4 divided doses
Long-acting preparations	Theophylline anhydrous (100% theophylline)	Theo-Dur, Theobid, Theoclear-LA, Theolair-SR	PO 150–300 mg q8–12h; Maximal dose, 13 mg/kg or 900 mg daily, whichever is less	PO 100–200 mg q8–12h; Maximal dose, 24 mg/kg/day
Theophylline mixtures	Theophylline 130 mg ephedrine sulfate 25 mg hydroxyzine hydrochloride 10 mg	Marax	PO 1 tablet 2–4 times daily	Age over 5 years, PO ½ tablet 2–4 times daily
	Theophylline 150 mg guaifenesin 90 mg	Quibron	Tablets, PO 1–2 capsules q6–8h Elixir, PO 15–30 ml q6–8h	PO 4–6 mg/kg q6–8h
	Theophylline 130 mg ephedrine hydrochloride 24 mg phenobarbital 8 mg	Tedral	PO 1–2 tablets q4h	Weight over 60 lb, PO ½–1 tablet q4h

micronized powder to be inhaled. The solution is for use with a power-operated nebulizer; hand-operated nebulizers are not suitable.

Occasionally, a person may experience cough or bronchospasm following cromolyn inhalation. If a significant amount of bronchospasm occurs, the drug should be discontinued. Also, the drug should be discontinued if a therapeutic response is not obtained within 4 weeks of therapy.

A nasal solution (Nasalcrom) is available for prevention and treatment of allergic rhinitis; an ophthalmic solution (Opticrom) is available for prevention and treatment of allergic conjunctivitis and keratitis.

Routes and dosage ranges

Intal

Adults: 20 mg (capsule or solution) inhaled 4 times daily

Children 5 years and older for capsules, 2 years and older for nebulizer solution: Same as adults

Nasalcrom

Adults: 1 spray in each nostril 3–6 times daily at regular intervals

Children 6 years and older: Same as adults

Opticrom

Adults: 1–2 drops (cromolyn 1.6 mg/drop) in each eye 4–6 times daily at regular intervals

Children: Same as adults

Beclomethasone, flunisolide, and **triamcinolone** are topical corticosteroids for inhalation. Topical administration minimizes systemic absorption and adverse effects. These preparations may substitute for or allow reduced dosage of systemic corticosteroids.

In asthmatics taking an oral corticosteroid, the oral dosage is reduced slowly (over several months, at 1- to 2-week intervals) when an inhaled corticosteroid is added. The goal is to give the lowest oral dose necessary to control symptoms. Beclomethasone and flunisolide are also available in nasal solutions for treatment of allergic rhinitis that does not respond to other treatment.

Routes and dosage ranges

Beclomethasone

Adults: Oral inhalation, 2 inhalations (0.84 mg/dose) 3–4 times daily; maximal dose of 20 inhalations in 24 hours. Nasal inhalation (Vanceril nasal inhaler), 1 inhalation (0.42 mg) in each nostril 2–4 times daily

Children 6–12 years: Oral inhalation, 1–2 inhalations 3–4 times daily; maximal dose of 10 inhalations in 24 hours.

Children over 12 years: Nasal inhalation, same as adults

Flunisolide

Adults: Oral inhalation, 2 inhalations (0.50 mg/dose) twice daily, morning and evening; maximal dose, 4 inhalations twice daily (2 mg). Nasal inhalation (Nasalide), 2 sprays in each nostril twice daily; maximal daily dose, 8 sprays in each nostril

Children 6–15 years: Oral inhalation, 2 inhalations twice daily. Nasal inhalation, 1 spray in each nostril 3 times daily or 2 sprays twice daily; maximal daily dose, 4 sprays in each nostril

Triamcinolone

Adults: Oral inhalation, 2 inhalations 3–4 times daily; maximal dose, 16 inhalations in 24 hours

Children 6–12 years: 1–2 inhalations 3–4 times daily to a maximum of 12 inhalations/24 hours

Hydrocortisone, prednisone and **methylprednisolone** (Solu-Medrol) are systemic corticosteroids that are given to clients who do not respond adequately to bronchodilator therapy. Corticosteroids are given intravenously in acute, severe attacks of asthma or bronchospasm; they are given orally or topically in chronic asthma or bronchospasm.

Routes and dosage ranges

Hydrocortisone sodium phosphate and sodium succinate

Adults: IV 100–200 mg q4–6h initially, then decreased or switched to an oral dosage form

Children: IV 1–5 mg/kg q4–6h

Methylprednisolone sodium succinate

Adults: IV 2–60 mg q4–6h

Children: IV 1–4 mg/kg q4–6h

Prednisone

Adults: PO 20–60 mg/day

Children: PO 2 mg/kg/day initially

Principles of therapy: bronchodilating and antiasthmatic drugs

ASSESSMENT GUIDELINES

Assess the client's pulmonary function.

1. General assessment factors include rate and character of respiration, skin color, arterial blood gas

analysis, and pulmonary function tests. Abnormal breathing patterns (*e.g.*, rate below 12 or above 24 per minute, dyspnea, cough, orthopnea, wheezing, "noisy" respirations) may indicate respiratory distress. Severe respiratory distress is characterized by tachypnea, dyspnea, use of accessory muscles of respiration, and hypoxia. Early signs of hypoxia include mental confusion, restlessness, anxiety, and increased blood pressure and pulse rate. Late signs include cyanosis and decreased blood pressure and pulse. Hypoxemia is confirmed if arterial blood gas analysis shows Po_2 under 50 mm Hg.

2. Acute bronchospasm is a medical emergency. The client is in obvious and severe respiratory distress. A characteristic feature of bronchospasm is forceful expiration or wheezing.
3. If the client has chronic asthma, try to determine frequency and severity of acute attacks; factors that precipitate or relieve acute attacks; antiasthmatic medications taken occasionally or regularly; allergies; and condition between acute attacks, such as restrictions in activities of daily living due to asthma.
4. If the client has chronic bronchitis or emphysema, assess for signs of respiratory distress, hypoxia, cough, amount and character of sputum, exercise tolerance (*e.g.*, dyspnea on exertion, dyspnea at rest), medications, nondrug treatment measures (*e.g.*, breathing exercises, chest physiotherapy).

NURSING INTERVENTIONS

Use measures to prevent, relieve, or decrease bronchospasm when possible. General measures include those to prevent respiratory disease or promote an adequate airway. Some specific measures include the following:

1. Encourage clients to drink 2000 to 3000 ml of fluids daily. This helps keep respiratory tract secretions relatively thin and easy to remove.
2. Use mechanical measures for removing respiratory tract secretions and preventing their retention. Effective measures include coughing, deep breathing, percussion, and postural drainage. Expectorant drugs may be irritating and have not been shown to be of therapeutic value.
3. Assist the client to identify and avoid exposure to conditions that precipitate acute asthma or bronchospasm. For example, allergens may be removed from the home, school, or work environment. When bronchospasm is precipitated by exercise, prevention of bronchospasm by prior inhalation of bronchodilating agents is preferable to avoidance of exercise, especially in children.
4. Encourage the client to stop smoking and to avoid other bronchial irritants (*e.g.*, aerosol hair sprays, antiperspirants, and cleaning products) when possible.
5. Try to prevent or reduce anxiety. Anxiety may cause or aggravate bronchospasm. Stay with the client during an acute asthma attack or bronchospasm if feasible. Clients experiencing severe and prolonged bronchospasm (status asthmaticus) should be admitted or transferred to a hospital intensive care unit.

DRUG SELECTION AND ADMINISTRATION

Choice of drug and route of administration are determined largely by severity of the disease process and the client's response to therapy. Some guidelines include the following:

1. Epinephrine, administered subcutaneously, is the initial drug of choice for an acute attack of bronchospasm.
2. Aerosol products act directly on the lungs. Drugs given by inhalation can usually be given in smaller doses and produce fewer adverse effects than oral drugs.
3. When adrenergic bronchodilators are prescribed for clients who are elderly or who have heart disease or a history of cardiac arrhythmias, the more selective $beta_2$ agonists (*e.g.*, albuterol, metaproterenol, terbutaline) are preferred.
4. Theophylline preparations are most often given by the oral route. Aminophylline may be given intravenously for rapid drug action. Rectal preparations are not recommended because they are irritating to tissues and absorption is erratic.
5. Cromolyn is used prophylactically; it is not effective in treating acute attacks of asthma.
6. Adrenal corticosteroids should be used only when other bronchodilating and antiasthmatic drugs are ineffective. In acute asthma, a corticosteroid is often given for approximately 1 week. A continuous intravenous infusion may be used initially; oral therapy is substituted when feasible. In chronic asthma, inhaled corticosteroids are preferred. These drugs may be effective when used alone or with relatively small doses of an oral corticosteroid.
7. Using several drugs concurrently may be more effective than using a single agent. One advantage of a multiple drug regimen is that smaller doses of each agent can usually be given. This may decrease adverse effects and allow dosages to be increased when exacerbation of symptoms occurs.

8. Combination products are not generally recommended, because they do not allow adequate titration of dosage for individual components. In addition, they may contain drugs that have not been proved effective (*e.g.*, expectorants such as guaifenesin).

DOSAGE FACTORS

Dosage of bronchodilator and antiasthmatic drugs must be individualized so that the smallest effective amounts are given. With theophylline preparations, guidelines include the following:

1. Dosage should be individualized to maintain serum drug concentrations of 10 to 20 μg/ml. Serum levels should be monitored because of individual differences in hepatic metabolism. Serum levels above 20 μg/ml are associated with a high incidence of toxicity. Blood for serum levels should be drawn 1 to 2 hours after immediate-release dosage forms and 4 hours after sustained-release forms.
2. Children and clients who smoke cigarettes usually need higher doses to maintain therapeutic blood levels because they metabolize theophylline rapidly.
3. Clients who have liver disease, congestive heart failure, chronic pulmonary disease, or acute viral infections usually need smaller doses because these conditions impair theophylline metabolism.
4. For clients who are obese, theophylline dosage should be calculated on the basis of lean or ideal body weight, since theophylline is not highly distributed in fatty tissue.
5. Other factors, such as absorption and bioavailability of particular dosage forms, also affect serum drug levels and therefore affect drug toxicity.
6. A rational way to optimize dosage is to start with a low dose and gradually increase the amount according to serum theophylline levels.

NURSING ACTIONS: BRONCHODILATING AND ANTIASTHMATIC DRUGS

Nursing Actions	*Rationale/Explanation*
1. Administer accurately	
a. Give oral theophylline preparations at regular intervals around the clock.	To maintain therapeutic serum drug levels
b. Give oral theophylline preparations before meals and with a full glass of water. If gastrointestinal upset occurs, give with food.	To promote dissolution and absorption. Taking with food may help to decrease nausea and vomiting. However, these symptoms are primarily due to stimulation of the vomiting center in the brain rather than to local irritation of the gastrointestinal tract.
c. For a continuous intravenous infusion of aminophylline, dilute the drug in 5% dextrose in water or 0.9% sodium chloride injection to a concentration of 1 or 2 mg/ml (*e.g.*, 500 mg of aminophylline in 500 ml of intravenous fluid). Infuse a loading dose (about 6 mg/kg) over 20 to 30 minutes; infuse a maintenance dose of 0.5 to 0.9 mg/kg/hour.	Dosage for maintenance therapy is based on serum drug concentrations and appearance of adverse effects (*e.g.*, tachycardia, premature ventricular contractions, nausea, vomiting, seizures).
2. Observe for therapeutic effects	Relief of bronchospasm and wheezing should be evident within a few minutes after giving subcutaneous epinephrine, intravenous aminophylline, or aerosolized adrenergic bronchodilators.
a. Decreased dyspnea and wheezing	
b. Reduced rate and improved quality of respirations	
c. Reduced anxiety and restlessness	
d. Therapeutic serum levels of theophylline (10 to 20 μg/ml)	

Nursing Actions	Rationale/Explanation
e. Improved arterial blood gases (normal values: Po_2—80 to 100 mm Hg; Pco_2—35 to 45 mm Hg; *p*H—7.35 to 7.45)	
f. Improved exercise tolerance	
g. Decreased incidence and severity of acute attacks of bronchospasm with chronic administration of drugs	
3. Observe for adverse effects	
a. Cardiac stimulation—tachycardia, palpitations, arrhythmias	This is the major adverse effect of bronchodilator therapy and results from stimulation of beta-adrenergic receptors in the heart.
b. Convulsive seizures	Theophylline stimulates the CNS. Seizures occur at toxic serum concentrations (above 20 μg/ml). They may occur without preceding symptoms of toxicity and may result in death. Diazepam (Valium) or phenytoin (Dilantin) may be used to control seizures.
c. Nausea and vomiting	Theophylline stimulates the chemoreceptor trigger zone in the medulla oblongata. This effect is usually related to high serum concentration; however, it may appear after a single dose.
d. Muscle tremor	This effect is mediated through the $beta_2$ receptors in the periphery. Decreasing the dose or switching to another agent may decrease this effect.
e. Other CNS symptoms—agitation, insomnia, restlessness, headache	
4. Observe for drug interactions	
a. Drugs that *increase* effects of bronchodilators	
(1) Monoamine oxidase (MAO) inhibitors	These drugs inhibit the metabolism of catecholamines. The subsequent administration of bronchodilators may increase blood pressure. Severe hypertensive reactions have been reported with ephedrine.
(2) Erythromycin, clindamycin, cimetidine	These drugs may decrease theophylline clearance and thereby increase the plasma levels.
b. Drugs that *decrease* effects of bronchodilators	
(1) Lithium	Lithium may increase excretion of theophylline and therefore decrease therapeutic effectiveness.
(2) Phenobarbital	This drug may increase the metabolism of theophylline by way of enzyme induction.
(3) Propranolol, other nonselective beta blockers	These drugs may cause bronchoconstriction and oppose effects of bronchodilators.
5. Teach clients	
a. Take only as prescribed. If desired effects are not achieved or if symptoms worsen, inform the physician. Do not increase dosage or frequency of taking medication.	Tolerance may develop to bronchodilators after repeated use or abuse. It is most commonly seen with the inhalers. Continued use in this manner may lead to serious cardiac side-effects.
b. Use inhalers correctly, as follows:	
(1) Shake well immediately before each use.	To disperse medication evenly
(2) Remove the cap from the mouthpiece.	
(3) Exhale fully, expelling as much air from the lungs as possible.	To increase drug effectiveness

Nursing Actions	Rationale/Explanation
(4) With the inhaler in the upright position, place the mouthpiece just inside the mouth, and use the lips to form a tight seal. (5) While inhaling deeply, fully depress the top of the inhaler with the index finger. (6) Hold the breath as long as possible. Before exhaling, remove the mouthpiece from the mouth and the finger from the canister. (7) Wait 3 to 5 minutes before taking a second inhalation of the drug.	
(8) Rinse the mouthpiece and store the inhaler away from heat.	Inhaler contents are pressurized and may explode if heated.
c. If a bronchodilator and a corticosteroid are prescribed for inhalation, use the bronchodilator first.	To increase penetration of the cortocosteroid
d. Avoid excessive intake of coffee, tea, and cola drinks.	These caffeine-containing beverages may increase nervousness and insomnia during bronchodilator therapy.

Selected References

American Medical Association (AMA) Division of Drugs: AMA Drug Evaluations, 5th ed. New York, John Wiley & Sons, 1983

Au WYW, Dutt AK, DeSoyza N: Theophylline kinetics in chronic obstructive airway disease in the elderly. Clin Pharmacol Ther 37:472–478, April 1985

Bitolterol—a new bronchodilator. Med Lett Drugs Ther 27:46–47, May 1985

Bukowskyj M, Nakatsu K, Munt PW: Theophylline reassessed. Ann Intern Med 101:63–73, July 1984

Cherniak RM: Current Therapy of Respiratory Disease 1984–1985. Philadelphia, BC Decker, 1984

Corticosteroid aerosols for asthma. Med Lett Drugs Ther 27:5–6, January 1985

Dunlap CI, Marchionno P: Help your COPD patient take a better breath—with inhalers. Nursing 13:42–43, May 1983

Facts and Comparisons. St. Louis, J B Lippincott (Updated monthly)

Guidelines for nursing care of the pulmonary patient. Los Angeles, California Thoracic Society, 1984

Hansten PD: Drug Interactions: Clinical Significance of Drug–Drug Interactions, 5th ed. Philadelphia, Lea & Febiger, 1985

Herrold RK: Mechanical ventilation: The drug connection. Am J Nurs 84:1389–1391, November 1984

Kirilloff LH, Tibbals SC: Drugs for asthma: A complete guide. Am J Nurs 83:55–61, January 1983

Middleton E, Reed CE, Ellis EF (eds): Allergy Principles and Practice. St. Louis, C V Mosby, 1983

Rodman MJ, Karch AM, Boyd EH, Smith DW: Pharmacology and Drug Therapy in Nursing, 3rd ed. Philadelphia. J B Lippincott, 1985

Shapiro GG, Konic P: Cromolyn sodium: A review. Pharmacotherapy 5:156–170, May–June 1985.

Sustained-release theophylline. Med Lett Drugs Ther 26:1–3, January 1984

Tobin MJ: Use of bronchodilator aerosols. Arch Intern Med 145:1659–1663, September 1985

Wang VA, Dworetzky M: How to manage your asthmatic patient: Recent advances. Drug Ther 13:79–102, September 1983

Weiner N: Norepinephrine, epinephrine and the sympathomimetic amines. In Gilman AG, Goodman LS, Rall TW, Murad F (eds): The Pharmacological Basis of Therapeutics, 7th ed, pp 145–180. New York, Macmillan, 1985

Wiener MB, Simkins RA: Respiratory disorders. In Wiener MB, Pepper GA (eds): Clinical Pharmacology and Therapeutics in Nursing, 2d ed, pp 420–442. New York, McGraw-Hill, 1985

48

ANTIHISTAMINES

Description and uses

Antihistamines are pharmacologic agents that antagonize the action of histamine. To understand the use of antihistamines, it is first necessary to understand the action of histamine in the body. Histamine is an important chemical mediator that is stored in almost every type of body tissue, particularly in mast cells and basophils. It is discharged from mast cells into the vascular system in response to certain stimuli (*e.g.*, antigen–antibody reactions, tissue injury, extreme cold, and specific drugs). Once released, histamine exerts various effects on body tissues, as listed below:

1. Histamine contracts smooth muscle such as those of the bronchi, gastrointestinal tract, and uterus. Histamine-induced bronchoconstriction may play a role in the cause of bronchial asthma.
2. Histamine acts on capillaries to cause vasodilation and subsequent hypotension. In addition, the skin on the face and upper parts of the body may become flushed.
3. Histamine increases capillary permeability to fluid, resulting in outflow of fluid into subcutaneous tissues and edema formation. Local edema in nasal mucosa produces the nasal congestion characteristic of allergic reactions and the common cold.
4. Histamine causes dilation of cerebral blood vessels, which may cause severe headache.
5. Histamine stimulates secretion of gastric juice in large amounts and with high acidity. It also increases bronchial, intestinal, and salivary secretions.
6. Histamine stimulates sensory nerve endings to cause pain and itching.

Antihistamine drugs prevent histamine from acting on target tissues. Because antihistamines are structurally related to histamine, the drugs occupy the same receptor sites as histamine and competitively antagonize its actions. They do not prevent histamine release or reduce the amount released. There are two types of histamine receptors, called H_1 and H_2 receptors. Conventional antihistamines act on H_1 receptors and may be called H_1 blockers. These are the antihistamines discussed in this chapter. Cimetidine (Tagamet) and ranitidine (Zantac) are H_2 blocking agents that are used to prevent or treat peptic ulcer disease. They are discussed in Chapter 60.

Antihistamines are effective in inhibiting vascular permeability, edema formation, bronchoconstriction, and pruritus associated with histamine release. They are partially effective in histamine-induced hypotension; they are ineffective in antigen-induced bronchoconstriction and increased gastric acid secretion. Antihistamines also exert depressant effects on the central nervous system (CNS) to produce sedation and drowsiness. In a few people, particularly children, antihistamines may produce paradoxic restlessness and hyperactivity.

Many antihistamines are available for clinical use (Table 48-1). These agents are similar in effectiveness

(Text continues on p. 456.)

TABLE 48-1. COMMONLY USED ANTIHISTAMINES

	Generic name	Trade name	Routes and dosage ranges: Adults	Routes and dosage ranges: Children	Comments
Ethylenediamines	Tripelennamine citrate	PBZ elixir	PO 25–50 mg q4–6h; maximal daily dose, 300 mg	PO 5 mg/kg/24h in 4–6 divided doses or 150 mg/m²/day in divided doses	Elixir contains 37.5 mg of tripelennamine citrate per 5 ml. Dosages are based on the hydrochloride salt. Each milliliter of elixir is equal to 5 mg of tripelennamine hydrochloride. Citrate is more palatable than hydrochloride. Low incidence of adverse effects, which include moderate sedation, mild gastrointestinal distress, paradoxic excitation, hyperirritability. Dizziness is common.
	Tripelennamine hydrochloride	PBZ hydrochloride	PO 25–50 mg q4–6h; Maximal daily dose, 600 mg	PO 5 mg/kg/24h in 4–6 divided doses or, for children over 5 years old, 50 mg b.i.d.–t.i.d.; maximal daily dose, 300 mg	See tripelennamine citrate.
	Pyrilamine maleate		PO 75–200 mg daily in 3–4 divided doses	Age 6–12 years, PO 12.5–25 mg q.i.d.	Low incidence of drowsiness.
Ethanolamines	Carbinoxamine maleate	Clistin	PO 12–32 mg daily in divided doses Long-acting preparation, PO 8–12 mg q6–12h	PO 0.2 mg/kg in 3–4 divided doses or 2–4 mg t.i.d.–q.i.d.	Lowest incidence of drowsiness of the ethanolamines. Anticholinergic effect very weak. Causes some drowsiness, dizziness, dryness of mouth, and gastrointestinal distress.
	Clemastine fumarate	Tavist	PO 2.68 mg 1–3 times daily, not to exceed 8.04 mg/day Long-acting preparation, initially, PO 1.34 mg b.i.d., not to exceed 8.04 mg/day	Safety and efficacy in children under 12 years of age have not been established	Drowsiness is the most frequent side-effect, but central sedative effects are generally low in occurrence. Anticholinergic effect very weak.
	Dimenhydrinate	Dramamine	PO 50–100 mg q4h Rectal 100 mg q.d.–b.i.d. IM, IV 50 mg	Age 8–12 years, 25–50 mg t.i.d.	Often used to prevent motion sickness. May cause drowsiness. May mask ototoxicity caused by aminoglycoside antibiotics.
	Diphenhydramine hydrochloride	Benadryl	PO 25–50 mg t.i.d.–q.i.d. IM, IV 10–50 mg up to a maximal single dose	PO 12.5–25 mg t.i.d. or 5 mg/kg/day IM, IV 5 mg/kg or 150 mg/	Topical preparation also available. May affect blood pressure when given parenterally. Also used

TABLE 48-1. COMMONLY USED ANTIHISTAMINES (*Continued*)

	Generic name	Trade name	Routes and dosage ranges: Adults	Routes and dosage ranges: Children	Comments
			of 100 mg; maximal daily dose, 400 mg	m^2/day in 4 divided doses during a 24-hour period, up to a maximum of 300 mg/day	in motion sickness and for emotionally disturbed children. Drowsiness decreases with continued usage. Protect from light.
Alkylamines	Chlorpheniramine maleate	Chlor-Trimeton	PO 2–4 mg t.i.d.–q.i.d. Sustained-release preparation, PO 8–12 mg q.d.–t.i.d. IM, IV, SC 5–40 mg	Age 6–12 years, PO, SC 0.35 mg/kg/day in 4 divided doses Age 7 years and over, sustained-release preparation, PO 8 mg q12h Not recommended for children under 6 years of age	Overall, low incidence of adverse effects, with drowsiness being the most common. Given parenterally for amelioration of allergic reactions to blood or plasma and in anaphylaxis. Only preparations without preservatives may be given IV, and the drug should be injected over 1 minute. A common ingredient in over-the-counter products for cold and allergy symptoms.
	Brompheniramine maleate	Dimetane	PO 4–8 mg t.i.d.–q.i.d. Sustained-release preparation, PO 8–12 mg b.i.d. IM, IV, SC 10 mg q6–12h; maximal daily dose, 40 mg	Infant to 6 years, PO 0.5 mg/kg/day or 15 mg/m^2/day in divided doses Age over 6 years, PO, half of adult dose Age under 12, IM, IV, SC 0.5 mg/kg/day or 15 mg/m^2/day in divided doses	Mild drowsiness is the most common reaction. Do not use solution containing preservatives for IV injection.
	Dexchlorpheniramine maleate	Polaramine	PO 1–2 mg t.i.d. or q.i.d. Sustained-release preparation, PO 4–6 mg b.i.d.	Infants, PO, one fourth of adult dose or 0.15 mg/kg/day in 4 divided doses Under 12 years, PO, half of adult dose Do not use sustained-release preparation	Incidence of adverse effects is low. Most common reaction is a mild drowsiness.
	Triprolidine hydrochloride	Actidil	PO 2.5 mg t.i.d.–q.i.d.	Age over 6 years, PO 1.25 mg t.i.d.–q.i.d. Age 4–6 years, PO 0.9 mg t.i.d.–q.i.d. Age 2–4 years, 0.6 mg t.i.d.–q.i.d.	Rapid onset with low incidence of adverse effects; drowsiness is the most common. Others include dizziness, gastrointestinal distress, paradoxic excitation, hyperirritability.

TABLE 48-1. COMMONLY USED ANTIHISTAMINES (*Continued*)

	Generic name	Trade name	Routes and dosage ranges: Adults	Routes and dosage ranges: Children	Comments
				Age 4 months–2 years, 0.3 mg t.i.d.–q.i.d. In children up to 6 years, use syrup only	
Phenothiazines	Methdilazine, methdilazine hydrochloride	Tacaryl, Tacaryl hydrochloride	PO 8 mg b.i.d.–q.i.d.	Infants, PO 2 mg b.i.d. Age over 3 years, PO 4 mg b.i.d.–q.i.d.	Used as an antipruritic in allergic and nonallergic pruritus. Drowsiness less prominent than with other phenothiazines used as antihistamines. Most serious adverse reactions seen with antipsychotic phenothiazines have not been reported with this agent. Chewable tablet must be chewed and swallowed promptly.
	Promethazine hydrochloride	Phenergan	PO 25 mg at bedtime or 12.5 mg q.d.–b.i.d. Rectal 25 mg, may be repeated in 4–6 hours IM, IV 12.5–25 mg, may be repeated in 2 hours	PO 0.13 mg/kg in AM and, when necessary, 0.5 mg/kg at bedtime; or 25 mg at bedtime and 6.25–12.5 mg t.i.d. IM no more than half of adult dose	Very potent antihistamine with pronounced sedative effects that limit its use in ambulatory clients. Also used as sedative and in motion sickness. Photosensitization is a contraindication to further use. All precautions applicable to phenothiazines should be observed (see Chap. 9).
	Trimeprazine tartrate	Temaril	PO 2.5 mg q.i.d. Sustained-release preparation, PO 5 mg q12h	Age under 3 years, PO, 1.25 mg t.i.d., maximal daily dose, 5 mg Age 3–12 years, PO 2.5 mg q.i.d.; maximal daily dose, 10 mg	Used for symptomatic relief of acute and chronic pruritus. Drowsiness is the most common reaction. Dizziness and dry mouth may also occur (see also phenothiazines in Chap. 9).
Piperazines	Meclizine hydrochloride	Antivert	Motion sickness, PO 25–50 mg q.d. 1 hour before traveling Vertigo, 25–100 mg daily in divided doses		Used mostly in motion sickness. May cause drowsiness, dry mouth, blurred vision.
	Cyclizine hydrochloride	Marezine hydrochloride	PO 50 mg ½ hour before travel; repeat q4–6h; maximal daily dose, 300 mg IM 50 mg t.i.d.–q.i.d. or as required	Age 6–10 years, PO, half of adult dose, IM 1 mg/kg t.i.d.	Widely used as an antiemetic. Contraindicated in pregnancy. May cause drowsiness, dizziness, irritability.

TABLE 48-1. COMMONLY USED ANTIHISTAMINES (*Continued*)

	Generic name	Trade name	Routes and dosage ranges: *Adults*	Routes and dosage ranges: *Children*	Comments
Miscellaneous antihistamines	Cyproheptadine	Periactin	PO 4 mg t.i.d., not to exceed 0.5 mg/kg/day	Age 2–6 years, PO 2 mg b.i.d.–t.i.d., not to exceed 12 mg daily Age 6–14 years, 4 mg t.i.d., not to exceed 16 mg daily	Particularly used in treatment of pruritic dermatoses, angioedema, and migraine. Weight gain has been reported. The drug is sometimes used therapeutically as an appetite stimulant in children. May cause drowsiness and dry mouth. Contraindicated in glaucoma, urinary retention, and premature and full-term infants.
	Azatadine maleate	Optimine	PO 1–2 mg b.i.d. Use lower dosage in elderly.	Dosage not established	Chemically similar to cyproheptadine. Has prolonged action. Used in allergic rhinitis and chronic urticaria. Drowsiness is the most common side-effect. Should not be used in clients with asthma, in children under 12 years of age, or during pregnancy or lactation.
	Diphenylpyraline hydrochloride	Hispril	PO 2 mg t.i.d.–q.i.d. Sustained-release preparation, 5 mg q.d.–b.i.d.	Age 6–12 years, PO 2 mg t.i.d.–q.i.d. Age under 6 years, PO 1–2 mg q.d.–b.i.d. Do not exceed 4 mg daily; do not use sustained-release preparation	Low incidence of adverse effects, which include drowsiness, dizziness, headache, dry mouth.
	Hydroxyzine hydrochloride, hydroxyzine pamoate	Atarax, Vistaril	PO 75–100 mg daily in 3–4 divided doses Preoperative and postoperative sedation, prepartum and postpartum sedation, IM 25–100 mg as a single dose Serious psychiatric conditions, IM 50–100 mg q4–6h PRN	PO 2 mg/kg/day in 4 divided doses Preoperative and postoperative sedation, IM 0.6 mg/kg in a single dose	Has antihistaminic, antiemetic, antianxiety, and sedative effects and is used for all these actions. Low incidence of adverse effects; drowsiness is usually transient.
	Terfenadine	Seldane	PO 60 mg q12h	Safety and efficacy in children under 12 years have not been established	Chemically different from other antihistamines. Reportedly causes less sedation than other antihistamines; other adverse effects are similar.

as histamine antagonists but differ in potency, dosage, incidence of adverse effects, and dosage forms available. Antihistamines can be subdivided into the following six groups:

1. *Ethylenediamines* have weak CNS depressant effects and therefore cause less drowsiness than most other antihistamines. However, they often cause gastrointestinal distress. The prototype of the ethylenediamines is pyrilamine.
2. *Ethanolamines* are strong CNS depressants and cause a high incidence of drowsiness. Gastrointestinal distress is low in incidence. The prototype of this group is diphenhydramine (Benadryl).
3. *Alkylamines* are effective in relatively low dosage and are the most suitable agents for daytime use. The members of this group are among the most commonly used antihistamines. Individual responses to these drugs vary, and either CNS depression or stimulation may occur. The prototypical agent is chlorpheniramine (Chlor-Trimeton).
4. *Phenothiazines* are used mainly for CNS depressant and antiemetic effects. They are related to the phenothiazine antipsychotic drugs discussed in Chapter 9. The prototype of this group is promethazine (Phenergan).
5. *Piperazines* have prolonged antihistaminic activity with a relatively low incidence of drowsiness. However, mental alertness is decreased, and operation of machinery may be hazardous.
6. *Miscellaneous* agents include hydroxyzine (Vistaril), which is often used as an antiemetic and preoperative sedative, and cyproheptadine (Periactin), which is used in pruritic dermatoses, angioedema, and migraine.

Antihistamines are well absorbed following oral and parenteral administration. They are primarily metabolized by the liver and excreted within 24 hours by the kidneys. When given orally, effects occur within 15 to 60 minutes and last about 4 to 6 hours. Enteric-coated or sustained-release preparations last 8 to 12 hours. Long-acting dosage forms may be less effective owing to inadequate dissolution and absorption. When given parenterally, antihistaminic effects occur more rapidly. Some topical preparations of antihistamines are available, but they should be avoided because they are inactive when applied to intact skin, they act as local anesthetics rather than antihistamines on denuded skin, and they may cause sensitization.

Clinical indications for use of antihistamines include the following:

1. Upper respiratory disorders. From 75% to 95% of people with hay fever (seasonal allergic rhinitis) experience some relief of sneezing, rhinorrhea, nasal airway obstruction, and conjunctivitis with the use of antihistamines. People with perennial allergic rhinitis (nonseasonal) usually experience decreased nasal congestion and drying of nasal mucosa. Antihistamines are generally ineffective in the treatment of asthma.
2. Dermatologic conditions. Antihistamines are the drugs of choice for treatment of acute urticaria but are less effective in chronic urticaria. Other indications for use include contact dermatitis, atopic dermatitis, drug-induced allergic skin reactions, pruritus ani, and pruritus vulvae.
3. Vascular disorders. Antihistamines may be useful in treating angioedema, but they are second-choice drugs, after epinephrine.
4. Hypersensitivity phenomena. Antihistamines are helpful in treating urticaria and pruritus associated with allergic reactions. However, they are less effective in treating bronchoconstriction and hypotension. Epinephrine is the drug of choice for treating these serious allergic reactions (anaphylactic shock). Antihistamines may be given to prevent allergic reactions to blood transfusions.
5. Miscellaneous uses. The anticholinergic effects of some antihistamines (*e.g.*, diphenhydramine) are sometimes used in treatment of Parkinson's disease and drug-induced extrapyramidal reactions that simulate parkinsonism. The drugs decrease rigidity and improve speech and voluntary movement. The sedative effect of some antihistamines is used for preoperative sedation. In addition, many over-the-counter products for sleep or daytime sedation contain an antihistamine as the active ingredient, (*e.g.*, Compoz, Sominex). Antihistamines may be useful in motion sickness, Meniere's disease, and other types of vertigo. These agents may also be used to prevent allergic reactions to contrast media (*e.g.*, iodine preparations) used for various diagnostic tests.

Antihistamines are contraindicated or must be used with caution in clients with hypersensitivity to the drugs, narrow-angle glaucoma, prostatic hypertrophy, stenosing peptic ulcer, bladder neck obstruction, and during pregnancy.

Principles of therapy: antihistamines

1. Assess the client's condition in relation to disorders in which antihistamines are used. For the client

with known allergies, try to determine factors that precipitate or relieve allergic reactions and specific signs and symptoms experienced during a reaction.
2. When specific allergens or precipitating factors are identified, allergic reactions may be prevented by avoiding exposure to them.
3. Antihistamines are more effective when given before exposure to allergens because the drugs can then occupy receptor sites before histamine is released.
4. Choice of antihistamine is based on the desired effect, duration of action, and adverse effects.
   a. For treatment of acute allergic reactions, a rapid-acting agent of short duration is preferred.
   b. For chronic allergic symptoms (*e.g.*, allergic rhinitis), long-acting preparations provide more consistent relief.
   c. For clients who are sensitive to the sedative effects of antihistamines or who must stay alert, an antihistamine with a relatively low sedative effect is indicated.
   d. Some antihistamines have relatively specific indications for use. For example, dimenhydrinate (Dramamine) and meclizine (Antivert) are often used to prevent or treat motion sickness; trimeprazine (Temaril) and cyproheptadine (Periactin) are especially effective in treatment of pruritus; promethazine (Phenergan) and hydroxyzine (Vistaril) are often used in nausea and vomiting.
   e. Some clients respond better to certain antihistamines than to others. Consequently, if one antihistamine does not relieve symptoms or produces excessive sedation, another may be effective.
   f. Several combination products (*e.g.*, Actifed, Dimetapp), containing one or more antihistamines, adrenergic agents, and perhaps other ingredients, are often used to relieve symptoms of the common cold and other upper respiratory disorders. Like other fixed-dose drug combinations, these products may not contain the optimum amount of each component drug.

USE IN PREGNANCY

During pregnancy, antihistamines should not be used unless expected benefits clearly outweigh potential adverse effects. They should not be used at all during the third trimester; both full-term and premature infants may have severe reactions.

PEDIATRIC CONSIDERATIONS

In pediatric drug therapy, there is a higher risk of adverse effects. Therapeutic doses may decrease mental alertness or cause paradoxic excitation. Overdoses may cause hallucinations, convulsions, and death.

GERIATRIC CONSIDERATIONS

In geriatric drug therapy, antihistamines may cause dizziness, sedation, syncope, hypotension, and toxic confusional states.

NURSING ACTIONS: ANTIHISTAMINES

Nursing Actions	*Rationale/Explanation*
1. Administer accurately	
a. Give oral antihistamines with meals.	To decrease gastrointestinal effects of the drugs
b. Give intramuscular antihistamines deeply into a large muscle mass.	To decrease tissue irritation
c. Inject intravenous antihistamines slowly, over a few minutes.	Severe hypotension may result from rapid intravenous injection.
d. When a drug is used to prevent motion sickness, give 30 to 60 minutes before travel.	

Nursing Actions	Rationale/Explanation
2. Observe for therapeutic effects	Therapeutic effects depend on the reason for use.
a. A verbal statement of therapeutic effect (relief of symptoms)	
b. Decreased nausea and vomiting when given for antiemetic effects	
c. Decreased dizziness and nausea when taken for motion sickness	
d. Drowsiness or sleep when given for sedation	
3. Observe for adverse effects	
a. Sedation—ranging from mild drowsiness to deep sleep	Due to CNS depression, which occurs with most antihistamines. Sedation is the most common adverse effect.
b. Paradoxic excitation—restlessness, insomnia, tremors, nervousness, and palpitations	This reaction is more likely to occur in children. It may result from the anticholinergic effects of antihistamines.
c. Convulsive seizures	Antihistamines, particularly the phenothiazines, may lower the seizure threshold.
d. Dryness of the mouth, nose and throat, blurred vision, urinary retention, and constipation	Due to anticholinergic effects of antihistamines
e. Gastrointestinal distress—anorexia, nausea, vomiting	These symptoms are especially likely to occur with the ethylenediamine group of antihistamines.
f. Allergic reactions—skin rashes, photosensitivity	These are more likely to occur with topical antihistamine preparations.
g. Teratogenicity	Piperazine antihistamines are teratogenic.
4. Observe for drug interactions	
Drugs that *increase* effects of antihistamines	
(1) Ethyl alcohol, CNS depressants (*e.g.,* antianxiety and antipsychotic agents, narcotic analgesics, sedative–hypnotics)	Additive CNS depression. Concomitant use may lead to drowsiness, lethargy, stupor, respiratory depression, coma, and death.
(2) Monoamine oxidase (MAO) inhibitors	Inhibit metabolism of antihistamines, leading to an increased duration of action; increased incidence and severity of anticholinergic adverse effects
(3) Tricyclic antidepressants	Additive anticholinergic side-effects
5. Teach clients	
a. Take antihistamines only as prescribed or as instructed on packages of over-the-counter preparations.	To maximize therapeutic benefit and minimize adverse effects
b. Do not drink alcohol or take other drugs without the physician's knowledge and consent.	To avoid adverse effects and dangerous drug interactions. Alcohol and other drugs with CNS-depressant effects may cause excessive sedation, respiratory depression, and death.
c. Do not smoke, drive a car, or operate machinery until drowsiness has worn off.	To avoid injury. Drowsiness usually decreases after a few days of continuous drug administration.
d. Report adverse effects such as excessive drowsiness.	The physician may be able to change drugs or dosages to decrease adverse effects.
e. Store antihistamines out of reach of children.	To avoid accidental ingestion

Selected References

American Medical Association (AMA) Division of Drugs: AMA Drug Evaluations, 5th ed. New York, John Wiley & Sons, 1983

Anderson PD: Basic Human Anatomy and Physiology: Clinical Implications for the Health Professions. Monterey, CA, Wadsworth, 1984

Douglas WW: Histamine and 5-hydroxytryptamine (serotonin) and their antagonists. In Gilman AG, Goodman LS, Rall TW, Murad F (eds): The Pharmacological Basis of Therapeutics 7th ed, pp 605–638. New York, Macmillan, 1985

Facts and Comparisons. St. Louis, J B Lippincott (Updated monthly)

Guyton AC: Textbook of Medical Physiology, 7th ed. Philadelphia, W B Saunders, 1986

Hansten PD: Drug Interactions: Clinical Significance of Drug–Drug Interactions, 5th ed. Philadelphia, Lea & Febiger, 1985

Malseed RT: Pharmacology: Drug Therapy and Nursing Considerations, 2d ed. Philadelphia, J B Lippincott, 1985

49

NASAL DECONGESTANTS, ANTITUSSIVES, MUCOLYTICS, AND COLD REMEDIES

Description and uses

Common signs and symptoms of several respiratory disorders are nasal congestion, cough, and increased secretions. Characteristics of these signs and symptoms include the following:

1. Nasal congestion is manifested by obstructed nasal passages ("stuffy nose") and nasal drainage ("runny nose"). It is a prominent symptom of the common cold and allergic rhinitis. Nasal congestion results from dilation of the blood vessels in the nasal mucosa and engorgement of the mucous membranes with blood. At the same time, nasal membranes are stimulated to increase mucus secretion. Related symptomatic terms are *rhinorrhea* (the discharge of mucus from the nose), *rhinitis* (inflammation of the mucous membrane of the nose), and *coryza* (profuse discharge from the mucous membrane of the nose).
2. Cough is a forceful expulsion of air from the lungs. It is normally a protective reflex for removing foreign bodies, environmental irritants, or accumulated secretions from the respiratory tract. The cough reflex involves both central and peripheral mechanisms. Centrally, the cough center in the medulla oblongata receives stimuli and initiates the reflex response (deep inspiration, closed glottis, build-up of pressure within the lungs and forceful exhalation). Peripherally, "cough receptors" in the pharynx, larynx, trachea, or lungs may be stimulated by air, dryness of mucous membranes, or excessive secretions. A cough is described as "productive" when secretions are expectorated; it is "nonproductive" when it is dry and no sputum is expectorated.

   Cough is a prominent symptom of respiratory tract infections (*e.g.*, influenza, bronchitis, pharyngitis) and chronic obstructive pulmonary diseases (*e.g.*, emphysema, chronic bronchitis).
3. Increased secretions may result from excessive production or decreased ability to cough or otherwise remove secretions from the respiratory tract. Secretions may seriously impair respiration by obstructing airways and preventing air flow to and from alveoli, where gas exchange occurs. Secretions may also cause atelectasis and cause or aggravate infections by supporting bacterial growth.

Respiratory disorders characterized by retention of secretions include influenza, pneumonia, upper respiratory infections, acute and chronic bronchitis, emphysema, and acute attacks of bronchial asthma. Nonrespiratory conditions that predispose to secretion retention include immobility, debilitation, cigarette smoking, and postoperative status. Surgical procedures involving the chest or abdomen are most likely to be associated with retention of secretions because pain may decrease the client's ability to cough, breathe deeply, and ambulate.

Individual decongestants, antitussives, expectorants, and mucolytics are listed in Table 49-1; combination cold, cough, and allergy remedies are listed in Table 49-2.

NASAL DECONGESTANTS

Nasal decongestants are used to relieve nasal obstruction and discharge. Adrenergic (sympathomimetic) drugs are most often used for this purpose (see Chap. 18). These agents relieve nasal congestion by constricting arterioles and reducing blood flow to nasal mucosa. Most nasal decongestants are applied topically to the nasal mucosa as nasal sprays or solutions. Some (*e.g.*, ephedrine, phenylephrine) may be used orally or topically; phenylpropanolamine is prepared only for oral use. Nasal decongestants are most often used to relieve rhinitis associated with respiratory infections or allergies. They may also be used to reduce local blood flow before nasal surgery and to aid visualization of the nasal mucosa during diagnostic examinations.

ANTITUSSIVES

Antitussive agents suppress cough by depressing the cough center in the medulla oblongata or the cough receptors in the throat, trachea, or lungs. Centrally acting antitussives include narcotics (codeine, hydrocodone, hydromorphone, and morphine) and nonnarcotics (benzonatate, dextromethorphan, and noscapine). Peripherally acting agents (*e.g.*, glycerin, ammonium chloride) usually contain demulcents or local anesthetics to decrease irritation of pharyngeal mucosa. These agents are used as gargles, lozenges, and syrups. Flavored syrups are often used as vehicles for other drugs. Lozenges and hard candy increase the flow of saliva, which also soothes pharyngeal mucosa and may suppress cough.

The major clinical indication for use of antitussives is a dry, hacking, nonproductive cough that interferes with rest and sleep. It is usually not desirable to suppress a productive cough.

EXPECTORANTS

Expectorants are agents given orally to liquefy respiratory secretions and allow for their easier removal. Objective tests have failed to demonstrate the effectiveness of these drugs. However, they are still commonly used. They are available as single-drug preparations or as ingredients in many combination cough and cold remedies.

MUCOLYTICS

Mucolytics are agents administered by inhalation in order to liquefy mucus in the respiratory tract. Solutions of mucolytic drugs may be nebulized into a face mask or mouthpiece or instilled directly into the respiratory tract through a tracheostomy. Sodium chloride solution and acetylcysteine (Mucomyst) are the only agents currently recommended for use as mucolytics. Acetylcysteine is effective within 1 minute after inhalation, and maximal effects occur within 5 to 10 minutes. It is effective immediately after direct instillation. Acetylcysteine is also widely used in the treatment of acetaminophen overdosage (see Chap. 6).

COLD REMEDIES

Many combination products are available for treating symptoms of the common cold. Most of the products contain an antihistamine, a nasal decongestant, and an analgesic. Some contain antitussives, expectorants, and other agents as well. These products are also used to treat allergic rhinitis. Although some cold remedies require a physician's prescription, many are proprietary, over-the-counter (OTC) formulations.

Commonly used ingredients include chlorpheniramine maleate (antihistamine), phenylephrine or phenylpropanolamine (adrenergic nasal decongestants), acetaminophen or aspirin (analgesics), codeine or dextromethorphan (antitussives), and guaifenesin (expectorant). Specific ingredients and amounts of each vary; several proprietary products come in several formulations. For example, see Novahistine, Phenergan, and Robitussin in Table 49-2.

Principles of therapy: nasal decongestants, antitussives, mucolytics, and cold remedies

ASSESSMENT GUIDELINES

Assess the client's condition in relation to disorders for which the drugs are used.

1. With nasal congestion, observe for decreased ability to breathe through the nose. If a nasal discharge is present, note the amount, color, and thickness. Question the person about the duration and extent of nasal congestion as well as factors that precipitate or relieve the symptom.

TABLE 49-1. NASAL DECONGESTANTS, ANTITUSSIVES, AND EXPECTORANTS

	Generic name	Trade name	Routes and dosage ranges: Adults	Routes and dosage ranges: Children
Nasal decongestants	Ephedrine sulfate		PO 25–50 mg q3–4h Topically, 1–2 drops of 1%–3% solution as needed	
	Naphazoline hydrochloride	Privine hydrochloride	Topically, 1–2 drops or 2 spray inhalations no more often than q4–6h	Age over 6 years, topically, same as adults Age under 6 years, not recommended
	Oxymetazoline hydrochloride	Afrin	Topically, 2–4 drops or 2–3 spray inhalations in each nostril, morning and bedtime	Age over 6 years, topically, same as adults Age under 6 years, 2–3 drops of 0.025% solution twice daily
	Phenylephrine hydrochloride	Neo-Synephrine	PO 10 mg 3 times daily Topically, 2–3 drops of 0.25%–1% solution in each nostril as needed	Age over 6 years, PO 5 mg 3 times daily; topically, same as adults Infants, topically, 1–2 drops of 0.125% solution as needed
	Phenylpropanolamine hydrochloride	Propagest	PO 25 mg q3–4h or 50 mg q6–8h	Age 8–12 years, PO 20–25 mg 3 times daily
	Propylhexedrine	Benzedrex	Topically, 2 inhalations (0.6–0.8 mg) in each nostril as needed	
	Pseudoephedrine hydrochloride	Sudafed	PO 60 mg 3–4 times daily Sustained-release preparations, PO 120 mg twice daily	Age over 6 years, PO 60 mg 3–4 times daily Age 4 months–6 years, PO 30 mg 3–4 times daily
	Tetrahydrozoline hydrochloride	Tyzine	Topically, 2–3 drops or 1–2 sprays of 0.1% solution instilled in each nostril, no more often than q3h	Age 6 years and over, topically, 1–3 drops of 0.05% solution in each nostril q4–6h Age under 6 years, not recommended
	Xylometazoline hydrochloride	Otrivin hydrochloride	Topically, 2–4 drops or inhalations of 0.1% solution in each nostril 2–3 times daily	Age 6 months–12 years, topically, 2–3 drops of 0.05% solution in each nostril 2–3 times daily Age under 6 months, topically, 1 drop of 0.05% solution in each nostril 2–3 times daily
Narcotic antitussives	Codeine phosphate or sulfate		PO 15 mg q4h as needed; maximal dose, 120 mg/24 hour	PO 1–1.5 mg/kg/day in 6 divided doses as necessary
	Hydrocodone bitartrate		PO 5–10 mg 3–4 times daily	PO 0.6 mg/kg/day in 3–4 divided doses
	Hydromorphone hydrochloride	Dilaudid	PO 1 mg q3–4h	
	Morphine sulfate		PO 2–4 mg 3–4 times daily	Age over 1 year, PO 0.06 mg/kg 3–4 times daily
Nonnarcotic antitussives	Benzonatate	Tessalon	PO 100 mg 3 times daily; Maximal daily dose, 600 mg	Age over 10 years, PO same as adults Age under 10 years, PO 8 mg/kg/day in 3–6 divided doses
	Dextromethorphan	Romilar CF	PO 15–30 mg 3–4 times daily	Age 2–5 years, PO 1 tsp of 7.5 mg/5 ml or $\frac{1}{2}$ tsp of 15 mg/5 ml q4h, up to 4 doses in 24 hours

TABLE 49-1. NASAL DECONGESTANTS, ANTITUSSIVES, AND EXPECTORANTS (*Continued*)

	Generic name	Trade name	Routes and dosage ranges	
			Adults	*Children*
				Age 6–12 years, PO 2 tsp of 7.5 mg/5 ml or 1 tsp of 15 mg/5 ml q4h, up to 4 doses in 24 hours
Expectorants	Guaifenesin (glyceryl guaiacolate)	Robitussin	PO 200 mg (2 tsp) q4h	Age 12 years or over, PO 200 mg (2 tsp) q4h Age 6–12 years, PO 100 mg (1 tsp) q4h Age 2–6 years, PO 50 mg ($\frac{1}{2}$ tsp) q4h
	Iodinated glycerol	Organidin	PO 60 mg (2 30-mg tablets, 20 drops of 5% solution, or 5 ml of elixir) 4 times daily	PO 30 mg or less 4 times daily, depending on age and weight
	Potassium iodide, saturated solution	SSKI	PO 300–600 mg (0.3–0.6 ml) in a full glass of fluid (water, milk, or fruit juice) 3–4 times daily	PO 150–300 mg (0.15–0.3 ml) well diluted in water, milk, or fruit juice 3–4 times daily
Mucolytic	Acetylcysteine	Mucomyst	Nebulization, 1–10 ml of a 20% solution or 2–20 ml of a 10% solution 3–4 times daily Instillation, 1–2 ml of a 10% or 20% solution q1–4h Acetaminophen overdosage: PO 140 mg/kg initially, then 70 mg/kg q4h for 17 doses; dilute a 10% or 20% solution to a 5% solution with cola, fruit juice, or water	

2. With coughing, a major assessment factor is whether the cough is productive of sputum or dry and hacking. If the cough is productive, note the color, odor, viscosity and amount of sputum. In addition, assess factors that stimulate or relieve cough and the client's ability and willingness to cough effectively.

NURSING INTERVENTIONS

Encourage clients to use measures to prevent or minimize incidence and severity of symptoms.

1. With allergic disorders, avoid exposure to allergens, when possible. Common allergens include plant pollens, dust, animal dander, and medications.
2. Avoid smoking cigarettes. Cigarette smoke irritates respiratory tract mucosa. This irritation causes cough, increased secretions, and decreased effectiveness of cilia in cleaning the respiratory tract.
3. Avoid exposure to crowds, especially during winter months when the incidence of influenza is high.
4. Avoid contact with persons who have colds or other respiratory infections. This is especially important for clients with chronic lung disease, since upper respiratory infections may precipitate acute attacks of asthma or bronchitis.
5. Maintain a fluid intake of 2000 to 3000 ml daily unless contraindicated by cardiovascular or renal disease.
6. Maintain nutrition, rest, activity, and other general health measures.
7. Practice good handwashing techniques.
8. Annual vaccination for influenza is recommended for clients who are elderly or have chronic respiratory, cardiovascular, or renal disorders.

DRUG SELECTION AND ADMINISTRATION

Choice of drugs and routes of administration is influenced by several client- and drug-related variables. Some guidelines include the following:

1. Single-drug formulations are usually preferred over combination products because they allow flexibility and individualization of dosage. Combi-

TABLE 49-2. REPRESENTATIVE COMBINATION COLD, COUGH, AND ALLERGY REMEDIES*

Trade name	Ingredients						Comments
	Antihistamine	*Nasal decongestant*	*Analgesic*	*Antitussive*	*Expectorant*	*Other*	
Actifed	Triprolidine HCl 2.5 mg/tab or cap; 1.25 mg/5 ml of syrup	Pseudoephedrine HCl 60 mg/tab or cap; 30 mg/5 ml of syrup					A commonly prescribed product; now available OTC
Actifed with codeine cough syrup	Triprolidine HCl 1.25 mg/5 ml	Pseudoephedrine HCl 30 mg/5 ml		Codeine 10 mg/5 ml		Alcohol 4.3%	
Allerest	Chlorpheniramine maleate 2 mg/tab	Phenylpropanolamine HCl 18.7 mg/tab					OTC
Allerest (children's preparation)	Chlorpheniramine maleate 1 mg/tab	Phenylpropanolamine HCl 9.4 mg/tab					OTC
Cheracol Syrup				Codeine 10 mg/5 ml	Guaifenesin 100 mg/5 ml	Alcohol 4.75%	
Cheracol D Cough Liquid				Dextromethorphan 10 mg/5 ml	Guaifenesin 100 mg/5 ml	Alcohol 4.75%	OTC
Comtrex	Chlorpheniramine maleate 1 mg/tab or cap	Phenylpropanolamine HCl 12.5 mg/tab or cap	Acetaminophen 325 mg/tab or cap	Dextromethorphan 10 mg/tab or cap			OTC
Contac	Chlorpheniramine maleate 8 mg/cap	Phenylpropanolamine HCl 75 mg/cap					OTC, long-acting (timed-release capsule)
Coricidin	Chlorpheniramine maleate 2 mg/tab		Acetaminophen 325 mg/tab				OTC
Coricidin D	Chlorpheniramine maleate 2 mg/tab	Phenylpropanolamine 12.5 mg/tab	Acetaminophen 325 mg/tab				OTC
CoTylenol cold formula	Chlorpheniramine maleate 2 mg/tab or cap	Pseudoephedrine HCl 30 mg/tab or cap	Acetaminophen 325 mg/tab or cap	Dextromethorphan 15 mg/tab or cap			OTC
CoTylenol liquid (children's preparation)	Chlorpheniramine maleate 1 mg/5 ml	Phenylpropanolamine HCl 6.25 mg/5 ml	Acetaminophen 160 mg/5 ml			Alcohol 8.5%	OTC
Dimetapp Elixir	Brompheniramine maleate 2 mg/5 ml	Phenylpropanolamine HCl 12.5 mg/5 ml				Alcohol 2.3%	
Dimetapp Extentabs	Brompheniramine maleate 12 mg/tab	Phenylpropanolamine HCl 75 mg/tab					OTC, frequently prescribed, long-acting (10–12 hours) preparation
Dristan	Chlorpheniramine maleate 2	Phenylephrine HCl 5 mg/cap or tab	Acetaminophen 325 mg/cap or tab				OTC

TABLE 49-2. REPRESENTATIVE COMBINATION COLD, COUGH, AND ALLERGY REMEDIES* (*Continued*)

Trade name	Ingredients: Antihistamine	Nasal decongestant	Analgesic	Antitussive	Expectorant	Other	Comments
	mg/cap or tab						
Drixoral	Dexbrompheniramine maleate 6 mg/tab	Pseudoephedrine sulfate 120 mg/tab					OTC, timed-release tablets, long-acting
Novahistine Elixir	Chlorpheniramine maleate 2 mg/5 ml	Phenylephrine HCl 5 mg/5 ml				Alcohol 5%	OTC
Novahistine DH	Chlorpheniramine maleate 2 mg/5 ml	Pseudoephedrine HCl 30 mg/5 ml		Codeine 10 mg/5 ml		Alcohol 5%	
Novahistine DMX		Pseudoephedrine HCl 30 mg/5 ml		Dextromethorphan 10 mg/5 ml	Guaifenesin 100 mg/5 ml	Alcohol 10%	OTC
Novahistine Expectorant		Pseudoephedrine HCl 30 mg/5 ml		Codeine 10 mg/5 ml	Guaifenesin 100 mg/5 ml	Alcohol 7.5%	
Phenergan VC	Promethazine HCl 6.25 mg/5 ml	Phenylephrine HCl 5 mg/5 ml				Alcohol 7%	
Phenergan VC with codeine	Promethazine HCl 6.25 mg/5 ml	Phenylephrine HCl 5 mg/5 ml		Codeine 10 mg/5 ml		Alcohol 7%	
Robitussin A-C				Codeine 10 mg/5 ml	Guaifenesin 100 mg/5 ml	Alcohol 3.5%	
Robitussin CF		Phenylpropanolamine HCl 12.5 mg/5 ml		Dextromethorphan 10 mg/5 ml	Same as Robitussin A-C	Alcohol 4.75%	OTC
Robitussin DAC		Pseudoephedrine HCl 30 mg/5 ml		Codeine 10 mg/5 ml	Same as Robitussin A-C	Alcohol 1.4%	
Robitussin DM				Dextromethorphan 15 mg/5 ml	Same as Robitussin A-C	Alcohol 1.4%	OTC
Robitussin PE		Pseudoephedrine HCl 30 mg/5 ml			Same as Robitussin AC	Alcohol 1.4%	OTC
Sine-Off	Chlorpheniramine maleate 2 mg/tab	Phenylpropanolamine HCl 12.5 mg/tab	Aspirin 325 mg/tab				OTC
Sinutab	Chlorpheniramine maleate 2 mg/tab	Pseudoephedrine HCl 30 mg/tab	Acetaminophen 325 mg/tab				OTC
Sinutab II		Pseudoephedrine HCl 30 mg/tab or cap	Acetaminophen 500 mg/tab or cap				OTC

* OTC indicates nonprescription products.

nation products may contain unneeded or ineffective components as well as less than optimum dosages of individual ingredients.

2. Most nasal decongestants are applied topically as nasal solutions or sprays. These are rapidly effective because they come into direct contact with nasal mucosa. If used longer than 10 days or in excessive amounts, these products may produce rebound nasal congestion. Therefore, topical preparations are usually preferred for short-term use. For long-term use (more than 10 days), oral drugs are preferred. Phenylephrine (Neo-Synephrine), phenylpropanolamine, and pseudoephedrine (Sudafed) are commonly used nasal decongestants, in both prescription and over-the-counter products.

   For clients with cardiovascular disease, topical nasal decongestants are preferred. Oral agents are generally contraindicated because of cardiovascular effects (*e.g.*, increased force of myocardial contraction, increased heart rate, and increased blood pressure).

   In children, especially infants, the imidazole derivatives should not be used. If absorbed systemically, these drugs may cause central nervous system (CNS) depression with resultant coma and hypothermia. Imidazole derivatives are naphazoline (Privine), oxymetazoline (Afrin), and tetrahydrozoline (Tyzine).

3. Most antitussives are given orally as tablets or "cough syrups." Syrups serve as vehicles for antitussive drugs and may exert antitussive effects of their own by soothing irritated pharyngeal mucosa.

   Narcotic antitussives are Schedule II agents under the Controlled Substances Act. Strong narcotic agents (*e.g.*, morphine, hydromorphone) should be used as antitussives only in severe, painful cough that cannot be controlled by milder narcotics (*e.g.*, codeine, hydrocodone) or nonnarcotic antitussives.

   Dextromethorphan (Romilar) is probably the antitussive drug of choice in most circumstances. Compared to codeine, dextromethorphan is similarly effective without the disadvantages of a narcotic preparation. Dextromethorphan has no analgesic effect, does not produce tolerance or dependence, and does not depress respiration. Further, dextromethorphan is the only nonnarcotic antitussive whose efficacy has been demonstrated by extensive research studies.

4. If a combination product is used, the ingredients should be effective and indicated for the symptoms being treated. Ingredients should also be present in therapeutic dosages. For nasal congestion accompanying the common cold and allergic rhinitis, probably the most rational combination products are those containing an adrenergic nasal decongestant and an antihistamine. However, these agents may cause excessive drying of respiratory tract secretions and make them more difficult to expectorate.

5. For treatment of excessive respiratory tract secretions, mechanical measures (*e.g.*, coughing, deep breathing, ambulation, chest physiotherapy, forcing fluids) are more likely to be effective than expectorant drug therapy.

NURSING ACTIONS: NASAL DECONGESTANTS, ANTITUSSIVES, AND COLD REMEDIES

Nursing Actions	*Rationale/Explanation*
1. Administer accurately	
a. With topical nasal decongestants	
(1) Use only preparations labeled for intranasal use.	Intranasal preparations are usually dilute, aqueous solutions prepared specifically for intranasal use. Some agents (*e.g.*, phenylephrine) are available in ophthalmic solutions as well. The two types of solutions cannot be used interchangeably.
(2) Use the drug concentration ordered.	Some drug preparations are available in several concentrations. For example, phenylephrine preparations may contain 0.125%, 0.25%, 0.5%, or 1% of drug.
(3) For instillation of nose drops, have the client lie down or sit with the neck hyperextended. Instill medication without touching the dropper to the nares. Rinse the medication dropper after each use.	To avoid contamination of the dropper and medication

Nursing Actions	***Rationale/Explanation***
(4) For nasal sprays, have the client sit, squeeze the container once to instill medication, avoid touching the spray tip to the nares, and rinse the spray tip after each use.	Most nasal sprays are designed to deliver one dose when used correctly. If necessary, secretions may be cleared and a second spray used. Correct usage and cleansing prevents contamination and infection.
(5) Give nasal decongestants to infants 20 to 30 minutes before feeding.	Nasal congestion interferes with an infant's ability to suck.
b. With cough syrups, administer them undiluted and instruct the client to avoid eating and drinking for about 30 minutes.	Part of the therapeutic benefit of cough syrups stems from soothing effects on pharyngeal mucosa. Food or fluid removes the medication from the pharynx.
c. Instruct clients to swallow benzonatate perles without chewing.	If perles are chewed, local anesthetic effects numb oral mucosa.
2. Observe for therapeutic effects	Therapeutic effects depend on the reason for use.
a. When nasal decongestants are given, observe for decreased nasal obstruction and drainage.	
b. With antitussives, observe for decreased coughing.	The goal of antitussive therapy is to suppress nonpurposeful coughing, not productive coughing.
c. With cold and allergy remedies, observe for decreased nasal congestion, rhinitis, muscle aches, and other symptoms.	
3. Observe for adverse effects	
a. With nasal decongestants, observe for	
(1) Tachycardia, cardiac arrhythmias, hypertension	These effects may occur with any of the adrenergic drugs (see Chap. 18). When adrenergic drugs are used as nasal decongestants, cardiovascular effects are more likely to occur with oral agents. However, topically applied drugs may also be systemically absorbed through the nasal mucosa or by being swallowed and absorbed through the gastrointestinal tract.
(2) Rebound nasal congestion, chronic rhinitis and possible ulceration of nasal mucosa	Adverse effects on nasal mucosa are more likely to occur with excessive or long-term (more than 10 days) use.
b. With antitussives, observe for	
(1) Excessive suppression of the cough reflex (inability to cough effectively when secretions are present)	This is a potentially serious adverse effect because retained secretions may lead to atelectasis, pneumonia, hypoxia, hypercarbia, and respiratory failure.
(2) Nausea, vomiting, constipation, dizziness, drowsiness, pruritus, and drug dependence	These are adverse effects associated with narcotic agents (see Chap. 5). When narcotics are given for antitussive effects, however, they are given in relatively small doses and are unlikely to cause adverse reactions.
(3) Nausea, drowsiness and dizziness with nonnarcotic antitussives.	Adverse effects are infrequent and mild with these agents.
c. With combination products (*e.g.,* cold remedies), observe for adverse effects of individual ingredients (*i.e.,* antihistamines, adrenergics, analgesics, and others)	Adverse effects are rarely significant when the products are used as prescribed. There may be subtherapeutic doses of one or more component drugs, especially in over-the-counter formulations. Also, the drowsiness associated with antihistamines may be offset by stimulating effects of adrenergics. Ephedrine, for example, has CNS-stimulating effects.
4. Observe for drug interactions	
a. Drugs that *increase* effects of nasal decongestants	These interactions are more likely to occur with oral decongestants than topically applied drugs.
(1) Cocaine, digitalis, general anesthetics, monoamine oxidase (MAO) inhibitors, other adrenergic drugs, thyroid preparations, and xanthines	Increased risks of cardiac arrhythmias

Nursing Actions	Rationale/Explanation
(2) Antihistamines, epinephrine, ergot alkaloids, MAO inhibitors, methylphenidate	Increased risks of hypertension due to vasoconstriction
b. Drugs that *increase* antitussive effects of codeine CNS depressants (alcohol, antianxiety agents, barbiturates, and other sedative–hypnotics)	Additive CNS depression. Codeine is given in small doses for antitussive effects, and risks of significant interactions are minimal.
c. Drugs that alter effects of dextromethorphan MAO inhibitors	This combination is contraindicated. Apnea, muscular rigidity, hyperpyrexia, laryngospasm, and death may occur.
d. Drugs that may alter effects of combination products for coughs, colds, and allergies. (1) Adrenergic (sympathomimetic) agents (see Chap. 18) (2) Antihistamines (see Chap. 48) (3) CNS depressants (see Chaps. 5, 7, 8, 13) (4) CNS stimulants (see Chap. 16)	Interactions depend on the individual drug components of each formulation. Risks of clinically significant drug interactions are increased with usage of combination products.
5. Teach clients	
a. Do not use nose drops more often than recommended or for longer than 10 consecutive days.	Excessive or prolonged use may damage nasal mucosa and produce chronic nasal congestion.
b. Blow the nose gently before instilling nasal solutions or sprays.	To clear nasal passages and increase effectiveness of medications
c. Do not touch the dropper tip to the nostrils when instilling nasal solutions.	To prevent contamination of the solution
d. Rinse the dropper or spray tip after each use.	To prevent bacterial contamination of the medication
e. Report palpitations, dizziness, drowsiness, rapid pulse.	These effects may occur with nasal decongestants and "cold remedies" and may indicate excessive dosage.
f. Consult a physician or pharmacist before taking over-the-counter cold, cough, and allergy medications.	Many products are available, with different amounts of ingredients. Consultation can assist in choosing the most appropriate product.

Selected References

American Medical Association (AMA) Division of Drugs: AMA Drug Evaluations, 5th ed. New York, John Wiley & Sons, 1983

Anderson PD: Basic Human Anatomy and Physiology: Clinical Implications for the Health Professions. Monterey, CA, Wadsworth, 1984

Culbertson VC, Burton BA: Symptoms of "cold" and allergy. In Wiener MB, Pepper GA (eds): Clinical Pharmacology and Therapeutics in Nursing, 2d ed, pp 282–298. New York, McGraw-Hill, 1985

Facts and Comparisons. St. Louis, J B Lippincott (Updated monthly)

Guyton AC: Textbook of Medical Physiology, 7th ed. Philadelphia, W B Saunders, 1986

Hansten PD: Drug Interactions: Clinical Significance of Drug–Drug Interactions, 5th ed. Philadelphia, Lea & Febiger, 1985

Rodman MJ, Karch AM, Boyd EH, Smith DW: Pharmacology and Drug Therapy in Nursing, 3rd ed. Philadelphia, J B Lippincott, 1985

VIII

DRUGS AFFECTING THE CARDIOVASCULAR SYSTEM

50

PHYSIOLOGY OF THE CARDIOVASCULAR SYSTEM

The cardiovascular or circulatory system is composed of the heart, blood vessels, and blood. The general functions of the system are to carry oxygen, nutrients, hormones, and antibodies to all body cells and to remove waste products of cell metabolism (CO_2 and others). Efficiency of the system depends on the heart's ability to pump blood, the patency of blood vessels, and the quality and quantity of blood.

Heart

The heart is a hollow, muscular organ that functions as a double pump to circulate 5 to 6 liters of blood through the body every minute.

1. The heart has four chambers: two atria and two ventricles. The *atria* are receiving chambers. The right atrium receives deoxygenated blood from the upper part of the body by way of the superior vena cava, from the lower part of the body by way of the inferior vena cava, and from veins and sinuses within the heart itself. The left atrium receives oxygenated blood from the lungs through the pulmonary veins. The *ventricles* are distributing chambers. The right ventricle sends deoxygenated blood through the pulmonary circulation. It is small and thin walled because it contracts against minimal pressure. The left ventricle pumps oxygenated blood through the systemic circuit. It is much more muscular and thick walled because it contracts against relatively high pressure. The right atrium and right ventricle form one pump, and the left atrium and left ventricle form another. The right and left sides of the heart are separated by a strip of muscle called the *septum.*
2. The layers of the heart are the endocardium, myocardium, and epicardium. The *endocardium* is the membrane lining the heart chambers. It is continuous with the lining of blood vessels entering and leaving the heart and covers the heart valves. The *myocardium* is the strong muscular layer of the heart that provides the pumping power of the circulation. The *epicardium* is the outer, serous layer of the heart. The heart is enclosed in a fibroserous sac called the *pericardium.*
3. Heart valves function to guide the one-way flow of blood and prevent backflow. The *mitral* valve separates the left atrium and left ventricle. The *tricuspid* valve separates the right atrium and right ventricle. The *pulmonic* valve separates the right ventricle and pulmonary artery. The *aortic* valve separates the left ventricle and aorta.
4. The heart contains special cells that are able to carry electrical impulses much more rapidly than ordinary muscle fibers. This special conduction system consists of the sinoatrial (SA) node, the atrioventricular (AV) node, bundle of His, right and

left bundle branches, and Purkinje fibers. The SA node is the normal pacemaker of the heart. It can be compared to a battery. It originates a burst of electrical energy approximately 70 to 80 times each minute under normal circumstances. The electrical current flows over the heart in an orderly way to produce contraction of both atria, then both ventricles.

A unique characteristic of the heart is that each part can generate its own electrical impulse to contract. For example, the ventricles can beat independently but at a rate of only 30 to 40 beats per minute. In addition, the heart does not require nervous stimulation to contract. However, the autonomic nervous system does influence heart rate. Sympathetic nerves increase heart rate; parasympathetic nerves (by way of the vagus nerve) decrease heart rate.

5. The heart receives its blood supply from the coronary arteries. Coronary arteries branch off the aorta and fill during *diastole,* the resting or filling phase of the cardiac cycle. Coronary arteries branch into "end-arteries," which supply certain parts of the myocardium without an overlapping supply from other branches. However, there are many artery-to-artery anastomoses between adjacent vessels. The anastomotic arteries do not supply sufficient blood to the heart if a major artery is suddenly occluded. However, they may dilate into arteries of considerable size when disease (usually coronary atherosclerosis) develops slowly. The resultant *collateral circulation* may provide sufficient blood for myocardial function, at least during rest.

Blood vessels

The three types of blood vessels are arteries, veins, and capillaries. Arteries and veins are similar in that they have three layers. The *intima* is the smooth inner lining of endothelium. The *media* is the middle layer of muscle and elastic tissue. The *adventitia* is the outer layer of connective tissue.

1. *Arteries* and *arterioles* have a thick media and control peripheral vascular resistance. They are sometimes called "resistance" vessels. Their efficiency depends on patency and ability to constrict or dilate in response to various stimuli. The degree of constriction or dilation (vasomotor tone) determines peripheral vascular resistance, which is a major determinant of blood pressure.
2. *Veins* have a thin media and valves that assist blood flow against gravity. They are sometimes called "capacitance" vessels, since blood may accumulate in various parts of the venous system. Their efficiency depends on patency, competency of valves, and the pumping action of muscles around veins.
3. *Capillaries* are very thin-walled vessels. Exchange of gases, nutrients, and waste products occurs across capillary walls.
4. *Lymphatic vessels* parallel the veins and drain tissue fluids. They carry lymphocytes and large molecules of protein and fat. They empty into the venous system.

Blood

Blood generally functions to nourish and oxygenate all body cells, protect the body from invading microorganisms, and initiate hemostasis upon injury to a blood vessel. Specific functions and components include the following:

1. Functions
   a. Transports oxygen to cells and carbon dioxide from cells to lungs for removal from the body
   b. Carries absorbed food products from the gastrointestinal tract to tissues; at the same time, it carries metabolic wastes from tissues to the kidneys, skin, and lungs for excretion
   c. Carries hormones from endocrine glands to other parts of the body
   d. Carries leukocytes and antibodies to sites of injury, infection, and inflammation
   e. Helps regulate body temperature by transferring heat produced by cell metabolism to the skin, where it can be released
   f. Carries platelets to injured areas for hemostasis
2. Components
   a. Plasma composes approximately 55% of the total blood volume. Plasma is more than 90% water. Other ingredients are the following:
      (1) Serum albumin, which helps maintain blood volume by exerting colloid osmotic pressure
      (2) Fibrinogen, which is necessary for hemostasis
      (3) Gamma globulin, which is necessary for defense against microorganisms
      (4) Less than 1% antibodies, nutrients, metabolic wastes, respiratory gases, enzymes, and inorganic salts
   b. Solid particles compose approximately 45% of total blood volume. Solid particles are erythrocytes, also called red blood cells (RBCs); leu-

kocytes, also called white blood cells (WBCs); and thrombocytes, also called platelets. The bone marrow produces all RBCs, 60% to 70% of WBCs, and all platelets. Lymphatic tissues (spleen and lymph nodes) produce 20% to 30%, and reticuloendothelial tissues (spleen, liver, lymph nodes) produce 4% to 8%, of WBCs. Characteristics of solid particles include the following:

(1) Erythrocytes function mainly to transport oxygen. Almost all oxygen (95% to 97%) is transported in combination with hemoglobin; very little is dissolved in blood. The life span of a normal RBC is about 120 days.
(2) Leukocytes function mainly as a defense mechanism against microorganisms. They leave the bloodstream to enter injured tissues and phagocytize the injurious agent. They also produce antibodies. The life span of a normal WBC is a few hours.
(3) Platelets are fragments of large cells, called megakaryocytes, found in the red bone marrow. Platelets are essential to blood coagulation.

Drug therapy in cardiovascular disorders

Cardiovascular disorders are leading causes of morbidity and mortality. They may involve any structure or function of the cardiovascular system. Generally, a disorder in one part of the system eventually disturbs the function of all other parts. Cardiovascular disorders that are usually responsive to drug therapy include congestive heart failure, cardiac arrhythmias, angina pectoris, hypertension, hypotension, and shock. Disorders that are relatively unresponsive to drug therapy include atherosclerosis, peripheral vascular disease, and valvular disease. Blood disorders that respond to drug therapy include certain types of anemia and coagulation disorders.

Cardiovascular drugs may be given to increase or decrease cardiac output, blood pressure, and heart rate; to alter heart rhythm; to increase or decrease blood clotting; to alter the quality of blood; and to decrease chest pain of cardiac origin. Cardiovascular drugs are often given for palliation of symptoms. For example, in disorders caused or aggravated by atherosclerosis (*e.g.*, angina pectoris, hypertension, congestive heart failure), the drugs relieve symptoms but do not alter the underlying disease process.

Selected References

Anderson PD: Basic Human Anatomy and Physiology: Clinical Implications for the Health Professions. Monterey, CA, Wadsworth, 1984

Guyton AC: Textbook of Medical Physiology, 7th ed. Philadelphia, W B Saunders, 1986

Rodman MJ, Karch AM, Boyd EH, Smith DW: Pharmacology and Drug Therapy in Nursing, 3rd ed. Philadelphia, J B Lippincott, 1985

51

CARDIOTONIC–INOTROPIC AGENTS USED IN CONGESTIVE HEART FAILURE

Description and uses

Cardiotonic–inotropic agents increase the force of myocardial contraction and thereby improve the pumping ability of the heart. Drugs with cardiotonic–inotropic effects include adrenergics, digitalis glycosides, amrinone, and milrinone. Adrenergics (*e.g.*, epinephrine) also increase cardiac workload and oxygen consumption; they are discussed further in Chapter 18. Digitalis glycosides, amrinone, and milrinone are the focus of this chapter. The major clinical use of these agents is the treatment of congestive heart failure (CHF). To facilitate understanding of drug effects, characteristics and drug therapy of CHF are discussed.

CONGESTIVE HEART FAILURE

Congestive heart failure is a common condition that occurs when the heart is unable to pump enough blood to meet tissue needs for oxygen and nutrients. Most CHF is caused by hypertension, coronary artery disease, or valvular disorders. Other causative factors include hyperthyroidism, excessive intravenous fluids or blood transfusions, and drugs that decrease the force of myocardial contraction (*e.g.*, beta-adrenergic blocking agents) or cause retention of sodium and water (*e.g.*, corticosteroids, estrogens, nonsteroidal anti-inflammatory agents). These factors impair the pumping ability or increase the workload of the heart so that an adequate cardiac output cannot be maintained. When cardiac output falls, a number of compensatory mechanisms occur in the body's attempt to maintain blood flow to tissues. One mechanism is increased sympathetic activity, which increases the force of myocardial contraction, increases heart rate, and causes vasoconstriction. Another mechanism involves increased volume of blood and increased pressure within the heart chambers, which stretches muscle fibers and results in ventricular hypertrophy. A third mechanism is activation of the renin-angiotensin-aldosterone system. Renin is an enzyme produced in the kidney. When released into the bloodstream, it stimulates the production of angiotensin II, a powerful vasoconstrictor. Increased production of aldosterone by the adrenal cortex is also stimulated, and aldosterone increases reabsorption of sodium and water in renal tubules.

As a result of these compensatory mechanisms, there is increased preload (amount of venous blood returning to the heart), increased workload of the heart, and increased afterload (amount of resistance in the aorta and peripheral blood vessels that the heart must overcome to pump effectively). All these mechanisms act to increase blood pressure. Although initially effective, the compensatory mechanisms themselves increase the workload of the heart, and they are limited in extent and duration of action. Eventually, signs and symptoms of CHF occur when, despite these compensatory mechanisms, an adequate cardiac output can no longer be maintained and failure or decompensation occurs.

Drug therapy of CHF is aimed toward altering the compensatory mechanisms. In addition to cardiotonic–inotropic agents, diuretics, vasodilators, and angiotensin-converting enzyme inhibitors are used.

Diuretics. Diuretics are often used in the treatment of CHF. They act to decrease plasma volume (extracellular fluid volume) and increase excretion of sodium and water, thereby decreasing preload. Intravenous furosemide (Lasix) also has a vasodilatory effect that helps to relieve vasoconstriction (afterload) in acute CHF (pulmonary edema). Diuretics are discussed in greater detail in Chapter 56.

Vasodilators. Although vasodilator drugs have long been used for other therapeutic purposes, their use in CHF is relatively recent. Venous dilators (*e.g.*, nitroglycerin and other nitrates) act to decrease preload; arterial dilators (*e.g.*, hydralazine [Apresoline]) decrease afterload; and prazosin (Minipress) dilates both veins and arteries to decrease both preload and afterload. Nitrates are discussed in Chapter 53; other vasodilators are discussed primarily in Chapter 55.

Angiotensin-converting enzyme inhibitors. Captopril (Capoten) and enalapril (Vasotec) are enzyme inhibitors that prevent the pharmacologically inactive angiotensin I from being converted to the powerful vasoconstrictor, angiotensin II. Although the mechanism of action differs, the overall effect of these agents is that of vasodilation. Captopril is approved for the treatment of hypertension and CHF. Enalapril is currently approved for hypertension.

DIGITALIS GLYCOSIDES

Digitalis glycosides are among the most frequently prescribed drugs. They are derived from various species of the foxglove plant (*Digitalis purpurea* and *Digitalis lanata*). (Glycosides are substances derived from plants that yield a sugar and one or more other products when hydrolyzed.) In CHF, the drugs exert a cardiotonic or positive inotropic effect. Increased myocardial contractility allows the ventricles to empty more completely with each heart beat. With improved cardiac output, heart size, heart rate, end-systolic and end-diastolic pressures, vasoconstriction, sympathetic nerve stimulation, and venous congestion decrease. The mechanism by which digitalis increases the force of myocardial contraction is not completely clear. One explanation is that the drug inhibits Na,K-ATPase, an enzyme that decreases movement of sodium out of myocardial cells after contraction has occurred. This results in an increased intracellular concentration of sodium. The sodium displaces bound calcium, thereby increasing the intracellular concentration of free calcium ions. The calcium then enhances the excitation–contraction coupling of the contractile proteins, actin and myosin, of myocardial cells.

Another clinical use of digitalis preparations is in the management of atrial arrhythmias (*e.g.*, atrial fibrillation, atrial flutter). Atrial arrhythmias are disturbances of the cardiac conduction system in which atrial muscle tissue functions as pacemaker rather than the sinoatrial (SA) node. The abnormal pacemaker usually initiates and transmits electrical impulses to the ventricles at a rapid rate. The resulting ventricular tachycardia increases cardiac workload. If tachycardia is severe or prolonged, diastole is shortened, and heart chambers do not have adequate filling time. This causes reduced cardiac output, impaired circulation, and inadequate blood flow to tissues. In atrial arrhythmias, digitalis acts to slow the rate of ventricular contraction (negative chronotropic effect). Negative chronotropic effects are probably caused by several factors. First, digitalis has a direct depressant effect on cardiac conduction tissues, especially the atrioventricular (AV) node. This action decreases the number of electrical impulses allowed to reach the ventricles from supraventricular sources. Second, digitalis indirectly stimulates the vagus nerve. Third, increased efficiency of myocardial contraction and vagal stimulation both act to decrease compensatory tachycardia resulting from the sympathetic nervous system response to inadequate circulation.

Digitalis glycosides are distributed to most body tissues, including red blood cells, skeletal muscle, and the heart. To achieve therapeutic effects, cardiac tissue must maintain an adequate concentration of digitalis. Maximum drug effect is exerted when a steady-state tissue concentration has been achieved. This occurs in about five drug half-lives when "loading doses" are not given (approximately 1 week for digoxin, 1 month for digitoxin). If more rapid drug effects are required by the client's condition, a "loading dose" may be given.

Traditionally, a loading dose is called a "digitalizing" dose. Digitalization (administration of an amount sufficient to produce therapeutic effects) may be accomplished rapidly by giving approximately 0.75 to 1 mg of digoxin over a 24-hour period. Since rapid digitalization engenders higher risks of toxicity, the current trend is slow digitalization in nonemergency situations. Slow digitalization may be accomplished by initiating digitalis therapy with a maintenance dose.

Digitalis has a low therapeutic index; that is, a dose adequate for therapeutic effect may be accompanied by signs of toxicity. Digitalis intoxication or toxicity may result from many contributing factors, such as the following:

1. Accumulation of larger than necessary maintenance doses
2. Rapid loading or digitalization, whether by one or more large doses or frequent administration of small doses
3. Impaired liver or renal function, which prolongs drug metabolism and excretion
4. Age extremes (young or old)
5. Electrolyte imbalance (*e.g.*, hypokalemia, hypomagnesemia, hypercalcemia)
6. Hypoxia, whether resulting from heart or lung disease, which increases myocardial sensitivity to digitalis
7. Hypothyroidism, which slows metabolism and causes drug accumulation
8. Concurrent treatment with other drugs affecting the heart, such as quinidine, verapamil, or nifedipine

All digitalis glycosides have the same pharmacologic actions (*i.e.*, therapeutic and adverse effects). However, digitalis preparations used clinically vary in potency, rate of absorption, onset of action, and rate of elimination.

Individual cardiotonic/inotropic agents

DIGITALIS PREPARATIONS

Commonly used preparations

Digoxin (Lanoxin) is the most prescribed digitalis preparation in the United States. The drug is a purified cardiac glycoside of the *D. lanata* plant. Digoxin is used in the treatment of CHF and atrial tachyarrhythmias. Digoxin is a versatile drug that may be used in acute or chronic conditions, for digitalization, or for maintenance therapy. It can be given by oral or parenteral routes. Specific characteristics of digoxin include the following:

1. Digoxin has a rapid onset of action. When given intravenously, onset of action occurs within 10 to 30 minutes and maximal effects occur in $1\frac{1}{2}$ to 3 hours. This rapid onset of action allows digoxin to be used in emergency situations when rapid digitalization is desired. When given orally, onset of action occurs in $1\frac{1}{2}$ to 6 hours and maximal effects occur in 4 to 6 hours.
2. Digoxin has a relatively short duration of action, with a serum half-life of 1 to 2 days. When digoxin therapy is initiated with maintenance doses, therapeutic serum levels and maximal drug benefit are achieved in approximately 1 week. When digoxin is discontinued, the drug is eliminated from the body in approximately 1 week. This characteristic is advantageous in titrating dosage to achieve optimal therapeutic effects without toxicity. In addition, if toxicity does occur, toxic effects are not prolonged.
3. Absorption of oral digoxin preparations is influenced by several factors, as follows:
   a. The most efficiently absorbed oral digoxin preparations are the liquid-filled capsules (Lanoxicaps) and the elixir used for children. Lanoxicaps are reportedly close to intravenous digoxin in bioavailability. Capsules containing 0.1 mg are equivalent to 0.125-mg tablets, and 0.2-mg capsules are equivalent to 0.25-mg tablets. The elixir dosage form is approximately 90% absorbed.
   b. Digoxin tablets vary in rate of absorption from 40% to 75%. Differences in bioavailability may be a significant clinical problem because a person may be stabilized on a particular brand of digoxin but underdosed or overdosed if another brand is taken. Differences are attributed to rate and extent of tablet dissolution rather than amounts of digoxin.
   c. Digoxin absorption is delayed or decreased by the presence of food in the gastrointestinal tract, by delayed gastric emptying, by malabsorption syndromes, and by concurrent administration of some drugs (*e.g.*, antacids, cholestyramine, colestipol).
4. Digoxin is excreted unchanged by the kidneys. Dosage must be reduced in the presence of renal failure to prevent drug accumulation and toxicity.
5. Therapeutic serum levels of digoxin are 0.5 to 2 ng/ml; toxic serum levels are those above 2 ng/ml. However, toxicity may occur at virtually any serum level.

6. The preferred routes of administration for digoxin are oral and intravenous. Although the parenteral solution can be given intramuscularly, this route may cause severe pain and muscle necrosis at the site of injection.
7. Available preparations of digoxin include *tablets* containing 0.125 mg, 0.25 mg, or 0.5 mg; *capsules* (Lanoxicaps) containing 0.05 mg, 0.1 mg or 0.2 mg; *solutions for injection* containing 0.1 mg/ml in a 1-ml ampule or 0.25 mg/ml in a 2-ml ampule; and a *pediatric elixir* containing 0.05 mg/ml.

Routes and dosage ranges

Adults: Digitalizing dose, PO 1–1.5 mg in divided doses over 24 hours; IV 0.5–1 mg in divided doses over 24 hours
Maintenance dose, PO, IV 0.125–0.5 mg daily

Children over 10 years: Same as adults

Children 2–10 years: Digitalizing dose, PO 0.02–0.04 mg/kg in 4 divided doses q6h; IV 0.015–0.035 mg/kg in 4 divided doses q6h
Maintenance dose, PO, IV approximately 20%–35% of the digitalizing dose

Children 1 month–2 years: Digitalizing dose, PO 0.035–0.06 mg/kg in 4 divided doses q6h; IV 0.035–0.05 mg/kg in 4 divided doses q6h
Maintenance dose, PO, IV approximately 20%–35% of the digitalizing dose

Newborns: Digitalizing dose, PO 0.025–0.035 mg/kg in 4 divided doses q6h; IV 0.02–0.03 mg/kg in 4 divided doses q6h
Maintenance dose, PO, IV approximately 20%–35% of the digitalizing dose

Digitoxin (Crystodigin, Purodigin) is the second most prescribed digitalis preparation. It is the most cardioactive glycoside of the *D. purpurea* plant. Digitoxin has the slowest onset of action, the longest interval to reach peak action time, and the longest half-life of all digitalis glycosides. Consequently, it is more often used for maintenance therapy than for rapid digitalization. Compared to digoxin, digitoxin has the following characteristics:

1. Digitoxin has a slower onset of action. When given intravenously, onset of action occurs in 30 to 120 minutes with maximal effects in 4 to 8 hours. When given orally, onset of action occurs in 3 to 6 hours with maximal effects in 8 to 12 hours.
2. Digitoxin has a longer duration of action and a half-life of 7 days. If digitoxin therapy is initiated with maintenance doses, therapeutic serum levels and maximal effects do not occur for approximately 1 month. This delay may be somewhat minimized by initiating therapy with loading doses. When digitoxin is discontinued, approximately 1 month is required for elimination of the drug from the body. The longer duration of action may be an advantage for clients who are unable or unwilling to take digitoxin daily because therapeutic effects persist for several days after a dose. However, if toxicity occurs, the delay in drug elimination prolongs toxic effects.
3. Digitoxin tablets are well absorbed from the intestinal tract (90% to 100%), and bioavailability has not been a problem. However, absorption is delayed or decreased by the presence of food in the gastrointestinal tract, by delayed gastric emptying, and by malabsorption syndromes.
4. Digitoxin is metabolized in the liver, excreted in bile, reabsorbed from the gastrointestinal tract, and eventually excreted in the urine as inactive metabolites. For this reason, digitoxin may be the digitalis preparation of choice in clients with renal failure.
5. Therapeutic serum levels of digitoxin are 10–35 ng/ml. Toxic serum levels are those above 35 ng/ml.
6. The oral route of administration is preferred.
7. Available preparations of digitoxin are *tablets* containing 0.05 mg, 0.1 mg, 0.15 mg, or 0.2 mg and a *solution for injection* containing 0.2 mg/ml.

Routes and dosage ranges

Adults: Digitalizing dose, PO, IV 0.8–1.2 mg in divided doses over 24 hours
Maintenance dose, PO, IV 0.05–0.2 mg daily (average, 0.1 mg)

Children over 12 years: Same as adults

Children 2–12 years: Digitalizing dose, PO, IV, IM 0.02–0.03 mg/kg in 3–4 divided doses q4–6h
Maintenance dose, PO, IV, IM approximately 10% of the digitalizing dose

Children 2 weeks–2 years: Digitalizing dose PO, IV, IM 0.04 mg/kg in 3–4 divided doses q4–6h
Maintenance dose, PO, IV, IM approximately 10% of the digitalizing dose

Newborns: Digitalizing dose, PO, IV, IM 0.022 mg/kg in 3–4 divided doses q4–6h
Maintenance dose, PO, IV, IM approximately 10% of the digitalizing dose

Rarely used preparations

Digitalis leaf (Digifortis) is obtained from dried leaves of the *D. purpurea* plant. The preparation contains three cardioactive glycosides. These are digitoxin, which exerts most pharmacologic action, gitalin, and gitoxin.

Routes and dosage ranges

Adults: Digitalizing dose, PO 1.2–1.8 g, in divided doses over 24 hours
Maintenance dose, PO 100–200 mg daily

Deslanoside (Cedilanid D) is derived from the *D. lanata* plant. It is occasionally used for rapid digitalization (onset of action, 10 to 30 minutes; maximal effects, 2 to 3 hours) but offers no advantage over digoxin. If used, another digitalis glycoside must be used for maintenance therapy, since no oral dosage form is available.

Routes and dosage ranges

Adults: Digitalizing dose IM, IV 0.8–1.6 mg in divided doses over 24 hours

AMRINONE AND MILRINONE

Amrinone (Inocor) is a newer cardiotonic–inotropic agent used in short-term management of CHF that is not controlled by digitalis and diuretic therapy. Its inotropic effects are attributed to increased levels of cyclic adenosine monophosphate (cyclic AMP) or calcium in myocardial cells. Amrinone also relaxes vascular smooth muscle to produce vasodilation and decrease preload and afterload. In CHF, amrinone increases cardiac output by both inotropic and vasodilator effects. Amrinone is usually given as an intravenous bolus followed by a continuous infusion.

Milrinone is an analog of amrinone with similar actions and effects. Although not yet released for general use, studies indicate that milrinone is more potent than amrinone and that it can be given orally.

Route and dosage range

Amrinone

Adults: IV injection (loading dose), 0.75 mg/kg slowly, over 2 to 3 minutes
IV infusion (maintenance dose), 5 to 10 μg/kg/minute, diluted in 0.9% or 0.45% NaCl solution to a concentration of 1 mg/ml–3 mg/ml. The maximal recommended dosage is 10 mg/kg/day.

Principles of therapy: cardiotonic–inotropic agents

ASSESSMENT GUIDELINES

1. Assess the client's condition for current or potential CHF.
   a. Identify risk factors for CHF:
      (1) Cardiovascular disorders—atherosclerosis, hypertension, coronary artery disease, myocardial infarction, cardiac arrhythmias, cardiac valvular disease. Hypertension is one of the most frequent causes of CHF, especially if longstanding and inadequately treated.
      (2) Noncardiovascular disorders—severe infections, hyperthyroidism, pulmonary disease (*e.g.,* cor pulmonale—right-sided heart failure resulting from lung disease)
      (3) Other factors—excessive amounts of intravenous fluids, rapid infusion of intravenous fluids or blood transfusions, advanced age
      (4) A combination of any of the above factors
   b. Interview and observe for signs and symptoms of chronic CHF. Within the clinical syndrome of CHF, clinical manifestations vary from few and mild to many and severe, depending on the pumping ability of the heart. Specific signs and symptoms include the following:
      (1) Common signs and symptoms of mild CHF are ankle edema, dyspnea on exertion, and easy fatigue with exercise. Edema results from increased venous pressure, which allows fluids to leak into tissues; dyspnea and fatigue result from tissue hypoxia.
      (2) With moderate or severe CHF, more extensive edema, dyspnea, and fatigue at rest are likely to occur. Additional signs and symptoms include orthopnea, postnocturnal dyspnea, and cough (from congestion of the respiratory tract with venous blood); mental confusion (from cerebral hypoxia); oliguria and decreased renal function (from decreased blood flow to the kidneys); and anxiety.
   c. Observe for signs and symptoms of acute heart failure. Acute pulmonary edema indicates acute heart failure and is a medical emergency. Causes include acute myocardial infarction, cardiac arrhythmias, severe hypertension, acute fluid or salt overload, and certain drugs (*e.g.,* quinidine and other cardiac depressants, guanethidine, propranolol and other antiadrenergics, and phenylephrine, norepinephrine and other alpha-adrenergic stimulants).

      Pulmonary edema occurs when left ventricular failure causes blood to accumulate in pulmonary veins and tissues. As a result, the person experiences severe dyspnea, hypoxia, hypertension, tachycardia, hemoptysis, frothy respiratory tract secretions, and anxiety.

2. With digitalis preparations, observe for signs and symptoms of atrial arrhythmias.
   a. Record the rate and rhythm of apical and radial pulses. Atrial fibrillation, the most common atrial arrhythmia, is characterized by tachycardia, pulse deficit (faster apical rate than radial rate), and a very irregular rhythm. Fatigue, dizziness, and fainting may occur.
   b. Check the electrocardiogram for abnormal P waves, rapid rate of ventricular contraction, and QRS complexes of normal configuration but irregular intervals.

PREVENTIVE NURSING INTERVENTIONS

Use measures to prevent or minimize CHF and atrial arrhythmias. In the broadest sense, preventive measures include sensible eating habits (a balanced diet, avoiding excess saturated fat and salt, weight control), avoiding cigarette smoking, and regular exercise. In the client at risk for developing CHF and arrhythmias, preventive measures include the following:

1. Treatment of hypertension
2. Avoidance of hypoxia
3. Weight control
4. Avoidance of excess sodium in the diet
5. Avoidance of fluid overload, especially in elderly clients
6. Maintenance of treatment programs for CHF, atrial arrhythmias, and other cardiovascular or noncardiovascular disorders

TREATMENT OF CONGESTIVE HEART FAILURE

The main treatment measures for CHF consist of drug therapy and diet therapy.

1. Traditional drug therapy for CHF involves a digitalis preparation and, frequently, a diuretic. This regimen is usually effective in relieving the fatigue, dyspnea, edema, and other signs and symptoms of CHF. During the past several years, because of the high incidence of adverse drug effects, greater understanding of the basic pathophysiology of CHF, and the development of new drugs or new uses for older drugs, many previous assumptions and practices are being challenged. As a result, drug therapy for CHF is somewhat controversial in relation to choice of drug and duration of administration. Some opinions include the following:
   a. Some authorities continue to recommend digitalis alone or in combination with a diuretic for initial treatment. Vasodilators and other drugs are added only if signs and symptoms persist or recur despite treatment.
   b. Some authorities suggest that digitalis is indicated when CHF is accompanied by atrial tachyarrhythmias (to slow ventricular response and decrease the workload of the heart), but it may not be needed with normal sinus rhythm. These physicians may use a diuretic as the initial drug of choice, with digitalis as a second choice if needed or even as a third choice drug, after a vasodilator.
   c. Another challenge to traditional therapy is whether digitalis should be continued throughout life or whether it can be safely stopped. Some studies indicate that digitalis can be discontinued in some clients without recurrence of heart failure. However, no clear-cut criteria exist for selecting these clients.
   d. At present, amrinone is indicated only for short-term treatment of CHF that does not respond to other measures. If milrinone is approved and satisfactory for oral administration, long-term administration may be feasible.
2. Dietary sodium restriction may reduce edema and allow a decrease in dosage of diuretics. For most clients, sodium restriction need not be severe. A common order is "no added salt." This may be accomplished by avoiding obviously salty food (*e.g.*, ham, potato chips, snack foods) and not adding salt during cooking or eating. The main source of sodium intake is probably table salt (a level teaspoonful contains 2300 mg of sodium).

GUIDELINES FOR DIGITALIS THERAPY

1. **Choice of digitalis preparation** and the route of administration depends primarily on the client's condition and the rapidity with which therapeutic effects are desired.
   a. Digoxin is the drug of choice in most situations because it can be used for rapid or slow digitalization, and, if toxicity occurs, it leaves the body within a few days. It is the most commonly used digitalis preparation for both adults and children.
   b. Digitoxin may be the drug of choice in clients with renal disease, since it is excreted primarily by the liver rather than by the kidneys.

c. Deslanoside may be given parenterally for rapid digitalization, but it offers no significant advantage over digoxin.
d. Preferred routes of digitalis administration are oral and intravenous. The intramuscular route is not recommended because pain and muscle necrosis may occur at intramuscular injection sites.

2. **Dosage of digitalis preparations** must be individualized. Dosage guidelines include the following:
   a. Digitalis dosages are usually stated as the average amounts needed for digitalization and maintenance therapy. These dosages must be interpreted with consideration of specific client characteristics. Digitalizing or loading doses are safe *only* for a short period, usually 24 hours. In addition, loading doses should be used cautiously in clients who have taken digitalis preparations within the previous 2 or 3 weeks. Maintenance doses, which are quite small in relation to digitalizing doses, may be safely used to initiate digitalis therapy and are always used for long-term digitalis therapy.
   b. Generally, larger doses are needed to slow the heart rate in atrial arrhythmias than to increase myocardial contractility in CHF.
   c. Smaller doses (loading and maintenance) should be given to clients who are elderly or who have hypothyroidism. Because metabolism and excretion of digitalis preparations are delayed in such people, the drugs may accumulate and cause toxicity if dosage is not reduced.

      Dosage should also be reduced in clients with hypokalemia, extensive myocardial damage, or cardiac conduction disorders. These conditions increase risks of digitalis-induced arrhythmias.
   d. Dosage can be titrated according to client response. In CHF, severity of symptoms, electrocardiograms, and serum drug concentrations are useful. In atrial fibrillation, dosage can be altered to produce the desired decrease in the ventricular rate of contraction. Optimal dosage is the lowest amount that relieves signs and symptoms of heart failure or alters heart rate and rhythm toward normal without producing toxicity.
   e. Intravenous dosage of digoxin should be 20% to 30% less than oral dosage.
   f. Dosage of digoxin must be significantly reduced in the presence of renal failure or when certain drugs are given concurrently.
      (1) With renal failure, digoxin dosage should be based on signs and symptoms of toxicity, creatinine clearance, and serum levels. Because digoxin is excreted renally, failure to reduce dosage in renal failure leads to drug accumulation in the body, with resultant toxicity.
      (2) When quinidine (an antiarrhythmic drug) or calcium channel blockers are given concurrently, they increase serum digoxin levels. As a result, digoxin may accumulate and cause toxicity.

3. **Maintenance therapy in the hospitalized client.** When clients are hospitalized, they may be unable to take a daily maintenance dose of digitalis at the scheduled time owing to diagnostic tests, certain treatment measures, or other valid reasons. As a general rule, the dose should be given later rather than omitted. If the client is having surgery, the nurse often must ask the physician whether the drug should be given on the day of surgery (*i.e.*, orally with a small amount of water or parenterally) and whether the drug should be reordered postoperatively. Many clients require continued digitalis therapy. However, if a dose is missed, probably no ill effects will occur, since pharmacologic actions of both digoxin and digitoxin persist longer than 24 hours.

4. **Electrolyte balance** must be monitored and maintained during digitalis therapy, particularly normal serum levels of potassium (3.5 to 5 mEq/liter), magnesium (1.5 to 2.5 mg/100 ml), and calcium (8.5 to 10 mg/100 ml). Hypokalemia and hypomagnesemia increase cardiac excitability and ectopic pacemaker activity, leading to arrhythmias; hypercalcemia enhances digitalis effects. These electrolyte abnormalities increase the risk of digitalis toxicity. Hypocalcemia increases excitability of nerve and muscle cell membranes and causes myocardial contraction to be weak (leading to a decrease in digitalis effect). The most common electrolyte abnormality is hypokalemia because potassium-losing diuretics are often given concurrently with digitalis preparations in the treatment of CHF. Supplemental potassium may be given to maintain normal serum levels.

5. **Identification and treatment of digitalis toxicity** require attention to several factors, including the following:
   a. A persistent difficulty in digitalis therapy is the similarity between the signs and symptoms of heart disease for which digitalis is given and the signs and symptoms of digitalis intoxication. Cardiac arrhythmias may indicate either

inadequate or excessive dosage of digitalis. (Toxicity is more likely to occur, however.) Serum drug levels and electrocardiograms may be helpful in verifying suspected toxicity.

b. When signs and symptoms of digitalis toxicity occur, digitalis should be discontinued, not just reduced in dosage. Most clients with mild or early toxicity recover completely within a few days after the drug is discontinued. If serious cardiac arrhythmias are present, more aggressive treatment measures may be indicated.

c. Drugs used to treat cardiac arrhythmias resulting from digitalis intoxication include potassium chloride, lidocaine, phenytoin (Dilantin), and atropine sulfate.

(1) Potassium chloride is a myocardial depressant that acts to decrease myocardial excitability. The dose depends on the severity of toxicity, serum potassium level, and client response. Potassium is contraindicated in renal failure and should be used with caution in the presence of cardiac conduction defects.

(2) Lidocaine, an antiarrhythmic–local anesthetic agent, is commonly used in the treatment of digitalis-induced arrhythmias. It acts to decrease myocardial irritability.

(3) Phenytoin is an anticonvulsant drug that may be effective in treating digitalis-induced arrhythmias. It is not clear whether phenytoin relieves arrhythmias by direct effects on the myocardium or by CNS-depressant effects.

(4) Atropine or isoproterenol may be used in the treatment of bradycardia or conduction defects. Other antiarrhythmic drugs may be used, but these are generally less effective in digitalis-induced arrhythmias than in arrhythmias due to other causes.

NURSING ACTIONS: CARDIOTONIC–INOTROPIC DRUGS

Nursing Actions	*Rationale/Explanation*
1. Administer accurately	
a. With digitalis preparations	
(1) Read the drug label and the physician's order very carefully when preparing a dose of any digitalis preparation.	Owing to name similarity, especially digoxin and digitoxin, special care must be taken to avoid giving one for the other, since dose and potency differ.
(2) Check the apical pulse before each dose. If the rate is below 60, omit the dose and notify the physician.	Bradycardia is an adverse effect.
(3) Have the same nurse give digitalis to the same clients when possible, since it is important to detect *changes* in rate and rhythm (see *Observe for therapeutic effects* and *Observe for adverse effects,* below)	
(4) Give oral digitalis preparations with food or after meals.	This may minimize gastric irritation and symptoms of anorexia, nausea, and vomiting. However, these symptoms probably arise from drug stimulation of chemoreceptors in the medulla rather than a direct irritant effect of the drug on the gastrointestinal tract.
(5) Inject intravenous digitalis preparations slowly (over at least 5 minutes).	Digoxin should be given slowly because the diluent, propylene glycol, has toxic effects on the cardiac conduction system if given too rapidly. Digoxin may be given undiluted or diluted with a fourfold or greater volume of sterile water for injection, 0.9% sodium chloride injection, or 5% dextrose injection. If diluted, use the solution immediately.
b. With amrinone	
(1) Give undiluted or diluted to a concentration of 1 mg/ml to 3 mg/ml	

Nursing Actions	Rationale/Explanation
(2) Dilute with 0.9% or 0.45% sodium chloride solution and use the diluted solution within 24 hours. Do not dilute with solutions containing dextrose.	Amrinone may be injected into intravenous tubing containing a dextrose solution because contact is brief. However, a chemical interaction occurs with prolonged contact.
(3) Give bolus injections into the tubing of an intravenous infusion, over 2 to 3 minutes	
(4) Administer maintenance infusions at a rate of 5 to 10 μg/kg/minute.	
2. Observe for therapeutic effects	
a. When the drugs are given in CHF, observe for	
(1) Fewer signs and symptoms of pulmonary congestion (dyspnea, orthopnea, cyanosis, cough, hemoptysis, rales, anxiety, restlessness)	The pulmonary symptoms that develop with CHF are a direct result of events initiated by inadequate cardiac output. The left side of the heart is unable to accommodate incoming blood flow from the lungs. The resulting back pressure in pulmonary veins and capillaries causes leakage of fluid from blood vessels into tissue spaces and alveoli. Fluid accumulation may result in severe respiratory difficulty and pulmonary edema, a life-threatening development. The improved strength of myocardial contraction resulting from cardiotonic–inotropic drugs reverses this potentially fatal chain of events.
(2) Decreased edema—absence of pitting, decreased size of ankles or abdominal girth, decreased weight	Diuresis and decreased edema result from improved circulation and increased renal blood flow.
(3) Increased tolerance of activity	Indicates a more adequate supply of blood to tissues
b. When digitalis is given in atrial arrhythmias, observe for	
(1) Gradual slowing of the heart rate to 70 to 80 beats per minute	
(2) Elimination of the pulse deficit	In clients with atrial fibrillation, slowing of the pulse rate and elimination of the pulse deficit are rough guides that digitalization has been achieved.
(3) Change in rhythm from irregular to regular	
3. Observe for adverse effects	
a. With digitalis, observe for	There is a high incidence of adverse effects with digitalis therapy. Therefore, every client receiving a digitalis preparation requires close observation. Severity of adverse effects can be minimized with early detection and treatment.
(1) Cardiac arrhythmias	Digitalis toxicity may cause any type of cardiac arrhythmia. These are the most serious adverse effects associated with digitalis therapy. They are detected as abnormalities in electrocardiograms and in pulse rate or rhythm.
(a) Premature ventricular contractions (PVCs)	PVCs are among the most common digitalis-induced arrhythmias. They are not specific for digitalis toxicity, since there are many possible causes. They are usually perceived as "skipped" heartbeats.
(b) Bradycardia	Excessive slowing of the pulse rate is an extension of the drug's therapeutic action of slowing conduction through the AV node and probably depressing the SA node as well.
(c) Paroxysmal atrial tachycardia with heart block	
(d) AV nodal tachycardia	
(e) AV block (second- or third-degree heart block)	
(2) Anorexia, nausea, and vomiting	These gastrointestinal effects commonly occur with digitalis therapy. Since they are caused, at least in part, by stimulation

Nursing Actions	Rationale/Explanation
	of the vomiting center in the brain, they occur with parenteral as well as oral administration. The presence of these symptoms raises suspicion of digitalis toxicity, but they are not specific, since many other conditions may cause anorexia, nausea, and vomiting. Also, clients receiving digitalis are often taking other medications that cause these side-effects, such as diuretics and potassium supplements.
(3) Headache, drowsiness, confusion	These CNS effects are most common in the elderly.
(4) Visual disturbances (*e.g.,* blurred vision, photophobia, altered perception of colors, flickering dots)	These are due mainly to drug effects on the retina and may indicate acute toxicity.
b. With amrinone, observe for	
(1) Thrombocytopenia	Thrombocytopenia is more likely to occur with prolonged therapy and is usually reversible if dosage is reduced or the drug is discontinued.
(2) Anorexia, nausea, vomiting, abdominal pain	Gastrointestinal symptoms can be decreased by reducing drug dosage.
(3) Hypotension	Hypotension probably results from vasodilatory effects of amrinone.
(4) Hepatotoxicity	If marked changes in liver enzymes occur in conjunction with clinical symptoms, the drug should be discontinued.
4. Observe for drug interactions	Most significant drug interactions increase risks of toxicity. Some alter absorption or metabolism to produce underdigitalization and decreased therapeutic effect.
a. Drugs that *increase* effects of digitalis glycosides	
(1) Adrenergic drugs (*e.g.,* ephedrine, epinephrine, isoproterenol), succinylcholine	Increase risks of cardiac arrhythmias
(2) Anticholinergics	Increase absorption of oral digitalis preparations by slowing transit time through the gastrointestinal tract
(3) Calcium preparations	Increase risks of cardiac arrhythmias. Intravenous calcium salts are contraindicated in digitalized clients.
(4) Quinidine, verapamil, nifedipine	Increase serum digoxin level and thereby increase risks of digitalis toxicity. Dosage of digoxin should be reduced if given concurrently with one of these drugs.
b. Drugs that *decrease* effects of digitalis glycosides	
(1) Antacids, cholestyramine, colestipol, laxatives, oral aminoglycosides (*e.g.,* neomycin)	Decrease absorption of oral digitalis preparations
(2) Barbiturates, phenylbutazone, phenytoin	Activate liver enzymes and accelerate metabolism of digitoxin
5. Teach clients about digitalis	
a. Name of drug, dose, reason receiving	
b. Teach the client or a family member to check the radial pulse at least once daily. Omit digitalis and report to the physician if the pulse is below 60.	Changes in the pulse may indicate adverse drug effects and a need to discontinue the drug.
c. How important it is to take as prescribed—*Do not* miss a dose. *Do not* take an extra dose. *Do not* take other medications without consulting the physician.	Owing to the relatively large number of drug interactions and risk of drug toxicity
d. If the client is taking other drugs such as diuretics and potassium, instruct about the importance of the balance between these drugs and digitalis. Also, instruct not to alter the dose of these drugs or stop taking them without consulting the physician.	A major risk develops if the diuretic is continued and potassium discontinued. This circumstance may lead to hypokalemia and digitalis toxicity. If the diuretic is stopped, edema is likely to recur. If the diuretic is discontinued but potassium is still taken, hyperkalemia can result.
e. Teach important side-effects, especially those to be reported to the physician or nurse such as change in	To promote early detection of toxicity and discontinuance of digitalis before serious problems develop

Nursing Actions	***Rationale/Explanation***
pulse rate or rhythm, gastrointestinal upset, visual problems.	
f. *Do not* use salt substitutes without consulting the physician.	Most salt substitutes contain potassium, which may be contraindicated, especially if a potassium supplement is being taken. Excessive potassium is cardiotoxic.
g. *Do not* use over-the-counter (nonprescription) drugs without checking with the physician.	A number of nonprescription drugs, including laxatives and antacids, contain significant amounts of sodium. Other drugs alter absorption of oral digitalis preparations.

Selected References

Algeo SS, Nolan PE, Fenster PE: Amrinone: A new therapy for heart failure. Drug Ther 8:81–89, November 1983

American Medical Association (AMA) Division of Drugs: AMA Drug Evaluations, 5th ed. New York, John Wiley & Sons, 1983

Cody RJ: Chronic heart failure: Specific therapy for vasoconstrictor mechanisms. Drug Ther 8:88–102, May 1983

Confino E, Zbella E, Elkayam U, Gleicher N: Using cardiac drugs during pregnancy. Drug Ther 15:131–145, March 1985

Elenbaas RM: Congestive heart failure. In Herfindal ET, Hirschman JL (eds): Clinical Pharmacy and Therapeutics, 3rd ed, pp 380–401. Baltimore, Williams & Wilkins, 1984

Facts and Comparisons. St. Louis, J B Lippincott (Updated monthly)

Fenster PE, Bressler R: Treating cardiovascular disease in the elderly. I. Digitalis glycosides and beta blockers. Drug Ther 14:125–132, February 1984

Fenster PE, Kern KB: Common drug interactions with digoxin. Drug Ther 8:91–94, February 1983

Friedman WF, George BL: New concepts and drugs in the treatment of congestive heart failure. Pediatr Clin North Am 31:1197–1227, December 1984

Guyton AC: Textbook of Medical Physiology, 7th ed. Philadelphia, W B Saunders, 1986

Hansten PD: Drug Interactions: Clinical Significance of Drug–Drug Interactions, 5th ed. Philadelphia, Lea & Febiger, 1985

Herfindal ET, Hirschman JL (eds): Clinical Pharmacy and Therapeutics, 3rd ed, Baltimore, Williams & Wilkins, 1984

Hoffman BF, Bigger JT Jr: Digitalis and allied cardiac glycosides. In Gilman AG, Goodman LS, Rall TW, Murad F (eds): The Pharmacological Basis of Therapeutics, 7th ed, pp 716–747. New York, Macmillan, 1985

Intravenous amrinone for congestive heart failure. Med Lett Drugs Ther 26:104–105, November 1984

Kleinhenz TJ: The inside story on preload and afterload. Nursing 15:50–55, May 1985

McCauley K, Burke K: Your detailed guide to drugs for CHF. Nursing 14:46–50, May 1984

Norsen LH, Fox GB: Understanding cardiac output—and the drugs that affect it. Nursing 15:34–41, April 1985

Rodman MJ, Karch AM, Boyd EH, Smith DW: Pharmacology and Drug Therapy in Nursing, 3rd ed. Philadelphia, J B Lippincott, 1985

Vasodilators for chronic congestive heart failure. Med Lett Drugs Ther 26:115–116, December 1984

52 ANTIARRHYTHMIC DRUGS

Description and uses

Antiarrhythmic agents are diverse drugs used for prevention and treatment of cardiac arrhythmias. Arrhythmias, also called dysrhythmias, are irregularities in heart rate or rhythm resulting from disturbances in electrical impulse formation, conduction, or both.

CHARACTERISTICS OF CARDIAC TISSUE

To understand arrhythmias and antiarrhythmic drug therapy, it is necessary to review some unique characteristics of cardiac muscle tissues, which normally regulate heart rate and rhythm. These characteristics are listed as follows:

1. Rhythmicity—each heart beat or cardiac cycle occurs at regular intervals and consists of four phases: *stimulation* from an electrical impulse, transmission or *conductivity* of the electrical impulse to adjacent cardiac tissues, *contraction* of atria and ventricles, and *relaxation* of atria and ventricles during which they refill with blood in preparation for the next contraction.
2. Excitability or irritability—the ability of cardiac muscle cells to respond to stimuli. To elicit contraction of myocardial cells, the stimulus must reach a certain intensity or threshold.
3. Refractoriness—decreased excitability. This property prevents myocardial response to a new stimulus while in a state of contraction from the previous stimulus.
4. Conductivity—the ability of heart muscle fibers to transmit electrical impulses. Under normal circumstances, electrical impulses originate in the sinoatrial (SA) node and are transmitted to atrial muscle, where they cause atrial contraction, then to the atrioventricular (AV) node, bundle of His, bundle branches, Purkinje fibers, and ventricular muscle where they cause ventricular contraction. The cardiac conduction system is depicted in Figure 52-1.

   Electrical activity in the heart can be graphically recorded as an electrocardiogram (ECG). Electrical "events" in the cardiac cycle are represented by waves or deflections, which were arbitrarily labeled P, QRS, and T. One cardiac cycle, as represented by the ECG, is shown in Figure 52-2. The P wave indicates atrial contraction. The PR interval indicates the time required for the electrical current to reach the ventricles. The QRS complex indicates ventricular contraction (depolarization or discharge of electrical current). The T wave indicates repolarization (preparation or electrical recovery for the next ventricular contraction).
5. Automaticity—the ability of the heart to generate an electrical impulse. Each cardiac cell is able to conduct impulses or contract independently of other cells. The characteristic of automaticity allows myocardial cells outside the normal conduction tissue to depolarize and initiate the

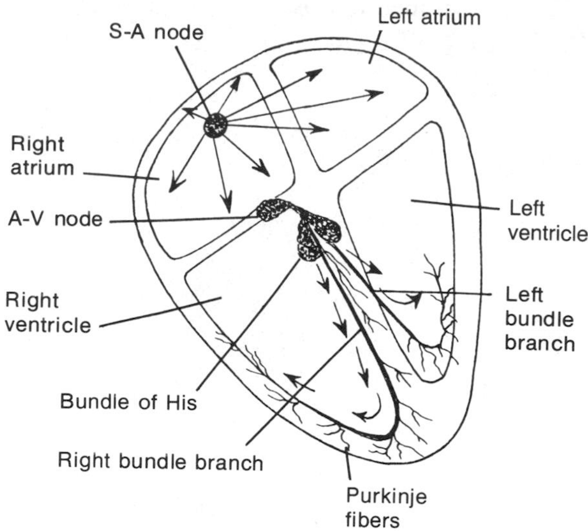

Figure 52-1. *The conducting system of the heart. Impulses originating in the S-A node are transmitted through the atria, into the A-V node to the bundle of His, and by way of the Purkinje fibers through the ventricles.*

electrical impulse, which culminates in atrial or ventricular contraction. When the impulse arises anywhere other than the SA node, it is called an *ectopic* impulse or focus. If the ectopic focus depolarizes at a rate faster than the SA node, the ectopic focus becomes the dominant pacemaker. Ectopic foci indicate myocardial irritability (increased responsiveness to stimuli).

CHARACTERISTICS OF CARDIAC ARRHYTHMIAS

Arrhythmias are usually categorized by rate, location, or patterns of conduction. They may originate in the SA node (sinus arrhythmias), atria, AV node (nodal arrhythmias), bundle branches, or ventricles.

Commonly occurring arrhythmias include sinus tachycardia, sinus bradycardia, premature atrial contractions (PACs), paroxysmal atrial tachycardia (PAT), atrial fibrillation, atrial flutter, AV nodal rhythm, paroxysmal nodal tachycardia, heart block, premature ventricular contractions (PVCs), ventricular fibrillation, and bundle branch blocks. Arrhythmias may be mild or severe, acute or chronic, episodic or relatively continuous. They are clinically significant if they interfere with cardiac function (*i.e.*, ability of the heart to pump sufficient blood to all body tissues). The normal heart is able to maintain an adequate cardiac output with ventricular rates ranging from 40 to 180 beats per minute. The diseased heart, however, may not be able to maintain an adequate cardiac output with heart rates below 60 or above 120. General characteristics of selected arrhythmias include:

1. Sinus arrhythmias are usually significant only if severe or prolonged. Tachycardia increases the workload of the heart and may lead to congestive heart failure or angina pectoris. Sinus tachycardia may cause anginal pain (myocardial ischemia) by two related mechanisms. One mechanism involves increased myocardial oxygen consumption. The other mechanism involves a shortened diastole so that coronary arteries may not have adequate filling time between heart beats. Thus, additional blood flow to the myocardium is required at the same time that a decreased blood supply is delivered.
2. Atrial arrhythmias are usually significant only in the presence of underlying heart disease. In coronary artery disease, atrial tachycardia increases myocardial oxygen consumption and shortens diastole. As a result, anginal pain may occur. In aortic valvular disease or hypertrophic myopathies, atrial fibrillation or flutter may decrease ventricular filling by as much as 30%, so that cardiac output may be severely impaired. Atrial fibrillation and flutter may also lead to the formation of thrombi in the atria.
3. Nodal arrhythmias may involve tachycardia and increased workload of the heart or bradycardia from heart block. Either tachycardia or bradycardia may decrease cardiac output. Heart block involves impaired conduction of the electrical impulse through the AV node. With first-degree heart block, conduction is slowed but not significantly. With second-degree heart block, every second, third, or fourth atrial impulse is blocked and does not reach the ventricles (2:1, 3:1, or 4:1 block).

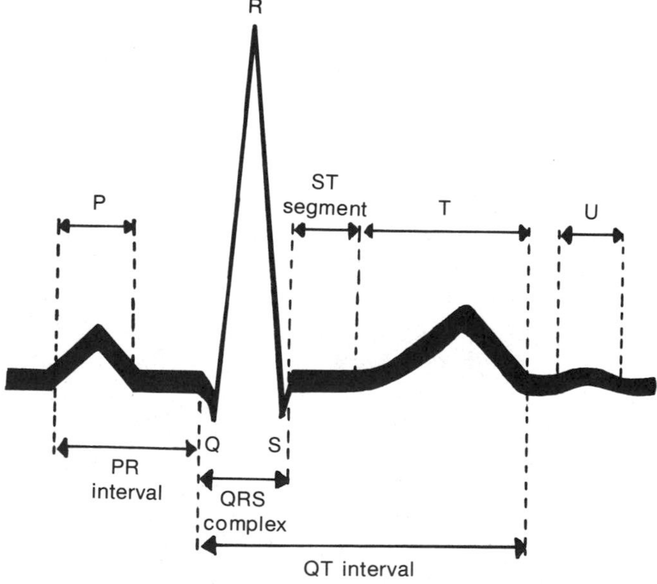

Figure 52-2. *ECG waves, complexes, and intervals.*

Thus, atrial and ventricular rates differ. Second-degree heart block may interfere with cardiac output or progress to third-degree block. Third-degree is the most serious type of heart block because no impulses reach the ventricles. As a result, ventricles beat independently at a rate of 30 to 40 per minute. This slow ventricular rate severely reduces cardiac output.

4. Ventricular arrhythmias are the most serious. These include PVCs, ventricular tachycardia, and ventricular fibrillation. PVCs may occasionally occur in anyone, and these are rarely significant. However, PVCs often occur after acute myocardial infarction and with ischemic heart disease. These may be life threatening or may lead to tachycardia, fibrillation, or asystole. PVCs are considered serious if they occur more than five times per minute, are coupled or grouped, are multifocal, or occur during the resting phase of the cardiac cycle.

   Ventricular tachycardia increases myocardial oxygen consumption and shortens diastole. Ventricular fibrillation produces ineffective myocardial contraction. As a result, there is no cardiac output. Death results unless effective cardiopulmonary resuscitation or defibrillation is instituted within approximately 4 to 6 minutes.

TREATMENT OF ARRHYTHMIAS

Arrhythmias may or may not require drug therapy. In emergencies, serious arrhythmias may be more effectively treated by electrical cardioversion or countershock. Less serious arrhythmias may be treated by removing the underlying cause (*e.g.*, electrolyte imbalance, digitalis intoxication, febrile illness, hyperthyroidism). Although not always required or desirable, antiarrhythmic drug therapy is usually indicated under the following conditions:

1. When the ventricular beat is so fast or irregular that cardiac output is impaired. Decreased cardiac output leads to symptoms of decreased systemic, cerebral, and coronary circulation.
2. When PVCs may develop into serious episodes of ventricular tachycardia.
3. When dangerous arrhythmias have already developed and may be fatal if not quickly terminated. For example, ventricular tachycardia may cause cardiac arrest.

The goals of antiarrhythmic drug therapy are to abolish the abnormal rhythm, restore normal sinus rhythm, and prevent recurrence of the arrhythmia.

Drugs used to prevent or abort arrhythmias belong to several therapeutic classifications. Antiarrhythmic drugs emphasized in this chapter are those used in treatment of tachyarrhythmias. Drugs used in bradyarrhythmias (*e.g.*, atropine and isoproterenol) are discussed primarily in Chapters 21 and 18, respectively. Digitalis glycosides are discussed in Chapter 51. Drugs used in tachyarrhythmias act mainly to prolong the refractory period (the time interval between one contraction and myocardial ability to respond to the next stimulus), decrease electrical impulse conduction, and decrease myocardial excitability.

Individual antiarrhythmic drugs

Quinidine is the prototype of antiarrhythmic drugs. It is also called a cardiac depressant drug. Quinidine is used primarily for chronic therapy. For clients with atrial fibrillation or flutter who have converted to normal sinus rhythm with digitalis glycosides or electrical cardioversion, quinidine may be used to maintain normal sinus rhythm. It is also used to prevent frequent PVCs, paroxysmal tachycardia, and postcountershock arrhythmias.

Quinidine exerts therapeutic effects in these arrhythmias by the following means:

1. Decreasing excitability or automaticity of both normal and abnormal (ectopic) pacemakers. Ectopic foci are more sensitive to the drug's inhibitory effect than is the SA node.
2. Decreasing the rate of impulse conduction through the myocardium. This action is caused by a direct effect on the atria, AV node, and ventricles.
3. Prolonging the refractory period of the myocardium. As a result, the myocardium does not contract with every impulse generated by an abnormal pacemaker.

Quinidine is well absorbed after oral administration. Therapeutic serum levels (approximately 3 to 6 μg/ml) are attained within 1 hour and persist for 6 to 8 hours. Quinidine is highly bound to serum albumin, which probably accounts for its relatively long duration of action and its half-life of approximately 6 hours. Quinidine is metabolized by the liver (about 80%) and excreted in the urine (about 20%). In alkaline urine (*i.e.*, *p*H above 7), renal excretion of quinidine decreases and serum levels may rise. Serum levels greater than 8 μg/ml are toxic.

Quinidine has a low therapeutic ratio and a high incidence of adverse effects that limit its clinical usefulness. The drug is usually contraindicated in clients with severe, uncompensated congestive heart failure or with heart block because it depresses myocardial contractility and conduction through the AV node.

Quinidine salts used clinically include quinidine gluconate (Duraquin), quinidine sulfate (Cin-Quin, Quinora), and quinidine polygalacturonate (Cardioquin). These salts differ in the amount of active drug (quinidine base) they contain and the rate of absorption with oral administration. The sulfate salt contains 83% quinidine base, and peak effects occur in 0.5 to 1.5 hours (4 hours for sustained-release forms). The gluconate salt contains 62% active drug, and peak effects occur in 3 to 4 hours. The polygalacturonate salt contains 60% active drug, and peak effects occur in about 6 hours. Quinidine gluconate may be given intramuscularly or intravenously, but such use is rare. The polygalacturonate salt is given orally. The gluconate and polygalacturonate salts reportedly cause less gastrointestinal irritation than quinidine sulfate. This is probably related to lower quinidine content. Oral extended-action preparations of quinidine (Quinidex Extentabs, Quinaglute Dura-Tabs) are also available.

Routes and dosage ranges

Adults: PO 200–600 mg q6h; maximal daily dose, 3–4 g
Maintenance dose, PO 200–600 mg q6h, or 1–2 extended-action tablets, 2–3 times daily
IM (quinidine gluconate) 600 mg initially, then 400 mg q4–6h
IV (quinidine gluconate) 200 mg in 100 ml of solution, given over 20–30 minutes with continuous electrocardiography and blood pressure monitoring
Children: PO 6 mg/kg q4–6h

Amiodarone (Cordarone) is chemically unrelated to other available antiarrhythmic drugs. It acts to prolong repolarization and refractoriness in all cardiac tissues, especially with chronic administration. More specifically, it impairs function of the SA node and slows the sinus rate; depresses AV node conduction; prolongs the refractory period of the accessory pathway in Wolfe-Parkinson-White (WPW) syndrome; alters automaticity of ectopic impulses in the Purkinje system; and antagonizes alpha and beta responses to catecholamine stimulation (antiadrenergic effect).

Amiodarone may be effective in several tachyarrhythmias including supraventricular tachycardia, atrial fibrillation and flutter, and ventricular tachycardia. A disadvantage, however, is that the drug has a long serum half-life, and therapeutic effects may be delayed 5 to 30 days unless loading doses are given. Effects may persist for several weeks after the drug is discontinued. Because of its adverse effects, amiodarone may be most useful in the management of arrhythmias resistant to other methods of treatment. Adverse effects include pulmonary fibrosis, myocardial depression, hypotension, bradycardia, hepatic dysfunction, central nervous system (CNS) disturbances (depression, insomnia, nightmares, hallucinations), peripheral neuropathy and muscle weakness, bluish discoloration of skin and corneal deposits that may cause photosensitivity, appearance of colored halos around lights, and reduced visual acuity. Most adverse effects are considered dose dependent and reversible.

Route and dosage ranges

Adults: Loading dose, PO 800–1600 mg daily for 1 to 3 weeks, with a gradual decrease to 600–800 mg daily for 1 month
Maintenance dose, PO 400 mg daily

Bretylium tosylate (Bretylol) is approved for parenteral administration in life-threatening arrhythmias (*e.g.*, ventricular tachycardia and ventricular fibrillation) when other antiarrhythmic drugs are ineffective. Its use should be limited to the intensive care setting. Bretylium prolongs the refractory period, but its exact mechanism of antiarrhythmic action is unknown. Bretylium is excreted almost entirely by the kidney. Therefore drug half-life (6 to 10 hours) is prolonged with renal insufficiency, and dosage must be reduced.

Routes and dosage ranges

Adults: IM 5 mg/kg, repeated in 1–2 hours; then q6–8h
IV 5–10 mg/kg, diluted (10-ml ampule of drug solution in a minimum of 50 ml of intravenous fluid) and infused over 10–20 minutes
During cardiopulmonary resuscitation, IV 5 mg/kg given by direct injection (undiluted). This dose may be repeated q15–30 minutes to a maximal total dose of 30 mg/kg

Disopyramide phosphate (Norpace) is an antiarrhythmic drug approved for oral administration to adults with ventricular arrhythmias. Disopyramide is similar to quinidine and procainamide in pharmacologic actions. It is well absorbed after oral administration and reaches peak serum levels (2–6 μg/ml) within 30–60 minutes (toxic levels, >9 μg/ml). Drug half-life is 5 to 8 hours. Disopyramide is excreted by the kidneys and the liver in almost equal proportions. Dosage must be reduced in renal insufficiency.

Route and dosage range

Adults: PO 300 mg loading dose, followed by 150 mg q6h. Usual dose, PO 400–800 mg/day, in 4 divided doses

Lidocaine hydrochloride (Xylocaine), a local anesthetic (see Chap. 14), is the drug of choice for treating serious ventricular arrhythmias associated with acute myocardial infarction, cardiac surgery, cardiac catheterization, and electrical cardioversion. Lidocaine exerts its antiarrhythmic action by decreasing myocardial irritability (automaticity) in the ventricles. It has little effect on atrial tissue and is not useful in treating atrial arrhythmias. Compared to quinidine and procainamide, lidocaine is described as follows:

1. It does not decrease AV conduction or myocardial contractility with usual therapeutic doses.
2. It has a rapid onset and short duration of action. After intravenous administration of a bolus dose, therapeutic effects occur within 1 to 2 minutes and last approximately 20 minutes. This characteristic is advantageous in emergency treatment but limits lidocaine usage to intensive care settings.
3. It is metabolized in the liver. Dosage must be reduced in clients with hepatic insufficiency or congestive heart failure to avoid drug accumulation and toxicity.
4. It is less likely to cause heart block, cardiac asystole, ventricular arrhythmias, and congestive heart failure.

Therapeutic serum levels of lidocaine are 2 to 5 μg/ml (toxic levels, >7 μg/ml). Lidocaine may be given intramuscularly in emergencies when intravenous administration is not possible. When given intramuscularly, therapeutic effects occur in approximately 15 minutes and last about 90 minutes. Lidocaine is contraindicated in people who are allergic to related local anesthetics (*e.g.*, procaine). Anaphylactic reactions may occur in sensitized persons.

Routes and dosage ranges

Adults: IV 1–2 mg/kg, usually not to exceed 50–100 mg, as a single bolus injection over 2 minutes. This is followed by a continuous infusion (1 g of lidocaine in 500 ml of 5% dextrose in water) at a rate to deliver 1–4 mg/minute. Maximal dose, 300 mg/hour
IM 4–5 mg/kg as a single dose. May repeat in 60–90 minutes

Phenytoin (Dilantin), an anticonvulsant drug (see Chap. 11), is useful in treatment of various cardiac arrhythmias, especially arrhythmias produced by digitalis intoxication. Phenytoin decreases automaticity and improves conduction through the AV node. Decreased automaticity helps control arrhythmias, while enhanced conduction may improve cardiac function. Further, since heart block may result from digitalis, quinidine, or procainamide, phenytoin may relieve arrhythmias without intensifying heart block. Phenytoin is not a cardiac depressant. Its only quinidinelike action is to suppress automaticity; otherwise, it counteracts the effects of quinidine and procainamide largely by increasing the rate of conduction. Phenytoin also has a longer half-life (22 to 36 hours) than other antiarrhythmic drugs. Given intravenously, a therapeutic plasma level (10 to 20 μg/ml) can be obtained rather rapidly (toxic levels, >20 μg/ml). Given orally, however, the drug may not reach a steady-state concentration for approximately 1 week unless loading doses are given initially.

Routes and dosage ranges

Adults: PO Loading dose 13 mg/kg (about 1000 mg) first day; 7.5 mg/kg second and third days; maintenance dose 4–6 mg/kg/day (average amount 400 mg), in 1–2 doses, starting on the fourth day of phenytoin therapy
IV 100 mg every 5 minutes until the arrhythmia is reversed or toxic effects occur; maximal dose, 1 g/24 hours
IM, not recommended for treatment of serious arrhythmias because absorption is delayed

Procainamide (Pronestyl, others) is similar to quinidine in actions and uses. Quinidine may be preferred for long-term use because procainamide produces a high incidence of adverse effects, including a syndrome resembling lupus erythematosus. Procainamide has a short duration of action (3 to 4 hours); sustained-release tablets (Procan SR) prolong action to approximately 6 hours. Therapeutic serum levels are 4 to 8 μg/ml; toxic levels, >16 μg/ml.

Routes and dosage ranges

Adults: PO 1 g loading dose initially, then 250–500 mg q3–4h (q6h for sustained-release tablets)
IM 500–1000 mg as a single loading dose for rapid drug action, followed by oral maintenance doses
IV 25–50 mg/minute to a maximal dose of 1000 mg
Children: PO 50 mg/kg/day in 4–6 divided doses

Propranolol (Inderal) is a nonselective beta-adrenergic blocking agent (see Chap. 19). Propranolol is a versatile and frequently prescribed drug used to treat hypertension and angina pectoris as well as cardiac arrhythmias. Propranolol exerts antiarrhythmic effects by blocking sympathetic nervous system stimulation of beta receptors in the heart. Blockage of receptors in the SA node (the normal cardiac pacemaker) and ectopic foci (abnormal pacemakers in atrial or ventricular tissue) decreases automaticity, and blockage of receptors in the AV node increases the refractory period.

Propranolol is most often used to slow the ventricular rate of contraction in supraventricular tachyarrhythmias (*e.g.*, atrial fibrillation, atrial flutter, paroxysmal supraventricular tachycardia). Propranolol may also be useful in long-term therapy to prevent ventricular arrhythmias, especially those precipitated by exercise or emotional upset. Despite its relatively wide spectrum of antiarrhythmic effectiveness, propranolol is rarely the drug of first choice for treating an acute arrhythmia. Propranolol is contraindicated in the presence of congestive heart failure unless the arrhythmia being treated is the cause of the heart failure.

Routes and dosage ranges

Adults: PO 40–120 mg/day in 2–4 divided doses
IV 1–3 mg, not to exceed 1 mg/minute

Tocainide (Tonocard) is an oral analog of lidocaine with similar pharmacologic actions. It is used to suppress ventricular arrhythmias, including frequent PVCs and ventricular tachycardia. It is well absorbed, and peak serum levels are obtained in 0.5 to 3 hours. Taking with food delays but does not decrease absorption. Therapeutic serum levels are 4 to 10 μg/ml, with toxic levels above 10 μg/ml.

Route and dosage range

Adults: PO 400 mg q8h initially, increased up to 1800 mg daily in 3 divided doses if necessary

Verapamil (Calan, Isoptin) is a calcium antagonist that slows conduction through the AV node. It is approved for use in paroxysmal supraventricular tachycardias and in atrial fibrillation and flutter. In atrial fibrillation and flutter, verapamil slows the rate of ventricular response rather than terminating the arrhythmia. When verapamil is given intravenously, therapeutic serum levels are achieved within 2 to 5 minutes, reach peak levels in 10 to 15 minutes and last up to 6 hours. Verapamil is metabolized by the liver; its metabolites are primarily excreted by the kidneys. Verapamil is contraindicated in digitalis toxicity because it may worsen heart block. If verapamil is used with propranolol or digitalis, caution must be exercised to avoid further impairment of myocardial contractility. Do *not* use intravenous verapamil with intravenous propranolol; potentially fatal bradycardia and hypotension may occur.

Routes and dosage ranges

Adults: PO 40–120 mg q6–8h
IV 5–10 mg initially; then 10 mg 30 minutes later if necessary

Principles of therapy: antiarrhythmic drugs

ASSESSMENT GUIDELINES

Assess the client's condition in relation to cardiac arrhythmias.

1. Identify conditions or risk factors that may precipitate arrhythmias. These include the following:
   a. Hypoxia
   b. Electrolyte imbalances
   c. Acid–base imbalances
   d. Myocardial infarction, coronary artery disease
   e. Cardiac valvular disease
   f. Febrile illness
   g. Respiratory disorders (*e.g.*, chronic lung disease
   h. Exercise
   i. Emotional upset
   j. Excessive ingestion of caffeine-containing beverages (*e.g.*, coffee, tea, colas)
   k. Cigarette smoking
   l. Drug therapy with digitalis glycosides, antiarrhythmic drugs, CNS stimulants, anorexiants, and tricyclic antidepressants
   m. Hyperthyroidism
2. Observe for clinical signs and symptoms of arrhythmias. Mild or infrequent arrhythmias may be perceived by the client as palpitations or skipped heart beats. More severe arrhythmias may produce manifestations that reflect decreased cardiac output and other hemodynamic changes as follows:
   a. Hypotension, bradycardia or tachycardia, irregular pulse
   b. Shortness of breath, dyspnea, and cough from impaired respiration
   c. Syncope or mental confusion from reduced cerebral blood flow
   d. Chest pain from decreased coronary artery blood flow. Angina pectoris or myocardial infarction may occur.
   e. Oliguria from decreased renal blood flow
3. When ECGs are available (*e.g.*, 12-lead ECG or continuous ECG monitoring), assess for indications of arrhythmias.

PREVENTIVE NURSING INTERVENTIONS

Use measures to prevent or minimize arrhythmias.

1. Treat underlying disease processes that contribute to arrhythmia development. These include both cardiovascular (*e.g.,* acute myocardial infarction) and noncardiovascular (*e.g.,* chronic lung disease) disorders.
2. Prevent or treat other conditions that predispose to arrhythmias (*e.g.,* hypoxia, electrolyte imbalance).
3. Encourage the client to avoid cigarette smoking, overeating, excessive coffee drinking, and other lifestyle habits that may cause or aggravate arrhythmias. Long-term supervision and counseling may be needed.
4. For the client receiving antiarrhythmic drugs, implement the above measures to minimize incidence and severity of acute arrhythmias and assist the client to comply with drug therapy.

GUIDELINES FOR DRUG THERAPY OF ARRHYTHMIAS

1. In several arrhythmias, drug therapy is not the first treatment choice. For example, the initial treatment of choice for ventricular fibrillation is immediate defibrillation by electrical countershock. In paroxysmal supraventricular tachycardias, measures to increase vagal tone (*e.g.,* carotid sinus massage, Valsalva's maneuver) or sleep are usually preferred.
2. Rational drug therapy for cardiac arrhythmias requires accurate identification of the arrhythmia, understanding of the basic mechanisms causing the arrhythmia, observation of the hemodynamic and electrocardiographic effects of the arrhythmia, and knowledge of the pharmacologic actions of specific antiarrhythmic drugs.
3. In symptomatic arrhythmias that require drug therapy, choice of antiarrhythmic drug is largely empirical. Although some arrhythmias usually respond to particular drugs, different drugs or combinations of drugs are often required. Some guidelines for drug choice include the following:
   a. Atropine and isoproterenol (Isuprel) are drugs of choice for sinus bradycardia or heart block.
   b. A digitalis glycoside is the initial drug of choice in atrial fibrillation and atrial flutter.
   c. Quinidine, procainamide (Pronestyl), and disopyramide (Norpace) are useful in long-term prevention or acute treatment of atrial and ventricular arrhythmias (*e.g.,* PACs, PAT, atrial fibrillation, atrial flutter, AV nodal premature contractions, AV nodal tachycardia, PVCs, ventricular tachycardia).
   d. Lidocaine or phenytoin is the drug of choice for treating digitalis-induced arrhythmias.
   e. Lidocaine is the drug of choice for treating PVCs and ventricular tachycardia. Tocainide may be useful because it can be given orally.
   f. Propranolol and other beta blockers are not drugs of choice for initial treatment of most arrhythmias. However, they may be useful in treating a variety of arrhythmias, often in combination with other antiarrhythmic drugs.
   g. Bretylium and amiodarone are approved for use only in refractory arrhythmias.
   h. Verapamil is more effective in atrial arrhythmias than in ventricular arrhythmias.
4. Quinidine, procainamide, and lidocaine all have a vagal blocking action on the AV node and should not be used to treat atrial fibrillation unless digitalis has been given. Without the digitalis action of blocking AV conduction, these drugs may allow a 1:1 ventricular response at a dangerously rapid rate. One of these drugs may be used to treat ventricular tachyarrhythmias without first treating the patient with digitalis, however.

NURSING ACTIONS: ANTIARRHYTHMIC DRUGS

Nursing Actions	*Rationale/Explanation*
1. Administer accurately	
a. Check apical and radial pulses before each dose. Withhold the dose and report to the physician if marked changes are noted in rate, rhythm, or quality of pulses.	Bradycardia may indicate impending heart block or cardiovascular collapse.

Nursing Actions	Rationale/Explanation
b. Check blood pressure at least once daily in hospitalized clients.	To detect hypotension. Hypotension is most likely to occur when antiarrhythmic drug therapy is being initiated or altered.
c. During intravenous administration of antiarrhythmic drugs, maintain continuous cardiac monitoring and check blood pressure about every 5 minutes.	For early detection of hypotension and impending cardiac collapse. These drug side-effects are more likely to occur with intravenous use.
d. Give oral drugs at evenly spaced time intervals.	To maintain adequate blood levels
e. Follow undiluted intravenous phenytoin with an injection of sterile saline through the same needle or catheter. *Do not* mix parenteral phenytoin with any other drug, and *do not* add to intravenous solutions other than normal saline (0.9% NaCl) for intermittent intravenous infusion.	Phenytoin is strongly alkaline, with a *p*H of 11 to 12. Saline is used to "flush" the vein and avoid local venous irritation. Solubility of the drug is very *p*H dependent, and mixing with other drugs or solutions other than normal saline causes a white precipitate. Intramuscular injection is not recommended owing to pain and delayed absorption.
f. Give lidocaine parenterally only, as a bolus injection or a continuous drip. Use only solutions labeled "For Cardiac Arrhythmias" and *do not* use solutions containing epinephrine. Give an intravenous bolus over 2 minutes.	Lidocaine solutions that contain epinephrine are used for local anesthesia only. They should never be given intravenously in cardiac arrhythmias, since the epinephrine can cause or aggravate arrhythmias. Rapid injection (within about 30 seconds) produces transient blood levels several times greater than therapeutic range limits. Therefore, there is increased risk of toxicity without a concomitant increase in therapeutic effectiveness.
g. Give in a peripheral vein.	To allow mixing with blood. Injection into the central circulation (through a central venous pressure line, for example), is hazardous because a high drug concentration develops locally within the heart.
h. *Do not* add to a blood transfusion assembly.	
2. Observe for therapeutic effects **a.** Conversion to normal sinus rhythm **b.** Improvement in rate, rhythm, and quality of apical and radial pulses and the ECG **c.** Signs of increased cardiac output—blood pressure near normal range, urine output more adequate, no complaints of dizziness	After a single oral dose, peak plasma levels are reached in about 1 to 4 hours with quinidine, procainamide, and propranolol and in 6 to 12 hours with phenytoin. A state of equilibrium between plasma and tissue levels is reached in 1 or 2 days with quinidine, procainamide, and propranolol; in about 1 week with phenytoin; in several weeks with amiodarone (unless loading doses are given); and in just a few minutes with intravenous lidocaine. Although this information may be helpful in determining when therapeutic effects are most likely to appear, remember that many other factors influence therapeutic effects, such as dose, frequency of administration, presence of conditions that alter drug metabolism, arterial blood gases, serum electrolyte levels, and myocardial status.
d. Serum drug levels within therapeutic ranges (1) Quinidine 3 to 6 μg/ml (2) Disopyramide 2 to 6 μg/ml (3) Procainamide 4 to 8 μg/ml (4) Lidocaine 2 to 5 μg/ml (5) Phenytoin 8 to 20 μg/ml (6) Propranolol 0.05 to 0.1 μg/ml (7) Tocainide 4 to 10 μg/ml	Serum drug levels must be interpreted in light of the client's clinical status.
3. Observe for adverse effects **a.** Heart block—may be indicated on the ECG by a prolonged PR interval, prolonged QRS complex, or absence of P waves.	Owing to depressant effects on the cardiac conduction system

Nursing Actions	Rationale/Explanation
b. Arrhythmias—aggravation of existing arrhythmia, tachycardia, bradycardia, PVCs, ventricular tachycardia or fibrillation	Tachycardia is probably caused by the anticholinergic effect of the drugs plus the response of the sympathetic nervous system to the mild hypotension induced by the drug. Bradycardia may occur with propranolol.
c. Hypotension	Owing to decreased cardiac output
d. Additional adverse effects with specific drugs	
(1) Disopyramide—mouth dryness, blurred vision, urinary retention, and other anticholinergic effects	These effects commonly occur.
(2) Lidocaine—drowsiness, paresthesias, muscle twitching, convulsions, changes in mental status (*e.g.,* confusion), hypersensitivity reactions (*e.g.,* urticaria, edema, anaphylaxis)	Most adverse reactions result from drug effects on the CNS. Convulsions are most likely to occur with high doses. Hypersensitivity reactions may occur in people who are allergic to related local anesthetic agents.
(3) Phenytoin—nystagmus, ataxia, slurring of speech, tremors, drowsiness, confusion, gingival hyperplasia	CNS changes are caused by depressant effects.
(4) Propranolol—weakness or dizziness, especially with activity or exercise	The beta-adrenergic blocking action of propranolol blocks the normal sympathetic nervous system response to activity and exercise. Clients may have symptoms caused by deficient blood supply to body tissues.
(5) Quinidine—hypersensitivity and cinchonism (tinnitus, vomiting, severe diarrhea, vertigo, headache)	
(6) Tocainide—lightheadedness, dizziness, nausea, paresthesia, tremor	These are the most frequent adverse effects. They may be reversed by decreasing dosage, administering with food, or discontinuing the drug.
4. Observe for drug interactions	
a. Drugs that *increase* effects of antiarrhythmics	These drugs may potentiate therapeutic effects or increase risk of toxicity.
(1) Antiarrhythmic agents	When antiarrhythmic drugs are combined, there are additive cardiac depressant effects.
(2) Anticholinergics	Additive anticholinergic effects
(3) Antihypertensives, diuretics, phenothiazine antipsychotic agents	Additive hypotension
(4) Digitalis preparations	Additive bradycardia with propranolol
(5) Chloramphenicol (Chloromycetin), isoniazid (INH)	These drugs inhibit metabolism of phenytoin and may produce phenytoin toxicity
b. Drugs that *decrease* effects of antiarrhythmic agents	
Atropine sulfate	Atropine is used to reverse propranolol-induced bradycardia.
5. Teach clients	
a. Name, dose, reason for receiving drug	
b. Report ankle edema, fatigue, dyspnea, weight gain.	These symptoms may indicate drug-induced congestive heart failure, since these cardiac depressant drugs decrease myocardial contractility.
c. Space activities and rest at intervals.	With these drugs, there is decreased tolerance of activity and exercise.
d. Check pulse at least once daily for irregularity or excessive slowness.	Antiarrhythmic drugs may themselves cause arrhythmias. Bradycardia is a side-effect of propranolol.
e. Maintain regular time intervals in taking medication.	To maintain therapeutic blood levels
f. Phenytoin may color urine pink to reddish brown.	This is a harmless color change.

Selected References

American Medical Association (AMA) Division of Drugs: AMA Drug Evaluations, 5th ed. New York, John Wiley & Sons, 1983

Bigger JT Jr, Hoffman BF: Antiarrhythmic drugs. In Gilman AG, Goodman LS, Rall TW, Murad F (eds): The Pharmacological Basis of Therapeutics, 7th ed, pp 748–783. New York, Macmillan, 1985

Breckenridge AM: When should plasma levels of cardioactive drugs be monitored? Drug Ther 14:177–196, May 1984

Confino E, Zbella E, Elkayam U, Gleicher N: Using cardiac drugs during pregnancy. Drug Ther 15:131–145, March 1985

Fenster PE, Bressler R: Treating cardiovascular disease in the elderly. II. Antiarrhythmics, diuretics and calcium channel blockers. Drug Ther 14:209–215, March 1984

Garson A Jr: Arrhythmias in pediatric patients. Med Clin North Am 68:1171–1210, September 1984

Gill MA, Noguchi JK: Cardiac arrhythmias. In Herfindal ET, Hirschman JL (eds): Clinical Pharmacy and Therapeutics, 3rd ed, pp 419–441. Baltimore, Williams & Wilkins, 1984

Guyton AC: Textbook of Medical Physiology, 7th ed. Philadelphia, W B Saunders, 1986

Hansten PD: Drug Interactions: Clinical Significance of Drug–Drug Interactions, 5th ed. Philadelphia, Lea & Febiger, 1985

Hasegawa GR: Tocainide: A new oral antiarrhythmic. Drug Intell Clin Pharmacol 19:514–517, July–August 1985

Moser SA: Get ready: The new antiarrhythmics are coming. Nursing 15:56–58, September 1985

Pasquale FN, DePace NL, Morganroth J: Therapy with conventional antiarrhythmic drugs for ventricular arrhythmias. Med Clin North Am 68:1295–1319, September 1984

Rodman MJ, Karch AM, Boyd EH, Smith DW: Pharmacology and Drug Therapy in Nursing, 3rd ed. Philadelphia, J B Lippincott, 1985

Rotmensch HH, Elkayam U, Frishman W: Antiarrhythmic drug therapy during pregnancy. Ann Intern Med 98:487–497, April 1983

53

ANTIANGINAL DRUGS

Description and uses

Angina pectoris is a clinical syndrome characterized mainly by chest pain. It occurs when there is a deficit in myocardial oxygen supply (myocardial ischemia) in relation to myocardial oxygen demand. It is most often caused by atherosclerotic plaque formation in the coronary arteries. Atherosclerotic plaque narrows the lumen, decreases elasticity, and impairs dilation of coronary arteries. The result is impaired blood flow to the myocardium, especially with exercise or other factors that increase the cardiac workload and need for oxygen.

Angina pectoris is generally described as a dull, heavy substernal pain that radiates into the left shoulder and down the left arm. The pain may also radiate to the back, neck, or lower jaw. Several types of angina pectoris have been described. *Stable angina* is the typical chest pain that is usually precipitated by exercise and relieved by rest or nitroglycerin. It may also be precipitated by stress, anxiety, cigarette smoking, or cold weather. Recurrent episodes of stable angina usually have the same pattern of onset, duration, and intensity of symptoms. *Unstable angina* results from progressive atherosclerosis and produces increased frequency, intensity, and duration of symptoms. Unstable angina is less responsive to rest, nitroglycerin, and other medical therapy. In *vasospastic angina* (also called Prinzmetal's or variant angina), chest pain occurs at rest. It is attributed to spasm in a coronary artery.

Drugs used in angina pectoris are the organic nitrates, the beta-adrenergic blocking agents, and the calcium antagonists. Generally, these drugs relieve anginal pain by decreasing myocardial demand for oxygen or increasing blood supply to the myocardium. Another drug, dipyridamole (Persantine), is a coronary artery vasodilator that has been used for long-term treatment of angina pectoris. However, there is no reliable evidence that the drug is effective in decreasing the incidence or severity of acute anginal attacks.

ORGANIC NITRATES

Organic nitrates (*e.g.,* nitroglycerin) act to relax smooth muscle in blood vessel walls. This action produces vasodilation, which relieves anginal pain by several mechanisms. First, dilation of veins reduces venous pressure and venous return to the heart. This decreases blood volume and pressure within the heart (preload), which in turn decreases cardiac workload and oxygen demand. Second, organic nitrates dilate coronary arteries and can increase blood flow to ischemic areas of the myocardium. Third, organic nitrates dilate arterioles, which lowers peripheral vascular resistance (afterload). This results in lower systolic blood pressure and, consequently, reduced cardiac workload. The prototype of organic nitrates is nitroglycerin.

Clinical indications for nitroglycerin and other organic nitrates are treatment and prevention of acute anginal attacks. Sublingual preparations have a rapid onset (1 to 3 minutes) and short duration of action (1 to 2 hours). They are used to relieve acute anginal pain or to prevent pain during activities known to precipitate acute anginal attacks. For prevention, sublingual preparations are taken immediately before the activity. Oral preparations are used in long-term management of angina pectoris to decrease the frequency and severity of acute anginal attacks. Relatively high oral doses are required because first-pass metabolism in the liver prevents a portion of each dose from reaching the systemic circulation.

BETA-ADRENERGIC BLOCKING AGENTS

Beta-adrenergic blocking agents, of which propranolol is the prototype, are among the most frequently prescribed drugs. They are used in a variety of clinical conditions. Their actions, uses, and adverse effects are discussed in Chapter 19. In this chapter, the drugs are discussed only in relation to their use in angina pectoris.

Sympathetic stimulation of beta receptors in the heart increases heart rate and force of myocardial contraction, both of which increase myocardial oxygen demand and may precipitate acute anginal attacks. Beta-blocking drugs block or inhibit sympathetic stimulation. Thus, the drugs reduce heart rate and myocardial contractility, particularly when there is increased sympathetic output during exercise. Beta blockers also reduce blood pressure, which in turn decreases myocardial workload and oxygen demand. In angina pectoris, propranolol and other beta-adrenergic blocking agents are used in long-term management to decrease frequency and severity of anginal attacks, decrease the need for sublingual nitroglycerin, and increase exercise tolerance.

CALCIUM CHANNEL BLOCKING AGENTS

Calcium channel blocking agents act on contractile and conductive tissues of the heart and on vascular smooth muscle. For these cells to function normally, the concentration of intracellular calcium must be increased. This is usually accomplished by movement of extracellular calcium into the cell and release of bound calcium from the sarcoplasmic reticulum in the cell. Thus, calcium plays an important role in maintaining vasomotor tone, myocardial contractility, and conduction. Calcium channel blocking agents prevent the movement of extracellular calcium into the cell. As a result, coronary and peripheral arteries are dilated, myocardial contractility is decreased, and the conduction system is depressed in relation to impulse formation (automaticity) and conduction velocity. In angina pectoris, the drugs improve the blood supply to the myocardium by dilating coronary arteries and decrease the workload of the heart by dilating peripheral arteries. Currently three calcium blockers are approved for use in the United States: nifedipine (Procardia), verapamil (Calan, Isoptin), and diltiazem (Cardizem). Although these agents have the same pharmacologic actions, they vary in their effects on the designated tissues. Thus, nifedipine is the most potent vasodilator of the three drugs, but verapamil and diltiazem have a greater effect on the conduction system. Cardiovascular effects are summarized in Table 53-1.

Clinical indications for use stem directly from pharmacologic actions of the drugs. All three may be used in the management of angina pectoris, and verapamil is used in the treatment of supraventricular tachyarrhythmias. Numerous studies have indicated that the drugs are also effective in the treatment of hypertension, and they have been used in Europe for this purpose for several years.

Individual antianginal drugs

ORGANIC NITRATES

Nitroglycerin (Nitro-Bid, Nitrospan, and others), the prototype of the organic nitrate antianginal drugs, is used to relieve acute angina pectoris, prevent exercise-induced angina, and decrease frequency and severity of acute anginal episodes. Nitroglycerin is available in several dosage forms for different routes of administration. When administered sublingually, nitroglycerin is absorbed directly into the systemic circulation. It acts within 1 to 3 minutes and lasts about 30 to 60 minutes. When applied topically to the skin, nitroglycerin is also absorbed directly into the systemic circulation. However, absorption occurs at a slower rate, and topical nitroglycerin has a longer duration of action than other forms. It is available in an ointment, which is effective for 4 to 8 hours, and a transdermal disc, which is effective for about 18 to 24 hours. An intravenous form of nitroglycerin is used to relieve acute anginal

TABLE 53-1. CARDIOVASCULAR EFFECTS OF CALCIUM CHANNEL BLOCKERS

	Nifedipine (Procardia)	Verapamil (Calan)	Diltiazem (Cardizem)
Dilate coronary arteries	Yes	Yes	Yes
Dilate peripheral arteries	Yes	Yes	Yes
Slow conduction through SA and AV nodes	No	Yes	Yes
Effect on heart rate	Increase	Increase or decrease	Decrease
Effect on myocardial contractility	Minimal	Decrease	Decrease

pain that does not respond to other agents. Although oral dosage forms of nitroglycerin are available, orally administered drug is extensively metabolized in the liver, and relatively small proportions of normal doses reach the systemic circulation. As a result, oral nitroglycerin is unlikely to be effective in preventing acute anginal pain.

Routes and dosage ranges

Adults: PO 2.5–9 mg 2–3 times daily
SL 0.15–0.6 mg PRN for chest pain
Topical ointment, $\frac{1}{2}$–2 inches q4–8h; do not rub in
Topical transdermal disc, applied once daily
IV 5–10 μg/minute initially, increased in 10- to 20-μg/minute increments up to 100 μg/minute or more if necessary to relieve pain

Amyl nitrite (Vaporole) is dispensed in a container that is crushed to release vapors. The vapors are inhaled. Onset of action and pain relief are rapid, but amyl nitrite is more likely to cause headache and hypotension than other nitrates used in angina pectoris.

Route and dosage range

Adults: Inhalation, 0.18–0.3 ml (one container)

Erythrityl tetranitrate (Cardilate) is an organic nitrate used for the long-term management or prophylaxis of angina pectoris. The drug is not suitable for acute episodes of anginal pain, since onset of action occurs after 5 to 10 minutes. Beneficial effects last 3 to 4 hours.

Routes and dosage ranges

Adults: SL 10 mg 3 times daily or before stress
PO 5–15 mg 3 times daily

Isosorbide dinitrate (Isordil, Sorbitrate) is widely used to reduce frequency and severity of acute anginal episodes. When given sublingually, isosorbide dinitrate acts in about 2 minutes, and its effects last about 1 to 2 hours. When higher doses are given orally, more drug escapes metabolism in the liver and produces systemic effects in about 30 minutes. Lower doses may be relatively ineffective. Therapeutic effects last about 4 hours after oral administration. The effective oral dose is usually determined by increasing the dose until headache occurs, indicating the maximal tolerable dose. Sustained-release capsules are also available.

Routes and dosage ranges

Adults: SL 2.5–10 mg PRN or q2–4h
PO 10–60 mg q4–6h
Sustained-release, PO 40 mg q6–12h

Pentaerythritol tetranitrate (Peritrate, PETN) is similar to erythrityl tetranitrate in actions and uses. It is used prophylactically in long-term management of angina pectoris. It is available in short-acting and sustained-release dosage forms.

Route and dosage range

Adults: PO 10–80 mg 2–4 times daily

BETA-ADRENERGIC BLOCKING AGENTS

Propranolol (Inderal) is the prototype beta blocker. It is used in treatment of angina pectoris to reduce frequency and severity of acute attacks. Propranolol is usually added to the antianginal drug regimen when maximal doses of isosorbide dinitrate do not prevent anginal episodes. Propranolol is especially useful in preventing exercise-induced tachycardia, which can precipitate anginal attacks.

Following oral administration, propranolol is well absorbed in the intestine. It is then metabolized extensively in the liver; a relatively small proportion of an oral dose (about 30%) reaches the systemic circulation. For this reason, oral doses of propranolol are much higher than intravenous doses. Onset of action is 30 minutes after oral administration and 1 to 2 minutes after intravenous injection. Because of variations in the degree of hepatic metabolism, clients vary widely in the dosages required to maintain a therapeutic response.

Routes and dosage ranges

Adults: PO 10–80 mg 2–4 times daily
IV 0.5–3 mg q4h until the desired response is obtained

Nadolol (Corgard) has the same actions, uses, and adverse effects as propranolol. However, nadolol has a longer half-life than propranolol. As a result, nadolol is given once daily. Dosage must be reduced with renal failure, since the kidneys are the major route of elimination.

Route and dosage range

Adults: PO 40–240 mg daily in a single dose

CALCIUM CHANNEL BLOCKING AGENTS

Diltiazem (Cardizem) is approved for treatment of vasospastic and chronic stable angina. It is reportedly intermediate in effects, between nifedipine and verapamil, and well tolerated. Diltiazem is well absorbed with oral administration and is moderately bound to plasma proteins (70% to 85%). It is metabolized in the liver to a metabolite that is approximately half as active as the parent drug. A small amount is excreted in the urine. Onset of action is about 30 minutes, and peak plasma levels occur in 2 to 3 hours.

Route and dosage range

Adults: PO 30 mg 4 times daily, before meals and at bedtime. Dosage may be gradually increased to 240 mg daily, in 3–4 divided doses, if needed for optimal effects.

Nifedipine (Procardia) is approved for treatment of vasospastic and chronic stable angina. It has more potent vasodilating effects than diltiazem and verapamil but does not affect the conduction system of the heart. Nifedipine is highly bound to plasma proteins and is metabolized to an inactive compound. Onset of action occurs in about 20 minutes, and peak plasma levels occur in about 30 minutes.

Route and dosage range

Adults: PO 10 mg 3 times daily initially, increased to 20–30 mg 3–4 times daily if necessary

Verapamil (Isoptin, Calan) is approved for oral administration in the treatment of angina pectoris and for intravenous administration in the treatment of supraventricular tachyarrhythmias. In arrhythmias, verapamil decreases SA node function and AV node conduction to reduce the rate of ventricular response. Verapamil is highly bound to plasma proteins and is metabolized to norverapamil, a metabolite about 20% as active as the parent drug. With oral administration, onset of action occurs in about 30 minutes, and peak plasma levels occur in 1 to 2 hours. With intravenous administration, peak effects occur within 3 to 5 minutes.

Routes and dosage range

Adults: PO 80 mg q6–8h initially, increased to a maximal dose of 480 mg daily if necessary.
IV 5–10 mg over 2 minutes initially. A repeat dose of 10 mg may be given in 30 minutes if the initial response is not adequate.

Elderly adults: IV 5–10 mg over at least 3 minutes. Repeat in 30 minutes if necessary.

Children up to 1 year: IV 0.1–0.2 mg/kg (usual single dose range 0.75–2 mg) as bolus injection over 2 minutes, with continuous electrocardiogram monitoring.

Children 1–15 years: 0.1–0.3 mg/kg (usual single dose range 2–5 mg) over 2 minutes. Maximal dose, 5 mg. Repeat dose in 30 minutes if necessary.

Principles of therapy: antianginal drugs

ASSESSMENT GUIDELINES

Assess the client's condition in relation to angina pectoris. Specific assessment data vary with each person but usually should include the following:

1. During the initial nursing history interview, try to answer the following questions:
   a. How long has the client been taking antianginal drugs? For what purpose are they being taken (prophylaxis, treatment of acute attacks, or both)?
   b. What is the frequency and duration of acute anginal attacks?
   c. Do symptoms other than chest pain occur during acute attacks (*e.g.*, sweating, nausea)?
   d. Are there particular activities or circumstances that provoke acute attacks? Do attacks ever occur when the client is at rest?
   e. What relieves symptoms of acute angina?
   f. If the client takes nitroglycerin, ask how often it is required, how many tablets are needed for relief of pain, how often the supply is replaced, and where the client stores or carries the drug.
2. During an acute attack, assess the following:
   a. Location and quality of the pain. Chest pain is nonspecific. It may be a symptom of numerous disorders, such as pulmonary embolism, esophageal spasm or inflammation (heartburn), costochondritis, and anxiety. Chest pain of cardiac origin is caused by myocardial ischemia and may indicate angina pectoris or myocardial infarction. In a client with known coronary artery disease or angina pectoris, it is probably safer to assume that any chest pain is of cardiac origin and that nitroglycerin and rest are indicated. If chest pain is severe, prolonged (longer than approximately 30 minutes), and unrelieved by rest and nitroglycerin, assume that a myocardial infarction has occurred until proved otherwise. Keep the client at rest, and notify the physician immediately.
   b. Other parameters of client status, such as blood pressure, heart rate, presence of symptoms other than chest pain, posture, and facial expression.

PREVENTIVE NURSING INTERVENTIONS

Use the following measures to prevent acute anginal attacks:

1. Assist in preventing, recognizing, and treating contributory disorders, such as atherosclerosis, hypertension, hyperthyroidism, hypoxia, and anemia.
2. Assist the client to recognize and avoid precipitating factors (*e.g.*, heavy meals, cigarette smoking, strenuous exercise) when possible. If anxiety is a factor, relaxation techniques or psychologic counseling may be helpful.
3. Assist the client to develop a more healthful life style in terms of diet, adequate rest and sleep, and regular exercise. A supervised exercise program helps to develop collateral circulation.

GUIDELINES FOR NITROGLYCERIN USE

1. Nitroglycerin is the drug of choice in acute angina. Three sublingual tablets may be used, 5 minutes apart, if necessary. If chest pain is not relieved, keep the client at rest and notify the physician immediately. A myocardial infarction or other problem may be causing the chest pain.
2. Leave sublingual nitroglycerin at the bedside of hospitalized clients. The tablets should be within reach so they can be used immediately. Record the number of tablets used daily, and be sure an adequate supply is available.

NURSING ACTIONS: ANTIANGINAL DRUGS

Nursing Actions	*Rationale/Explanation*
1. Administer accurately	
a. Check blood pressure and heart rate before each dose of an antianginal drug. Withhold the drug if systolic blood pressure is below 90 mm Hg. If the dose is omitted, record and report to the physician.	Hypotension is an adverse effect of antianginal drugs. Bradycardia is an adverse effect of propranolol and nadolol. Dosage adjustments may be necessary if these effects occur.
b. Give antianginal drugs on a regular schedule, at evenly spaced intervals.	To increase effectiveness in preventing acute attacks of angina
c. If oral nitrates and topical nitroglycerin are being used concurrently, stagger times of administration.	To minimize risks of additive hypotension and headache
d. For sublingual nitroglycerin and isosorbide dinitrate, instruct the client to place the tablets under the tongue until they dissolve.	
e. For oral isosorbide dinitrate, both regular and chewable tablets are available. Be sure each type of tablet is taken appropriately.	
f. For sublingual nitroglycerin, check the expiration date on the container.	Sublingual tablets of nitroglycerin are volatile. Once the bottle has been opened, they become ineffective after about 6 months and should be replaced.
g. To apply nitroglycerin ointment, use the special paper to measure the dose. Place the ointment on a nonhairy part of the body and apply with the applicator paper. Cover the area with plastic wrap or tape. Rotate application sites.	The measured paper must be used for accurate dosage. The paper is used to apply the ointment because the drug is readily absorbed through the skin. Skin contact should be avoided except on the designated area of the body. Plastic wrap or tape aids absorption and prevents removal of the drug. It also prevents soiling of clothes and linens. Application sites should be rotated because the ointment can irritate the skin.
h. For nitroglycerin patches, apply at the same time each day to clean, dry, hairless areas on the upper body or arms. Rotate sites. Avoid applying below the knee or elbow or in areas of skin irritation or scar tissue.	To promote effective and consistent drug absorption. The drug is not as well absorbed from distal portions of the extremities because of decreased blood flow. Rotation of sites decreases skin irritation.
i. For intravenous nitroglycerin, dilute the drug and give by continuous infusion, with frequent monitoring of	The drug should not be given by direct intravenous injection. The drug is potent and may cause hypotension. Dosage (flow

Nursing Actions	Rationale/Explanation
blood pressure and heart rate. Use only with the special administration set supplied by the manufacturer to avoid drug adsorption onto tubing.	rate) is adjusted according to response (pain relief or drop in systolic blood pressure of 20 mm Hg).
j. With intravenous verapamil, inject slowly, over 2 to 3 minutes.	To decrease hypotension and other adverse effects
2. Observe for therapeutic effects	
a. Relief of chest pain with acute attacks	Sublingual nitroglycerin usually relieves pain within 5 minutes. If pain is not relieved, two additional tablets may be given, 5 minutes apart. If pain is not relieved after 3 tablets, report to the physician.
b. Reduced incidence and severity of acute attacks with prophylactic antianginal drugs	
c. Increased exercise tolerance	
3. Observe for adverse effects	
a. With nitrates, observe for (1) Hypotension, dizziness, lightheadedness, tachycardia, palpitations, headache	Adverse effects are extensions of pharmacologic action. Vasodilation causes hypotension, which in turn causes dizziness from cerebral hypoxia and tachycardia from compensatory sympathetic nervous system stimulation. Hypotension can decrease blood flow to coronary arteries and precipitate angina pectoris or myocardial infarction. Hypotension is most likely to occur within an hour after drug administration. Vasodilation also causes headache, the most common adverse effect of nitrates.
b. With beta-adrenergic blocking agents, observe for (1) Hypotension, bradycardia, bronchospasm, congestive heart failure	Beta blockers lower blood pressure by decreasing myocardial contractility and cardiac output. Excessive bradycardia may contribute to hypotension and cardiac dysrhythmias. Bronchospasm is more likely to occur in clients with asthma or other chronic respiratory problems.
c. With calcium channel blockers, observe for (1) Hypotension, dizziness, lightheadedness, weakness, peripheral edema, headache, congestive heart failure, pulmonary edema, nausea, constipation. Bradycardia may occur with verapamil and diltiazem.	Adverse effects result primarily from reduced smooth muscle contractility. These effects, except constipation, are much more likely to occur with nifedipine. Nifedipine may cause profound hypotension, which activates the compensatory mechanisms of the sympathetic nervous system and the renin–angiotensin–aldosterone system. Peripheral edema may require the administration of a diuretic. Constipation is more likely to occur with verapamil. Diltiazem reportedly causes the fewest adverse effects of the three drugs.
4. Observe for drug interactions	
a. Drugs that *increase* effects of antianginal drugs	
(1) Antiarrhythmics, antihypertensive drugs, diuretics, phenothiazine antipsychotic agents	Additive hypotension
(2) Cimetidine	May increase beta-blocking effects of propranolol by slowing its hepatic clearance and elimination
(3) Digitalis glycosides	Additive bradycardia when given with beta-blocking agents
b. Drugs that *decrease* effects of antianginal drugs	
(1) Adrenergic drugs (*e.g.,* epinephrine, isoproterenol)	Adrenergic drugs, which stimulate beta receptors, can reverse bradycardia induced by beta blockers.
(2) Anticholinergic drugs	Drugs with anticholinergic effects can increase heart rate, offsetting slower heart rates produced by beta blockers.
(3) Calcium salts	May decrease therapeutic effectiveness of calcium channel blockers.

Nursing Actions	***Rationale/Explanation***
5. Teach clients	
a. Take the drugs only as prescribed. Do not increase dosage or discontinue the drugs without specific instructions from the physician.	Dosage of antianginal drugs must be individualized to maximize therapeutic effects and minimize adverse effects. Discontinuing antianginal drugs abruptly has been associated with increased anginal episodes and possibly myocardial infarctions.
b. With sublingual nitroglycerin, store tablets in the original glass container, in a cool place. Check the expiration date periodically and carry tablets so that they are always within reach but not where they will be exposed to body heat.	Nitroglycerin sublingual tablets lose their potency after 6 to 12 months or more rapidly if exposed to light and heat. Tablets should be readily accessible if an acute attack of angina occurs.
c. Record the number and severity of anginal episodes daily, along with the number of nitroglycerin tablets required to relieve the attack and the total number of tablets taken daily.	Antianginal drugs are most often given on an outpatient basis. Information from the client is necessary to monitor both therapeutic and adverse effects of drug therapy.
d. Headaches and dizziness may occur when antianginal drugs are started. These effects are usually transient and dissipate with continued therapy. If they persist or prevent normal activities of daily living, report to the physician.	Dosage may need to be reduced.
e. If dizziness occurs, avoid strenuous activity and assume an upright position slowly for about 1 hour after taking the drugs.	Dizziness is caused by a temporary decrease in blood pressure. It is most likely to occur when changing position from lying or sitting to standing and during the first hour after drug administration.

Selected References

American Medical Association (AMA) Division of Drugs: AMA Drug Evaluations, 5th ed. New York, John Wiley & Sons, 1983

Boden WE: Calcium antagonists. I. New roles in angina therapy. Drug Ther 15:49–61, October 1985

Burden LL, Atwell K: The treacherous waters of unstable angina pectoris. Nursing 13:50–55, July 1983

Butler JD, Harrison BL: Keeping up with calcium channel blockers. Nursing 13:38–43, July 1983

Connor WE, Bristow JD: Coronary Heart Disease: Prevention, Complications, and Treatment. Philadelphia, J B Lippincott, 1985

Hansten PD: Drug Interactions: Clinical Significance of Drug–Drug Interactions, 5th ed. Philadelphia, Lea & Febiger, 1985

Harralson AF: Angina pectoris. In Herfindal ET, Hirschman JL (eds): Clinical Pharmacy and Therapeutics, 3rd ed, pp 366–379. Baltimore, Williams & Wilkins, 1984

Johnson GP, Johanson BC: Beta blockers. Am J Nurs 82:1034–1043, July 1983

Katy RJ: New approaches to angina. Drug Ther 14:102–108, June 1984

Lute EJ: Calcium blockers: The important differences. RN 47:36–39, June 1984

Malseed RT: Pharmacology: Drug Therapy and Nursing Considerations, 2d ed. Philadelphia, J B Lippincott, 1985

Needleman P, Corr PB, Johnson EM Jr: Drugs used for the treatment of angina; organic nitrates, calcium channel blockers, and beta-adrenergic antagonists. In Gilman AG, Goodman LS, Rall TW, Murad F (eds): The Pharmacological Basis of Therapeutics, 7th ed, pp 806–826. New York, Macmillan, 1985

Nitroglycerin patches. Med Lett Drugs Ther 26:59–60, June 1984

Rossi L, Antman E: Calcium channel blockers: New treatment for cardiovascular disease. Am J Nurs 83:382–387, March 1983

Touloukian JE: Calcium channel blocking agents: Physiologic basis of nursing interventions. Heart Lung 14:342–349, July 1985

54

DRUGS USED IN HYPOTENSION AND SHOCK

Description and uses

Shock is a clinical syndrome characterized by decreased blood supply to tissues. Clinical symptoms depend on the degree of impaired perfusion of vital organs (*e.g.*, brain, heart, and kidneys). Common signs and symptoms include oliguria, heart failure, disorientation, clouded sensorium, mental confusion, seizures, cool extremities, and coma. Most, but not all, people in shock are hypotensive. In a previously hypertensive person, shock may be present if a drop in blood pressure of greater than 50 mm Hg has occurred, even if current blood pressure readings are "normal."

Drugs used in the treatment of shock are primarily the adrenergic agents. Adrenergic (sympathomimetic) drugs are discussed more extensively in Chapter 18. In this chapter, the drugs are discussed only in relation to their usage in hypotension and shock. In hypotension and shock, drugs with alpha-adrenergic activity (*e.g.*, norepinephrine, phenylephrine, methoxamine) are used to increase peripheral vascular resistance and raise blood pressure. Drugs with beta-adrenergic activity (*e.g.*, dobutamine, isoproterenol) are used to increase myocardial contractility and heart rate, which in turn raises blood pressure. Several drugs have both alpha- and beta-adrenergic activity (*e.g.*, dopamine, epinephrine, levarterenol, metaraminol). The goal of therapy with these agents is to increase tissue perfusion.

Adrenergic drugs with beta activity may be relatively contraindicated in shock states precipitated or complicated by cardiac arrhythmias. Beta-stimulating drugs should also be used cautiously in cardiogenic shock following myocardial infarction, since increased contractility and heart rate can increase myocardial oxygen consumption and extend the area of infarction.

Individual drugs used in hypotension and shock

Dopamine (Intropin) is a naturally occurring catecholamine that is a precursor to the neurotransmitter norepinephrine. Dopamine is also a central nervous system (CNS) neurotransmitter. Dopamine exerts its actions by stimulating either alpha, beta, or dopaminergic receptors, depending on the dose being used. In addition, dopamine acts indirectly by releasing norepinephrine from sympathetic nerve endings and the adrenal glands. Peripheral dopamine receptors are located in splanchnic and renal vascular beds. Stimulation of dopamine receptors produces vasodilation in the renal circulation and increases urine output. At low doses of 2 to 5 μg/kg/minute, dopamine stimulates dopaminergic receptors. At moderate doses (5 to 10 μg/kg/minute), dopamine also stimulates beta receptors and increases heart rate, myocardial contractility, and blood pressure. At rates higher than 10 μg/kg/minute, beta activity remains, but increasing alpha stimulation overcomes the dopaminergic actions.

Dopamine is particularly useful in hypovolemic and cardiogenic shock. Adequate fluid therapy is necessary for maximal pressor effect of dopamine. Acidosis decreases the effectiveness of dopamine.

Route and dosage ranges

Adults: IV 2 μg/kg/minute initially, gradually increasing to 20 μg/kg/minute if necessary. Prepare by adding 200 mg of dopamine (one 5-ml ampule) to 250 ml of intravenous fluid for a final concentration of 800 μg/ml or to 500 ml intravenous fluid for a final concentration of 400 μg/ml.

Children: Same as adults

Dobutamine (Dobutrex) is a synthetic catecholamine developed to provide an agent with little vascular activity. Dobutamine acts mainly on $beta_1$ receptors in the heart to increase the force of myocardial contraction with minimal increase in heart rate. Dobutamine may also increase blood pressure with large doses. Dobutamine is less likely to induce tachycardia and arrhythmias than dopamine and isoproterenol. It is most useful in cases of shock that require increases in cardiac output without the need for blood pressure support. Dobutamine has a short plasma half-life and therefore must be administered by continuous intravenous infusion. It is rapidly metabolized to inactive metabolites. It is recommended for short-term use only (a few hours).

Route and dosage ranges

Adults: IV 2.5–10 μg/kg/minute, increased to 40 μg/kg/minute if necessary. Reconstitute the 250-mg vial with 10 ml of sterile water or 5% dextrose injection. The resulting solution should be diluted to at least 50 ml with intravenous solution before administering (5000 μg/ml). Add 250 mg of drug to 500 ml of diluent for a concentration of 500 μg/ml.

Epinephrine (Adrenalin) is a naturally occurring hormone produced by the adrenal glands. At low doses, epinephrine stimulates beta receptors, which results in increased cardiac output and bronchodilation. Larger doses act on alpha receptors to increase blood pressure. Epinephrine is the drug of choice for treatment of anaphylactic shock. However, its use in other types of shock is limited because it may produce excessive cardiac stimulation, ventricular arrhythmias, and reduced renal blood flow. In addition, more potent vasoconstrictors are available (*e.g.*, levarterenol). Epinephrine is rapidly inactivated to metabolites, which are excreted by the kidneys. It is usually given by continuous intravenous infusion in treatment of shock. A single intravenous dose may be given in emergencies, such as cardiac arrest.

Routes and dosage ranges

Adults: IV 1–4 μg/minute. Prepare the solution by adding 2 mg (2 ml) of epinephrine injection 1:1000 to 250 or 500 ml of intravenous fluid. The final concentration is 8 or 4 μg/ml, respectively.
IV direct injection, 100–1000 μg of 1:10,000 injection, q 5–15 minutes, injected slowly. Prepare the solution by adding 1 ml epinephrine 1:1000 to 9 ml sodium chloride injection. The final concentration is 100 μg/ml.

Children: IV infusion, 0.025–0.3 μg/kg/minute
IV direct injection, 5–10 μg/kg, slowly

Isoproterenol (Isuprel) is a synthetic catecholamine that acts exclusively on beta receptors to increase heart rate, myocardial contractility, and systolic blood pressure. However, it also stimulates vascular $beta_2$ receptors, which cause vasodilation and may decrease diastolic blood pressure. For this reason, isoproterenol has limited usefulness as a pressor agent. It may also increase myocardial oxygen consumption and decrease coronary artery blood flow, which in turn causes myocardial ischemia. Cardiac arrhythmias may result from excessive beta stimulation. Owing to these limitations, use of isoproterenol is limited to shock associated with slow heart rates and myocardial depression.

Route and dosage ranges

Adults: IV infusion, 0.5–10 μg/minute. Prepare solution by adding 2 mg to 250 ml of intravenous fluid. Final concentration is 8 μg/ml.

Children: IV infusion, 0.05–0.3 μg/kg/minute

Levarterenol (Levophed) is a commercial preparation of the naturally occurring catecholamine, norepinephrine. Levarterenol increases blood pressure primarily by vasoconstriction. It also increases heart rate and force of myocardial contraction. It is useful in cardiogenic and septic shock, but reduced renal blood flow limits its prolonged use.

Route and dosage ranges

Adults: IV infusion, 1–4 μg/minute, up to a maximum of 15 μg/minute. Prepare solution by adding 2 mg to 500 ml of intravenous fluid. Final concentration is 4 μg/ml.

Children: IV infusion, 0.03–0.1 μg/kg/minute

Metaraminol (Aramine) is occasionally used in hypotensive states. Metaraminol acts indirectly by releasing norepinephrine from sympathetic nerve endings. Actions are similar to those of norepinephrine except that metaraminol is less potent and has a longer duration of action.

Routes and dosage ranges

Adults: IM 2–10 mg
IV injection 2–5 mg
IV infusion, add 100–500 mg of metaraminol to 500 ml of intravenous fluid. Adjust flow rate (dosage) to maintain the desired blood pressure.
Children: IM 0.1 mg/kg
IV injection, 0.01 mg/kg
IV infusion, 1 mg/25 ml of diluent. Adjust flow rate to maintain the desired blood pressure.

Methoxamine (Vasoxyl) acts on alpha-adrenergic receptors to cause vasoconstriction, increase peripheral vascular resistance, and raise blood pressure. The drug acts similarly to phenylephrine and is used occasionally in hypotension.

Routes and dosage ranges

Adults: IM 10–20 mg
IV 3–5 mg, slowly
Children: IM 0.25 mg/kg
IV 0.08 mg/kg, slowly

Phenylephrine (Neo-Synephrine) is an adrenergic drug that stimulates alpha-adrenergic receptors. As a result, phenylephrine constricts arterioles and raises both systolic and diastolic blood pressures. Phenylephrine resembles epinephrine but has fewer cardiac effects and a longer duration of action. Reduction of renal and mesenteric blood flow limits prolonged usage.

Routes and dosage ranges

Adults: IV infusion, 100–180 μg/minute initially, then 40–60 μg/minute. Prepare solution by adding 10 or 20 mg of phenylephrine to 500 ml of intravenous fluid. Final concentration is 20 or 40 μg/ml, respectively.
IV injection 100–500 μg
Children: SC, IM 0.1 mg/kg

Principles of therapy: drugs used in hypotension and shock

ASSESSMENT GUIDELINES

Assess the client's condition in relation to hypotension and shock.

1. Identify clients at risk for developing hypotension and shock.
   a. *Hypovolemic shock* is characterized by a decreased circulating blood volume and may occur with acute blood loss, severe burns, or dehydration.
   b. *Cardiogenic shock* is characterized by decreased cardiac output and may result from myocardial infarction, arrhythmias, or valvular disease.
   c. *Septic shock* is characterized by decreased peripheral vascular resistance. It most often results from gram-negative bacterial infections but may occur with gram-positive infections as well.
   d. *Anaphylactic shock* is characterized by decreased peripheral vascular resistance. It may result from a hypersensitivity (allergic) reaction to drugs or other substances (see Chap. 18).
2. Assess high-risk clients for signs and symptoms.
   a. Check blood pressure, heart rate, urine output, skin temperature of extremities, level of consciousness, orientation to person, place, and time, and adequacy of respiration. Abnormal values are not specific indicators of hypotension and shock, but they may indicate a need for further evaluation. Generally, report blood pressure below 90/60, heart rate above 100, and urine output below 50 ml/hour.
   b. Check electrocardiographic and other assessment data if available.

PREVENTIVE NURSING INTERVENTIONS

Use measures to prevent or minimize hypotension and shock.

1. General measures include those to maintain fluid balance, control hemorrhage, treat infections, prevent hypoxia, and control other causative factors.
2. Learn to recognize *impending* shock so that treatment can be initiated early. *Do not wait* until symptoms are severe.

GUIDELINES FOR TREATMENT OF HYPOTENSION AND SHOCK

1. Vasopressor drugs are less effective in the presence of inadequate blood volume, electrolyte abnormalities, and acidosis. These conditions must also be treated if present.
2. Septic shock requires appropriate antibiotic therapy in addition to other treatment measures. If an

abscess is the source of infection, it must be surgically drained.

3. Hypovolemic shock is most effectively treated by intravenous fluids that replace the type of fluid lost; that is, blood loss should be replaced with whole blood, and gastrointestinal losses should be replaced with solutions containing electrolytes (*e.g.*, Ringer's lactate or sodium chloride solutions with added potassium chloride).
4. Cardiogenic shock may be complicated by pulmonary congestion, in which diuretic drugs are indicated.

NURSING ACTIONS: DRUGS USED IN HYPOTENSION AND SHOCK

Nursing Actions	*Rationale/Explanation*
1. Administer accurately	
a. Use a large vein for the venipuncture site (*e.g.*, the antecubital vein). Tape the needle or catheter securely. Use arm boards and other devices to restrict movement if necessary.	To decrease risks of extravasation
b. Dilute drugs for continuous infusion in 250 or 500 ml of intravenous fluid. A 5% dextrose injection is compatible with all of the drugs and is most often used. For use of other intravenous fluids, consult drug manufacturers' literature. Dilute drugs for bolus injections to at least 10 ml with sodium chloride or water for injection.	To avoid adverse effects, which are more likely to occur with concentrated drug solutions.
c. Use a separate intravenous line or a "piggyback" intravenous setup.	This allows the adrenergic drug solution to be regulated or discontinued without disruption of other intravenous lines.
d. Use an infusion pump.	To administer the drug at a consistent rate. This helps to prevent wide fluctuations in blood pressure and other cardiovascular functions.
e. Discard any solution with a brownish color or precipitate.	Most of the solutions are stable for 24 to 48 hours. Epinephrine and isoproterenol decompose on exposure to light, producing a brownish discoloration.
f. Start the adrenergic drug slowly and increase as necessary to obtain desired responses in blood pressure and other parameters of cardiovascular function.	Flow rate (dosage) is titrated according to client response.
g. Stop the drug gradually.	Abrupt discontinuance of pressor drugs may cause "rebound" hypotension.
2. Observe for therapeutic effects	
a. Systolic blood pressure of 80 to 100 mm Hg	These levels are adequate for tissue perfusion. Higher levels may increase cardiac workload, resulting in reflex bradycardia and decreased cardiac output. However, higher levels may be necessary to maintain cerebral blood flow in the elderly.
b. Heart rate of 60 to 100; improved quality of peripheral pulses	These indicate improved tissue perfusion and cardiovascular function.
c. Improved urine output	Increased urine output indicates improved blood flow to the kidneys.
d. Improved skin color and temperature	

Nursing Actions	Rationale/Explanation
e. Pulmonary–capillary wedge pressure between 15 and 20 mm Hg in cardiogenic shock	Normal pulmonary–capillary wedge pressure is 6 to 12 mm Hg. Higher levels are required to maintain cardiac output in cardiogenic shock.
3. Observe for adverse effects	
a. Bradycardia	Reflex bradycardia may occur with levarterenol, metaraminol, methoxamine, and phenylephrine.
b. Tachycardia	This is most likely to occur with isoproterenol but may occur with dopamine and epinephrine.
c. Arrhythmias	Fatal arrhythmias due to excessive adrenergic stimulation of the heart may occur with any of the agents used in hypotension and shock.
d. Hypertension	This is most likely to occur with high doses of levarterenol, metaraminol, methoxamine, and phenylephrine.
e. Hypotension	This is most likely to occur with low doses of dopamine and isoproterenol, owing to vasodilation.
f. Angina pectoris—chest pain, dyspnea, palpitations	All pressor agents may increase myocardial oxygen consumption and induce myocardial ischemia.
g. Tissue necrosis if extravasation occurs	This may occur with extravasation of solutions containing dopamine, levarterenol, metaraminol, and phenylephrine, owing to local vasoconstriction and impaired blood supply. Tissue necrosis may be prevented by injecting 5 to 10 mg of phentolamine (Regitine), subcutaneously, around the area of extravasation. Regitine is most effective if injected within 12 hours after extravasation.
4. Observe for drug interactions	
a. Drugs that *increase* effects of pressor agents	
(1) General anesthetics (*e.g.,* halothane)	Halothane and other halogenated anesthetics increase cardiac sensitivity to sympathomimetic drugs and increase the risks of cardiac arrhythmias.
(2) Anticholinergic drugs (*e.g.,* atropine)	Atropine and other drugs with anticholinergic activity may potentiate the tachycardia that often occurs with pressor agents, especially isoproterenol.
(3) Monoamine oxidase (MAO) inhibitors (*e.g.,* tranylcypromine)	All effects of exogenously administered adrenergic drugs are magnified in clients taking MAO inhibitors, since MAO is the circulating enzyme responsible for metabolism of adrenergic agents.
(4) Oxytocics (*e.g.,* oxytocin)	The risk of severe hypertension is increased.
b. Drugs that *decrease* effects of pressor agents	
(1) Beta-blocking agents (*e.g.,* propranolol)	Beta-blocking agents antagonize the cardiac stimulation produced by some pressor agents (*e.g.,* dobutamine, isoproterenol). Decreased heart rate, myocardial contractility and blood pressure may result.
5. Teach clients	
a. Report pain, edema, or cool skin around the venipuncture site.	These symptoms may indicate leakage of the drug solution into surrounding tissues. If extravasation occurs, prompt treatment may prevent severe tissue damage.
b. That frequent measurements of blood pressure, pulse and other observations are necessary.	Knowing what to expect will decrease the client's anxiety.

Selected References

Barrows JJ: Shock demands drugs—but which one's best for your patient? Nursing 12:34–41, February 1982.

Cantwell R, Hollis R, Rogers MP: Think fast—what do you know about cardiac drugs for a code? Nursing 12:34–41, October 1982.

Guyton AC: Textbook of Medical Physiology, 7th ed. Philadelphia, W B Saunders, 1986

Hansten PD: Drug Interactions: Clinical Significance of Drug–Drug Interactions, 5th ed. Philadelphia, Lea & Febiger, 1985

Malseed RT: Pharmacology: Drug Therapy and Nursing Considerations, 2d ed. Philadelphia, J B Lippincott, 1985

Nursing care of the patient in shock. I. Pharmacotherapy. Am J Nurs 82:943–964, June 1982

Purcell JA: Shock drugs: Standardized guidelines. Am J Nurs 82:965–974, June 1982

55

ANTIHYPERTENSIVE DRUGS

Description and uses

Antihypertensive drugs are used to treat hypertension (high blood pressure), a common, chronic disorder affecting an estimated 60 million people in the United States. Hypertension increases risks of congestive heart failure, cerebral infarction and hemorrhage, coronary artery disease, and renal disease. To understand hypertension and antihypertensive drug therapy, one must first understand the physiologic mechanisms that normally control blood pressure, characteristics of hypertension, and characteristics of antihypertensive drugs.

REGULATION OF ARTERIAL BLOOD PRESSURE

Arterial blood pressure reflects the force exerted on arterial walls by blood flow. Blood pressure normally stays relatively constant because of homeostatic mechanisms that are able to adjust blood flow. The two major determinants of arterial blood pressure are cardiac output and peripheral vascular resistance. Cardiac output equals the product of the heart rate and stroke volume ($CO = HR \times SV$). Stroke volume is the amount of blood ejected with each heartbeat (approximately 60 to 90 ml). Thus, cardiac output depends on blood volume and other cardiovascular factors. Peripheral vascular resistance is determined by the degree of constriction or dilation in arterioles (vascular tone). Any condition that affects heart rate, stroke volume, or peripheral resistance affects systemic arterial blood pressure.

Regulation of blood pressure involves a complex network of nervous, hormonal, and renal mechanisms. The nervous and hormonal mechanisms act rapidly; renal mechanisms act more slowly. When hypotension occurs, the sympathetic nervous system (SNS) is stimulated, the hormones epinephrine and norepinephrine are secreted by the adrenal medulla, angiotensin II and aldosterone are formed, and the kidneys retain fluid. These compensatory mechanisms act to raise the blood pressure. Specific effects include the following:

1. Constriction of arterioles, which increases peripheral vascular resistance
2. Constriction of veins and increased venous tone
3. Stimulation of cardiac beta-adrenergic receptors, which increases heart rate and force of myocardial contraction
4. Secretion of renin by the kidneys. In the bloodstream, renin acts on a plasma protein to produce angiotensin I, which is converted to angiotensin II by the enzyme peptidyl dipeptidase. Angiotensin II is a potent vasoconstrictor. It constricts arterioles and increases peripheral resistance. It also stimulates secretion of aldosterone by the adrenal cortex. Aldosterone causes the kidneys to retain sodium and water.
5. Retention of fluid by the kidneys, which increases blood volume and cardiac output

When arterial blood pressure is elevated, the following sequence of events occurs:

1. Kidneys excrete more fluid (increase urine output).
2. Fluid loss reduces both extracellular fluid volume and blood volume.
3. Decreased blood volume reduces venous blood flow to the heart and therefore decreases cardiac output.
4. Decreased cardiac output reduces arterial blood pressure.

HYPERTENSION

Hypertension is a persistently high blood pressure that results from abnormalities in the regulatory mechanisms described above. It is usually defined as a systolic pressure above 140 mm Hg or a diastolic pressure above 90 mm Hg on multiple blood pressure measurements.

Primary or essential hypertension, that for which no cause can be found, comprises about 90% of known cases. Secondary hypertension may result from renal, endocrine, or central nervous system (CNS) disorders as well as drugs that stimulate the SNS or cause retention of sodium and water. Primary hypertension can be controlled with appropriate therapy, but it cannot be cured. Secondary hypertension can sometimes be cured by surgical therapy, but the number of clients involved is small (5% to 10%). Hypertension is also described as mild (diastolic pressure 90 to 104), moderate (diastolic pressure 105 to 114), and severe (diastolic pressure above 115). A diastolic pressure below 90 with a systolic pressure of 160 or above is usually called isolated systolic hypertension.

Hypertension profoundly alters cardiovascular function by increasing the workload of the heart and causing thickening and sclerosis of arterial walls. As a result of increased cardiac workload, the myocardium hypertrophies as a compensatory mechanism. However, heart failure eventually occurs. As a result of arterial changes, the lumen is narrowed, blood supply to tissues is decreased, and risks of thrombosis are increased. In addition, necrotic areas may develop in arteries, and these may rupture with sustained high blood pressure. The areas of most serious damage are the heart, brain, kidneys, and eyes. These are often called "target organs."

Initially and perhaps for years, primary hypertension may produce no symptoms. If symptoms occur, they are usually vague and nonspecific. Hypertension may go undetected or it may be incidentally discovered when blood pressure measurements are done as part of a routine physical examination, screening test, or assessment of other disorders. Eventually, symptoms reflect target organ damage. Not infrequently, hypertension is discovered after a person experiences angina pectoris, myocardial infarction, congestive heart failure, stroke, or renal disease. In some people, a syndrome called malignant or accelerated hypertension occurs in which severe hypertension and target organ damage develop rapidly and may cause death within 1 to 2 years.

Hypertensive crisis is a severely elevated blood pressure that may be an extension of malignant hypertension or caused by cerebral hemorrhage, dissecting aortic aneurysm, renal disease, pheochromocytoma, or eclampsia. Hypertensive crisis is a medical emergency that requires immediate lowering of blood pressure. Symptoms include severe headache, nausea, vomiting, visual disturbances, neurologic disturbances, disorientation, and decreased level of consciousness (drowsiness, stupor, coma).

ANTIHYPERTENSIVE DRUGS

Drugs used in the treatment of primary hypertension belong to four groups: diuretics, antiadrenergics, vasodilators, and angiotensin-converting enzyme (ACE) inhibitors. These drugs generally act to decrease blood pressure by decreasing cardiac output, peripheral vascular resistance, blood volume, or renin release from the kidneys.

Diuretics

The exact mechanism by which diuretics decrease blood pressure is not known. Antihypertensive effects are usually attributed to sodium and water depletion. In fact, diuretic drugs generally produce the same effects as severe dietary sodium restriction. In many cases of mild hypertension, diuretic therapy alone may lower blood pressure. When diuretic therapy is begun, blood volume and cardiac output decrease. With long-term administration of a diuretic, cardiac output returns to normal, but there is a persistent decrease in peripheral vascular resistance. This has been attributed to a persistent small reduction in extracellular water and plasma volume, decreased receptor sensitivity to vasopressor substances such as angiotensin, direct arteriolar vasodilatation, and arteriolar vasodilatation secondary to electrolyte depletion in the vessel wall.

In moderate or severe hypertension that does not respond to diuretics alone, the diuretic is continued and another antihypertensive drug is added. Most nondiuretic antihypertensive agents cause retention of sodium and water. Diuretics are given to prevent sodium and water retention. Diuretics therefore potentiate the antihypertensive effects of other agents.

The most commonly used diuretics are the thiazides (*e.g.,* hydrochlorothiazide [HydroDiuril]). Others are useful in particular circumstances. See Chapter 56 for more information regarding diuretic drugs.

Antiadrenergics

Antiadrenergic (sympatholytic) drugs inhibit activity of the SNS. When the SNS is stimulated (see Chap. 17), the nerve impulse travels from the brain and spinal cord to the ganglia. From the ganglia, the impulse travels along postganglionic fibers to effector organs (*e.g.*, heart, blood vessels). Although SNS stimulation produces widespread effects in the body, the effects relevant to this discussion are the increases in heart rate, force of myocardial contraction, cardiac output, and blood pressure that occur. When the nerve impulse is inhibited or blocked at any location along its pathway, the result is decreased blood pressure.

Antiadrenergic antihypertensive drugs are often subclassified as centrally or peripherally acting agents. Some drugs have both central and peripheral actions. The centrally active drugs, methyldopa, clonidine, and guanabenz, block SNS impulses in the brain. Propranolol and reserpine may also have central actions but are primarily peripherally acting agents. Peripherally active drugs include trimethaphan camsylate, which acts at ganglionic sites; guanethidine, guanadrel, and reserpine, which act at postganglionic nerve endings; prazosin, an alpha-adrenergic blocking agent that acts to dilate blood vessels and decrease peripheral vascular resistance; and beta-adrenergic blocking agents (*e.g.*, propranolol, others) that act to decrease heart rate, force of myocardial contraction, cardiac output, and renin release from the kidneys.

Two other alpha-adrenergic blocking agents, phentolamine and phenoxybenzamine, are occasionally used in hypertension resulting from catecholamine excess. These drugs are discussed in Chapter 19.

Vasodilators

Vasodilator antihypertensive drugs act directly on blood vessels to cause dilation and decreased peripheral vascular resistance. Hydralazine, diazoxide, and minoxidil act mainly on arterioles; nitroprusside and prazosin act on both arterioles and venules. These drugs have limited effect on hypertension when used alone because the vasodilating action that lowers blood pressure also stimulates the SNS and arouses reflexive compensatory mechanisms (vasoconstriction, tachycardia, and increased cardiac output), which raise blood pressure. This effect can be prevented during long-term therapy by also giving a drug that prevents excessive sympathetic stimulation (*e.g.*, propranolol). These drugs also cause sodium and water retention, which may be minimized by giving a diuretic concomitantly.

Angiotensin-converting enzyme inhibitors

Captopril (Capoten) and enalapril (Vasotec) represent a newer group of antihypertensive drugs. They act by interfering with the renin–angiotensin system of blood pressure control. More specifically, they block the enzyme that normally converts the physiologically inactive angiotensin I to the potent vasoconstrictor angiotensin II.

In clients with normal renal function, ACE inhibitors may be used alone or in combination with other antihypertensive agents such as thiazide diuretics. In clients with impaired renal function, the drugs are recommended for those who fail to respond or who experience intolerable adverse effects with other antihypertensive agents.

Captopril is also used in the treatment of congestive heart failure, in which it decreases vasoconstriction and cardiac workload. Enalapril is approved for use in the treatment of hypertension and is being studied for use in congestive heart failure. It has a slightly different chemical structure than captopril and reportedly causes fewer adverse effects.

Other antihypertensive drugs

Drugs from a number of groups have become obsolete in the treatment of hypertension. One such group includes sedatives and tranquilizers. Although they are still included in some treatment protocols, these drugs do not lower peripheral vascular resistance or cardiac output and have no place in the treatment of hypertension. Another group is the ganglionic blocking agents. Since these drugs block both sympathetic and parasympathetic functions, their side-effects limit their usefulness. Trimethaphan or other ganglionic blockers may be used parenterally in treating hypertensive crises, but they have largely been replaced by the parenteral vasodilators diazoxide and nitroprusside or by oral minoxidil or captopril.

A third group is the antihypertensive monoamine oxidase (MAO) inhibitors. Pargyline (Eutonyl) is the only commercially available MAO inhibitor used in hypertension. Pargyline may interact with many foods and drugs to cause hypertensive crisis. This characteristic, plus the availability of other agents that are safer and more effective, has rendered pargyline obsolete in hypertension. However, other MAO inhibitors (isocarboxazid [Marplan], phenelzine [Nardil], and tranylcypromine [Parnate]) are occasionally used in treatment of depression (see Chap. 10). A fourth group, the veratrum alkaloids (*e.g.*, cryptenamine [Unitensin]), were formerly important antihypertensive drugs. They are no longer used clinically because of a high incidence of adverse reactions and the availability of safer and more effective drugs.

Individual drugs

Diuretics are discussed in Chapter 56 and listed in Table 56-1. Antihypertensive agents are shown in Table 55-1; antihypertensive-diuretic combination products are listed in Table 55-2.

Principles of therapy: antihypertensive drugs

ASSESSMENT GUIDELINES

Assess the client's condition in relation to hypertension.

1. Identify conditions and risk factors that may lead to hypertension. These include the following:
   a. Obesity
   b. Elevated serum cholesterol and triglycerides
   c. Cigarette smoking
   d. Sedentary lifestyle
   e. Family history of hypertension or other cardiovascular disease
   f. Black race
   g. Renal disease (*e.g.*, renal artery stenosis)
   h. Adrenal disease (*e.g.*, hypersecretion of aldosterone, pheochromocytoma)
   i. Other cardiovascular disorders (*e.g.*, arteriosclerosis, left ventricular hypertrophy)
   j. Diabetes mellitus
   k. Oral contraceptives, corticosteroids, appetite suppressants, decongestants, nonsteroidal anti-inflammatory agents
   l. Neurologic disorders (*e.g.*, brain damage)
2. Observe for signs and symptoms of hypertension.
   a. Check blood pressure accurately and repeatedly. As a rule, multiple measurements in which systolic pressure is above 140 mm Hg or diastolic pressure is above 90 mm Hg, or both, are necessary to establish a diagnosis of hypertension. Single measurements provide little useful information.

      The importance of accurate blood pressure measurements cannot be overemphasized because there are many possibilities for errors. Some ways to improve accuracy and validity include using correct equipment (*e.g.*, proper cuff size), having the client in the same position each time blood pressure is measured (*e.g.*, sitting or supine with arm at heart level), using the same arm for repeated measurements, and having the same person do successive recordings on a particular client.
   b. In most cases of early hypertension, elevated blood pressure is the only clinical manifestation. If symptoms do occur, they are usually nonspecific (*e.g.*, headache, weakness, fatigue, tachycardia, dizziness, palpitations, epistaxis).
   c. Eventually, signs and symptoms occur as target organs are damaged. Heart damage is often reflected as angina pectoris, myocardial infarction, or congestive heart failure. Chest pain, tachycardia, dyspnea, fatigue, and edema may occur. Brain damage may be indicated by transient ischemic attacks (TIAs) or strokes of varying severity with symptoms ranging from syncope to hemiparesis. Renal damage may be reflected by proteinuria, increased blood urea nitrogen (BUN), and increased serum creatinine. Ophthalmoscopic examination may reveal hemorrhages, sclerosis of arterioles, and inflammation of the optic nerve (papilledema). Since arterioles can be visualized in the retina of the eye, damage to retinal vessels may indicate damage to arterioles in the heart, brain, and kidneys.

NURSING INTERVENTIONS

Implement measures to prevent or minimize hypertension. Preventive measures are mainly lifestyle changes to reduce risk factors. These measures must be started in childhood and continued throughout life. Once hypertension is diagnosed, lifetime adherence to a therapeutic regimen may be necessary to control the disease and prevent complications. The role of the nurse is important in the prevention, early detection, and treatment of hypertension. Some guidelines for intervention at community, family, and personal levels include the following:

1. Participate in community programs to promote proper nutrition; avoid obesity; avoid excessive ingestion of salt, meat, and dairy products; and decrease cigarette smoking.
2. Participate in screening programs and make appropriate referrals when abnormal blood pressures are detected. If hypertension develops in women

TABLE 55-1. ANTIHYPERTENSIVE DRUGS

	Generic name	Trade name	Routes and dosage ranges: Adults	Routes and dosage ranges: Children
Antiadrenergic agents				
Centrally active drugs	Clonidine	Catapres	PO 0.1 mg 2 times daily initially, gradually increased if necessary up to 2.4 mg/day. Average daily maintenance dose, 0.2–0.8 mg	
	Guanabenz	Wytensin	PO 4 mg twice daily, increased by 4–8 mg daily every 1–2 weeks if necessary to a maximal dose of 32 mg twice daily	
	Methyldopa	Aldomet	PO 250 mg 2–3 times daily initially, increased gradually at intervals of not less than 2 days until blood pressure is controlled or a daily dose of 3 g is reached	PO 10 mg/kg/day in 2–4 divided doses initially, increased or decreased according to response. Maximal dose, 65 mg/kg/day or 3 g daily, whichever is less
Ganglionic blocking agent	Trimethaphan camsylate	Arfonad	Hypertensive crisis, IV diluted in 5% dextrose injection to a concentration of 1 mg/ml and given as a continuous infusion at an initial flow rate of 3–4 mg/minute, then individualize rate depending on blood pressure. Rates vary from 0.3–6 mg/minute	
Postganglionic-active drugs	Guanadrel	Hylorel	PO 10 mg daily initially. Usual dosage range, 20–75 mg daily in divided doses	
	Guanethidine sulfate	Ismelin	PO 10 mg daily initially, increased every 5–7 days to a maximal daily dose of 300 mg if necessary. Usual daily dose, 25–50 mg. For hospitalized clients, therapy may be initiated with 25–50 mg daily and increased every 1–2 days	PO 0.2 mg/kg/day initially, increased by the same amount every 7–10 days if necessary to a maximum dose of 3 mg/kg/day
	Reserpine	Serpasil	PO 0.25–0.5 mg daily initially for 1–2 weeks, reduced slowly to 0.1–0.25 mg daily for maintenance	Safety has not been established for use in children
Alpha-adrenergic blocking agent	Prazosin	Minipress	PO 1 mg 2–3 times daily initially, increased if necessary to a total daily dose of 20 mg in divided doses. Average daily maintenance dose, 6–15 mg/day.	
Beta-adrenergic blocking agents	Acebutolol	Sectral	PO 400 mg once daily initially, increased to 800 mg daily if necessary	
	Atenolol	Tenormin	PO 50 mg once daily initially, increased in 1–2 weeks to 100 mg once daily, if necessary	
	Metoprolol	Lopressor	PO 50 mg twice daily, gradually increased in weekly or longer intervals, if necessary, to a maximal daily dose of 450 mg	
	Nadolol	Corgard	PO 40 mg daily initially, gradually increased, if necessary, by 40–80 mg daily. Average daily dose, 80–320 mg	
	Pindolol	Visken	PO 5 mg 2–3 times daily initially, increased by 10 mg/day at 3- to 4-week intervals to a maximal daily dose of 60 mg	
	Propranolol	Inderal	PO 40 mg twice daily initially gradually increased to 160–640 mg daily	PO 1 mg/kg/day initially, gradually increased to a maximum daily dose of 10 mg/kg

	Generic name	Trade name	Routes and dosage ranges: Adults	Routes and dosage ranges: Children
	Timolol	Blocadren	PO 10 mg twice daily initially, increased gradually if necessary. Average daily dose, 20–40 mg; maximal daily dose, 60 mg	
Alpha–beta-adrenergic blocking agent	Labetalol	Trandate, Normodyne	PO 100 mg twice daily, increased by 100 mg twice daily every 2–3 days if necessary. Usual maintenance dose, 200–400 mg twice daily. Severe hypertension may require 1200–2400 mg daily. IV injection, 20 mg slowly over 2 minutes, followed by 40–80 mg every 10 minutes until the desired blood pressure is achieved or 300 mg has been given IV infusion, add 200 mg to 250 ml of 5% dextrose or 0.9% sodium chloride solution (concentration 2 mg/3 ml) and infuse at a rate of 3 ml/minute. Adjust flow rate according to blood pressure and substitute oral labetalol when blood pressure is controlled.	
Direct-acting vasodilators	Diazoxide	Hyperstat	Hypertensive crisis, IV 1–3 mg/kg (up to 150 mg) by rapid injection (within 30 seconds), repeated as necessary at 5- to 15-minute intervals	Hypertensive crisis, same as for adults
	Hydralazine	Apresoline	Chronic hypertension, PO 10 mg 4 times daily for 2–4 days, increase to 25 mg 4 times daily for 2–4 days if necessary, then increase to 50 mg 4 times daily if necessary, to a maximal daily dose of 300 mg Hypertensive crisis, IM, IV 10–20 mg, increased to 40 mg if necessary. Repeat dose as needed	Chronic hypertension, 0.75 mg/kg/day initially in 4 divided doses. Gradually increased over 3–4 weeks to a maximal dose of 7.5 mg/kg/day if necessary. Hypertensive crisis, IM, IV 0.1–0.2 mg/kg/dose every 4–6 hours as needed
	Minoxidil	Loniten	PO 5 mg once daily initially, increased gradually until blood pressure is controlled. Average daily dose, 10–40 mg; maximal daily dose, 100 mg in single or divided doses	Age under 12 years, PO 0.2 mg/kg/day initially as a single dose, increased gradually until blood pressure is controlled. Average daily dose, 0.25–1.0 mg/kg; maximal daily dose, 50 mg
	Sodium nitroprusside	Nipride	IV infusion at a flow rate to deliver 0.5–10 μg/kg/minute. Average dose is 3 μg/kg/minute. Prepare solution by adding 50 mg of sodium nitroprusside to 250–1000 ml of 5% dextrose in water and wrap promptly in aluminum foil to protect from light	Same as for adults
Angiotensin-converting enzyme inhibitors	Captopril	Capoten	PO 25 mg 2–3 times daily initially, increased after 1–2 weeks, if necessary, to 50 mg 2–3 times daily, then to 100 mg 2–3 times daily, then to 150 mg 2–3 times daily. Maximal daily dose, 450 mg	
	Enalapril	Vasotec	PO 5 mg once daily, increased to 10–40 mg daily, in 1 or 2 doses, if necessary	

TABLE 55-2. REPRESENTATIVE ANTIHYPERTENSIVE–DIURETIC COMBINATION PRODUCTS

Trade name	Antihypertensive component	Diuretic component	Route and dosage range
Aldoril-15	Methyldopa 250 mg	Hydrochlorothiazide 15 mg	PO 1 tablet 2–3 times daily for 48 hours, then increased or decreased according to response
Aldoril-25	Methyldopa 250 mg	Hydrochlorothiazide 25 mg	Same as Aldoril-15
Aldoril-D30	Methyldopa 500 mg	Hydrochlorothiazide 30 mg	Same as Aldoril-15
Aldoril-D50	Methyldopa 500 mg	Hydrochlorothiazide 50 mg	Same as Aldoril-15
Capozide	Captopril 25 mg	Hydrochlorothiazide 15 mg	PO 1 tablet 2–3 times daily
	Captopril 25 mg	Hydrochlorothiazide 25 mg	PO 1 tablet 2–3 times daily
	Captopril 50 mg	Hydrochlorothiazide 15 mg	PO 1 tablet 2–3 times daily
	Captopril 50 mg	Hydrochlorothiazide 25 mg	PO 1 tablet 2–3 times daily
Combipres 0.1 mg	Clonidine 0.1 mg	Chlorthalidone 15 mg	PO 1 tablet twice daily
Combipres 0.2 mg	Clonidine 0.2 mg	Chlorthalidone 15 mg	PO 1 tablet twice daily
Combipres 0.3 mg	Clonidine 0.3 mg	Chlorthalidone 15 mg	PO 1 tablet twice daily
Corzide 40/5	Nadolol 40 mg	Bendroflumethazide 5 mg	PO 1 tablet daily
Corzide 80/5	Nadolol 80 mg	Bendroflumethazide 5 mg	PO 1 tablet daily
Hydropres 25	Reserpine 0.125 mg	Hydrochlorothiazide 25 mg	PO 1 tablet 1–4 times daily
Hydropres 50	Reserpine 0.125 mg	Hydrochlorothiazide 50 mg	PO 1 tablet 1–2 times daily
Inderide 40/25	Propranolol 40 mg	Hydrochlorothiazide 25 mg	PO 1–2 tablets twice daily
Inderide 80/25	Propranolol 80 mg	Hydrochlorothiazide 25 mg	PO 1–2 tablets twice daily
Minizide 1	Prazosin 1 mg	Polythiazide 0.5 mg	PO 1 capsule 2–3 times daily
Minizide 2	Prazosin 2 mg	Polythiazide 0.5 mg	PO 1 capsule 2–3 times daily
Minizide 5	Prazosin 5 mg	Polythiazide 0.5 mg	PO 1 capsule 2–3 times daily
Regroton	Reserpine 0.25 mg	Chlorthalidone 50 mg	PO 1–2 tablets daily in a single dose
Demi-Regroton	Reserpine 0.125 mg	Chlorthalidone 25 mg	PO 1–2 tablets daily in a single dose
Serpasil-Esidrix #1	Reserpine 0.1 mg	Hydrochlorothiazide 25 mg	PO 2 tablets daily in single or divided doses
Serpasil-Esidrix #2	Reserpine 0.1 mg	Hydrochlorothiazide 50 mg	PO 2 tablets daily in single or divided doses
Ser-Ap-Es	Reserpine 0.1 mg Hydralazine 25 mg	Hydrochlorothiazide 15 mg	PO 1–2 tablets 2–3 times daily
Tenoretic 50	Atenolol 50 mg	Chlorthalidone 25 mg	PO 1 tablet daily
Tenoretic 100	Atenolol 100 mg	Chlorthalidone 25 mg	PO 1 tablet daily
Timolide	Timolol 10 mg	Hydrochlorothiazide 25 mg	PO 1–2 tablets 1–2 times daily

taking oral contraceptives, the drug is usually discontinued for 3 to 6 months to see whether blood pressure decreases without antihypertensive drugs.

3. Assist the hypertensive client to comply with prescribed therapy. Noncompliance is high among clients with hypertension. Reasons often given for noncompliance include lack of symptoms, lack of motivation and self-discipline to make needed lifestyle changes (*e.g.*, lose weight, stop smoking, restrict salt intake), perhaps experiencing more symptoms from medications than from hypertension, cost of therapy, and failure to realize the importance of treatment, especially as related to prevention of major cardiovascular diseases (myocardial infarction, stroke, and death). In addition, several studies have shown that compliance decreases as the number of drugs and number of doses increase.

The nurse can help increase client compliance by teaching about hypertension, assisting to make necessary lifestyle changes, and maintaining close personal supervision. Losing weight, stopping smoking, and other changes are most likely to be effective if attempted one at a time.

THERAPEUTIC REGIMENS

Once the diagnosis of hypertension is established, a therapeutic regimen must be designed and implemented. For clients with mild or borderline hypertension (blood pressure 140/90 or slightly above), weight loss and salt restriction alone may lower blood pressure. For most clients, however, drug therapy is required. One effective regimen is called the "stepped-care" approach, in which drugs are added in a stepwise fashion as necessary to control blood pressure. The steps are outlined as follows:

Step I. A thiazide diuretic (*e.g.*, hydrochlorothiazide) or a beta blocker (*e.g.*, propranolol) is begun at minimal dosage and increased if necessary. This regimen may be adequate to control blood pressure.

Step II. If the diuretic or beta blocker does not lower blood pressure sufficiently, it is continued and a second antihypertensive drug is added. Step II drugs include beta blockers, captopril, clonidine, guanabenz, methyldopa, prazosin, and reserpine. The chosen drug is started at low dosage and increased if necessary. If a beta-blocking agent was the step I drug, a diuretic may be added for step II.

Step III. If blood pressure is still not lowered sufficiently, the above drugs are continued and hydralazine or captopril is added as the third drug.

Step IV. For resistant hypertension, guanethidine, minoxidil, or captopril may be added as a fourth drug.

Several weeks may be necessary before optimal drugs and dosages are known. The goal of drug therapy for most clients is achievement and maintenance of normal blood pressure range (below 140/90) without intolerable adverse effects. If this goal cannot be achieved, lowering blood pressure to any extent is still considered beneficial in decreasing incidence of coronary artery disease and stroke.

DRUG SELECTION

Choice of antihypertensive drugs depends primarily on client characteristics and responses. Some guidelines include the following:

1. Diuretics are preferred for initial therapy in clients aged 50 years or older, those who are black, those with peripheral vascular disease, those with asthma or other forms of chronic obstructive pulmonary disease, those with low renin hypertension, or those with labile diabetes. Thiazide and related diuretics are equally effective in lowering blood pressure. Hydrochlorothiazide (HydroDiuril) is commonly used.
2. Beta-blocking agents are increasingly being used alone or as step I therapy. They are especially likely to be effective in clients under 50 years of age with high renin hypertension, tachycardia, palpitations, ischemic heart disease, or left ventricular hypertrophy.
    a. Most beta blockers are approved for use in hypertension and are probably equally effective. However, acebutolol (Sectral), atenolol (Tenormin), or metoprolol (Lopressor) is preferred for clients with asthma, peripheral vascular disease, or insulin-dependent diabetes mellitus. These drugs act more specifically to block beta-adrenergic receptors in the heart, have less effect on bronchial and vascular smooth muscle, and have less potentiation of insulin-induced hypoglycemia.
    b. Beta-blocking agents are contraindicated in bradycardia, congestive heart failure, heart block, severe bronchospastic disease, and labile diabetes mellitus, since they produce or aggravate these conditions.
3. Methyldopa (Aldomet) is often used as a step II drug. If not effective, clonidine (Catapres), guanabenz (Wytensin), or captopril (Capoten) may be substituted for methyldopa. The latter drugs may cause more adverse effects than methyldopa. Clonidine and guanabenz often cause drowsiness, dry mouth, and fatigue. Clonidine may also cause severe hypertension if discontinued abruptly. Captopril may cause infrequent but potentially serious renal and hematologic problems.
4. Calcium channel blockers are being investigated for use in hypertension and are probably effective as step II or step III drugs.
5. Hydralazine (Apresoline) is often used as a step III drug. It is most effective when combined with a beta blocker and a diuretic to prevent hypotension-induced compensatory mechanisms (cardiovascular stimulation and fluid retention) that act to raise blood pressure. Minoxidil (Loniten) may be substituted for hydralazine in resistant cases, but it causes more severe adverse effects.
6. Few newly diagnosed hypertensive clients are given reserpine. Most usage involves clients undergoing long-term maintenance regimens.
7. Several drugs are used in the treatment of hypertensive emergencies. Diazoxide (Hyperstat) and nitroprusside (Nipride) have often been used, but newer agents such as labetalol (Trandate), captopril (Capoten), and minoxidil (Loniten) are also effective. Nifedipine (Procardia), a calcium channel blocker, has been given orally (by having the client chew the capsule) and sublingually (by piercing the capsule and placing the contents under the client's tongue).
8. Numerous combination products are available for treatment of hypertension. Most contain a beta blocker, methyldopa, reserpine, clonidine, hydralazine, or prazosin as the antihypertensive component and a thiazide or related diuretic as the diuretic component. Most of these products are available in several formulations in which the amounts of the diuretic and the antihypertensive agent vary (see Table 55-2).

    Combination products are not recommended for use in initial treatment of hypertension because the dosage of each ingredient should be individualized. However, if individualized dosages of ingredients are compatible with a combination product, the combination product may be used for long-term maintenance therapy. A combination product may aid compliance with the treatment regimen by reducing the number of tablets or capsules taken daily.

DOSAGE FACTORS

1. Dosage of antihypertensive drugs must be titrated according to individual response. Generally, dosage is started at minimal levels and increased if necessary. Several drugs, including thiazide diuretics, have been found effective at lower doses than formerly used. Lower doses decrease the incidence and severity of adverse effects.
2. For many clients, it may be more beneficial to add another drug rather than increase dosage. Two or three drugs in small doses may be effective and cause fewer adverse effects than a single drug in large doses. When two or more drugs are given, dosage of each drug may need to be reduced.

DURATION OF THERAPY

Clients who are able to achieve and maintain control of their blood pressure for a year or so may be candidates for "step-down" adjustments in their drug therapy; that is, dosages and numbers of drugs may be reduced, and some drugs may even be discontinued. Of course, any such adjustments must be gradual and carefully supervised by a physician. Expected benefits include fewer adverse effects and greater compliance. This concept represents a departure from former thinking that drug therapy was required throughout the client's lifetime.

SODIUM RESTRICTION

Any therapeutic regimen for hypertension includes sodium restriction. Severe restrictions are not generally acceptable to clients; however, moderate restrictions (avoiding heavily salted foods such as cured meats, sandwich meats, pretzels, and potato chips and not adding salt to food at the table) are beneficial and more easily implemented. These statements are based on research studies that indicate the following:

1. Sodium restriction alone reduces blood pressure.
2. Sodium restriction potentiates the antihypertensive actions of diuretics and other antihypertensive drugs. Conversely, excessive sodium intake decreases the antihypertensive actions of all antihypertensive drugs. Patients with unrestricted salt intake who are taking thiazides may lose excessive potassium and become hypokalemic.
3. Sodium restriction may decrease dosage requirements of antihypertensive drugs, thereby decreasing the incidence and severity of adverse effects.

ANTIHYPERTENSIVE DRUGS IN THE PERIOPERATIVE PERIOD

Although opinions differ on continuing or stopping antihypertensive drugs before surgery, the Joint National Committee on Detection, Evaluation, and Treatment of High Blood Pressure recommends that drug therapy be continued until surgery and restarted as soon as possible after surgery. If clients are unable to take drugs orally, parenteral diuretics, antiadrenergic agents, or vasodilators may be given. The anesthesiologist must be informed about the client's medication status.

ANTIHYPERTENSIVE DRUGS IN RENAL IMPAIRMENT

In hypertensive clients with primary renal disease or diabetic nephropathy, drug therapy may slow progression of renal impairment. Sodium retention may be a causative factor, so that diuretics are important in treatment. Thiazides should be used cautiously if at all; relatively large doses of furosemide (Lasix), bumetanide (Bumex), or metolazone (Zaroxolyn) may be required. Antiadrenergics, vasodilators, and ACE inhibitors are usually effective in renal disease. Dosage of captopril and enalapril should be reduced in clients with renal impairment.

ANTIHYPERTENSIVE DRUGS IN PREGNANCY

Few clear-cut guidelines exist for using antihypertensive drugs during pregnancy. However, some factors to be considered include the following:

1. For the hypertensive woman who becomes pregnant, general principles of drug therapy are the same as those for the nonpregnant hypertensive woman. In addition, blood pressure should be lowered gradually, nonpharmacologic measures should be emphasized (*i.e.,* weight control and salt restriction), and serum electrolytes should be closely monitored with diuretic drugs.
2. Although potential adverse effects on the fetus are a concern with any drug therapy during pregnancy, there is no evidence of teratogenicity with antihypertensive drugs given throughout pregnancy. Beta blockers and methyldopa have been used effectively and apparently improve fetal survival. Captopril is contraindicated because of increased fetal mortality in tests with pregnant animals.

3. For women who develop preeclampsia (a syndrome characterized by hypertension, edema, and proteinuria, formerly called toxemia of pregnancy), treatment is controversial. Some physicians use small doses of diuretics and other antihypertensive drugs; others rely mainly on bedrest and magnesium sulfate. Magnesium sulfate depresses the CNS and is given to prevent eclamptic convulsions. However, it also lowers blood pressure to some extent.

PEDIATRIC CONSIDERATIONS

Most principles of managing adult hypertension apply to managing childhood and adolescent hypertension; some additional elements that should be considered include the following:

1. Until the past 10 or 15 years, it was not common practice to measure blood pressure in children. As a result, normal ranges have not been established, incidence of hypertension is not known, and treatment is not well defined.
2. Blood pressure is probably more labile in children and adolescents. Therefore, multiple measurements are especially important in diagnosis of hypertension.
3. Young people have a greater incidence of secondary hypertension than adults. Diagnostic tests may be needed to rule out renovascular disease or coarctation of the aorta in those under 18 years of age with blood pressure above 140/90 and young children with blood pressures above the ninety-fifth percentile for their age group. Oral contraceptives may cause secondary hypertension in adolescents.
4. Once primary or essential hypertension is diagnosed, a therapeutic program must be instituted. Long-term effects of antihypertensive drugs on growth and development are unknown. Therefore, sodium restriction and weight reduction, if needed, may be preferred initially. If this approach is unsuccessful, diuretics, antiadrenergics, and vasodilators are indicated, especially for those with significantly elevated blood pressures or target organ involvement. The fewest drugs and the lowest doses should be used. Thus, if a step I drug is not effective, it may be better to give another single drug than to add a second drug to the regimen.
5. Some guidelines for choosing drugs are as follows:
   a. Thiazide diuretics do not commonly produce hyperglycemia, hyperuricemia, or hypercalcemia in children as they do in adults.
   b. Spironolactone (Aldactone) may alter menstrual cycles and cause emotional stress in adolescents. The drug commonly produces gynecomastia in young males, requiring cessation of the drug.
   c. Propranolol (Inderal) and other beta-adrenergic blocking agents should probably not be given to young children with resting pulse rates below 60.
   d. Hydralazine (Apresoline) seems to be less effective in childhood and adolescent hypertension than in adult disease.
6. Although all clients with primary hypertension need regular supervision and assessment of blood pressure, this is especially important with young children and adolescents because of growth and developmental changes.

GERIATRIC CONSIDERATIONS

Management of hypertension in elderly clients (over 65 years) requires consideration of the following factors:

1. There are basically two types of hypertension in elderly people. One is systolic hypertension, in which systolic blood pressure is above 160 mm Hg but diastolic pressure is below 95 mm Hg or normal. The other type, systolic–diastolic hypertension, involves elevations of both systolic and diastolic pressures.

   Until recently, systolic hypertension was considered a normal aspect of aging that did not require treatment. Increasing evidence indicates that both types of hypertension increase cardiovascular morbidity and mortality, especially congestive heart failure and stroke, and therefore such patients may benefit from treatment.
2. If the hypertensive geriatric client is obese and hypertension is not severe, weight reduction and perhaps moderate salt restriction may be the initial treatment of choice.
3. If antihypertensive drug therapy is required, the stepped-care approach used for other age groups is rational, based on the following considerations:
   a. The goal of drug therapy may be partial reduction of blood pressure rather than achievement of normal levels.
   b. Elderly clients may be especially susceptible to adverse effects of antihypertensive drugs. One reason is that homeostatic mechanisms are less efficient. For example, if hypotension occurs, the mechanisms that raise blood pressure are less efficient. Therefore, syncope may

occur. In addition, renal and liver function may be reduced, making accumulation of drugs more likely. Also, an elderly patient already prone to mental depression could be more sensitive to this adverse effect of antihypertensive drugs.

c. Lower drug doses are often effective in elderly clients. Generally, treatment should be started with smaller doses and increases should be smaller and spaced at longer intervals.

d. Blood pressure should be reduced *slowly* to facilitate adequate blood flow through arteriosclerotic vessels. Rapid lowering of blood pressure may produce cerebral insufficiency (syncope, transient ischemic attacks, stroke).

NURSING ACTIONS: ANTIHYPERTENSIVE DRUGS

Nursing Actions	*Rationale/Explanation*
1. Administer accurately	
a. Check blood pressure before each dose, preferably with the client in both supine and standing positions.	To monitor both therapeutic and adverse responses to drug therapy. This is especially important when initiating drug therapy, changing medications, or changing dosages.
b. Give oral captopril on an empty stomach.	Food decreases drug absorption.
c. Give other oral antihypertensive agents with or after food intake.	To decrease gastric irritation
d. For intravenous injection of propranolol or labetalol, the client should be attached to a cardiac monitor. In addition, parenteral atropine and isoproterenol (Isuprel) must be readily available.	For early detection and treatment of excessive myocardial depression and arrhythmias. Atropine may be used to treat excessive bradycardia. Isoproterenol may be used to stimulate myocardial contractility and increase cardiac output.
e. Inject diazoxide into an established peripheral intravenous line. Monitor the client closely for 15 minutes after the injection; observe for excessive hypotension, cerebral ischemia, or myocardial ischemia.	Diazoxide is a potent drug, and constant supervision is required initially to detect adverse reactions. After about 15 minutes, blood pressure gradually increases to the original level.
Discontinue the drug immediately if extravasation occurs.	The solution is very alkaline and irritating to tissues.
f. For nitroprusside administration, consult the manufacturer's instructions.	Nitroprusside is unstable in solution. It requires special mixing procedures and additional dilution in intravenous fluids.
2. Observe for therapeutic effects Decreased blood pressure. The usual goal is a normal blood pressure, that is, below 140/90.	Thiazide diuretics require 3 to 4 weeks to exert optimal antihypertensive effects. Reserpine requires about 2 to 3 weeks, and guanethidine requires about 2 to 7 days.
3. Observe for adverse effects	Adverse effects are most likely to occur in clients who are elderly, who have impaired renal function, and who are receiving multiple antihypertensive drugs or large doses of antihypertensive drugs.
a. Postural hypotension, dizziness, weakness	This is an extension of the expected pharmacologic action. Postural hypotension results from drug blockage of compensatory reflexes (vasoconstriction, decreased venous pooling in extremities, and increased venous return to the heart) that normally maintain blood pressure in the upright position. This adverse reaction may be aggravated by other conditions that cause vasodilation (*e.g.,* exercise, heat or hot weather, and alcohol consumption). Postural hypotension is more likely to occur with guanethidine, methyldopa, and reserpine.

Nursing Actions	Rationale/Explanation
b. Sodium and water retention, increased plasma volume, perhaps edema and weight gain	These effects result from decreased renal perfusion. This reaction can be prevented or minimized by concurrent administration of a diuretic.
c. Prolonged atrioventricular conduction, bradycardia.	Owing to increased vagal tone and stimulation
d. Gastrointestinal disturbances, including nausea, vomiting, and diarrhea	These effects are more likely to occur with hydralazine, methyldopa, propranolol, and captopril.
e. Mental depression with reserpine	Apparently caused by decreased levels of catecholamines and serotonin in the brain.
f. Bronchospasm or cardiac failure with propranolol and other beta-adrenergic blocking agents.	Caused by bronchoconstriction and depression of myocardial contractility. These drugs are contraindicated in asthma, other bronchoconstrictive lung diseases, and congestive heart failure.
g. Hypertensive crisis with abrupt withdrawal of clonidine or guanabenz	This may be prevented by tapering the prescribed dosage over a period of at least 2 to 4 days before discontinuing the drug.
4. Observe for drug interactions	
a. Drugs that *increase* effects of antihypertensives	
(1) Alcohol, phenothiazine antipsychotic agents, peripheral vasodilators	Because these drugs have hypotensive effects when used alone, additive hypotension occurs when they are combined with antihypertensive agents.
(2) Digitalis glycosides	Additive bradycardia with propranolol
b. Drugs that *decrease* effects of antihypertensives	
(1) Amphetamines	When given with guanethidine, amphetamines displace guanethidine from its site of action. When given with methyldopa, amphetamines decrease antihypertensive effects by increasing sympathetic activity.
(2) Tricyclic antidepressants	These drugs inhibit the action of clonidine and guanethidine.
(3) Monoamine oxidase inhibitors	Caused by antagonistic effects, which are apparently most significant with guanethidine
(4) Oral contraceptives	Oral contraceptives tend to increase blood pressure, probably by causing retention of sodium and water. When they are given concurrently with antihypertensive agents, dosage of antihypertensives may need to be increased.
5. Teach clients	In few other conditions is client education as important as with essential hypertension. Every effort must be made to aid understanding and compliance with the treatment regimen.
a. About the disease process	Although any teaching program should be individualized, the following are some useful points to include: (1) Essential hypertension is a chronic, lifelong problem that can be controlled but not cured. (2) The disease is rarely symptomatic unless complications occur. (3) Untreated hypertension may lead to myocardial infarction, stroke, and renal failure.
b. About nondrug measures	These are largely weight control and salt restriction. These measures may control mild hypertension and are useful adjuncts to drug therapy for moderate or severe hypertension.
c. About drug therapy	Antihypertensive drug therapy is usually long term, requires multiple drugs, and produces side-effects. Inform the client that he may not feel well when a medication is started or

Nursing Actions	***Rationale/Explanation***
	when dosage is increased, that several days or weeks of continuous drug therapy may be required for optimal antihypertensive effects, and that the drugs must be taken as prescribed for maximal benefit.
(1) Name and purpose of each drug	
(2) Adverse effects to be reported	Adverse effects can sometimes be prevented or minimized by nondrug measures, by changing drugs, or by reducing drug dosage.
(3) Measures to control orthostatic hypotension and dizziness. These include the following: move from supine or sitting positions to a standing position slowly; sleep with the head of the bed elevated; wear elastic stockings; exercise legs; avoid prolonged standing; avoid hot baths.	These measures allow adaptation of normal homeostatic mechanisms, avoid vasodilation, and avoid pooling of blood in the extremities. If symptoms still occur, the person should sit or lie down immediately to avoid a fall and possible injury.

Selected References

American Medical Association (AMA) Division of Drugs: AMA Drug Evaluations, 5th ed. New York, John Wiley & Sons, 1983

Confino E, Zbella E, Elkayam U, Gleicher N: Using cardiac drugs during pregnancy. Drug Ther 15:131–145, March 1985

Drugs for hypertension. Med Lett Drugs Ther 26:107–112, December 1984

Facts and Comparisons. St. Louis, J B Lippincott (Updated monthly)

Hansten PD: Drug Interactions: Clinical Significance of Drug–Drug Interactions, 5th ed. Philadelphia, Lea & Febiger, 1985

Joint National Committee on Detection, Evaluation, and Treatment of High Blood Pressure. The 1984 report. Arch Intern Med 144:1045–1057, May 1984

Labetalol for hypertension. Med Lett Drugs Ther 26:83–85, September 1984

Mirkin BL, Newman TJ: Efficacy and safety of captopril in the treatment of severe childhood hypertension: Report of the International Collaborative Study Group. Pediatrics 75:1091–1100, June 1985

Rocchini AP: Childhood hypertension: Etiology, diagnosis, and treatment. Pediatr Clin North Am 31:1259–1273, December 1984

Rodman MJ, Karch AM, Boyd EH, Smith DW: Pharmacology and Drug Therapy in Nursing, 3rd ed. Philadelphia, J B Lippincott, 1985

Rudd P, Blaschke TF: Antihypertensive agents and the drug therapy of hypertension. In Gilman AG, Goodman LS, Rall TW, Murad F (eds): The Pharmacological Basis of Therapeutics, 7th ed, pp 784–805. New York, Macmillan, 1985

Weibert RT: Hypertension. In Herfindal ET, Hirschman JL (eds): Clinical Pharmacy and Therapeutics, 3rd ed, pp 442–474. Baltimore, Williams & Wilkins, 1984

56
DIURETICS

Description and uses

Diuretics are drugs that increase renal excretion of water, sodium, and other electrolytes, thereby increasing urine formation and output. Diuretics are important therapeutic agents widely used in the treatment of edematous (*e.g.*, congestive heart failure, renal and hepatic disease) and nonedematous (*e.g.*, hypertension, ophthalmic surgery) conditions. To aid understanding of diuretic drug therapy, renal physiology related to drug action and characteristics of edema are reviewed before further discussion of the drugs. Individual diuretics are listed in Table 56-1.

RENAL PHYSIOLOGY

The primary function of the kidneys is to regulate the volume, composition, and *p*H of body fluids. The kidneys receive about 25% of the cardiac output. From this large amount of blood flowing through it, the normally functioning kidney is very efficient in retaining substances needed by the body and eliminating those not needed. The nephron is the functional unit of the kidney, and each kidney contains approximately 1 million nephrons.

Each nephron is composed of a glomerulus and a tubule (Fig. 56-1). The glomerulus is a network of capillaries that receives blood from the renal artery. Bowman's capsule is a thin-walled structure that surrounds the glomerulus, then narrows and continues as the tubule. The tubule is a thin-walled structure of epithelial cells surrounded by peritubular capillaries. The tubule is divided into three segments, the proximal tubule, loop of Henle, and distal tubule, which differ in structure and function. The tubules are often called "convoluted" tubules because of their many twists and turns. The convolutions provide a large surface area of close proximity between the blood flowing through the peritubular capillaries and the glomerular filtrate flowing through the tubular lumen. Consequently, substances can be readily exchanged through the walls of the tubules.

The nephron functions by three processes: glomerular filtration, tubular reabsorption, and tubular secretion. These processes normally maintain the fluid volume, electrolyte concentration, and *p*H of body fluids within a relatively narrow range. They also remove waste products of cellular metabolism. A minimum daily urine output of approximately 400 ml is required to remove normal amounts of metabolic end-products.

Glomerular filtration

Arterial blood enters the glomerulus, by the afferent arteriole, at the relatively high pressure of approximately 70 mm Hg. This pressure "pushes" water, electrolytes, and other solutes out of the capillaries into Bowman's capsule and thence to the proximal tubule. This fluid, called *glomerular filtrate,* contains the same components as blood except for blood cells, fats, and proteins.

TABLE 56-1. DIURETIC AGENTS

	Generic name	Trade name	Routes and dosage ranges: Adults	Routes and dosage ranges: Children
Thiazide and related diuretics	Bendroflumethiazide	Naturetin	PO 5 mg daily initially. For maintenance, 2.5–20 mg daily or intermittently	PO up to 0.4 mg/kg/day initially, in 2 divided doses. For maintenance, 0.05–0.1 mg/kg/day in a single dose.
	Benzthiazide	Aquatag	PO 50–200 mg daily for several days initially, depending on response. For maintenance, dosage is gradually reduced to the minimal effective amount.	PO 1–4 mg/kg/day initially, in 3 divided doses. For maintenance, dosage is reduced to the minimal effective amount
	Chlorothiazide	Diuril	PO 500–1000 mg 1–2 times daily, IV 500 mg twice daily	PO 22 mg/kg/day in 2 divided doses Infants under age 6 months, up to 33 mg/kg/day in 2 divided doses IV not recommended
	Chlorthalidone	Hygroton	PO 25–100 mg daily	3 mg/kg 3 times weekly, adjusted according to response
	Cyclothiazide	Anhydron	PO 1–5 mg daily initially. For maintenance, 1–2 mg every other day or 2–3 times weekly	PO 0.02–0.04 mg/kg/day
	Hydrochlorothiazide	HydroDiuril, Esidrix, Oretic	PO 25–100 mg 1–2 times daily	PO 2 mg/kg/day in 2 divided doses Infants under age 6 months, up to 3.3 mg/kg/day in 2 divided doses
	Hydroflumethiazide	Saluron	PO 25–200 mg daily	PO 1 mg/kg/day
	Indapamide	Lozol	PO 2.5–5 mg daily	Dosage not established
	Methyclothiazide	Enduron	PO 2.5–10 mg daily	PO 0.05–0.2 mg/kg/day
	Metolazone	Zaroxolyn, Diulo	PO 5–20 mg daily, depending on severity of condition and response	
	Polythiazide	Renese	PO 1–4 mg daily, depending on severity of condition and response.	PO 0.02–0.08 mg/kg/day
	Quinethazone	Hydromox	PO 50–200 mg daily	
	Trichlormethiazide	Metahydrin, Naqua	PO 2–4 mg 1–2 times daily initially. For maintenance, 1–4 mg once daily	PO 0.07 mg/kg/day in single or divided doses
Loop diuretics	Bumetanide	Bumex	PO 0.5–2 mg daily as a single dose. May be repeated q4–6h to a maximal daily dose of 10 mg, if necessary. Giving on alternate days or for 3–4 days with rest periods of 1–2 days is recommended for long-term control of edema. IV, IM 0.5–1 mg, repeated in 2–3 hours if necessary, to a maximal daily dose of 10 mg. Give IV injections over 1–2 minutes.	Not recommended for children under 18 years of age

TABLE 56-1. DIURETIC AGENTS (*Continued*)

	Generic name	Trade name	Routes and dosage ranges: Adults	Routes and dosage ranges: Children
	Ethacrynic acid	Edecrin	Edema, PO 50–100 mg daily, increased or decreased according to severity of condition and response. Maximal daily dose, 400 mg Rapid mobilization of edema, IV 50 mg or 0.5–1 mg/kg injected slowly to a maximum of 100 mg/dose	PO 25 mg daily No recommended parenteral dose in pediatric patients
	Furosemide	Lasix	Edema, PO 20–80 mg as a single dose initially. If an adequate diuretic response is not obtained, dosage may be gradually increased by 20- to 40-mg increments at intervals of 6–8 hours. For maintenance, dosage range and frequency of administration vary widely and must be individualized. Maximal daily dose, 600 mg Hypertension, PO 40 mg twice daily, gradually increased if necessary Rapid mobilization of edema, IV 20–40 mg initially, injected slowly. This dose may be repeated in 2 hours. With acute pulmonary edema, initial dose is usually 40 mg, which may be repeated in 60–90 minutes. Acute renal failure, IV 40 mg initially, increased if necessary. Maximum dose, 1–2 g/24 hours Hypertensive crisis, IV 40–80 mg injected over 1–2 minutes. With renal failure, much larger doses may be needed.	PO 2 mg/kg 1–2 times daily initially, gradually increased by increments of 1–2 mg/kg/dose if necessary at intervals of 6–8 hours. Maximal daily dose, 6 mg/kg IV 1 mg/kg initially. If diuretic response is not adequate, increase dosage by 1 mg/kg no sooner than 2 hours after previous dose. Maximal dose, 6 mg/kg
Potassium-sparing diuretics	Amiloride	Midamor	PO 5–20 mg daily	
	Spironolactone	Aldactone	PO 25–200 mg daily	PO 3.3 mg/kg/day in divided doses
	Triamterene	Dyrenium	PO 100–300 mg daily in divided doses	PO 2–4 mg/kg/day in divided doses
Osmotic agents	Glycerin	Osmoglyn	PO 1–1.5 g/kg of body weight, usually given as a 50% or 75% solution, 1–2 hours before ocular surgery	Same as adults
	Isosorbide	Ismotic	PO 1.5–3 g/kg, up to 4 times daily if necessary for glaucoma or ocular surgery	

TABLE 56-1. DIURETIC AGENTS (*Continued*)

	Generic name	Trade name	Routes and dosage ranges	
			Adults	*Children*
	Mannitol	Osmitrol	Diuresis, IV infusion 50–200 g over 24 hours, flow rate adjusted to maintain a urine output of 30–50 ml/hour Oliguria and prevention of renal failure, IV 50–100 g Reducton of intracranial or intraocular pressure, IV 1.5–2 g/kg, given as a 20% solution, over 30–60 minutes	Same as adults
Combination diuretic products	Hydrochlorothiazide 50 mg, and amiloride 5 mg	Moduretic	PO 1–2 tablets daily	
	Hydrochlorothiazide 25 mg and spironolactone 25 mg	Aldactazide 25/25	PO 1–8 tablets daily	
	Hydrochlorothiazide 50 mg and spironolactone 50 mg	Aldactazide 50/50	PO 1–4 tablets daily	
	Hydrochlorothiazide 25 mg and triamterene 50 mg	Dyazide	Hypertension, PO 1 capsule twice daily initially, then adjusted according to response Edema, 1–2 capsules twice daily	
	Hydrochlorothiazide 50 mg and triamterene 75 mg	Maxzide	PO 1 tablet daily	

The glomerular filtration rate (GFR) is approximately 180 liters per day, or 125 milliliters per minute. Most of this fluid is reabsorbed as the glomerular filtrate travels through the tubules. The end-product is approximately 2 to 3 liters of urine daily. Urine flows into collecting tubules, which carry it to the renal pelvis. From the renal pelvis, urine flows through the ureters, bladder, and urethra for elimination from the body.

Blood that does not become part of the glomerular filtrate travels out of the glomerulus through the efferent arteriole. The efferent arteriole branches into the peritubular capillaries, which eventually empty into veins and return the blood to the systemic circulation.

Tubular reabsorption

The term *reabsorption,* in relation to renal function, indicates movement of substances from the tubule (glomerular filtrate) to the blood in the peritubular capillaries. Most reabsorption occurs in the proximal tubule. Approximately 100% of glucose and amino acids is reabsorbed; approximately 80% of water, sodium, potassium, chloride, and most other substances is reabsorbed. As a result, only a portion of the glomerular filtrate (about 20%) enters the loop of Henle. In the descending limb of the loop of Henle, water is reabsorbed; in the ascending limb, sodium is reabsorbed. A large fraction of the total amount of sodium (up to 30%) filtered by the glomeruli is reabsorbed in the loop of Henle. Additional sodium is reabsorbed in the distal tubule, primarily by the exchange of sodium ions for potassium ions secreted by epithelial cells of tubular walls. Final reabsorption of water occurs in the distal tubule and small collecting tubules. The remaining water and solutes are now correctly called urine.

Antidiuretic hormone (ADH) from the posterior pituitary gland promotes reabsorption of water from the distal tubules and the collecting ducts of the kidneys. This conserves water needed by the body and

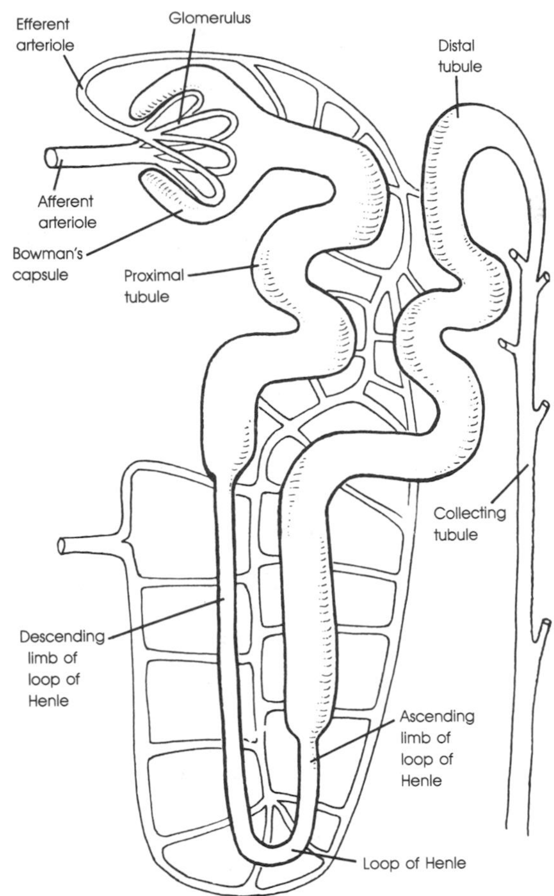

Figure 56-1. *The nephron, the functional unit of the kidney.*

produces a more concentrated urine. Aldosterone, a hormone from the adrenal cortex, promotes sodium–potassium exchange mainly in the distal tubule and collecting ducts. Thus, aldosterone promotes sodium reabsorption and potassium loss.

Tubular secretion

The term *secretion,* in relation to renal function, indicates movement of substances from blood in the peritubular capillaries to glomerular filtrate flowing through the renal tubules. Secretion occurs in the proximal and distal tubules, across the epithelial cells that line the tubules. In the proximal tubule, uric acid, creatinine, hydrogen ions, and ammonia are secreted; in the distal tubule, potassium ions, hydrogen ions, and ammonia are secreted. Secretion of hydrogen ions is important in maintaining acid–base balance in body fluids.

ALTERATIONS IN RENAL FUNCTION

Many clinical conditions alter renal function. In some conditions, excessive amounts of substances (*e.g.,* sodium and water) are retained; in others, needed substances (*e.g.,* potassium, proteins) are eliminated. These conditions include cardiovascular, renal, hepatic, and other disorders that may be treated with diuretic drugs.

Edema

Edema is the excessive accumulation of fluid in body tissues. It is a symptom of many disease processes and may occur in any part of the body. Additional characteristics include the following:

1. Edema formation results from one or more of the following mechanisms that allow fluid to leave the bloodstream (intravascular compartment) and enter interstitial spaces.
   a. *Increased capillary permeability* occurs as part of the response to tissue injury. Thus, edema may occur with burns and trauma or allergic and inflammatory reactions.
   b. Increased capillary hydrostatic pressure results from a sequence of events in which increased blood volume (from fluid overload or sodium and water retention) or obstruction of venous blood flow causes a high venous pressure and a high capillary pressure. This is the primary mechanism for edema formation in congestive heart failure, pulmonary edema, and renal failure.
   c. *Decreased plasma oncotic pressure* may occur with decreased synthesis of plasma proteins (caused by liver disease or malnutrition) or increased loss of plasma proteins (caused by burn injuries or the nephrotic syndrome). Plasma proteins are important in keeping fluids within the bloodstream. When plasma proteins are lacking, fluid leaves the capillaries and accumulates in tissues.
2. Edema interferes with blood flow to tissues. Thus, it interferes with delivery of oxygen and nutrients and removal of metabolic waste products. If severe, edema may distort body features, impair movement, and interfere with activities of daily living.
3. Specific manifestations of edema are determined by its location and extent. A common type of localized edema is that which occurs in the feet and ankles (dependent edema), especially with prolonged sitting or standing. A less common but more severe type of localized edema is pulmonary edema. This life-threatening condition occurs with circulatory overload (of intravenous fluids or blood transfusions, for example) or acute heart failure. Generalized massive edema (anasarca) interferes with the functions of many body organs and tissues.

DIURETIC DRUGS

Drugs with diuretic effects act directly on the kidneys to decrease reabsorption of sodium, chloride, water, and other substances. Major subclasses of diuretics are the thiazides and related diuretics, loop diuretics, and potassium-sparing diuretics. These groups differ from each other primarily because they act at different sites in the nephron.

Major clinical indications for diuretics are edema and hypertension. In edematous states, diuretics mobilize tissue fluids by decreasing plasma volume. In hypertension, the exact mechanism by which diuretics lower blood pressure is unknown. However, antihypertensive action is usually attributed to sodium depletion. Initially, diuretics decrease blood volume and cardiac output. With chronic use, cardiac output and plasma volume return to normal, but there is a persistent decrease in peripheral vascular resistance. Sodium depletion may have a vasodilating effect on arterioles. Use of diuretic agents in the treatment of congestive heart failure and hypertension is discussed further in Chapters 51 and 55, respectively.

Thiazide and related diuretics

Thiazide diuretics are synthetic drugs that are chemically related to the sulfonamides. Chlorothiazide (Diuril) is the prototype of thiazide diuretics, but hydrochlorothiazide (HydroDiuril), a more potent derivative, is more commonly used. Related diuretics are nonthiazides whose pharmacologic actions are essentially the same as those of the thiazides; they include chlorthalidone (Hygroton), metolazone (Zaroxolyn), and quinethazone (Hydromox).

Thiazides and related drugs are the most frequently prescribed diuretic agents. They decrease reabsorption of sodium and water in the ascending limb of the loop of Henle and in the distal tubule. They also decrease reabsorption of chloride and bicarbonate.

Thiazides and related drugs are well absorbed from the gastrointestinal tract following oral administration. They are widely distributed in body fluids but accumulate only in the kidneys. With most of the drugs, diuretic effects occur within 2 hours, peak at 4 to 6 hours, and last 6 to 24 hours. Most of the drugs are excreted unchanged by the kidneys in 3 to 6 hours. Some of the newer drugs (*e.g.*, polythiazide [Renese] and chlorthalidone [Hygroton]) have longer durations of action, approximately 48 to 72 hours, attributed to slower excretion.

These drugs are especially useful in long-term treatment of congestive heart failure and hypertension. They are not effective when immediate diuresis is required and are relatively ineffective with decreased renal function. They cross the placenta and may have adverse effects on the fetus. Thus, usage during pregnancy must be based on careful consideration of potential benefits versus potential harm. Thiazides and related drugs are contraindicated in clients who are allergic to sulfonamide drugs.

Loop diuretics

Loop diuretics exert their primary pharmacologic actions in the ascending limb of the loop of Henle. They are also called high-ceiling diuretics because they are the most effective diuretic agents available for clinical use. This class includes three pharmacologically similar drugs: furosemide (Lasix), ethacrynic acid (Edecrin), and bumetanide (Bumex).

Loop diuretics inhibit sodium and chloride reabsorption primarily in the loop of Henle. Their saluretic (sodium-losing) effect is up to ten times greater than that of thiazide diuretics. These drugs may be given orally or intravenously. After oral administration, diuretic effects occur within 30 to 60 minutes, peak in 1 to 2 hours, and last 6 to 8 hours. After intravenous administration, diuretic effects occur within 5 minutes, peak in 15 to 45 minutes, and last about 2 hours. They are rapidly excreted by the kidneys, and drug accumulation does not occur even with repeated doses.

The loop diuretics are the diuretics of choice when rapid effects are required (*e.g.*, pulmonary edema) and when renal function is impaired (creatinine clearance less than 30 ml/minute). The drugs are contraindicated during pregnancy unless absolutely necessary.

Although both drugs are effective diuretics, furosemide is used much more often than ethacrynic acid. Furosemide has a wider range of effective dosages. It also causes less ototoxicity and fewer gastrointestinal disturbances than ethacrynic acid. Bumetanide is a newer loop diuretic that may produce diuresis in some clients who no longer respond to furosemide or who are allergic to furosemide. In addition, larger doses can be given in smaller volumes because it is approximately 40 times as potent as furosemide on a weight basis.

Potassium-sparing diuretics

Potassium-sparing diuretics include three drugs. One drug is spironolactone (Aldactone), which is an aldosterone antagonist. Aldosterone is a hormone secreted by the adrenal cortex. It promotes retention of sodium and water and excretion of potassium by stimulating the sodium–potassium exchange mechanism in the distal tubule and collecting ducts. The other two drugs (triamterene and amiloride) are chemically unrelated to spironolactone but are similar to each other in diuretic activity.

Potassium-sparing diuretics are relatively weak diuretics when used alone; they are usually given in combination with potassium-losing diuretics to increase diuretic activity and decrease potassium loss. These drugs act in the distal renal tubule. Spironolactone blocks the sodium-retaining effects of aldosterone, and aldosterone must be present for spironolactone to be effective. Triamterene and amiloride act directly on the distal renal tubule to decrease the exchange of sodium for potassium. Their action is independent of aldosterone activity.

Potassium-sparing diuretics are contraindicated in the presence of renal insufficiency because their use in this situation may cause hyperkalemia. Hyperkalemia is the major adverse effect of these drugs; clients receiving potassium-sparing diuretics should *not* be given potassium supplements, encouraged to eat high potassium foods, or allowed to use salt substitutes. Salt substitutes contain potassium chloride rather than sodium chloride.

Osmotic diuretics

Osmotic agents produce rapid diuresis by increasing the solute load (osmotic pressure) of the glomerular filtrate. The increased osmotic pressure causes water to be pulled from extravascular sites into the bloodstream, thereby increasing blood volume and decreasing reabsorption of water and electrolytes in the renal tubules. Mannitol (Osmitrol) is useful in treating oliguria or anuria, and it may prevent acute renal failure during prolonged surgery, trauma, or infusion of cisplatinum (Cisplatin), an antineoplastic agent. Mannitol is effective even when renal circulation and glomerular filtration rate are reduced (*e.g.*, in hypovolemic shock, trauma, or dehydration). Other important clinical uses of hyperosmolar agents include reduction of intracranial pressure before or after neurosurgery, reduction of intraocular pressure before certain types of ophthalmic surgery, and promotion of urinary excretion of toxic substances. Other osmotic agents include urea (Ureaphil), glycerin (Osmoglyn), and isosorbide (Ismotic).

Principles of therapy: diuretics

ASSESSMENT GUIDELINES

Assess the client's status in relation to baseline data and conditions in which diuretic drugs are used.

1. Useful baseline data include serum electrolytes, uric acid, blood glucose, creatinine, and urea nitrogen, since diuretics may alter these values. Other data are blood pressure readings, weight, amount and appearance of urine output, and measurement of edematous areas such as ankles or abdomen.
2. Edema
   a. Visible edema often occurs in the feet and legs of ambulatory clients.
   b. Rapid weight gain may indicate fluid retention.
   c. With congestive heart failure, numerous signs and symptoms result from edema of various organs and tissues. For example, congestion in the gastrointestinal tract may cause nausea and vomiting; liver congestion may cause abdominal pain and tenderness; and congestion in the lungs (pulmonary edema) causes rapid, labored breathing, hypoxemia, frothy sputum, and other manifestations of severe respiratory distress.
   d. Cerebral edema may be manifested by confusion, headache, dizziness, convulsions, unconsciousness, bradycardia, or failure of the pupils to react to light.
   e. Ascites, which occurs with hepatic cirrhosis, is an accumulation of fluid in the abdominal cavity. The abdomen appears much enlarged.
3. Congestive heart failure. In addition to edema, fatigue and dyspnea are common symptoms of congestive heart failure.
4. Hypertension (blood pressure above 140/90 mm Hg on several measurements). This may be the only clinical manifestation present.

PREVENTIVE NURSING INTERVENTIONS

Promote measures to prevent or minimize conditions for which diuretic drugs are used.

1. With edema, helpful measures include the following:
   a. Decreasing dietary sodium intake
   b. Losing weight, if obese
   c. Elevating legs when sitting
   d. Avoiding prolonged standing or sitting
   e. Wearing support hose or elastic stockings
   f. Treating the condition causing edema
2. With congestive heart failure and in elderly clients, administer intravenous fluids or blood transfusions carefully to avoid fluid overload and pulmonary edema. Fluid overload may occur with rapid administration or excessive amounts of intravenous fluids.
3. With hypertension, helpful measures include the following:
   a. Decreasing dietary sodium intake
   b. Losing weight, if obese

DRUG SELECTION

Choice of diuretic drug depends primarily on the client's condition.

1. Thiazides and related diuretics are drugs of choice for most clients who require diuretic therapy. They are especially useful in conditions (*e.g.*, congestive heart failure and hypertension) that require long-term use of diuretics. Because all the drugs in this group have equal therapeutic effectiveness, there is little reason to choose one over another. However, use of drugs with a longer duration of action may increase client compliance by requiring less frequent administration.
2. Furosemide is the drug of choice when rapid diuretic effects are required or when renal insufficiency is present.
3. A potassium-sparing diuretic may be given concurrently with a potassium-losing diuretic to prevent or treat hypokalemia and to augment the diuretic effect.
4. Combination products containing a potassium-losing and a potassium-sparing diuretic (*e.g.*, Dyazide, Aldactazide, Maxzide, Moduretic) are not recommended for initial diuretic therapy. When a drug of each type is needed, dosage of each drug should be titrated separately. Then, if titrated doses are similar to the amounts in the combination products, the combination products may be used.

DOSAGE FACTORS

Dosage of diuretics depends largely on the client's condition and response. Thus, dosage should always be individualized to administer the minimal effective amount.

1. In liver disease, electrolyte imbalances produced by diuretics may precipitate or aggravate hepatic coma.
2. In renal disease, furosemide is often given in large doses to achieve a diuretic response. Bumetanide may be a useful alternative, since it can be given in smaller doses.

USE IN EDEMA

When diuretics are used to treat patients with edema, the underlying cause of the edema should be addressed, not just the edema itself. In treating such patients, it is preferable to aim for a weight loss of about 2 pounds (about 1 kg) per day. Rapid and excessive diuresis may cause dehydration and decreased blood volume with circulatory collapse.

USE WITH DIGITALIS

When digitalis preparations and diuretics are given concomitantly, as is common practice in treating patients with congestive heart failure, there is increased risk of digitalis toxicity.

1. Digitalis toxicity is related to diuretic-induced hypokalemia. Potassium is a myocardial depressant and antiarrhythmic; it has essentially opposite cardiac effects to those of digitalis. In other words, extracellular potassium decreases the excitability of myocardial tissue, but digitalis increases excitability. The higher the serum potassium, the less effective a given dose of digitalis. Conversely, decreased serum potassium increases the likelihood of digitalis-induced cardiac arrhythmias, even with "small" doses of digitalis.
2. Supplemental potassium chloride, a potassium-sparing diuretic, and other measures to prevent hypokalemia are often used to maintain normal serum potassium levels (3.5–5.0 mEq/liter).

PREVENTION AND TREATMENT OF POTASSIUM IMBALANCES

Potassium imbalances (see Chap. 32) may occur with diuretic therapy. Both hypokalemia and hyperkalemia are cardiotoxic and should be prevented when possible.

1. Hypokalemia (serum potassium level under 3.5 mEq/liter) may occur with potassium-losing diuretics (*e.g.*, hydrochlorothiazide, furosemide). Measures to prevent or treat hypokalemia include the following:
   a. Giving supplemental potassium, usually potassium chloride (KCl), in an average dosage range of 20 to 60 mEq daily.
   b. Giving a potassium-sparing diuretic along with the potassium-losing drug.
   c. Increasing food intake of potassium. Many texts advocate this approach as being preferable to supplemental potassium or combination diuretic therapy. However, the effectiveness of this approach is not clearly established. Although the minimal daily requirement of potassium is not known, usual recommendations are 40 to 50 mEq daily for the healthy adult. Potassium loss with diuretics may be several times this amount.

      Some foods (*e.g.*, bananas) have undeserved reputations for having high potassium content; actually, large amounts must be ingested. To provide 50 mEq of potassium daily, estimated amounts of certain foods include:

1000 ml of orange juice
1600 ml of apple or grape juice
1200 ml of pineapple juice
4 to 6 bananas
30 to 40 prunes

Some of these foods are high in calories and may be contraindicated, at least in large amounts, for obese clients.

d. Using salt substitutes. One teaspoonful of salt substitute contains approximately 60 to 70 mEq of potassium chloride.
e. Restricting dietary sodium intake. This reduces potassium loss by decreasing the amount of sodium available for exchange with potassium in renal tubules.

2. Hyperkalemia (serum potassium level above 5 mEq/liter) may occur with potassium-sparing diuretics (spironolactone, triamterene, amiloride). The following measures prevent hyperkalemia:
   a. Avoiding use of potassium-sparing diuretics and potassium supplements in clients with renal insufficiency.
   b. Avoiding excessive amounts of potassium chloride supplements and salt substitutes.
   c. Maintaining urine output, the major route for eliminating potassium from the body.

USE IN PREGNANCY

None of the diuretic drugs has been proved safe and effective for use during pregnancy.

1. Diuretics should not be given routinely to relieve edema during pregnancy. Edema in the lower extremities is quite common but may be caused by impaired venous blood flow from pressure exerted by the gravid uterus ("physiologic" edema) rather than a disease process ("pathologic" edema). If diuretics are necessary for "pathologic" edema or hypertension, small doses of thiazide diuretics plus sodium restriction are probably acceptable. One concern is decreased placental blood flow occurring as a result of decreased plasma volume. This may impair fetal nutrition and growth.
2. Thiazide diuretics cross the placenta and may cause fetal or neonatal jaundice, thrombocytopenia, hemolytic anemia, electrolyte imbalances, hypoglycemia, or altered carbohydrate metabolism.
3. Furosemide is contraindicated during pregnancy because of possible teratogenic effects; bumetanide is reportedly nonteratogenic.
4. During lactation, diuretics should not be given, since they enter breast milk. Breast-feeding should be discontinued if diuretic therapy is required.

GERIATRIC CONSIDERATIONS

Diuretic drug therapy must be used cautiously in elderly clients. Careful observation is needed. The elderly are especially sensitive to adverse effects such as electrolyte imbalance. Also, rapid or excessive diuresis may cause myocardial infarction, renal impairment, or cerebral thrombosis as a result of severe orthostatic hypotension.

NURSING ACTIONS: DIURETICS

Nursing Actions	Rationale/Explanation
1. Administer accurately	
a. Give in the early morning if ordered daily.	So that peak action will occur during waking hours and not interfere with sleep
b. Take safety precautions. Keep a bedpan or urinal within reach. Keep the call light within reach and be sure the client knows how to use it. Assist to the bathroom anyone who is elderly, weak, dizzy, or unsteady in walking.	Mainly to avoid falls
2. Observe for therapeutic effects	
Decrease or absence of edema, increased urine output, decreased blood pressure	Most oral diuretics start their action within about 2 hours; intravenous diuretics act within minutes. Antihypertensive effects may not be evident for several days.

Nursing Actions	**Rationale/Explanation**
(1) Weigh daily while edema is present, two or three times weekly thereafter. Weigh under standard conditions: early morning before eating or drinking, after urination, with the same amount of clothing, and using the same scales.	Body weight is a very good indicator of fluid gain or loss. A weight change of 2.2 lb (1 kg) may indicate a gain or loss of 1000 ml of fluid. Also, weighing assists in dosage regulation to maintain therapeutic benefit without excessive or too rapid fluid loss.
(2) Record fluid intake and output every shift.	Normally, oral fluid intake approximates urinary output (1500 ml/24 hours). With diuretic therapy, urinary output may exceed intake, depending on the amount of edema or fluid retention, renal function, and diuretic dosage. All sources of fluid gain, including intravenous fluids, must be included; all sources of fluid loss (perspiration, fever, wound drainage, gastrointestinal tract drainage) are important. Clients with abnormal fluid losses have less urine output with diuretic therapy. Oliguria (decreased excretion of urine) may require stopping the drug. Output greater than 100 ml/hour may indicate that side-effects are more likely to occur.
(3) Observe and record characteristics of urine.	Excessively dilute urine may indicate excessive fluid intake or greater likelihood of fluid and electrolyte imbalance due to rapid diuresis. Concentrated urine may mean oliguria or decreased fluid intake.
(4) Check daily for edema: ankles for the ambulatory client; sacral area and posterior thighs for clients at bedrest. Also, it is often helpful to measure abdominal girth, ankles, and calves to monitor gain or loss of fluid.	Expect a decrease in visible edema and size of measured areas. If edema reappears or worsens, a thorough reassessment of the client is in order. Questions to be answered include the following: (1) Is the prescribed diuretic being taken correctly? (2) What type of diuretic and what dosage is ordered? (3) Is there worsening of the underlying condition(s) that contributed to edema formation in the first place? (4) Has other disease developed?
(5) In clients with congestive heart failure or acute pulmonary edema, observe for decreased dyspnea, rales, cyanosis, and cough.	Decreased fluid in the lungs leads to dramatic improvement in respirations as more carbon dioxide and oxygen gas exchange takes place and greater tissue oxygenation occurs.
(6) Record blood pressure two to four times daily when diuretic therapy is initiated.	Although thiazide diuretics apparently do not lower normal blood pressure, other diuretics may, especially with excessive or rapid diuresis.
3. Observe for adverse effects	Major adverse effects are fluid and electrolyte imbalances.
a. With potassium-losing diuretics (thiazides, bumetanide, furosemide, ethacrynic acid), observe for	
(1) Hypokalemia (a) Serum potassium levels below 3.5 mEq/liter (b) Electrocardiographic changes (*e.g.,* low voltage, flattened T wave, depressed ST segment) (c) Cardiac arrhythmias; weak, irregular pulse. (d) Hypotension (e) Weak, shallow respirations (f) Anorexia, nausea, and vomiting (g) Decreased peristalsis or paralytic ileus (h) Skeletal muscle weakness (i) Confusion, disorientation	Potassium is required for normal muscle function. Thus, potassium depletion causes weakness of cardiovascular, respiratory, digestive, and skeletal muscles. Clients most likely to develop hypokalemia are those who are taking large doses of diuretics, potent diuretics (*e.g.,* furosemide), or adrenal corticosteroids; those who have decreased food and fluid intake; or those who have increased potassium losses through vomiting, diarrhea, chronic laxative or enema use, or gastrointestinal suction. Clinically significant symptoms are most likely to occur with a serum potassium level below 3 mEq/liter.
(2) Hyponatremia, hypomagnesemia, hypochloremic alkalosis, and changes in serum and urinary calcium	In addition to potassium, sodium, chloride, magnesium, and bicarbonate are also lost with diuresis. Thiazides and related diuretics cause hypercalcemia and hypocalciuria. They have been used to prevent calcium nephrolithiasis (kidney stones).

Nursing Actions	Rationale/Explanation
	Furosemide and other loop diuretics tend to cause hypocalcemia and hypercalciuria.
(3) Dehydration (a) Poor skin turgor, dry mucous membranes (b) Oliguria; urine of high specific gravity (c) Thirst (d) Tachycardia; hypotension (e) Decreased level of consciousness (f) Elevated hematocrit (above 45%)	Fluid volume depletion occurs with excessive or rapid diuresis. If it is prolonged or severe, hypovolemic shock may occur.
(4) Hyperglycemia—blood glucose above 120 mg/100 ml, polyuria, polydipsia, polyphagia, glycosuria	Hyperglycemia is more likely to occur in clients with known or latent diabetes mellitus. Larger doses of hypoglycemic agents may be required. The hyperglycemic effect may be reversible when diuretic therapy is discontinued.
(5) Hyperuricemia—serum uric acid above 7.0 mg/100 ml	Hyperuricemia is usually asymptomatic except for clients with gout, a predisposition toward gout, or chronic renal failure. Apparently, decreased renal excretion of uric acid allows its accumulation in the blood.
(6) Pulmonary edema with osmotic diuretics	Pulmonary edema is most likely to occur in clients with congestive heart failure who are unable to tolerate the increased blood volume produced by the drugs.
(7) Ototoxicity with furosemide and ethacrynic acid	Reversible or transient hearing impairment, tinnitus, and dizziness are more common, although irreversible deafness may occur. Ototoxicity is more likely to occur when the drugs are injected rapidly in clients with severe renal impairment, or when other ototoxic drugs (*e.g.,* aminoglycoside antibiotics) are being taken concurrently.
(8) Hypersensitivity reactions (skin rash, dermatitis) and hematologic reactions (leukopenia, thrombocytopenia)	These effects rarely occur.
b. With potassium-sparing diuretics (spironolactone, triamterene, amiloride) observe for	
Hyperkalemia (a) Serum potassium levels above 5 mEq/liter (b) Electrocardiographic changes (*i.e.,* prolonged PR interval, wide QRS complex; tall, peaked T wave; depressed ST segment) (c) Cardiac arrhythmias, which may progress to ventricular fibrillation and asystole	Hyperkalemia is most likely to occur in people with impaired renal function or who are ingesting additional potassium (*e.g.,* salt substitutes).
4. Observe for drug interactions	
a. Drugs that *increase* effects of diuretics	
(1) Aminoglycoside antibiotics	Additive ototoxicity with ethacrynic acid
(2) Antihypertensive agents	Additive hypotensive effects
(3) Corticosteroids	Additive hypokalemia
b. Drugs that *decrease* effects of diuretics	
Vasopressors (*e.g.,* epinephrine, norepinephrine)	These drugs may antagonize hypotensive effects of diuretics by decreasing responsiveness of arterioles.
5. Teach clients	
a. Take diuretics in the early morning.	To avoid nocturia
b. Expect increased frequency of urination, decreased edema, and weight loss.	Polyuria lasts only a few days or weeks in nonedematous clients.
c. Weigh periodically, under standardized conditions.	Weighing is most helpful in edematous conditions.

Nursing Actions	Rationale/Explanation
d. If the client is taking digitalis, a potassium-losing diuretic, and a potassium supplement, emphasize that these drugs must be taken as prescribed.	This is a frequently ordered combination of drugs for clients with congestive heart failure. To increase therapeutic effectiveness and avoid hypokalemia and digitalis toxicity, the balance among these drugs must be maintained.
e. Report adverse effects.	So that the treatment regimen can be altered, if indicated
f. Ask the physician about salt intake and the use of salt substitutes.	Severe salt restriction is usually not necessary. However, it is generally recommended that table salt and obviously salty foods (*e.g.*, ham, packaged sandwich meats, potato chips) be avoided. Salt substitutes should be used only on the advice of a physician. These preparations contain potassium rather than sodium, and hyperkalemia may occur.
g. Maintain regular medical supervision.	Diuretic therapy is often long term. Supervision is needed to monitor drug effects and adjust dosage when indicated.

Selected References

American Medical Association (AMA) Division of Drugs: AMA Drug Evaluations, 5th ed. New York, John Wiley & Sons, 1983

Facts and Comparisons. St. Louis, J B Lippincott (Updated monthly)

Fenster PE, Bressler R: Treating cardovascular disease in the elderly. II. Antiarrhythmics, diuretics, and calcium channel blockers. Drug Ther 14:209–215, March 1984

Hansten PD: Drug Interactions: Clinical Significance of Drug–Drug Interactions, 5th ed. Philadelphia, Lea & Febiger, 1985

Malseed RT: Pharmacology: Drug Therapy and Nursing Considerations, 2d ed. Philadelphia, J B Lippincott, 1985

Mudge GH: Agents affecting volume and composition of body fluids. In Gilman AG, Goodman LS, Rall TW, Murad F (eds): The Pharmacological Basis of Therapeutics, 7th ed, pp 846–878. New York, Macmillan, 1985

Rodman MJ, Karch AM, Boyd EH, Smith DW: Pharmacology and Drug Therapy in Nursing, 3rd ed. Philadelphia, J B Lippincott, 1985

Weiner IM, Mudge GH: Diuretics and other agents employed in the mobilization of edema. In Gilman AG, Goodman LS, Rall TW, Murad F (eds): The Pharmacological Basis of Therapeutics, 7th ed, pp 887–907. New York, Macmillan, 1985

57

ANTICOAGULANT, ANTIPLATELET, AND THROMBOLYTIC AGENTS

Description and uses

Anticoagulant, antiplatelet, and thrombolytic drugs are used in the prevention and treatment of thrombotic and thromboembolic disorders. Thrombosis involves the formation (thrombogenesis) or presence of a blood clot (thrombus) within the vascular system. Blood coagulation is a normal body defense mechanism to prevent blood loss. Thus, thrombogenesis may be lifesaving when it occurs as a response to hemorrhage. However, it may be a life-threatening process when it occurs at other times because the thrombus can obstruct a blood vessel and impair the blood supply of tissues beyond the clot. When a portion of a thrombus breaks off and travels to another part of the body, it is called an *embolus.* Ultimate consequences of thrombi and emboli depend primarily on location and size. Thrombi and emboli that lodge in vital organs are major causes of morbidity and mortality from such disorders as myocardial infarction, stroke, and pulmonary embolism.

Under normal circumstances, thrombi are constantly being formed and dissolved (thrombolysis), but the blood stays fluid and blood flow is not significantly obstructed. If the balance between thrombogenesis and thrombolysis is upset, thrombotic or bleeding disorders result. Thrombotic disorders occur much more often than bleeding disorders. To aid understanding of drug therapy for thrombotic disorders, normal blood coagulation and characteristics of arterial and venous thrombosis are discussed.

BLOOD COAGULATION

Normal blood coagulation is a complex process involving numerous interacting elements. It is initiated by injury to a blood vessel and followed by two successive phases or series of events that result in clot formation.

Platelet or vascular phase

Platelets, also called thrombocytes, are produced in the bone marrow and released into the bloodstream, where they circulate for approximately 10 days before their removal by the spleen. Platelets are fragments of large cells called *megakaryocytes;* they contain no nuclei and are therefore unable to repair or replicate themselves. Their only known function in the body is related to hemostasis (the control of bleeding by blood coagulation).

When injury occurs to a blood vessel wall, platelets elongate and become "sticky" so that they adhere to the vessel wall and to other platelets (platelet aggregation). At the same time, the fragile cell membrane disintegrates and allows leakage of platelet contents (*e.g.*, thromboplastin and other clotting factors, calcium, serotonin, epinephrine, adenosine diphosphate [ADP], and thromboxane A_2) that serve various functions to stop bleeding. Thromboplastin activates prothrombin. Serotonin and epinephrine cause vasoconstriction. Thromboxane A_2 (a prostaglandin synthesized by platelets) is a potent stimulus of both vasoconstriction and platelet aggregation.

Platelets act within seconds to form a platelet plug and stop bleeding. Platelets usually disappear from a blood clot within 24 hours, to be replaced by fibrin.

Blood coagulation phase

Blood coagulation acts more slowly (within 1 to 2 minutes) to cause hemostasis. It involves sequential activation of clotting factors that are normally present in blood and tissues as inactive precursors. Characteristics and functions of coagulation factors are listed in Table 57-1. Major steps in the coagulation process are the following:

1. Release of thromboplastin by disintegrating platelets and damaged tissue
2. Conversion of prothrombin to thrombin. This step requires thromboplastin and calcium ions.
3. Conversion of fibrinogen to fibrin by thrombin

THROMBOTIC AND THROMBOEMBOLIC DISORDERS

Thrombosis may occur in both arteries and veins. Arterial thrombosis is usually associated with atherosclerotic plaque, hypertension, and turbulent blood flow. These conditions damage the inner lining of the artery so that platelets adhere, aggregate, and release thromboplastin to initiate the coagulation process. Arterial thrombi cause disease by obstructing blood flow. If the obstruction is incomplete or temporary, local tissue ischemia (deficient blood supply) occurs. If the obstruction is complete or prolonged, local tissue death or infarction occurs.

Venous thrombosis is usually associated with venous stasis. When blood flows very slowly, thrombin and other coagulant substances present in the blood become sufficiently concentrated in local areas to initiate the clotting process. With a normal rate of blood flow, these substances are rapidly removed from the blood, primarily by Kupffer cells in the liver. A venous thrombus is less cohesive than an arterial thrombus. Consequently, an embolus can easily become detached and travel to other parts of the body.

Venous thrombi cause disease by two mechanisms. First, thrombosis causes local congestion, edema, and perhaps inflammation by impairing normal outflow of venous blood (*e.g.*, thrombophlebitis, deep vein thrombosis). Second, embolization causes obstruction of blood supply when the embolus becomes lodged. The pulmonary arteries are frequent sites of embolization.

TABLE 57-1. BLOOD COAGULATION FACTORS

Number	Name	Functions
I	Fibrinogen	Forms fibrin, the insoluble protein strands that compose the supporting framework of a blood clot. Thrombin and calcium are required for the conversion
II	Prothrombin	Forms thrombin, which catalyzes the conversion of fibrinogen to fibrin
III	Thromboplastin	Converts prothrombin to thrombin
IV	Calcium	Catalyzes the conversion of prothrombin to thrombin
V	Labile factor	Required for formation of active thromboplastin
VII	Proconvertin or Stable factor	Accelerates action of tissue thromboplastin
VIII	Antihemophilic factor (AHF)	Promotes breakdown of platelets and formation of active platelet thromboplastin
IX	Christmas factor	Similar to Factor VIII
X	Stuart factor	Promotes action of thromboplastin
XI	Plasma thromboplastin antecedent (PTA)	Promotes platelet aggregation and breakdown, with subsequent release of platelet thromboplastin
XII	Hageman factor	Similar to Factor XI
XIII	Fibrin-stabilizing factor (FSF)	Converts fibrin meshwork to the dense, tight mass of the completely formed clot

DRUGS USED IN THROMBOTIC AND THROMBOEMBOLIC DISORDERS

Drugs given to prevent or treat thrombosis exert pharmacologic action by altering some aspect of the blood coagulation process. Anticoagulants are the drugs most widely used in thrombotic disorders. They are more effective in preventing venous thrombosis than arterial thrombosis. Antiplatelet drugs are useful in certain conditions to prevent arterial thrombosis. Thrombolytic agents are occasionally used to dissolve thrombi in life-threatening thromboembolic disease.

Anticoagulants

Anticoagulant drugs are given to prevent the formation of new clots and the growth or extension of clots already present. They do not dissolve formed clots, improve blood flow in tissues around the clot, or prevent ischemic damage to tissues beyond the clot. The two most commonly used anticoagulants are heparin and warfarin sodium (Coumadin), a coumarin derivative. These drugs act by different mechanisms to interfere with certain coagulation factors and prevent thrombus formation (see discussions of the individual drugs). Other coumarin derivatives such as dicumarol (also called bishydroxycoumarin) and phenprocoumon (Liquamar) are used occasionally.

Clinical indications for anticoagulants include prevention or treatment of various thromboembolic disorders such as thrombophlebitis, deep vein thrombosis (DVT), and pulmonary embolism. Heparin is used for a number of other purposes as well.

Antiplatelet drugs

Antiplatelet drugs prevent platelet aggregation and thereby interfere with the initial phase of blood coagulation. Increased platelet aggregation is associated with atherosclerosis and thromboembolic disorders. For example, arterial thrombi, which are composed primarily of platelets, may embolize from abnormal heart valves, mural thrombi, or atherosclerotic plaque.

The drugs used clinically for antiplatelet effects (aspirin, dipyridamole [Persantine], and sulfinpyrazone [Anturane]) were introduced for other purposes. The effectiveness of the drugs in reducing cardiovascular morbidity and mortality is still under investigation. At present, antiplatelet drugs are recommended for clients with transient ischemic attacks (TIAs) who are not candidates for surgery (*e.g.*, carotid endarterectomy) and for clients with prosthetic heart valves, often in combination with an oral anticoagulant (*i.e.*, warfarin sodium). The drugs may also be useful in preventing repeated or subsequent myocardial infarctions in clients who have had a myocardial infarction.

Thrombolytic agents

Thrombolytic agents are given to help dissolve formed blood clots (thrombi). They act by stimulating conversion of plasminogen to plasmin (also called fibrinolysin). *Fibrinolysin* is a proteolytic enzyme that hydrolyzes fibrin, the framework of a thrombus.

The two thrombolytic agents currently available, streptokinase and urokinase, are recommended only for treatment of acute, severe thromboembolic disease (*e.g.*, myocardial infarction, pulmonary emboli, and iliofemoral thrombophlebitis).

Individual drugs

ANTICOAGULANTS AND THEIR ANTIDOTES

Heparin sodium (Lipo-Hepin, Liquamin) is a pharmaceutical preparation of the natural anticoagulant produced primarily by mast cells in pericapillary connective tissue. Endogenous heparin is found in various body tissues, most abundantly in the liver and lungs. Exogenous heparin is obtained from bovine lung or porcine intestinal mucosa and standardized in units of biologic activity.

Heparin acts in conjunction with antithrombin III to inactivate several clotting factors (IX, X, XI, and perhaps XII) and thrombin so that thrombus formation is prevented. Antithrombin III is an alpha globulin normally present in the blood as a natural anticoagulant substance. Antithrombin III must be present for heparin action.

Heparin sodium approaches the ideal anticoagulant; that is, it is fast acting (acts immediately after intravenous administration, within 20 to 30 minutes after subcutaneous injection), readily excreted, and almost nontoxic. It is metabolized in the liver and excreted in the urine, primarily as inactive metabolites. Heparin does not cross the placental barrier and is not secreted in breast milk. Disadvantages of heparin are the short duration of action and subsequent requirement for frequent administration, the necessity for parenteral injection because it is not absorbed from the gastrointestinal tract, its relatively high cost, and local tissue reactions at injection sites.

Heparin is widely used for prevention and treatment of thromboembolic diseases. Prophylactically, heparin may be given to prevent DVT and pulmonary embolism. The following clients may be candidates for low-dose heparin prophylaxis:

1. Those having abdominal or thoracic surgery who are over 40 years of age or have additional risk factors for DVT (*e.g.*, obesity, varicose veins)
2. Those with a history of thrombophlebitis or pulmonary embolism
3. Those having gynecologic surgery, especially if they have been taking estrogens or oral contraceptives or have other risk factors for DVT.
4. Those expected to be on bedrest or to have limited activity for longer than 5 days, especially if debilitating conditions are also present (*e.g.*, severe congestive heart failure, stroke, malignant disease)

Low-dose heparin prophylaxis is either not effective or contraindicated in major orthopedic surgery, abdominal prostatectomy, and brain surgery.

Therapeutically, heparin is used for treatment of acute thromboembolic disorders (*e.g.*, DVT, thrombophlebitis, pulmonary embolism). In these conditions, the aim of therapy is to prevent further thrombus formation and embolization. Heparin is also used in disseminated intravascular coagulation (DIC), a life-threatening condition characterized by widespread clotting, which depletes the blood of coagulation factors. The depletion of coagulation factors then produces widespread bleeding. The goal of heparin therapy in DIC is to prevent blood coagulation long enough for clotting factors to be replenished and thus be able to control hemorrhage. Although sometimes used in arterial occlusive disease, myocardial infarction and stroke, heparin therapy has not been proved effective in preventing further thromboembolic problems. However, heparin may be effective in preventing embolization from prosthetic heart valves.

Heparin is also used to prevent clotting during cardiac and vascular surgery, extracorporeal circulation, hemodialysis, and blood transfusions and in blood samples to be used in laboratory tests and intermittent intravenous infusion devices (*e.g.*, heparin lock). When heparin is used with intermittent intravenous infusion devices, a dilute solution of 10 units/ml or 100 units/ml is instilled periodically to maintain patency of the device.

Contraindications to heparin therapy include gastrointestinal ulcerations (*e.g.*, peptic ulcer disease, ulcerative colitis), blood dyscrasias, severe kidney or liver disease, severe hypertension, polycythemia vera, and recent surgery of the eye, spinal cord, or brain. It should be used with caution with mild hypertension, renal or hepatic disease, alcoholism, history of gastrointestinal ulcerations, drainage tubes (*e.g.*, nasogastric tubes, in-dwelling urinary catheters), and any occupation with high risks of traumatic injury.

Routes and dosage ranges

Adults: IV injection, 5000 units initially, followed by 5000–10,000 units q4–6h, up to a maximal daily dose of 25,000 units
DIC, IV injection, 50–100 units/kg, q4h
IV infusion, 20,000–40,000 units daily at initial rate of 0.25 unit/kg/minute, then adjusted according to blood clotting tests (activated partial thromboplastin time [APTT])
SC 10,000–12,000 units q8h or 14,000–20,000 units q12h
Low-dose prophylaxis, SC 5000 units 2 hours before surgery, then q12h until discharged from hospital or fully ambulatory

Children: DIC, IV injection, 25–50 units/kg q4h
IV infusion, 50 units/kg initially, followed by 100 units/kg q4h

Heparin sodium and dihydroergotamine mesylate (Embolex) is approved for the prevention of postoperative thromboembolic disorders (*e.g.*, DVT, pulmonary embolism) in clients over 40 years of age who are having major thoracic, abdominal, or pelvic surgery. The combination product is reportedly more effective than either drug alone.

Dihydroergotamine (DHE) is an alpha-adrenergic blocking agent (see Chap. 19) that acts on the smooth muscle of veins to cause constriction. As a result, it accelerates venous blood flow and decreases venous stasis. Venous stasis is a major risk factor for thromboembolic disorders.

Lidocaine, a local anesthetic, is added to this product to decrease pain and irritation at the injection site.

Contraindications include hypersensitivity to any of the three component drugs, peripheral vascular disease, coronary artery disease, angina pectoris, severe hypertension, impaired renal or hepatic function, sepsis, bleeding disorders, clients having surgery on the brain, spinal cord, or eye, those having spinal anesthesia, and those receiving oral anticoagulants or platelet-active drugs.

Route and dosage range

Adults: SC DHE 0.5 mg with heparin 5000 units 2 hours preoperatively, then q12h for 5–7 days postoperatively. Give by deep SC injection, usually into abdominal wall, with a 25- or 26-gauge needle.

Protamine sulfate is used only as an antidote or antagonist for heparin overdose. Heparin is an acid; protamine sulfate is a base. Thus, protamine neutralizes heparin activity. Protamine dosage depends on the amount of heparin administered during the previous 3 or 4 hours. Each milligram of protamine neutralizes 80 to 100 units of heparin. A single dose should not exceed 50 mg. The drug is injected intravenously over 1 to 3 minutes. Protamine effects occur immediately and last for approximately 2 hours. A second dose may be required, since heparin activity lasts about 4 hours.

Warfarin sodium (Coumadin, Panwarfin) is the prototype and most commonly used coumarin anticoagulant. Warfarin acts in the liver to prevent synthesis of vitamin K–dependent clotting factors (*i.e.*, factors II, VII, IX, and X). Warfarin is similar to vitamin K in structure and therefore acts as a competitive antagonist to hepatic utilization of vitamin K. Anticoagulant effects do not occur for approximately 3 to 5 days after warfarin is started because clotting factors already in the blood follow their normal pathway of elimination. Warfarin has no effect on circulating clotting factors or on platelet function.

Warfarin is well absorbed after oral administration. Although it can be given parenterally, there is no advantage in therapeutic effect. Warfarin is highly bound to plasma proteins. It is metabolized in the liver and primarily excreted as inactive metabolites by the kidneys.

Warfarin is most useful in long-term prevention or treatment of venous thromboembolic disorders. It is also used to prevent embolization from prosthetic heart valves. Warfarin has sometimes been advocated for use after myocardial infarction (to prevent reinfarction) and in strokes caused by cerebral thrombosis. However, the usefulness of anticoagulant therapy in these conditions is not clearly established. As a general rule, warfarin is not indicated in arterial thrombosis because arterial thrombi are composed primarily of platelets, and warfarin has no effect on platelet functions.

Contraindications to warfarin therapy include gastrointestinal ulcerations (*e.g.*, peptic ulcer disease, ulcerative colitis), blood dyscrasias (*e.g.*, hemophilia, thrombocytopenia), severe kidney or liver disease, severe hypertension, and recent surgery of the eye, spinal cord, or brain. Warfarin also crosses the placenta and is contraindicated during pregnancy. Warfarin should be used cautiously with mild hypertension, renal or hepatic disease, alcoholism, history of gastrointestinal ulcerations, drainage tubes (*e.g.*, nasogastric tubes, in-dwelling urinary catheters), and occupations with high risks of traumatic injury.

Routes and dosage ranges

Adults: PO 10–15 mg daily initially, then adjusted according to prothrombin time (PT). Average daily maintenance dose, 2–10 mg

IM, IV, same dosage as above (these routes are rarely used)

Phytonadione (Vitamin K, Mephyton) is the antidote for warfarin overdosage. An oral dose of 10 to 20 mg will usually stop minor bleeding and return the prothrombin time to a normal range within 24 hours.

Infrequently used coumarin anticoagulants

Dicumarol (bishydroxycoumarin) is a long-acting, orally administered coumarin anticoagulant. Peak effects occur 3 to 5 days after drug therapy is started. When discontinued, effects persist 2 to 10 days.

Route and dosage ranges

Adults: PO 200–300 mg initially, followed by 25–200 mg daily, based on prothrombin time

Phenprocoumon (Liquamar) is a long-acting, orally administered coumarin anticoagulant. Peak effects occur 48 to 72 hours after administration of the initial dose. Effects persist up to 7 days after the drug is discontinued.

Route and dosage range

Adults: PO 24 mg initially. Average maintenance dose 0.75–6 mg, adjusted according to prothrombin time

ANTIPLATELET AGENTS

Aspirin is a commonly used analgesic–antipyretic–anti-inflammatory drug (see Chap. 6) with potent antiplatelet effects. Aspirin exerts pharmacologic actions by inhibiting synthesis of prostaglandins. In this instance, aspirin acetylates the enzyme in platelets that normally synthesizes thromboxane A_2, a prostaglandin that causes platelet aggregation. Thus, aspirin prevents formation of thromboxane A_2, thereby preventing platelet aggregation and thrombus formation. Antithrombotic effects persist for the life of the platelet, approximately 10 days. Aspirin may be used as an antiplatelet agent for prevention of myocardial reinfarction and in clients with prosthetic heart valves or TIAs. Adverse effects are uncommon with dosages used for antiplatelet effects.

Route and dosage range

Adults: PO 150–325 mg daily

Dipyridamole (Persantine) is a vasodilator and antiplatelet drug that has little effect when used alone. High dosages are required to prevent platelet aggregation. Dipyridamole is recommended only for prevention of thromboemboli in clients with prosthetic heart valves. For this purpose, it is given in combination with aspirin.

Route and dosage range

Adults: PO 25–75 mg 3 times daily, 1 hour before meals

Sulfinpyrazone (Anturane) is a uricosuric agent that is most often used in the treatment of gout. It also prevents platelet aggregation. The clinical usefulness of sulfinpyrazone in thromboembolic disorders is not clearly established.

Route and dosage range

Adults: PO 600–800 mg daily, in 3–4 divided doses

THROMBOLYTIC AGENTS AND THEIR ANTIDOTE

Streptokinase (Streptase) is a protein derived from streptococci. It promotes dissolution of blood clots by interacting with a plasminogen proactivator. The resulting substance catalyzes the conversion of plasminogen to plasmin. Plasmin (fibrinolysin) breaks down fibrin. Streptokinase may be used for treatment of acute pulmonary emboli or iliofemoral thrombophlebitis when these conditions are severe and life threatening. Bleeding, fever, and allergic reactions may occur. Heparin and warfarin are given after streptokinase therapy is finished.

Streptokinase may also be injected directly into a coronary artery to dissolve a thrombus if done within 6 hours of onset of symptoms. An additional use is to dissolve clots in arterial or venous lines.

Route and dosage range

Adults: IV 250,000 units over 30 minutes, then 100,000 units hourly for 24–72 hours, depending on the thrombin time (therapeutic range is 2–5 times the control value). Recommended doses vary widely.

Urokinase (Abbokinase) is a proteolytic enzyme that catalyzes the conversion of plasminogen to plasmin. Plasmin breaks down fibrin and thereby promotes dissolution of blood clots. Urokinase is recommended for use in clients who are allergic to streptokinase. Urokinase is contraindicated in children, pregnant women, and clients with wounds, malignancies, and recent strokes. In addition, all other contraindications to heparin and warfarin therapy also apply to urokinase. Incidence of bleeding is high with urokinase. Heparin and warfarin are started after urokinase therapy is completed.

Route and dosage range

Adults: IV 4400 units/kg over 10 minutes, followed by continuous infusion of 4400 units/kg/hour for 12 hours

Aminocaproic acid (Amicar) is a specific antidote for an overdose of streptokinase or urokinase. The usual dose is 5 g, orally or intravenously, followed by 1.25 g/hour until bleeding is controlled. Maximal dose is 30 g/24 hours. Rapid intravenous administration should be avoided because it may cause hypotension or cardiac arrhythmias. Aminocaproic acid may also be used in other bleeding disorders caused by hyperfibrinolysis (*e.g.*, cardiac surgery, blood disorders, hepatic cirrhosis, prostatectomy, neoplastic disorders). The drug should *not* be used unless hyperfibrinolysis is present.

Principles of therapy: anticoagulant, antiplatelet, and thrombolytic agents

ASSESSMENT GUIDELINES

Assess the client's status in relation to thrombotic and thromboembolic disorders.

1. Risk factors for thromboembolism include:
   a. Immobility (*e.g.*, limited activity or bedrest for more than 5 days)
   b. Obesity
   c. Cigarette smoking
   d. History of varicose veins, thrombophlebitis, or pulmonary emboli
   e. Congestive heart failure
   f. Pedal edema
   g. Lower limb trauma
   h. Myocardial infarction
   i. Atrial fibrillation
   j. Mitral or aortic stenosis
   k. Prosthetic heart valves
   l. Abdominal, thoracic, pelvic, or major orthopedic surgery
   m. Atherosclerotic heart disease or peripheral vascular disease
   n. Oral contraceptive pills

2. Signs and symptoms of thrombotic and thromboembolic disorders depend on the location and size of the thrombus.
   a. DVT and thrombophlebitis usually occur in the legs. The conditions may be manifested by edema (the affected leg is often measurably larger than the other) and pain, especially in the calf when the foot is dorsiflexed (positive Homans' sign). If thrombophlebitis is superficial, it may be visible as a red, warm, tender area following the path of a vein.
   b. Pulmonary embolism, if severe enough to produce symptoms, is manifested by chest pain, cough, hemoptysis, tachypnea, and tachycardia. Massive emboli cause hypotension, shock, cyanosis, and death.
   c. DIC is usually manifested by bleeding. The bleeding may range from petechiae or oozing from a venipuncture site to massive internal bleeding or bleeding from all body orifices.

PREVENTIVE NURSING INTERVENTIONS

1. Use measures to prevent thrombotic and thromboembolic disorders.
   a. Have the client ambulate regularly, especially postoperatively.
   b. Instruct clients with limited mobility to exercise their legs. If the client is unable to perform active exercises, the nurse or physical therapist can do passive exercises.
   c. Have the client wear elastic stockings. Elastic stockings should be removed every 8 hours and replaced after inspecting the skin. Improperly applied elastic stockings can impair circulation rather than aid it.
   d. Instruct the client to avoid wearing tight girdles, garters, and stockings with tight elastic bands; crossing the legs at the knees; prolonged sitting, standing, and bedrest; and placing pads or pillows under the knees when in bed. These measures reduce or prevent venous stasis, a risk factor for clotting disorders.
   e. Avoid trauma to lower extremities.
   f. Maintain adequate fluid intake (1500 to 3000 ml daily) to avoid dehydration and hemoconcentration.
2. For the client receiving anticoagulant therapy, implement safety measures to prevent trauma and bleeding.
   a. For clients who are unable to ambulate safely owing to weakness, sedation, or other conditions, keep the call light within reach, keep bedrails elevated, and assist in ambulation.
   b. Provide an electric razor for shaving.
   c. Avoid intramuscular injections, venipunctures, and arterial punctures when possible.
   d. Avoid intubations when possible (*e.g.*, nasogastric tubes, in-dwelling urinary catheters).

DRUG SELECTION

Choice of anticoagulant or antiplatelet drug depends on the reason for use.

1. Heparin is the drug of choice in acute thromboembolic disorders because the anticoagulant effect begins immediately with intravenous administration.
2. Warfarin sodium is the drug of choice for long-term maintenance therapy (*i.e.*, several weeks or months), since it can be given orally.
3. Aspirin is probably the most widely used antiplatelet drug for prevention of myocardial reinfarction and arterial thrombosis in clients with TIAs and prosthetic heart valves.
4. When anticoagulation is required during pregnancy, heparin is used because it does not cross the placenta. Warfarin is contraindicated during pregnancy.

DOSAGE FACTORS

Dosage of anticoagulant drugs must be individualized, primarily according to blood coagulation tests, client characteristics, and concomitant drug therapy.

1. Heparin dosage is regulated by the APTT, which is a modification of the partial thromboplastin time (PTT). It is reportedly more sensitive than the PTT and requires less time to perform. The APTT is sensitive to changes in blood clotting factors, except factor VII. Thus, normal or control values indicate normal blood coagulation; therapeutic values indicate low levels of clotting factors and delayed blood coagulation. During heparin therapy, the APTT should be maintained at $1\frac{1}{2}$ to $2\frac{1}{2}$ times the control or baseline value. The normal control value is 16 to 25 seconds; therefore, therapeutic values are 24 to 50 seconds. For intermittent methods of administration, blood for the APTT should be drawn about 1 hour before a dose of heparin is scheduled. APTT is not necessary with low-dose heparin given subcutaneously for prophylaxis of thromboembolism.
2. Warfarin dosage is regulated according to PT,

which is sensitive to changes in several blood coagulation factors, especially three of the four vitamin K–dependent factors (*i.e.*, II, VII, and X). Thus, normal or control values indicate normal levels of these blood coagulation factors; therapeutic values indicate low levels of these factors and delayed blood coagulation. A normal baseline or control PT is about 12 seconds; a therapeutic value is approximately twice the control or 24 seconds. Therapeutic values may range from $1\frac{1}{2}$ to $2\frac{1}{2}$ times the control value.

When an oral anticoagulant is started, PT should be measured daily until a stable daily dose is reached (the dose that maintains PT within therapeutic values and does not cause bleeding). Often, the daily dose is ordered after the physician obtains the PT report. This process may require 1 to 2 weeks. Thereafter, PT is measured every 2 to 4 weeks for the duration of oral anticoagulant drug therapy.

The prothrombin time test is based on the one-stage prothrombin time. However, so many modifications of the test have been made that normal values vary among laboratories. Some laboratories report percent of normal prothrombin activity rather than prothrombin time in seconds. A value of 25% is approximately equal to 24 seconds; both are therapeutic levels. Because of these differences, the nurse must know the values used by a particular laboratory to interpret PT test results accurately. Also, the nurse must instruct the client receiving long-term therapy to use the same laboratory for PT tests or notify the physician when this is not possible.

3. Warfarin dosage may need to be reduced in clients with biliary tract disorders (*e.g.*, obstructive jaundice), liver disease (*e.g.*, hepatitis, cirrhosis), malabsorption syndromes (*e.g.*, steatorrhea), and hyperthyroidism or fever. These conditions increase anticoagulant drug effects by reducing absorption of vitamin K, decreasing hepatic synthesis of blood-clotting factors, or increasing the rate of degradation of clotting factors. Despite these influencing factors, however, the primary determinant of dosage is the prothrombin time.
4. Warfarin and other coumarin anticoagulants interact with many other drugs to cause increased, decreased, or unpredictable anticoagulant effects. Thus, warfarin dosage may need to be increased or decreased when other drugs are given concomitantly. Most drugs can be given if warfarin dosage is carefully titrated according to the prothrombin time. Prothrombin time measurements and vigilant observation are needed any time a drug is added to or removed from a drug therapy regimen containing an oral anticoagulant.

NURSING ACTIONS: ANTICOAGULANTS

Nursing Actions	*Rationale/Explanation*
1. Administer accurately	
a. With *heparin*	
(1) When transcribing a physician's order, write out "units" rather than using the abbreviation "U."	This is a safety precaution to avoid erroneous dosage. For example, 1000 U (1000 units) may be misread as 10,000 units.
(2) Check dosage carefully.	Although accurate dosage is important in all drug therapy, it is especially important with anticoagulants. A rather narrow range exists between therapeutic and toxic levels. Therefore, underdosage may cause thromboembolism, and overdosage may cause bleeding. In addition, heparin is available in several concentrations (1000, 2500, 5000, 10,000, 15,000, 20,000, and 40,000 units/ml).
(3) For subcutaneous heparin	
(a) Use a 26-gauge, $\frac{1}{2}$-inch needle.	To minimize trauma and risk of bleeding
(b) Use a tuberculin syringe and a drug volume of 0.5 ml or less.	To measure accurately and minimize trauma
(c) Cleanse injection site gently with an alcohol sponge.	To prevent infection

Nursing Actions	**Rationale/Explanation**
(d) Grasp a fold of tissue between thumb and fingers of the nondominant hand. Do not pinch tightly.	To give the drug in a deep subcutaneous or fat layer
(e) Insert the needle at a 90° angle into the skin fold, inject without aspirating, and withdraw the needle.	To minimize trauma and risk of bleeding
(f) Apply pressure to the site for 1 to 2 minutes.	To prevent bleeding
(g) Rotate injection sites (abdomen, upper arms, and lateral thighs may be used). Do not inject heparin within 2 inches of the umbilicus.	To minimize tissue irritation and trauma. Avoid the umbilical area to prevent inadvertent injection into umbilical veins.
(4) For intermittent intravenous administration	
(a) Give by direct injection into a heparin lock or tubing injection site.	These methods prevent repeated venipunctures.
(b) Dilute the dose in 50 to 100 ml of any intravenous fluid (usually 5% dextrose in water).	
(5) For continuous intravenous administration	This is usually the preferred method of administration because it maintains consistent serum drug levels rather than peak levels and trough levels.
(a) Use a volume-control device and an infusion control device.	To accurately regulate dosage and flow rate
(b) Add only enough heparin for a few hours. One effective method is to fill the volume-control set (*e.g.,* Volutrol) with 100 ml of 5% dextrose in water and add 5000 units of heparin to yield a concentration of 50 units/ml. Dosage is regulated by varying the flow rate. For example, administration of 1000 units/hour requires a flow rate of 20 ml/hour. Another method is to add 25,000 units of heparin to 500 ml of intravenous solution.	To avoid inadvertent administration of large amounts. Whatever method is used, it is desirable to standardize concentration of heparin solutions within an institution. Standardization is safer, since it reduces risks of errors in dosage.
b. After the initial dose of warfarin, check PT before subsequent dose. Do *not* give the dose if PT is more than $2\frac{1}{2}$ times the control value. Notify the physician.	Prothrombin time is measured daily until a maintenance dose is established, then periodically throughout warfarin therapy. Prolonged PT (*e.g.,* more than 30 seconds with a control value of 12 seconds) indicates high risk of bleeding.
2. Observe for therapeutic effects	
a. Absence of signs and symptoms when given prophylactically	
b. Decrease or improvement in signs and symptoms when given therapeutically (*e.g.,* less edema and pain with thrombophlebitis, less chest pain and respiratory difficulty with pulmonary embolism)	
c. PT (for warfarin) or APPT (for heparin) within therapeutic ranges ($1\frac{1}{2}$ to $2\frac{1}{2}$ the control value)	
3. Observe for adverse effects	
a. Bleeding	Bleeding is the major adverse effect of anticoagulant drugs. It may occur anywhere in the body, spontaneously or in response to minor trauma.
(1) Record vital signs regularly.	Hypotension and tachycardia may indicate internal bleeding.
(2) Check stools for blood (melena).	Gastrointestinal bleeding is fairly common; risks are increased with intubation. Blood in stools may be bright red, tarry (blood that has been digested by gastrointestinal secretions), or oc-

Nursing Actions	Rationale/Explanation
	cult (hidden to the naked eye but present with a guaiac test). Hematemesis may also occur.
(3) Check urine for blood (hematuria).	Genitourinary bleeding is also fairly common; risks are increased with catheterization or instrumentation. Urine may be red (indicating fresh bleeding), brownish or smoky gray (indicating old blood). Or, bleeding may be microscopic (red blood cells are visible only on microscopic examination during urinalysis).
(4) Inspect the skin and mucous membranes daily.	Bleeding may occur in the skin as petechiae, purpura, or ecchymoses. Surgical wounds, skin lesions, parenteral injection sites, the nose, and gums may be bleeding sites.
(5) Assess for excessive menstrual flow.	
b. Other adverse effects	
(1) With heparin, tissue irritation at injection sites, transient alopecia, reversible thrombocytopenia, paresthesias, hypersensitivity	These effects are uncommon. They are more likely to occur with large doses or prolonged administration.
(2) With warfarin, dermatitis, diarrhea, alopecia	These effects occur only occasionally. Warfarin has been given for prolonged periods without toxicity.
4. Observe for drug interactions	
a. Drugs that *increase* effects of heparin	
(1) Aspirin, dipyridamole	These drugs inhibit platelet function and therefore increase risks of bleeding.
(2) Warfarin sodium (Coumadin)	Additive anticoagulant effects and increased risks of bleeding
b. Drugs that *decrease* effects of heparin	
(1) Antihistamines, digitalis glycosides, tetracyclines	These drugs antagonize the anticoagulant effects of heparin. Mechanisms are not clear.
(2) Protamine sulfate	The antidote for heparin overdose
c. Drugs that *increase* effects of warfarin and other coumarins	
(1) Allopurinol, anabolic steroids (*e.g.,* methandrostenolone), cimetidine, tricyclic antidepressants (*e.g.,* amitriptyline), isoniazid (INH), methylphenidate	These drugs potentiate anticoagulant effects (and increase risks of bleeding) by inhibiting hepatic enzymes and slowing the rate of warfarin metabolism. Other mechanisms may also be involved.
(2) Antibiotics	Potentiate anticoagulant effects by decreasing production of vitamin K by intestinal bacteria. In addition, chloramphenicol and tetracyclines act by other mechanisms to increase risks of bleeding. Alternate antibiotics are preferred.
(3) Antidiabetic agents, oral	Displace anticoagulants from plasma protein binding sites
(4) Antilipemics (*e.g.,* clofibrate)	Displace oral anticoagulants from plasma protein binding sites; possibly other mechanisms
(5) Antineoplastics	Additive risks of bleeding because antineoplastic drugs depress bone marrow function and platelet counts
(6) Antiplatelet agents (*e.g.,* aspirin, dipyridamole, sulfinpyrazone)	Decrease platelet aggregation
(7) Aspirin, other salicylates and nonsteroidal antiinflammatory agents (*e.g.,* phenylbutazone, indomethacin)	These drugs greatly increase risks of bleeding. They displace warfarin from plasma protein binding sites, decrease platelet aggregation, and are ulcerogenic. None of these drugs should be given concurrently with oral anticoagulants.
(8) Heparin	Additive anticoagulant effects
(9) Thyroid preparations (*e.g.,* Synthroid)	Increase metabolism of clotting factors
d. Drugs that may *increase* or *decrease* effects of oral anticoagulants	
(1) Alcohol	Alcohol may induce liver enzymes, which *decrease* effects by accelerating the rate of metabolism of the anticoagulant drug.

Nursing Actions	***Rationale/Explanation***
	However, with alcohol-induced liver disease (*i.e.,* cirrhosis), effects may be *increased* owing to impaired metabolism of the anticoagulant.
(2) Corticosteroids	These drugs may *decrease* effects by stimulating synthesis of clotting factors or other mechanisms. They may *increase* risks of bleeding by their ulcerogenic effects.
e. Drugs that *decrease* effects of warfarin and other coumarins	
(1) Antacids and griseofulvin	May decrease gastrointestinal absorption of oral anticoagulants
(2) Barbiturates and other sedative–hypnotics, carbamazepine, disulfiram, rifampin	These drugs activate liver metabolizing enzymes, which accelerate the rate of metabolism of oral anticoagulant drugs.
(3) Cholestyramine	Decreases absorption
(4) Diuretics	Increase synthesis and concentration of blood clotting factors
(5) Estrogens, including oral contraceptives	Increase synthesis of clotting factors and have thromboembolic effect.
(6) Vitamin K	Restores prothrombin and other vitamin K–dependent clotting factors in the blood. Antidote for overdose of oral anticoagulants.
5. Teach clients receiving long-term anticoagulant therapy	
a. Take as directed.	This is crucial to avoid both underdosage (risks of thromboemboli) and overdosage (risks of bleeding).
b. Do not take any other drugs without the physician's knowledge and consent, especially over-the-counter cold remedies and analgesics.	Oral anticoagulant drugs interact with many other drugs with subsequent increased or decreased anticoagulant effects, either of which may be harmful to the client. Many nonprescription analgesics and cold remedies contain aspirin. Aspirin and any aspirin-containing products are contraindicated with oral anticoagulants because the risks of bleeding are greatly increased.
c. Inform any physician, surgeon, or dentist about anticoagulant drug therapy before any treatment measures are begun.	This is mainly a safety measure to prevent bleeding episodes.
d. Keep all appointments for PT tests.	These tests are required regularly throughout oral anticoagulant therapy for safety (prevention of bleeding) and titration of dosage.
e. Use safety precautions (1) Avoid walking barefoot. (2) Avoid contact sports. (3) Use an electric razor. (4) Avoid injections when possible.	To avoid injury and subsequent bleeding
f. Carry an identification card, necklace, or bracelet (*e.g.,* Medic Alert) stating the name of the drug and the physician's name and telephone number.	
g. Inspect skin, mucous membranes, urine, and feces for signs of bleeding. Report to the physician if bleeding occurs.	Pinprick hemorrhages, bruising, or frank bleeding may occur in the skin and mucous membranes. Urine may be bright red or smoky gray. Feces may be bright red or black (tarry).
h. Apply direct pressure to superficial bleeding sites for 3 to 5 minutes or longer if necessary.	To prevent excessive blood loss
i. Do not eat large amounts of leafy green vegetables (*e.g.,* spinach), tomatoes, bananas, or fish.	These foods contain vitamin K, which may decrease anticoagulant effects.

Selected References

American Medical Association (AMA) Division of Drugs: AMA Drug Evaluations, 5th ed. New York, John Wiley & Sons, 1983

Chesebro JH, Steele PM, Fuster V: Platelet-inhibitor therapy in cardiovascular disease. Postgrad Med 78:48–71, July 1985

Creager MA: Preventing and treating deep-vein thrombophlebitis. Drug Ther 15:51–71, May 1985

Dihydroergotamine-heparin to prevent post-operative deep vein thrombosis. Med Lett Drugs Ther 27:45–46, May 1985

Facts and Comparisons. St. Louis, J B Lippincott (Updated monthly)

Hansten PD: Drug Interactions: Clinical Significance of Drug–Drug Interactions, 5th ed. Philadelphia, Lea & Febiger, 1985

Hirsh J: The optimal antithrombotic dose of aspirin. Arch Intern Med 145:1582–1583, September 1985

Malseed RT: Pharmacology: Drug Therapy and Nursing Considerations, 2d ed. Philadelphia, J B Lippincott, 1985

Nissen MB: Streptokinase therapy in acute myocardial infarction. Heart Lung 13:223–230, May 1984

O'Reilly RA: Anticoagulant, antithrombotic, and thrombolytic drugs. In Gilman AG, Goodman LS, Rall TW, Murad F (eds): The Pharmacological Basis of Therapeutics, 7th ed, pp 1338–1359. New York, Macmillan, 1985

Young LC: Streptokinase therapy. Focus Crit Care 10:20–23, April 1983

58

ANTILIPEMICS AND VASODILATORS

Description and uses

Antilipemic drugs are used in the treatment of clients with elevated blood lipids, a major risk factor for atherosclerosis. Peripheral vasodilator drugs are used in the treatment of clients with arterial insufficiency caused by atherosclerosis or vasospasm.

Atherosclerosis is the major cause of angina pectoris, myocardial infarction, cerebral vascular accidents (CVAs, or strokes), and peripheral vascular disease. Atherosclerosis is characterized by deposition of blood lipids on the lining of the arteries. These fatty plaques (atheromas) interfere with nutrition of the blood vessel lining and lead to necrosis, scarring, and calcification. The normally smooth endothelium becomes roughened and constricted, and the lumen size is reduced. These changes predispose to decreased blood flow, thrombus formation, and eventual occlusion of the vessel. When an artery is gradually occluded by atheromatous plaque, collateral circulation may develop sufficiently to provide oxygen and nutrients at rest. However, tissue ischemia and infarction are likely to develop with strenuous exercise or other conditions that increase tissue demands for oxygen and nutrients.

From the foregoing, it is clear that drugs to prevent or treat atherosclerotic vascular disease are very desirable. Antilipemic drugs have been available for some years. However, they have not been widely used because there was little evidence of decreased morbidity or mortality related to atherosclerosis, coronary artery disease, cerebrovascular insufficiency, or peripheral vascular disease. Also, drug usage was associated with adverse effects. More recently, studies have demonstrated beneficial effects, and use of the drugs may increase. Peripheral vasodilators have also been available a long time and are used clinically despite their questionable efficacy. Although they increase blood flow in normal vessels, they have not been proved to increase flow in atherosclerotic vessels or to decrease ischemia in body tissues. In fact, by diverting blood flow to the skin and nonischemic tissues, they may actually decrease flow to ischemic tissues. Also, they may cause hypotension, with a resultant decrease in cerebral blood flow. A new type of drug, a hemorheologic agent, reportedly improves blood flow by decreasing blood viscosity. Although the drug reduces symptoms of intermittent claudication, it is not yet clear whether drug therapy is more beneficial than exercise.

Antilipemic drugs are used to treat hyperlipidemia or hyperlipoproteinemia. Blood lipids are cholesterol, phospholipids, and triglycerides. Lipids are transported into and out of plasma by specific proteins called lipoproteins. Each lipoprotein contains cholesterol, phospholipid, and triglyceride in different and characteristic amounts, which can be measured in the laboratory.

The plasma lipoproteins are chylomicrons, very low-density lipoproteins (VLDL), low-density lipoproteins (LDL) and high-density lipoproteins (HDL). When blood lipid levels are elevated, there is an accompanying increase in blood levels of lipoproteins (hyperlipoproteinemia). Hyperlipoproteinemia may be primary (*i.e.*, genetic or familial) or secondary to dietary habits or other diseases (*e.g.*, diabetes mellitus, alcoholism, hypothyroidism, obstructive liver disease). The five major types of hyperlipoproteinemia are listed as follows:

1. Type I is characterized by elevated or normal serum cholesterol, elevated triglycerides, and chylomicronemia. It is a rare condition that may occur in infancy and childhood.
2. Type II is characterized by elevated cholesterol, normal or elevated triglycerides, and increased LDL. This type may be present at birth if genetic in origin. Type II is associated with a high risk of premature ischemic heart disease.
3. Type III is characterized by elevations of both cholesterol and triglycerides plus abnormal LDL and VLDL. This type usually occurs in middle-aged adults (40 to 60 years) and is associated with accelerated coronary and peripheral vascular disease.
4. Type IV has normal or elevated cholesterol levels, elevated triglycerides, and increased levels of VLDL. This type usually occurs in adults and may be the most common form of hyperlipoproteinemia. Type IV is often secondary to other diseases or to excessive intake of alcohol or carbohydrates. People with type IV are often obese. Ischemic heart disease may occur at 40 to 50 years of age.
5. Type V is characterized by elevated cholesterol and triglyceride levels with increased VLDL and chylomicronemia. This type usually occurs in adults and is uncommon. Type V is not associated with ischemic heart disease. Instead, it is associated with fat and carbohydrate intolerance, abdominal pain, and pancreatitis, which are relieved by lowering triglyceride levels.

Antilipemic drugs decrease hyperlipoproteinemias by altering the production, metabolism, or removal of lipoproteins. No drugs currently available are effective in lowering all types of hyperlipoproteinemia. Antilipemic drugs should be used only after 3 to 6 months of dietary therapy has failed to decrease hyperlipoproteinemia to an acceptable level. Further, the drugs should be given only to clients with signs and symptoms of coronary heart disease, a strong family history of coronary heart disease or hyperlipoproteinemia, or other risk factors for atherosclerotic vascular disease (*e.g.*, hypertension, diabetes mellitus, cigarette smoking). Specific antilipemic drugs and indications for use are listed in Table 58-1. The drugs should generally be discontinued after 2 to 3 months of therapy if blood lipids and lipoproteins are not lowered by at least 10% beyond that occurring with diet alone. Specific vasodilators are listed in Table 58-2.

Individual drugs

HEMORHEOLOGIC AGENT

Pentoxifylline (Trental), a methylxanthine derivative, is a hemorheologic agent that improves blood flow by decreasing blood viscosity rather than by vasodilation. Specific effects include increased flexibility of red blood cells with subsequent decreases in red blood cell aggregation and local hyperviscosity; decreased platelet aggregation; and decreased fibrinogen concentration.

Pentoxifylline is approved for use in intermittent claudication caused by chronic occlusive arterial insufficiency. It is contraindicated in clients who are unable to take methylxanthines such as theophylline or caffeine. It is apparently well tolerated, with only a few adverse reactions (dyspepsia, nausea, vomiting, dizziness, and headache) reported to occur in 1% to 3% of recipients.

Route and dosage range

Adults: PO 400 mg 3 times daily with meals, reduced to 400 mg 2 times daily if gastrointestinal and central nervous system side-effects occur

Principles of therapy: antilipemics and vasodilators

ASSESSMENT GUIDELINES

Assess the client's status in relation to atherosclerotic vascular disease.

1. Identify risk factors.
   a. Hypertension
   b. Diabetes mellitus
   c. High intake of dietary fat and refined sugars
   d. Obesity
   e. Lack of exercise
   f. Cigarette smoking
   g. Family history of atherosclerotic disorders
   h. Hyperlipidemia
2. Signs and symptoms depend on the specific problem.

TABLE 58-1. ANTILIPEMIC AGENTS

Generic name	Trade name	Clinical indications (type of hyperlipoproteinemia)	Mechanism of action	Route and dosage ranges *Adults*	*Children*
Cholestyramine	Questran	Type II	Binds bile acids in the intestines, resulting in increased oxidation of cholesterol to bile acids and decreased LDL cholesterol in the blood.	PO 12–24 g daily, in 2–4 divided doses, before or during meals and at bedtime	
Clofibrate	Atromid S	Types III, IV, V	Decreases synthesis of triglycerides and reduces VLDL	PO 2 g daily, in 2–4 divided doses	
Colestipol	Colestid	Type II	Same as cholestyramine	PO 15–30 g daily, in 2–4 divided doses, before or during meals and at bedtime	
Dextrothyroxine	Choloxin	Type II	Decreases cholesterol by increasing the rate of cholesterol catabolism	PO 1 mg daily for 1 month, increased at monthly intervals until therapeutic effects or maximal daily doses of 8 mg are achieved	PO 0.05 mg/kg/day initially. Maximal daily dose, 4 mg
Gemfibrozil	Lopid	Types IV, V	Decreases hepatic production of triglycerides, decreases VLDL, increases HDL	PO 900–1500 mg daily, usually 1200 mg in 2 divided doses, 30 minutes before morning and evening meals	
Nicotinic acid (niacin)		Types II, III, IV, V	Decreases synthesis and increases catabolism to lower cholesterol, triglycerides, LDL, and VLDL	PO 2–6 g daily, in 3–4 divided doses, with or just after meals	PO 55–87 mg/kg/day, in 3–4 divided doses, with or just after meals
Probucol	Lorelco	Type II	Decreases cholesterol and LDL	PO 500 mg twice daily, with morning and evening meals	

TABLE 58-2. VASODILATORS

Generic name	Trade name	Routes and dosage ranges (adults)
Papaverine hydrochloride	Pavabid, others	PO 100–300 mg 3–5 times daily Timed-release capsules, PO 150 mg q12h
Cyclandelate	Cyclospasmol	PO 1.2–1.6 g daily, in 4 divided doses, before meals and at bedtime. Decreased to 400–800 mg daily, in 2–4 divided doses, for maintenance.
Isoxsuprine hydrochloride	Vasodilan	PO 10–20 mg, 3–4 times daily IM 5–10 mg, 2–3 times daily
Nylidrin hydrochloride	Arlidin	PO 3–12 mg, 3–4 times daily
Niacin	Nicocap, others	Timed-release capsules, PO 300–400 mg q12h
Nicotinyl alcohol	Roniacol	PO 50–100 mg 3 times daily Sustained-release tablets (150 mg), 1–2 tablets twice daily
Tolazoline	Priscoline	SC, IM, IV 10–50 mg 4 times daily

a. Hyperlipidemia is manifested by elevated serum cholesterol (above 250 mg/100 ml) or triglycerides (above 150 mg/100 ml) or both.
b. Coronary artery atherosclerosis is manifested by myocardial ischemia (angina pectoris, myocardial infarction).
c. Cerebral vascular insufficiency may be manifested by syncope, memory loss, transient ischemic attacks (TIAs) or CVAs. Impairment of blood flow to the brain is caused primarily by atherosclerosis in the carotid, vertebral, or cerebral arteries.
d. Peripheral arterial insufficiency is manifested primarily by impaired blood flow in the legs (weak or absent pulses, cool, pale extremities, intermittent claudication, leg pain at rest, and development of gangrene, usually in the toes because they are most distal to blood supply). This condition results from atherosclerosis in the distal abdominal aorta, the iliac arteries, and the femoral and smaller arteries in the legs.

PREVENTIVE NURSING INTERVENTIONS

Use measures to prevent, delay, or minimize atherosclerosis.

1. Assist clients to control risk factors. Ideally, primary prevention begins in childhood with healthful eating habits (*i.e.*, avoiding excessive fats, meat, and dairy products; obtaining adequate amounts of all nutrients, including dietary fiber; avoiding obesity), exercise, and avoiding cigarette smoking. However, changing habits to a more healthful lifestyle is probably helpful at any time, before or after disease manifestations appear. Weight loss often reduces blood lipids and lipoproteins to a normal range. Changing habits is very difficult for most people, even those with severe symptoms.
2. Use measures to increase blood flow to tissues.
   a. Exercise is helpful in developing collateral circulation in the heart and lower extremities. Collateral circulation involves use of secondary vessels in response to tissue ischemia related to obstruction of the principal vessels. Clients with angina pectoris or previous myocardial infarction require a carefully planned and supervised program of progressive exercises. Those with peripheral arterial insufficiency can usually increase exercise tolerance by walking regularly. Distances should be determined by occurrence of pain and must be individualized.
   b. Posture and position may be altered to increase blood flow to the legs in peripheral arterial insufficiency. Elevating the head of the bed and having the legs horizontal or dependent may be helpful. Elevating the feet is usually contraindicated unless edema is present or likely to develop.
3. At present, the major treatment of occlusive vascular disease is surgical removal of atherosclerotic plaque or revascularization procedures. Thus, severe angina pectoris may be relieved by a coronary artery bypass procedure that detours around occluded vessels. This procedure may also be done after a myocardial infarction. The goal is to prevent infarction or reinfarction. TIAs may be relieved by carotid endarterectomy. The goal is to prevent a CVA. Peripheral arterial insufficiency may be relieved by aortofemoral, femoral–popliteal, or other bypass grafts that detour around occluded vessels.
   a. Although these procedures increase blood flow to ischemic tissues, they do not halt progression of atherosclerosis.
   b. The nursing role in relation to these procedures is to provide excellent preoperative and postoperative nursing care to promote healing, prevent infection, maintain patency of grafts, and help the client to achieve optimum function.
4. The most effective treatment in hyperlipoproteinemia is diet therapy. Specific diets have been developed for each type. Any antilipemic drug therapy must be accompanied by an appropriate diet.

PREGNANCY AND LACTATION

None of the antilipemic drugs has been established as safe for use during pregnancy or lactation.

DRUG INTERACTIONS

Cholestyramine decreases absorption of many oral medications (*e.g.*, corticosteroids, digitalis glycosides, folic acid, iron preparations, phenobarbital, tetracyclines, thiazide diuretics, thyroid preparations, fat-soluble vitamins, warfarin). When one of these drugs is ordered concomitantly with cholestyramine, the drug should be given at least 1 hour before or 4 to 6 hours after cholestyramine administration. In addition, dosage of the interactive drug may need to be changed when cholestyramine is added or withdrawn.

NURSING ACTIONS: ANTILIPEMICS AND VASODILATORS

Nursing Actions	*Rationale/Explanation*
1. Administer accurately	
a. Give cholestyramine before meals; mix with 4 to 6 ounces of water, milk, fruit juice, or other noncarbonated beverage, let stand 1 to 2 minutes, then stir.	The drug is available in a dry form, which should not be swallowed dry because of irritation to mucous membranes and possible obstruction of the esophagus.
b. Give nicotinic acid and probucol preparations with or after meals.	To decrease gastric irritation. This is probably not necessary with timed-release forms.
2. Observe for therapeutic effects	
a. With antilipemic agents, observe for decreased or normal levels of serum cholesterol (normal range is approximately 150 to 250 mg/100 ml), serum triglycerides (normal range is approximately 50 to 150 mg/100 ml), and lipoproteins (LDL and VLDL).	With *nicotinic acid,* cholesterol and triglycerides are usually lowered within 1 week and LDL within 3 to 5 weeks. With *clofibrate,* triglycerides and VLDL are usually lowered within 2 to 5 days. Lipid-lowering effects can be canceled by weight gain. With *cholestyramine,* cholesterol and LDL are usually lowered within 4 to 7 days. When the drug is discontinued, blood lipid levels return to pretreatment values in approximately 3 to 4 weeks. With *probucol,* maximal decrease in cholesterol and LDL occurs after 1 to 3 months of treatment.
b. With vasodilators, observe for increased warmth and improved color of extremities.	
c. With pentoxifylline, observe for decreased leg pain with exercise.	Improvement in function and symptoms may occur in 2 to 4 weeks.
3. Observe for adverse effects	
a. Gastrointestinal problems—nausea, vomiting, flatulence, constipation or diarrhea, abdominal discomfort	Gastrointestinal symptoms are the most common adverse effects of both antilipemic and vasodilator drugs.
b. With clofibrate and gemfibrozil, observe for an influenzalike syndrome (weakness, severe muscle cramps and tenderness); indications of cholelithiasis and cholecystitis; increased angina, thromboembolic disorders, and cardiac arrhythmias.	The mechanism of the influenzalike syndrome is unknown. Increased incidence of gallbladder disease is related to increased lithogenicity of bile. Development or aggravation of cardiovascular symptoms occurs in clients with coronary artery disease. Although all these adverse effects have not been reported with gemfibrozil, they may occur, since gemfibrozil is pharmacologically similar to clofibrate.
c. With vasodilator drugs, tachycardia, hypotension, dizziness, and flushing of the face and neck may occur.	These effects result from vasodilation of nonatherosclerotic blood vessels, including the skin capillaries of the face and neck.
d. With nicotinic acid, flushing of the face and neck, pruritus, and skin rash may occur as well as tachycardia, hypotension, and dizziness.	These symptoms may be prominent when nicotinic acid is used to lower blood lipids because relatively high doses are required. Aspirin 325 mg, given 30 minutes before nicotinic acid, reportedly decreases the flushing reaction.
e. With pentoxifylline, observe for dyspepsia, nausea, vomiting, dizziness, and headache.	These are the more common adverse effects.
4. Observe for drug interactions	
a. Drugs that *increase* effects of clofibrate	
(1) Acidifying agents (*e.g.,* ascorbic acid)	Decrease urinary excretion of clofibrate
(2) Dextrothyroxine (Choloxin), neomycin	Additive hypolipidemic effects. These drugs are sometimes used alone for treatment of hyperlipoproteinemia.
(3) Probenecid (Benemid)	Impairs renal and metabolic clearance of clofibrate

Nursing Actions	Rationale/Explanation
b. Drugs that *decrease* effects of clofibrate	
(1) Estrogens and oral contraceptives that contain estrogens	Estrogens increase blood lipids and thus antagonize effects of clofibrate.
(2) Rifampin	Induces hepatic metabolism of clofibrate
c. Drugs that *increase* effects of nicotinic acid and other vasodilating drugs	
Alcohol and antihypertensive vasodilating drugs (*e.g.*, hydralazine [Apresoline])	Additive vasodilation with hypotension and dizziness
5. Teach clients	
a. The most effective measures for preventing or controlling hyperlipidemia and atherosclerosis are those related to a healthful lifestyle (correct diet, weight control, exercise, not smoking cigarettes).	These measures are much more effective but more difficult for most people to implement than drug therapy.
b. When antilipemic drugs are used, appropriate dietary therapy is required as well.	The drugs are generally ineffective without dietary therapy. Overeating or gaining weight may cancel drug effects.
c. When taking vasodilator drugs, assume an upright position slowly.	To prevent or decrease vertigo, syncope, and weakness

Selected References

American Medical Association (AMA) Division of Drugs: AMA Drug Evaluations, 5th ed. New York, John Wiley & Sons, 1983

Brown MS, Goldstein JL: Drugs used in the treatment of hyperlipoproteinemias. In Gilman AG, Goodman LS, Rall TW, Murad F (eds): The Pharmacological Basis of Therapeutics, 7th ed, pp 827–845. New York, Macmillan, 1985

Facts and Comparisons. St. Louis, J B Lippincott (Updated monthly)

Hansten PD: Drug Interactions: Clinical Significance of Drug–Drug Interactions, 5th ed. Philadelphia, Lea & Febiger, 1985

Herbert PN, Terpstra AHM: Diet and exercise in the treatment of hyperlipoproteinemia. Drug Ther 14:42–52, May 1984

Lees RS, Lees AM: Lipid-lowering drugs: Renewed enthusiasm. Drug Ther 14:57–74, May 1984

Lipid-lowering drugs. Med Lett Drugs Ther 27:74–76, August 1985

Pentoxifylline for intermittent claudication. Med Lett Drugs Ther 26:103–104, November 1984

IX

DRUGS AFFECTING THE DIGESTIVE SYSTEM

59

PHYSIOLOGY OF THE DIGESTIVE SYSTEM

The digestive system consists of the alimentary canal (a tube extending from the oral cavity to the anus, approximately 25 to 30 feet [7.5 to 9 meters] long) and the accessory organs (salivary glands, gallbladder, liver, and pancreas). The main function of the system is to provide the body with fluids, nutrients, and electrolytes in a form that can be used at the cellular level. The system also disposes of waste products that result from the digestive process.

The alimentary canal has the same basic structure throughout. The layers of the wall are mucosa, connective tissue, and muscle. Peristalsis propels food through the tract and mixes the food bolus with digestive juices. Stimulation of the parasympathetic nervous system (by vagus nerves) increases both motility and secretions. The tract has an abundant blood supply, which increases cell regeneration and healing. Blood flow increases during digestion and absorption. Blood flow decreases with strenuous exercise, sympathetic nervous system stimulation (*i.e.,* "fight or flight"), aging (secondary to decreased cardiac output and atherosclerosis), and conditions that shunt blood away from the digestive tract (*e.g.,* congestive heart failure, atherosclerosis).

Organs of the digestive system

1. In the *oral cavity,* chewing mechanically breaks food into smaller particles, which can be swallowed more easily and which provide a larger surface area for enzyme action. Food is also mixed with saliva, which lubricates the food bolus for swallowing and initiates digestion of starch.
2. The *esophagus* is a musculofibrous tube about 10 inches (25 cm) long whose main function is to convey food from the pharynx to the stomach. It secretes a small amount of mucus and has some peristaltic movement.
3. The *stomach* is a dilated area that serves as a reservoir. It churns and mixes the food with digestive juices, secretes mucus and enzymes, starts protein breakdown, and secretes intrinsic factor, which is necessary for absorption of vitamin B_{12} from the ileum. Although there is much diffusion of water and electrolytes through the gastric mucosa, in both directions, there is very little absorption of these substances. Carbohydrates and amino acids are also poorly absorbed. Only a few highly lipid soluble substances, such as alcohol and some drugs, are absorbed in moderate quantities from the stomach.

   The inlet of the stomach is the cardiac sphincter at the end of the esophagus, and the outlet is the pyloric sphincter at the beginning of the duodenum. The stomach normally holds about 1000 ml comfortably and empties in about 4 hours. Numerous factors influence the rate of gastric emptying, including size of the pylorus, gastric motility, type of food, fluidity of chyme (the material produced by gastric digestion of food), and the state of the duodenum. Generally, factors that cause rapid emptying include carbohydrate foods, increased motility, fluid chyme, and an empty duodenum. The stomach empties more slowly with decreased gastric tone and motility, fatty foods, chyme of excessive acidity, and a duodenum that contains fats, proteins, or chyme of excessive acidity. When fats are present, the duodenal mucosa produces a hormone, enterogastrone, which inhibits gastric secretion and motility. This allows a longer time for the digestion of fats in the small intestine.

4. The *small intestine* consists of the duodenum, jejunum, and ileum and is about 20 feet (6 meters) long. The duodenum comprises the first 10 to 12 inches (25 to 27 cm) of the small intestine. The pancreatic and bile ducts empty into the duodenum at the papilla of Vater. The small intestine contains numerous glands that secrete digestive enzymes, hormones, and mucus. For the most part, digestion and absorption occur in the small intestine, including absorption of most orally administered drugs.
5. The *large intestine* consists of the cecum, colon, rectum, and anus. The ileum opens into the cecum. The colon secretes mucus and absorbs water.
6. The *pancreas* secretes enzymes, which are necessary for digestion of carbohydrates, proteins, and fats. It also secretes insulin and glucagon, hormones that regulate glucose metabolism and blood sugar levels.
7. The *gallbladder* is a small pouch attached to the underside of the liver that stores and concentrates bile. It has a capacity of about 50 to 60 ml. The gallbladder releases bile when fats are present in the duodenum.
8. The *liver* is a vital organ that performs numerous functions. It receives approximately 1500 ml of blood per minute or 25% to 30% of the total cardiac output. About three fourths of the blood flow is venous blood from the stomach, intestines, spleen, and pancreas (portal circulation); the remainder is arterial blood through the hepatic artery. The hepatic artery carries blood to the connective tissue of the liver and bile ducts, then empties into the hepatic sinuses and mixes with blood from the portal circulation. Venous blood from the liver flows into the inferior vena cava for return to the systemic circulation. The ample blood flow facilitates specific hepatic functions, which include the following.
   a. *Blood reservoir.* The liver can eject approximately 500 to 1000 ml of blood into the general circulation in response to stress, decreased blood volume, and sympathetic nervous system stimulation (*e.g.*, hemorrhagic or hypovolemic shock).
   b. *Blood filter and detoxifier.* Kupffer cells in the liver phagocytize bacteria carried from the intestines by the portal vein. They also break down worn-out erythrocytes, saving iron for reuse in hemoglobin synthesis, and form bilirubin, a waste product excreted in bile. The liver metabolizes many body secretions and most drugs to prevent accumulation and harmful effects on body tissues.

      Essentially all steroid hormones, including both adrenal corticosteroids and sex hormones, are at least partially conjugated in the liver and secreted into the bile. When the liver is damaged, these hormones may accumulate in body fluids and cause symptoms of hormone excess.

      Most drugs are active as the parent compound and are metabolized in the liver to an inactive metabolite that is then excreted by the kidneys. However, some drugs become active only after formation of a metabolite in the liver.

      The liver detoxifies or alters substances by oxidation, hydrolysis, or conjugation. Conjugation involves combining a chemical substance with an endogenous substance to produce an inactive or harmless compound.
   c. *Metabolism of carbohydrate, fat, and protein.* In carbohydrate metabolism, the liver functions to convert glucose to glycogen for storage and reconvert glycogen to glucose when needed to maintain an adequate blood sugar concentration. Excess glucose that cannot be converted to glycogen is converted to fat. The liver also changes fructose and galactose, which cannot be used by body cells, to glucose, which provides energy for cellular metabolism. Fats are both synthesized and catabolized by the liver. Amino acids from protein breakdown may be used to form glycogen, plasma proteins, and enzymes.
   d. *Storage of nutrients.* In addition to glycogen, the liver also stores fat-soluble vitamins (*i.e.*, vitamins A, D, E, K), vitamin B_{12}, iron, phospholipids, cholesterol, and small amounts of protein and fat.
   e. *Synthesis* of bile, serum albumin and globulin, prothrombin, fibrinogen, blood coagulation factors V, VII, VIII, IX, XI, and XII, and urea. Formation of urea removes ammonia from body fluids. Large amounts of ammonia are formed by intestinal bacteria and absorbed into the blood. If the ammonia is not converted to urea by the liver, plasma ammonia

concentrations rise to toxic levels and cause hepatic coma and death.

f. *Production of body heat* by continuous cellular metabolism. The liver is the body organ with the highest rate of chemical activity during basal conditions, and it produces about 20% of total body heat.

Secretions of the digestive system

1. *Mucus* is secreted by mucous glands in every part of the gastrointestinal tract. The functions of mucus are to protect the lining of the tract from digestive juices, lubricate the food bolus for easier passage, promote adherence of the fecal mass, and neutralize acids and bases.
2. *Saliva* consists of mucus and salivary amylase. It is produced by the salivary glands and totals approximately 1000 ml daily. Saliva has a slightly acidic to neutral *p*H (6 to 7) and functions to lubricate the food bolus and start starch digestion.
3. *Gastric juice* consists of mucus, digestive enzymes, hydrochloric acid, and electrolytes. The gastric glands secrete approximately 2000 ml of gastric juice daily. The *p*H is highly acidic (*p*H 1 to 3). Secretion is stimulated by the parasympathetic nervous system (by the vagus nerve), by the hormone gastrin, by the presence of food in the mouth, and by seeing, smelling, or thinking about food.

   The major digestive enzyme in gastric juice is pepsin, a proteolytic enzyme that functions best at a *p*H of 2 to 3. Hydrochloric acid provides the acid medium to promote pepsin activity. The major function of gastric juice is to begin digestion of proteins. There is also a weak action on fats by gastric lipase and on carbohydrates by gastric amylase. A large amount of mucus is secreted in the stomach to protect the stomach wall from the proteolytic action of pepsin. When mucus secretion is absent, gastric ulceration occurs within hours.
4. *Pancreatic juices* are alkaline (*p*H of 8 or above) secretions that contain amylase for carbohydrate digestion, lipase for fat digestion, and trypsin and chymotrypsin for protein digestion. They also contain large amounts of sodium bicarbonate, a base (alkali) that neutralizes the acid chyme from the stomach by reacting with hydrochloric acid. This protects the mucosa of the small intestine from the digestive properties of gastric juice. The daily amount of pancreatic secretion is approximately 1200 ml.
5. *Bile* is an alkaline secretion (*p*H about 8) that is formed continuously in the liver, carried to the gallbladder by the bile ducts, and stored there. The liver secretes approximately 600 ml of bile daily. This amount is concentrated to the 50 to 60 ml capacity of the gallbladder. Bile contains bile salts, cholesterol, bilirubin, fatty acids, and electrolytes. Bile salts are required for digestion and absorption of fats, including fat-soluble vitamins. Most of the bile salts are reabsorbed and reused by the liver (enterohepatic circulation); some are excreted in feces.

Effects of drugs on the digestive system

The digestive system and drug therapy have a reciprocal relationship. Many common symptoms (*i.e.,* nausea, vomiting, constipation, diarrhea, abdominal pain) relate to gastrointestinal dysfunction. These symptoms may result from a disorder in the digestive system or disorders in other body systems or from drug therapy. Many gastrointestinal symptoms and disorders alter the ingestion, dissolution, absorption, and metabolism of drugs. Drugs may be administered to *relieve* these symptoms and disorders. Drugs administered for conditions unrelated to the digestive system may *cause* such symptoms and disorders. Gastrointestinal conditions may alter responses to drug therapy.

Drugs used in digestive disorders act primarily to alter gastrointestinal secretion, absorption, or motility. They may act systemically or locally within the gastrointestinal tract. The drug groups included in this section are drugs used for peptic ulcer disease, laxatives, antidiarrheals, and antiemetics. Other drug groups used in gastrointestinal disorders include cholinergics (see Chap. 20), anticholinergics (see Chap. 21), corticosteroids (see Chap. 24), and anti-infective drugs (see Part VI).

Selected References

Anderson PD: Basic Human Anatomy and Physiology: Clinical Implications for the Health Professions. Monterey, CA, Wadsworth, 1984

Groer MW, Shekleton ME: Basic Pathophysiology: A Conceptual Approach, 2d ed. St. Louis, Mosby, 1983

Guyton AC: Textbook of Medical Physiology, 7th ed. Philadelphia, W B Saunders, 1986

Rodman MJ, Karch AM, Boyd EH, Smith DW: Pharmacology and Drug Therapy in Nursing, 3rd ed. Philadelphia, J B Lippincott, 1985

60

DRUGS USED IN PEPTIC ULCER DISEASE

Description and uses

Peptic ulcer disease is a common condition characterized by ulcer formation in an area of the gastrointestinal tract that is exposed to gastric acid. Therefore, peptic ulcers may develop in the esophagus, stomach, or duodenum. Acute ulcers occur more often in the stomach and may be associated with stress (*e.g.*, surgery, shock, head injury, severe burn injuries, major medical illness). These are often called "stress" ulcers. Acute ulcers may also be caused by certain drugs (*e.g.*, aspirin and other nonsteroidal anti-inflammatory drugs, corticosteroids, antineoplastics, and potassium tablets). Chronic ulcers are more likely to occur in the duodenum.

Despite extensive study, the cause of peptic ulcer disease is not clear. One etiologic factor is that gastric acid must be present. Gastric acid is a strong acid that is capable of digesting the stomach wall. Normally, autodigestion is prevented by mucus secretion, dilution of the acid by food and secretions, prevention of diffusion of hydrochloric acid from the stomach lumen back into the cells of the stomach lining, and regulation of acid secretion by the hormone gastrin.

Peptic ulcers are often attributed to an imbalance between the protein-digesting effects of gastric acid and pepsin and the protective mechanisms. Treatment of peptic ulcer disease is directed toward combating oversecretion of gastric acid, relieving pain, promoting healing, preventing recurrent ulcers, and preventing complications. Drugs used for peptic ulcer disease include histamine antagonists, antacids (see Table 60-1), anticholinergics (see Chap. 21 and Table 21-1), and sucralfate. Most of the drugs act to inhibit secretion of or neutralize gastric acid.

HISTAMINE ANTAGONISTS

Histamine is a substance found in almost every body tissue and released in response to certain stimuli (*e.g.*, allergic reactions, tissue injury). Once released, histamine causes the following reactions: contraction of smooth muscle in the bronchi, gastrointestinal tract, and uterus; dilation and increased permeability of capillaries; dilation of cerebral blood vessels; and stimulation of sensory nerve endings to cause pain and itching. Another effect of histamine, and the most important effect in relation to peptic ulcer disease, is strong stimulation of gastric acid secretion. Vagal stimulation causes release of histamine from cells in the gastric mucosa. The histamine then acts on receptors located on the parietal cells to increase production of hydrochloric acid. This receptor is called the *histamine-2 (H_2) receptor* and is the major determinant of hydrochloric acid production.

Traditional histamine antagonists (antihistamines or H_1 receptor blocking agents) prevent or reduce other effects of histamine but do not block histamine effects on gastric acid production. A new class of histamine antagonists (H_2 receptor blocking agents) was developed to inhibit gastric acid secretion. At present, cimetidine (Tagamet) and ranitidine (Zantac) are the only H_2 blockers approved for clinical use. They are used for prevention and treatment of peptic ulcer disease and hypersecretory states such as Zollinger–Ellison syndrome, a rare condition in which a pancreatic tumor secretes large amounts of gastrin. They are also used to prevent stress ulcers during severe illnesses, to treat esophagitis resulting from gastroesophageal reflux, and to prevent aspiration pneumonitis in people undergoing general anesthesia and surgery. The latter uses are considered investigational.

ANTACIDS

Antacids are alkaline substances that neutralize acids. They are often differentiated as systemic and nonsystemic agents. Systemic antacids are absorbed into body fluids and may alter acid–base balance. Sodium bicarbonate is the most frequently used systemic alkalinizing agent, especially during cardiopulmonary resuscitation and treatment of metabolic acidosis. (Sodium bicarbonate is discussed more extensively in Chapter 32.) In this chapter, nonsystemic or poorly absorbed antacids are discussed. These antacids act primarily in the stomach and are used to prevent and treat peptic ulcer disease. They are also used in the treatment of reflux esophagitis, gastritis, and pyrosis ("heartburn"). They may be useful in the prevention of gastrointestinal bleeding and stress ulcers.

Nonsystemic or gastric antacids used clinically are aluminum, magnesium, and calcium compounds. They react with hydrochloric acid in the stomach to produce neutral, less acidic, or poorly absorbed salts and to raise the *p*H (alkalinity) of stomach secretions. Raising *p*H to approximately 3.5 neutralizes more than 90% of gastric acid and inhibits conversion of pepsinogen to pepsin.

Gastric antacids differ in the amounts needed to neutralize gastric acid (approximately 50 to 80 mEq of acid are produced hourly), in onset of action, and in adverse effects produced. Aluminum compounds generally have a low neutralizing capacity (*i.e.*, large doses are required) and a slow onset of action. They can cause constipation. People who ingest large amounts of aluminum-based antacids over a long period may develop hypophosphatemia and osteomalacia because aluminum combines with phosphates in the gastrointestinal tract and prevents phosphate absorption. Aluminum compounds are rarely used alone. Magnesium-based antacids have a relatively high neutralizing capacity and a rapid onset of action. They may cause diarrhea and hypermagnesemia. Calcium compounds are effective and have a rapid onset of action but may cause hypersecretion of gastric acid ("acid rebound"), and "milk–alkali syndrome," which includes alkalosis and azotemia. Consequently, calcium compounds are rarely used in peptic ulcer disease. Although gastric antacids are considered nonsystemic drugs, small amounts of aluminum, magnesium, and calcium are absorbed from the gastrointestinal tract. Although normally insignificant, these small amounts may cause serious adverse effects in the presence of renal disease.

The most commonly used antacids are mixtures of aluminum hydroxide and magnesium hydroxide (*e.g.*, Gelusil, Mylanta, Maalox). Some antacid mixtures contain other ingredients, such as simethicone. Simethicone is an antiflatulent drug available alone as Mylicon. When added to antacid mixtures, simethicone does not affect gastric acidity, and its effectiveness in decreasing flatus is unproved.

ANTICHOLINERGIC AGENTS

Anticholinergic drugs (see Chap. 21) have been used extensively in the treatment of gastrointestinal disorders, including peptic ulcer disease. They have become largely obsolete for this purpose, however, because other drugs are more effective in decreasing gastric acid and do not cause as many adverse reactions. Some of the synthetic anticholinergic agents, such as anisotropine methylbromide (Valpin) and glycopyrrolate (Robinul), are occasionally used for antispasmodic effects in persistent abdominal pain and to prolong the effects of an antacid by delaying gastric emptying.

Individual drugs

HISTAMINE ANTAGONISTS

Cimetidine (Tagamet) is a type of antihistamine that was developed specifically to reduce secretion of gastric acid without causing the widespread effects and adverse reactions characteristic of anticholinergic drugs. Cimetidine decreases both the amount and acidity (hydrogen ion concentration) of gastric juices. The drug acts by blocking the action of histamine at H_2 receptor sites on parietal cells. Parietal cells, located in the mucosal lining of the stomach, are gastric acid–secreting cells. Cimetidine is usually called an H_2 receptor antagonist or H_2 blocker to differentiate it from conventional antihistamines, which do not affect gastric acid secretion.

Cimetidine is well absorbed following oral administration. After a single dose, peak blood level is reached in 1 to $1\frac{1}{2}$ hours, and an effective concentra-

TABLE 60-1. REPRESENTATIVE ANTACID PRODUCTS

Trade name	Components					Route and dosage ranges (adults)
	Magnesium oxide or hydroxide	*Aluminum hydroxide*	*Calcium carbonate*	*Sodium*	*Other*	
AlkaSeltzer effervescent tablets				296 mg	Sodium bicarbonate 958 mg, citric acid 832 mg, potassium bicarbonate 312 mg	PO 1–2 tablets, dissolved in 2–3 ounces of water, q4h as needed. Maximal dose, 8 tablets/24 hours
Aludrox	83 mg/tab, 103 mg/5 ml	233 mg/tab, 307 mg/5 ml		1.6 mg/tab, 1.15 mg/5 ml		PO 2 tablets or 10 ml q4h or PRN
Amphojel		300 or 600 mg/tab, 320 mg/5 ml		<7 mg/5 ml		PO 10 ml or 600 mg 5–6 times daily
Camalox	200 mg/tab, 200 mg/5 ml	225 mg/tab, 225 mg/5 ml	250 mg/tab, 250 mg/5 ml	1.5 mg/tab, 2.5 mg/5 ml		PO 2–4 tsp or tab, 4–5 times daily or as directed by physician, to maximal dose of 16 tablets or tsp/24 hours
Delcid	665 mg/5 ml	600 mg/5 ml		<15 mg/5 ml		PO 5 ml q4h as needed or as directed by physician, to maximal dose of 6 tsp (30 ml)/24 hours
Di-Gel	85 mg/tab, 87 mg/5 ml	282 mg/5 ml		10.6 mg/tab, 8.5 mg/5 ml	Tablets: simethicone 25 mg/tab, aluminum hydroxide and magnesium carbonate, 282 mg/tab Liquid: simethicone 20 mg per 5 ml	PO 2 tablets, chewed, or 2 tsp of liquid q2h, after meals, or between meals, and at bedtime. Maximal dose, 20 tablets or 20 tsp in 24 hours. Do not use maximal dose longer than 2 weeks
Gelusil	200 mg/5 ml	200 mg/5 ml		0.7 mg/5 ml	Simethicone 25 mg/5 ml	PO 10 or more ml or 2 or more tablets after meals and at bedtime or as directed by physician to a maximum of 12 tabs or tsp/24 hours
Gelusil-M	200 mg/5 ml	300 mg/5 ml		1.2 mg/5 ml	Simethicone 25 mg/5 ml	Same as Gelusil
Kolantyl	170 mg/wafer, 150 mg/5 ml	180 mg/wafer, 150 mg/5 ml				PO 1–4 tsp or wafers after meals and at bedtime or as directed by physician, to maximal dose of 12 tsp or wafers/24 hours
Maalox suspension	200 mg/5 ml	225 mg/5 ml		1.35 mg/5 ml		PO 30 ml 4 times daily, after meals and at bedtime or as directed by physician. Maximal dose, 16 tsp/24 hours
Maalox #1 tablets	200 mg/tab	200 mg/tab		0.84 mg/tab		PO 2–4 tablets, 4 times daily after meals and at bedtime or as directed by physician. Maximal dose, 16 tablets/24 hours
Maalox #2 tablets	400 mg/tab	400 mg/tab		1.84 mg/tab		PO 1–2 tablets, 4 times daily, after meals and at bedtime or as directed by physician. Maximal dose, 8 tablets/24 hours

TABLE 60-1. REPRESENTATIVE ANTACID PRODUCTS (*Continued*)

Trade name	Components					Route and dosage ranges (adults)
	Magnesium oxide or hydroxide	*Aluminum hydroxide*	*Calcium carbonate*	*Sodium*	*Other*	
Maalox Plus	200 mg/tab, 200 mg/5 ml	200 mg/tab, 225 mg/5 ml		1 mg/tab, 1.3 mg/5 ml	Simethicone 25 mg/tab, 25 mg/5 ml	PO 2–4 tsp or tablets 4 times daily after meals and at bedtime, or as directed by physician
Mylanta	200 mg/tab, 200 mg/5 ml	200 mg/tab, 200 mg/5 ml		0.77 mg/tab, 0.68 mg/5 ml	Simethicone 20 mg/tab, 20 mg/5 ml	PO 5–10 ml or 1–2 tablets q2–4h, between meals and at bedtime or as directed by physician
Mylanta II	400 mg/tab, 400 mg/5 ml	400 mg/tab, 400 mg/5 ml		1.3 mg/tab, 1.14 mg/5 ml	Simethicone 30 mg/tab, 30 mg/5 ml	Same as Mylanta
Titralac			420 mg/tab, 1 g/5 ml	<0.3 mg/tab, 11 mg/5 ml	Glycine, 180 mg/tab, 300 mg/5 ml	PO 1 tsp or 2 tabs, after meals or as directed by physician, to maximal dose of 19 tablets or 8 tsp/24 hours
WinGel	160 mg/5 ml	180 mg/5 ml				PO 1–2 tsp or tabs up to 4 times daily, or as directed by physician. Children over age 6 years: same as adults

tion is maintained for about 4 hours. The drug is distributed in almost all body tissues. Most of an oral dose is excreted unchanged in the urine within 24 hours; some is excreted in bile and eliminated in feces.

The major clinical indication for use of cimetidine is peptic ulcer disease. When used therapeutically for gastric or duodenal ulcers, cimetidine promotes healing, usually within 6 to 8 weeks. It is also effective in controlling gastrointestinal bleeding due to peptic ulcer disease. When used prophylactically, cimetidine can prevent recurrence of chronic ulcers or development of stress ulcers associated with severe burns, trauma, and other serious illnesses. Cimetidine may also be used in the treatment of Zollinger–Ellison syndrome.

There are no known contraindications to the use of cimetidine. However, the drug should be used with caution in people with renal or hepatic impairment or who are elderly, because drug half-life is prolonged and accumulation may occur. It should also be used with caution during pregnancy because it crosses the placenta, and it should not be taken during lactation because it is excreted in breast milk. Experience with cimetidine in children has been very limited, and it is generally not recommended for children younger than 16 years of age.

Routes and dosage ranges

Adults: PO 300 mg 4 times daily, with meals and at bedtime or 800 mg once daily at bedtime

Prophylaxis of recurrent ulcer, PO 400 mg at bedtime

IV injection 300 mg, diluted in 20 ml of 5% dextrose or saline solution and infused over at least 2 minutes, q6h

IV intermittent infusion 300 mg diluted in 100 ml of dextrose or saline solution and infused over 15–20 minutes, q6h

IM 300 mg q6h (undiluted)

Impaired renal function, PO, IV 300 mg q8–12 hours

Ranitidine (Zantac) is a histamine H_2 receptor blocking agent with the same mechanism of action and clinical indications for use as cimetidine. Its effectiveness in the prevention and treatment of peptic ulcer disease is similar to that of cimetidine. Ranitidine is more potent than cimetidine, so that smaller doses can be given less frequently. In addition, ranitidine reportedly causes fewer drug interactions than cimetidine.

Oral ranitidine is 50% to 60% bioavailable, reaches peak blood levels 1 to 3 hours after administration, and is metabolized in the liver; about 30% is excreted unchanged in the urine. Parenteral ranitidine is 90% to 100% bioavailable and reaches peak blood levels in approximately 15 minutes; about 65% to 80% is excreted unchanged in the urine. Because of these pharmacokinetic differences, larger doses are required with oral than with parenteral administration. Ranitidine accumulates in the presence of renal impairment, and dosage should therefore be reduced. Ranitidine can be eliminated from the body by hemodialysis or peritoneal dialysis.

Routes and dosage ranges

Adults: PO 150 mg twice daily or 300 mg once daily at bedtime
IM 50 mg q6–8h (undiluted)
IV injection, 50 mg diluted in 20 ml of 5% dextrose or 0.9% sodium chloride solution and injected over at least 5 minutes q6–8h
IV intermittent infusion, 50 mg diluted in 100 ml of 5% dextrose or 0.9% sodium chloride solution and infused over 15 to 20 minutes
Impaired renal function (creatinine clearance <50 ml/minute), PO 150 mg q24h; IV, IM 50 mg q18–24h
Oral ranitidine may be given without regard to meals.

LOCAL ANTIULCER AGENT

Sucralfate (Carafate) is a unique, locally active drug for short-term treatment of duodenal ulcer. It is a preparation of sulfated sucrose and aluminum hydroxide that promotes healing of duodenal ulcers. The agent reportedly combines with ulcer exudate, adheres to the ulcer site, and forms a protective coating that decreases further damage by gastric acid, pepsin, and bile salts. In clinical trials sucralfate was comparable to cimetidine in effectiveness (*i.e.,* healing of duodenal ulcer). Incidence and severity of adverse effects are low, with constipation and dry mouth being most often reported.

Routes and dosage ranges

Adults: PO 1 g (1000 mg) 4 times daily on an empty stomach (before meals and at bedtime)

Principles of therapy: antiulcer drugs

ASSESSMENT GUIDELINES

Assess the client's status in relation to peptic ulcer disease and other conditions in which antiulcer drugs are used.

1. Identify risk factors for peptic ulcer disease.
   a. Cigarette smoking
   b. Physiologic stress—shock, sepsis, burns, surgery, head injury, severe trauma, or medical illness
   c. Psychologic stress
   d. Genetic influences—clients with blood type O are more likely to have duodenal ulcers; those with blood type A are more likely to have gastric ulcers. Also, close relatives of clients with peptic ulcer disease have an increased risk of developing ulcers.
   e. Male sex—men have a higher incidence of both duodenal (4 times) and gastric ($2\frac{1}{2}$ times) ulcers, compared to women.
   f. Drug therapy with aspirin and other nonsteroidal anti-inflammatory drugs (*e.g.,* indomethacin [Indocin], phenylbutazone [Butazolidin]), corticosteroids, and antineoplastics. Although aspirin is known to cause gastric irritation, bleeding, erosive gastritis, and peptic ulcers, some studies have failed to demonstrate that the other agents are ulcerogenic.
2. Signs and symptoms depend on the type and location of the ulcer.
   a. Periodic epigastric pain, which occurs 1 to 4 hours after eating or during the night and is often described as burning or gnawing, is a characteristic symptom of chronic duodenal ulcer.
   b. Gastrointestinal bleeding occurs with acute or chronic ulcers when the ulcer erodes into a blood vessel. Clinical manifestations may range from mild (*e.g.,* occult blood in feces and eventual anemia) to severe (*e.g.,* hematemesis, melena, hypotension, and shock).
3. Reflux esophagitis is often associated with hiatal hernia and is usually characterized by a substernal burning sensation ("heartburn" or indigestion). It may also occur with obesity and overeating as a result of gastric distention. Symptoms are caused by backward flow of gastric acid onto esophageal mucosa.

PREVENTIVE NURSING INTERVENTIONS

Use measures to prevent or minimize peptic ulcer disease and reflux esophagitis.

1. With peptic ulcer disease, few preventive measures have proved effective. Helpful measures may include the following:
   a. General health measures such as a well-balanced diet, adequate rest, and regular exercise
   b. Controlling risk factors. Avoidance of cigarette

smoking and gastric irritants (*e.g.*, alcohol, aspirin, probably caffeine) may be helpful. There is no practical way to avoid psychologic stress, since it is part of everyday life. However, it may be possible to reduce stress (*e.g.*, by changing environments) or learn healthful methods of handling stress (*e.g.*, relaxation techniques, physical exercise).

c. For clients known to have peptic ulcer disease, the goals of treatment are to prevent recurrence and complications. Long-term drug therapy with histamine-2 receptor antagonists and antacids may be helpful in preventing recurrence, possibly with increased dosage during times of increased stress. With "active" peptic ulcer disease, assisting the client to follow the prescribed therapeutic regimen helps to promote healing and prevent serious complications (*i.e.*, hemorrhage, perforation, obstruction).

d. Diet therapy probably has little role in prevention or treatment of peptic ulcer disease. It is mentioned here because of the traditional use of "ulcer diets" or bland diets, which usually contain large amounts of milk and milk products. Although many people consider milk an "antacid" or buffer of gastric acid, it actually has little effect on the *p*H of gastric juices. In addition, protein and calcium in milk products induce hypersecretion of gastric acid. Thus, a diet regimen including frequent feedings of milk or milk and cream may aggravate peptic ulcer disease.

   Because various studies have failed to demonstrate the effectiveness of "ulcer diets," some physicians prescribe no dietary restrictions for clients with peptic ulcer disease, while others suggest avoiding highly spiced foods, gas-forming foods, and caffeine-containing beverages.

2. With reflux esophagitis, helpful measures are those that prevent or decrease gastroesophageal reflux of gastric contents (*e.g.*, elevating the head of the bed, avoiding gastric distention by eating small meals, not lying down for about 1 hour after eating, and avoiding obesity, constipation, or other conditions that increase intra-abdominal pressure).

GUIDELINES FOR THERAPY WITH HISTAMINE ANTAGONISTS

1. In peptic ulcer disease, a histamine antagonist is the drug of choice for both prevention and treatment. Full dosage may be given up to 8 weeks if necessary. If an ulcer heals within 2 to 3 weeks, as confirmed by gastroscopy, the drug may be discontinued or reduced in dosage. To prevent recurrence of an ulcer, the drug may be continued at a lower dosage, usually taken at bedtime. Dosage of both cimetidine and ranitidine should be reduced in the presence of impaired renal function.
2. In choosing a histamine antagonist, ranitidine reportedly has some advantages over cimetidine. First, it is more potent on a weight basis and has a longer duration of action. Consequently, it can be given in smaller, less frequent doses. Second, it causes fewer adverse effects. For example, it penetrates the blood–brain barrier less readily and is therefore less likely to cause mental confusion and other central nervous system (CNS) effects. It also lacks the antiandrogenic effects that may occur with cimetidine. Third, and perhaps most important, ranitidine causes fewer drug interactions than cimetidine. Cimetidine inhibits the cytochrome P450 microsomal enzyme system in the liver. This interferes with elimination of drugs normally metabolized by this enzyme system and increases the risks of adverse effects. Specific drugs whose metabolism is inhibited include some benzodiazepines, beta-adrenergic blocking agents, lidocaine, phenytoin, quinidine, theophylline, and warfarin. Current evidence indicates that ranitidine is less likely to cause these interactions than cimetidine.
3. Antacids are often given concurrently with histamine antagonists to relieve pain. Histamine antagonists relieve pain after approximately 1 week of administration.

GUIDELINE FOR THERAPY WITH SUCRALFATE

When sucralfate is used, it should be administered for 4 to 8 weeks unless healing is confirmed by radiologic or endoscopic examination.

GUIDELINES FOR THERAPY WITH ANTACIDS

1. Choice of antacid depends on characteristics of both clients and drug preparations and should be individualized. Combination products containing aluminum hydroxide and magnesium oxide or hydroxide are commonly used. Some guidelines include the following:
   a. It is probably better to use an agent with high *in vitro* neutralizing capacity. However, the

clinical or *in vivo* capacity may be different, depending on the amount of gastric acid and rate of gastric emptying. In a fasting state, for example, the antacid leaves the stomach in about 30 minutes and thereafter becomes ineffective.

b. Another consideration is side-effects. Calcium carbonate has a high neutralizing capacity, but doses large enough and frequent enough to maintain neutralization of gastric acid may cause hypercalcemia and impaired renal function due to systemic absorption. Magnesium hydroxide has a higher buffering capacity than magnesium hydroxide–aluminum hydroxide mixtures, but it may cause diarrhea and hypermagnesemia. Aluminum hydroxide has the least buffering capacity.

c. If rapid action is desired, magnesium hydroxide, magnesium oxide, and calcium carbonate are effective. Sodium bicarbonate is rapidly effective but of short duration. It is contraindicated for long-term use because of systemic absorption and possible metabolic alkalosis. Effervescent antacids have a rapid onset but short duration of action, since they leave the stomach quickly.

d. Antacid liquid suspensions usually act faster than chewable tablets. However, suspensions have not been proved more effective in neutralization of gastric acid. Chewable tablets may be more convenient in some circumstances.

e. Simethicone (Mylicon) is added to several antacid mixtures. This agent has no effect on intragastric *p*H and is of questionable value in relieving flatulence or gastroesophageal reflux, the purposes for which it is promoted.

f. Antacids containing magnesium are contraindicated in renal disease because hypermagnesemia may result.

g. Antacids with high sodium content may be contraindicated in edematous states such as congestive heart failure.

h. Antacids with high sugar content may be contraindicated in diabetes mellitus.

i. Although sodium bicarbonate (baking soda) and calcium carbonate are generally contraindicated in the large amounts and long-term usage required for treatment of peptic ulcer disease, occasional use is not likely to be harmful.

j. Efforts should be made to find an antacid preparation that is acceptable to the client in terms of taste, dosage, and convenience of administration.

2. As a general rule, single drugs are preferable to mixtures. However, antacid combinations have several advantages, including the following:
   a. Combining an antacid with a laxative effect (*e.g.*, magnesium hydroxide) with one having a constipating effect (*e.g.*, aluminum hydroxide) tends to prevent or reduce the incidence of both symptoms.
   b. Combining fast-acting and slow-acting antacids can prolong gastric acid neutralization.
   c. Mixtures allow smaller dosages of individual ingredients, and adverse effects may be prevented or reduced.
   d. Client compliance with antacid therapy is usually improved.
3. Antacid dosage, including frequency of administration, depends primarily on the purpose for use, buffering capacity of the antacid, and client response. Some guidelines include the following:
   a. To prevent stress ulcers in critically ill clients and to treat acute gastrointestinal bleeding, nearly continuous neutralization of gastric acid is desirable. Dose and frequency of administration must be sufficient to neutralize approximately 50 to 80 mEq of gastric acid each hour. This can be accomplished by a continuous intragastric drip through a nasogastric tube or by hourly administration.
   b. When a client has a nasogastric tube in place, antacid dosage may be titrated by aspirating stomach contents, determining *p*H with Nitrazine paper, and then basing the dose on the *p*H. (Most gastric acid is neutralized at a *p*H above 3.5, and most pepsin activity is eliminated at a *p*H above 5).
   c. For most clients, the standard practice of giving an antacid 1 hour and 3 hours after meals and at bedtime is effective and rational, although gastric acid is buffered intermittently rather than continuously. When an antacid is given on an empty stomach, gastric acid is neutralized for about 30 minutes, depending on gastric emptying time. When an antacid is taken after meals, buffering effects last about 2 hours.
   d. When antacids are used to relieve pain, they may be taken as needed.
   e. The usual dose of a liquid antacid is 30 ml (6 tsp). This amount is higher than doses recommended by most manufacturers (5 to 20 ml or 1 to 4 tsp).

NURSING ACTIONS: ANTIULCER DRUGS

Nursing Actions	*Rationale/Explanation*
1. Administer accurately	
a. Give oral cimetidine with meals and at bedtime. Oral ranitidine may be given without regard to meals.	When cimetidine is taken with meals, peak serum drug level coincides with gastric emptying, when gastric acidity is usually highest. When taken at bedtime, cimetidine prevents secretion of gastric acid for several hours. Thus, correct timing of drug administration may promote faster healing of the ulcer.
b. To give cimetidine or ranitidine intravenously, dilute in 20 ml of 5% dextrose or normal saline solution and inject over at least 2 minutes. For intermittent infusion, dilute in 100 ml of 5% dextrose or normal saline solution and infuse over 15 to 20 minutes.	
c. Shake liquid antacids well before measuring the dose.	These preparations are suspensions. Drug particles settle to the bottom of the container on standing and must be mixed thoroughly to give the correct dose.
d. Instruct clients to chew antacid tablets thoroughly.	To increase the surface area of drug available to neutralize gastric acid.
e. Give sucralfate 1 hour before meals and at bedtime. Do not give an antacid within 30 minutes before or after sucralfate.	To allow the drug to form its protective coating over the ulcer before high levels of gastric acidity. Sucralfate requires an acidic environment. After it has adhered to the ulcer, antacids and food do not affect drug action.
2. Observe for therapeutic effects	Therapeutic effects depend on the reason for use.
a. Decreased epigastric pain	Antacids should relieve ulcer pain within a few minutes. Cimetidine relieves pain in about 1 week by its healing effects on the ulcer.
b. Decreased gastrointestinal bleeding (*e.g.,* absence of visible or occult blood in vomitus, gastric secretions, or feces)	
c. Higher *p*H of gastric contents	The minimum acceptable *p*H with antacid therapy is 3.5. In acute situations the goal may be a *p*H of 7 (neutral).
d. Radiologic or endoscopic reports of ulcer healing	
3. Observe for adverse effects	
a. With histamine antagonists, observe for diarrhea or constipation, headache, dizziness, muscle aches, fatigue, skin rashes, mental confusion, delirium, coma, depression, fever.	Adverse effects are uncommon and usually mild with recommended doses and duration of drug therapy (8 weeks). CNS effects have been associated with high doses in elderly clients or those with impaired renal function. With long-term administration of cimetidine, other adverse effects have been observed. These include decreased sperm count and gynecomastia in men and galactorrhea in women.
b. With antacids containing magnesium, observe for diarrhea and hypermagnesemia.	Diarrhea may be prevented by combining these antacids with other antacids containing aluminum or calcium. Hypermagnesemia is unlikely in most clients but may occur in those with impaired renal function. These antacids should not be given to clients with renal failure.
c. With antacids containing aluminum or calcium, observe for constipation.	Constipation may be prevented by combining these antacids with other antacids containing magnesium. A high-fiber diet

Nursing Actions	Rationale/Explanation
	and adequate fluid intake (2000 to 3000 ml daily) also help prevent constipation.
d. With sucralfate, observe for constipation.	Thus far, adverse effects observed with sucralfate have been few and minor. (The drug is not absorbed systemically.) The most common one was constipation (4.7% in 2500 people).
4. Observe for drug interactions	Most significant drug interactions alter the effect of the other drug rather than that of the antiulcer drug. For example, cimetidine may potentiate anticoagulants; antacids alter the absorption of many oral drugs.
a. Drugs that *decrease* effects of cimetidine and ranitidine Antacids	Antacids decrease absorption of cimetidine and probably ranitidine. The drugs should not be given at the same time.
b. Drugs that *increase* effects of antacids Anticholinergic drugs (*e.g.,* atropine)	May increase effects by delaying gastric emptying and by decreasing acid secretion themselves
c. Drugs that *decrease* effects of antacids Cholinergic drugs (*e.g.,* dexpanthenol [Ilopan])	May decrease effects by increasing gastrointestinal motility and rate of gastric emptying
d. Drugs that *decrease* effects of sucralfate Antacids	Antacids should not be given within ½ hour before or after administration of sucralfate.
5. Teach clients	
a. Characteristics of the disease process, nondrug measures to prevent or minimize the disease process, and drug therapy. Diet should also be discussed, since myths abound in this area.	Peptic ulcer disease and other conditions for which antacids and antiulcer drugs are used are often chronic. Treatment, when required, is often done on an outpatient basis. Clients who are knowledgable about their conditions can participate more effectively in prevention and treatment.
b. Choose antacids carefully.	Because antacids do not require a prescription, many products are readily available. However, these products are not equally safe or effective in all persons.
(1) Consult with a physician before choosing an antacid for peptic ulcer disease or when heart or kidney disease is present.	Some antacids are safer and more effective than others in the large doses and long-term usage required for peptic ulcer disease. Some antacids should not be taken with heart disease (because of high sodium content with potential fluid retention and edema) or kidney disease (because of drug accumulation and higher risks of toxicity).
(2) Do not take baking soda, Alka-Seltzer effervescent antacid tablets, Titralac, or Tums more often than occasionally.	These products may cause serious adverse effects if taken in large amounts or for prolonged periods. Baking soda and Alka-Seltzer effervescent tablets contain large amounts of sodium; the other products contain calcium carbonate.

Selected References

American Medical Association (AMA) Division of Drugs: AMA Drug Evaluations, 5th ed. New York, John Wiley & Sons, 1983

Douglas WW: Histamine and 5-hydroxytryptamine (serotonin) and their antagonists. In Gilman AG, Goodman LS, Rall TW, Murad F (eds): The Pharmacological Basis of

Therapeutics, 7th ed, pp 605–638. New York, Macmillan, 1985

Facts and Comparisons. St. Louis, J B Lippincott (Updated monthly)

Guyton AC: Textbook of Medical Physiology, 7th ed. Philadelphia, W B Saunders, 1986

Harvey SC: Gastric antacids, miscellaneous drugs for the treatment of peptic ulcers, digestants and bile acids. In Gilman AG, Goodman LS, Rall TW, Murad F (eds): The Pharmacological Basis of Therapeutics, 7th ed, pp 980–993. New York, Macmillan, 1985

Ippoliti AF: Evolution in the medical treatment of peptic ulcer disease. Drug Ther 13:97–112, July 1983

Jadhav GR, Freston JW: Peptic ulcers: Can maintenance therapy prevent relapse? Drug Ther 13:183–190, January 1983

McCarthy DM: Ranitidine or cimetidine. Ann Intern Med 99:551–553, October 1983

Sucralfate for peptic ulcer—a reappraisal. Med Lett Drugs Ther 26:43–44, April 1984

61

LAXATIVES AND CATHARTICS

Description and uses

Laxatives and cathartics are drugs used to promote bowel elimination (defecation). The term *laxative* implies mild effects and elimination of soft, formed stool. The term *cathartic* implies strong effects and elimination of liquid or semiliquid stool. Since the different effects depend more on the dose than on the particular drug used, the terms *laxative* and *cathartic* are often used interchangeably.

Defecation is normally stimulated by movements and reflexes in the gastrointestinal tract. When the stomach and duodenum are distended with food or fluids, gastrocolic and duodenocolic reflexes cause propulsive or "mass" movements in the colon, which move feces into the rectum and arouse the urge to defecate. When sensory nerve fibers in the rectum are stimulated by the fecal mass, the defecation reflex causes strong peristalis, deep breathing, closure of the glottis, contraction of abdominal muscles, contraction of the rectum, relaxation of anal sphincters, and expulsion of the fecal mass.

The cerebral cortex normally controls the defecation reflex so that defecation can occur at acceptable times and places. Voluntary control inhibits the external anal sphincter to allow defecation or contracts the sphincter to prevent defecation. When contraction of the external sphincter is maintained, the defecation reflex dissipates and the urge to defecate usually does not recur until additional feces enter the rectum or several hours later.

People who often inhibit the defecation reflex or fail to respond to the urge to defecate develop constipation as the reflex weakens. *Constipation* is the infrequent and painful expulsion of hard, dry stools. There is no "normal" number of stools because of variations in the amount and type of food ingested as well as other individual characteristics. However, normal bowel elimination should produce a soft, formed stool without pain.

Laxatives and cathartics are somewhat arbitrarily classified as bulk-forming laxatives, surfactant laxatives or stool softeners, saline cathartics, irritant or stimulant cathartics, and lubricant or emollient laxatives. Individual drugs are listed in Table 61-1.

BULK-FORMING LAXATIVES

Bulk-forming laxatives (*e.g.*, methylcellulose, psyllium seed) are substances that are largely unabsorbed from the intestine. When water is added, these substances swell and become gellike. The added bulk or size of the fecal mass stimulates peristalsis and defecation. The substances may also act by pulling water into the intestinal lumen. Bulk-forming laxatives are the most physiologic laxatives because they act similarly to increased intake of dietary fiber.

SURFACTANT LAXATIVES (STOOL SOFTENERS)

Surfactant laxatives (*e.g.*, docusate sodium) decrease surface tension of the fecal mass to allow water to penetrate into the stool. They also act as a detergent to facilitate admixing of fat and water in the stool. As a result, stools are softer and easier to expel. These agents have little, if any, laxative effect. Their main value is to prevent straining at stool.

SALINE CATHARTICS

Saline cathartics (*e.g.*, magnesium citrate, milk of magnesia, sodium phosphate) are not well absorbed from the intestine. Consequently, they increase osmotic pressure in the intestinal lumen and cause water to be retained. Distention of the bowel leads to increased peristalsis and decreased intestinal transit time for the fecal mass. The resultant stool is semifluid.

IRRITANT OR STIMULANT CATHARTICS

The irritant or stimulant cathartics are the strongest and most abused laxative products. These drugs act by irritating the gastrointestinal mucosa and pulling water into the bowel lumen. As a result, feces are moved through the bowel too rapidly to allow colonic absorption of fecal water, and so a watery stool is eliminated. These cathartics are subdivided into three groups, which differ in location and time of action but are similar in mechanism of action, pharmacokinetics, and adverse effects. The groups are castor oil, anthraquinones (senna products, cascara sagrada, danthron), and diphenylmethanes (bisacodyl, phenolphthalein). Phenolphthalein is the active ingredient in several over-the-counter laxatives (*e.g.*, Ex-Lax, Feen-A-Mint). In addition to the oral agents, glycerin is administered as a rectal suppository. Glycerin stimulates bowel evacuation by its irritant effects on rectal mucosa and hyperosmotic effects in the colon. (Glycerin is not given orally for laxative effects.)

LUBRICANT LAXATIVES

Mineral oil is the only lubricant laxative used clinically. It lubricates the intestine and is thought to soften stool by retarding colonic absorption of fecal water, but the exact mechanism of action is unknown. Mineral oil may cause several adverse effects and is not recommended for long-term use.

CLINICAL INDICATIONS

Laxatives and cathartics are widely available on a nonprescription basis. They are among the most frequently used and abused drugs. One reason for overuse is the common misconception that a daily bowel movement is necessary for health and well-being. This notion may lead to a vicious cycle of events in which a person fails to have a bowel movement, takes a strong laxative, again fails to have a bowel movement, and so takes another laxative before the fecal column has had time to become reestablished (2 to 3 days). Thus, a pattern of laxative dependence and abuse is established. Despite widespread abuse of laxatives and cathartics, there are several rational indications for use. These include the following:

1. To relieve constipation in pregnant women, in elderly clients whose abdominal and perineal muscles have become weak and atrophied, in children with megacolon, and in clients receiving drugs that decrease intestinal motility (*e.g.*, narcotic analgesics, anticholinergics, tricyclic antidepressants)
2. To prevent straining at stool in clients with coronary artery disease (*e.g.*, postmyocardial infarction), hypertension, cerebrovascular disease, hemorrhoids, and other rectal conditions
3. To empty the bowel in preparation for bowel surgery or diagnostic procedures (*e.g.*, proctoscopy, colonoscopy, barium enema)
4. To accelerate elimination of potentially toxic substances from the gastrointestinal tract (*e.g.*, orally ingested drugs or toxic compounds)
5. To prevent absorption of intestinal ammonia in clients with hepatic encephalopathy
6. To obtain a stool specimen for parasitologic examination or to accelerate excretion of parasites after anthelmintic drugs have been administered.

CONTRAINDICATIONS

Laxatives and cathartics should not be used in the presence of undiagnosed abdominal pain. The danger is that the drugs may cause an inflamed appendix to rupture and spill gastrointestinal contents into the abdominal cavity, with subsequent peritonitis, a life-threatening situation. The drugs are also contraindicated with intestinal obstruction and fecal impaction.

TABLE 61-1. LAXATIVES AND CATHARTICS

	Generic name	Trade name	Routes and dosage ranges: Adults	Routes and dosage ranges: Children
Bulk-forming laxatives	Methylcellulose	Cologel	PO 5–20 ml 2–3 times daily with water (8 oz or more)	PO 5–10 ml 1–2 times daily with water (8 oz)
	Psyllium preparations	Metamucil, Effersyllium, Serutan, Perdiem Plain	PO 4–10 g (1–2 tsp) 1–3 times daily, stirred in at least 8 oz of water or other liquid	
Surfactant laxatives (stool softeners)	Docusate sodium	Colace, Doxinate	PO 50–200 mg daily	Age over 12 years, same dosage as adults Age 3–12 years, 20–120 mg daily Age under 3 years, 10–40 mg daily
	Docusate calcium	Surfak	PO 50–240 mg daily	Age over 12 years, same dosage as adults Age 2–12 years, 50–150 mg daily Age under 2 years, 25 mg daily
	Docusate potassium	Dialose	PO 100–300 mg daily	Age 6–12 years, 100 mg at bedtime
Saline cathartics	Magnesium citrate solution		PO 200 ml at bedtime	
	Magnesium hydroxide (milk of magnesia, magnesia magma)		Regular liquid, PO 15–60 ml at bedtime Concentrated liquid, PO 10–20 ml at bedtime	Regular liquid, PO 2.5–5 ml
	Polyethylene glycol-electrolyte solution (PEG 3350, sodium sulfate, sodium bicarbonate, sodium chloride, potassium chloride)	GoLYTELY	For bowel cleansing before gastrointestinal examination: PO 240 ml (8 oz) every 10 minutes until 4 liters are consumed	No recommended children's dose
	Sodium phosphate and sodium biphosphate	Fleet Phospho-soda Fleet Enema	PO 20–40 ml in 8 oz of water Rectal enema, 60–120 ml	Age 10 years and over, PO 10–20 ml in 8 oz of water Age 5–10 years, PO 5–10 ml in 8 oz of water Rectal enema, 60 ml
Irritant or stimulant cathartics (Anthraquinones)	Cascara sagrada	Cas-Evac	PO, tablets, 325 mg; fluidextract, 0.5–1.5 ml; aromatic fluid extract, 5 ml	
	Danthron	Modane, Dorbane	PO 37.5–150 mg	
	Senna pod preparations	Senokot, Black-Draught	Granules, PO 1 level tsp. once or twice daily; geriatric, obstetric, gynecologic clients. PO 0.5 level tsp. once or twice daily Syrup, PO 2–3 tsp once or twice daily; geriatric, obstetric, gynecologic clients, 1–1½ tsp once or twice daily Tablets, PO 2 tablets once or twice daily; geriatric, obstetric, gynecologic clients, 1 tablet once or twice daily Suppositories, 1 suppository at bedtime	Weight over 27 kg: granules, syrup, tablets, suppositories–½ adult dose

TABLE 61-1. LAXATIVES AND CATHARTICS (*Continued*)

	Generic name	Trade name	Routes and dosage ranges: Adults	Routes and dosage ranges: Children
Diphenylmethane cathartics	Bisacodyl	Dulcolax	PO 10–15 mg Rectal suppository, 10 mg	Age 6 years and over, PO 5–10 mg Age under 2 years, rectal suppository 5 mg
	Phenolphthalein	Alophen, Feen-A-Mint, Ex-Lax	PO 30–194 mg daily	
Other irritant cathartics	Castor oil	Alphamul, Neoloid	PO 15–60 ml	Age 5–15 years, PO 5–30 ml depending on strength of emulsion Age under 2 years, PO 1.25–7.5 ml depending on strength of emulsion
	Glycerin		Rectal suppository, 3 g	Age under 6 years, rectal suppository 1–1.5 g
Lubricant laxative	Mineral oil	Agoral Plain, Nujol, Petrogalar, Milkinol, Fleet Mineral oil enema	PO 15–30 ml at bedtime Rectal enema, 60–120 ml	Age over 6 years, PO 5–15 ml at bedtime Rectal enema, 30–60 ml

Principles of therapy: laxatives and cathartics

ASSESSMENT GUIDELINES

Assess clients for current or potential constipation.

1. Identify risk factors
   a. Diet with minimal fiber (*i.e.*, small amounts of fruits, vegetables and whole-grain products)
   b. Low fluid intake (*e.g.*, less than 2000 ml daily)
   c. Immobility or limited activity
   d. Drug therapy with central nervous system depressant drugs (*e.g.*, narcotic analgesics), anticholinergics, and others that reduce intestinal motility. Overuse of antidiarrheal agents may also cause constipation.
   e. Hemorrhoids, anal fissures, or other conditions characterized by painful bowel elimination
   f. Elderly or debilitated clients
2. Signs and symptoms
   a. Decreased number and frequency of stools
   b. Passage of dry, hard stools
   c. Abdominal distention and discomfort
   d. Flatulence

PREVENTIVE NURSING INTERVENTIONS

Teach clients nondrug measures to prevent constipation.

1. Eat foods high in dietary fiber daily. Fiber is the portion of plant food that is not digested. It is contained in fruits, vegetables, whole-grain cereals, and bread. Bran, the outer coating of cereal grains such as wheat or oats, is an excellent source of dietary fiber and is available in numerous cereal products.
2. Drink at least 6 to 10 glasses (8 ounces each) of fluid daily if not contraindicated.
3. Exercise regularly. Walking and other activities aid movement of feces through the bowel.
4. Establish regular bowel habits. The defecation urge is usually strongest after eating or drinking. This knowledge may be helpful in establishing a regular time for defecation. The defecation reflex is weakened or lost if repeatedly ignored. The place chosen for defecation should allow adequate privacy.

DRUG SELECTION

Choice of a laxative or cathartic depends on the reason for use and the client's condition.

1. For long-term use of laxatives or cathartics in clients who are elderly, unable or unwilling to eat an adequate diet, or debilitated, bulk-forming laxatives (*e.g.*, Metamucil, Effersyllium) are usually preferred. However, these agents should not be given to clients with dysphagia, adhesions, or strictures in the gastrointestinal tract because obstruction may occur.
2. For clients in whom straining at stool is potentially harmful or painful, stool softeners (*e.g.*, docusate sodium [Colace]) are agents of choice.
3. For occasional use to cleanse the bowel for endoscopic or radiologic examinations, saline or stimulant cathartics are acceptable (*e.g.*, magne-

sium citrate, polyethylene glycol-electrolyte solution, castor oil, bisacodyl [Dulcolax]). These drugs should not be used more often than once per week. Frequent use is likely to produce laxative abuse.

4. Oral use of mineral oil may cause potentially serious adverse effects (decreased absorption of fat-soluble vitamins and some drugs, lipid pneumonia if aspirated into the lungs). Thus, mineral oil is not an oral laxative of choice in any condition, although occasional use in the alert client is probably not harmful. Mineral oil is probably most useful as a retention enema to soften hard, dry feces and aid their expulsion. Mineral oil should not be used regularly.
5. In fecal impaction, a rectal suppository (*e.g.*, bisacodyl [Dulcolax]) or an enema (*e.g.*, oil retention or Fleet's enema) is preferred. Oral laxatives are contraindicated when a fecal impaction is present but may be given after the rectal mass is removed. Once the impaction is relieved, measures should be taken to prevent recurrence. If dietary and other nonpharmacologic measures are ineffective or contraindicated, use of a bulk-forming agent daily or another laxative once or twice weekly may be necessary.
6. Saline cathartics containing magnesium, phosphate or potassium salts are contraindicated in clients with renal failure because hypermagnesemia, hyperphosphatemia, or hyperkalemia may occur.
7. Saline cathartics containing sodium salts are contraindicated in clients with edema or congestive heart failure because enough sodium may be absorbed to cause further fluid retention and edema. They also should not be used in clients with impaired renal function or those following a sodium-restricted diet for hypertension. Polyethylene glycol-electrolyte solution (GoLYTELY) causes less sodium absorption than other saline cathartics because it uses sodium sulfate as the major sodium source. In addition, the electrolyte concentrations in this preparation cause virtually no net absorption or secretion of ions. Thus, large volumes may be given without significant changes in water or electrolyte balance.
8. Irritant or stimulant laxatives should usually be avoided in children because of potency and likelihood of promoting laxative abuse.
9. During pregnancy, castor oil should not be used because its irritant effect may induce premature labor. During lactation, danthron or cascara sagrada should not be used because they are excreted in breast milk and may cause diarrhea in the nursing infant.

NURSING ACTIONS: LAXATIVES AND CATHARTICS

Nursing Actions	***Rationale/Explanation***
1. Administer accurately	
a. Give bulk-forming laxatives with at least 8 ounces of water or other fluid. Mix with fluid immediately before administration.	To prevent thickening and expansion in the gastrointestinal tract with possible obstruction. These substances absorb water rapidly and solidify into a gelatinous mass.
b. With bisacodyl tablets, instruct the client to swallow the tablets without chewing and not to take them within an hour after ingesting milk or gastric antacids or while receiving cimetidine therapy	The tablets have an enteric coating to delay dissolution until they reach the alkaline environment of the small intestine. Chewing or giving the tablets close to antacid substances or to cimetidine-treated clients causes premature dissolution and gastric irritation and results in abdominal cramping and vomiting.
c. Give saline cathartics on an empty stomach with 240 ml of fluid.	To increase effectiveness
d. Refrigerate magnesium citrate and polyethylene glycol-electrolyte solution before giving.	To increase palatability and retain potency
e. Castor oil may be chilled and followed by fruit juice or other beverage.	To increase palatability
f. Insert rectal suppositories to the length of the index finger, next to rectal mucosa.	These drugs are not effective unless they are in contact with intestinal mucosa.

Nursing Actions	***Rationale/Explanation***
2. Observe for therapeutic effects	
a. Soft to semiliquid stool	Therapeutic effects occur in approximately 1 to 3 days with bulk-forming laxatives and stool softeners; 6 to 8 hours with bisacodyl tablets, cascara sagrada, danthron, phenolphthalein, and senna products; 15 to 60 minutes with bisacodyl and glycerin suppositories.
b. Liquid to semiliquid stool	Effects occur in approximately 1 to 3 hours with saline cathartics and castor oil
c. Decreased abdominal pain when used in irritable bowel syndrome or diverticulosis	
d. Decreased rectal pain when used in clients with hemorrhoids or anal fissures	Pain results from straining to expel hard, dry feces.
3. Observe for adverse effects	
a. Diarrhea—several liquid stools, abdominal cramping. Severe, prolonged diarrhea may cause hyponatremia, hypokalemia, dehydration, and other problems.	Diarrhea is most likely to result from strong, stimulant cathartics (*e.g.,* castor oil, bisacodyl, phenolphthalein, senna preparations) or large doses of saline cathartics (*e.g.,* milk of magnesia).
b. With bulk-forming agents, impaction or obstruction	Impaction or obstruction of the gastrointestinal tract can be prevented by giving ample fluids with these agents and not giving the drugs to clients with known dysphagia or strictures anywhere in the alimentary canal.
c. With saline cathartics, hypermagnesemia, hyperkalemia, fluid retention, and edema	Hypermagnesemia and hyperkalemia are more likely to occur in clients with renal insufficiency because of impaired ability to excrete magnesium and potassium. Fluid retention and edema are more likely to occur in clients with congestive heart failure or other conditions characterized by edema. Polyethylene glycol-electrolyte solution produces the least change in water and electrolyte balance.
d. With mineral oil, lipid pneumonia, and decreased absorption of vitamins A, D, E, and K	Lipid pneumonia can be prevented by not giving mineral oil to clients with dysphagia or impaired consciousness. Decreased absorption of fat-soluble vitamins can be prevented by not giving mineral oil with or shortly after meals or for longer than 2 weeks.
4. Observe for drug interactions	
a. Drugs that *increase* effects of laxatives and cathartics	
Cholinergics (*e.g.,* dexpanthenol [Ilopan])	Additive stimulation of intestinal motility. There is probably no reason to use such a combination.
b. Drugs that *decrease* effects of laxatives and cathartics	
(1) Anticholinergic drugs (*e.g.,* atropine) and other drugs with anticholinergic properties (*e.g.,* phenothiazine antipsychotic drugs, TCAs, some antihistamines, and antiparkinsonism drugs)	These drugs act to slow intestinal motility. Clients receiving these agents are at risk for developing constipation and requiring laxatives, perhaps on a long-term basis.
(2) CNS depressants (*e.g.,* narcotic analgesics)	Narcotic analgesics commonly cause constipation.
5. Teach clients	
a. Do not use laxatives or cathartics regularly unless prescribed by a physician.	Regular, unsupervised use of laxatives may cause potentially serious adverse effects or delay treatment for conditions causing constipation.

Nursing Actions	Rationale/Explanation
b. Use nondrug measures to promote normal bowel elimination—diet, fluids, exercise.	These measures are healthful and prevent changes in normal bowel functioning due to chronic laxative use or abuse.
c. *Never* take laxatives when acute abdominal pain is present.	Acute abdominal pain may indicate conditions that need surgical correction (*e.g.,* acute appendicitis). Taking a laxative may cause serious complications.
d. When taking laxatives, do not exceed recommended doses.	To avoid adverse effects
e. Discoloration of the urine may occur with cascara sagrada, danthron, phenolphthalein, or senna preparations.	Color of the urine may be pink-red, red-violet, red-brown, or yellow-brown, depending on the acidity or alkalinity of the urine.

Selected References

American Medical Association (AMA) Division of Drugs: AMA Drug Evaluations, 5th ed. New York, John Wiley & Sons, 1983

Anderson PD: Basic Human Anatomy and Physiology: Clinical Implications for the Health Professions. Monterey, CA, Wadsworth, 1984

Brunton LL: Laxatives. In Gilman AG, Goodman LS, Rall TW, Murad F (eds): The Pharmacological Basis of Therapeutics, 7th ed, pp 994–1003. New York, Macmillan, 1985

Facts and Comparisons. St. Louis, J B Lippincott (Updated monthly)

Hoopes JM, Piggott KS, Gunnett AE: Constipation and diarrhea. In Wiener MB, Pepper GA (eds): Clinical Pharmacology and Therapeutics in Nursing, 2d ed., pp 265–281. New York, McGraw-Hill, 1985

Malseed RT: Pharmacology: Drug Therapy and Nursing Considerations, 2d ed. Philadelphia, J B Lippincott, 1985

Sparberg M: Practical pointers for treating constipation. Drug Ther 14:97–105, May 1984

62
ANTIDIARRHEALS

Description and uses

Antidiarrheal drugs are used in the treatment of diarrhea. Diarrhea is the frequent expulsion of liquid or semiliquid stools. Diarrhea is a symptom of numerous conditions that increase bowel motility, cause secretion or retention of fluids in the intestinal lumen, and cause inflammation or irritation of the gastrointestinal tract. As a result, bowel contents are rapidly propelled toward the rectum, and absorption of fluids and electrolytes is limited. Some causes of diarrhea include the following:

1. Excessive use of laxatives
2. Intestinal infections with viruses, bacteria, or protozoa. The most common source of infection is ingestion of food or fluid that is contaminated by *Salmonella, Shigella,* or *Staphylococcus* microorganisms. The so-called travelers' diarrhea is usually caused by an enteropathogenic strain of *Escherichia coli.*
3. Undigested, coarse, or highly spiced food in the gastrointestinal tract. The food acts as an irritant and attracts fluids in a defensive attempt to dilute the irritating agent. This may result from inadequate chewing of food or lack of digestive enzymes.
4. Lack of digestive enzymes. Deficiency of pancreatic enzymes inhibits digestion and absorption of carbohydrates, proteins and fats. Deficiency of lactase, a sugar-splitting intestinal enzyme, inhibits digestion of milk and milk products.
5. Inflammatory bowel disorders such as gastroenteritis, diverticulitis, ulcerative colitis, and regional enteritis (Crohn's disease). In these disorders, the inflamed mucous membrane secretes large amounts of fluids into the intestinal lumen. In addition, when the ileum is diseased or a portion is surgically excised, large amounts of bile salts reach the colon, where they act as cathartics and cause diarrhea. Bile salts are normally reabsorbed from the ileum.
6. Drug therapy. Many oral drugs may irritate the gastrointestinal tract and cause diarrhea. Antibacterial drugs do so frequently. Antibacterial drugs may also cause diarrhea by altering the normal bacterial flora in the intestine.
7. Intestinal neoplasms. Tumors may increase intestinal motility by occupying space and stretching the intestinal wall. Diarrhea is sometimes alternated with constipation in colon cancer.
8. Functional disorders. Diarrhea may be a symptom of stress or anxiety in some clients. No organic disease process can be found in such circumstances.
9. Hyperthyroidism. This condition increases bowel motility.
10. Surgical excision or bypass of portions of the intestine, especially the small intestine. Such procedures decrease the absorptive area and increase fluidity of stools.

Diarrhea may be acute or chronic, mild or severe. Most episodes of acute diarrhea are defensive mechanisms by which the body tries to rid itself of irritants, toxins, and infectious agents. These are usually self-limiting and subside within 24 to 48 hours without serious consequences. If severe or prolonged, acute diarrhea may lead to serious fluid and electrolyte depletion, especially in young children and elderly adults. Chronic diarrhea may cause malnutrition and anemia. It is often characterized by remissions and exacerbations.

Antidiarrheal drugs include a variety of agents, most of which are discussed in other chapters. When used for treatment of diarrhea, the drugs may be given to relieve the symptom (nonspecific therapy) or the underlying cause of the symptom (specific therapy).

For symptomatic treatment of diarrhea, opiates and opiate derivatives (see Chap. 5) are the most effective. These drugs decrease diarrhea by slowing propulsive movements in the small and large intestines. Morphine, codeine, and related drugs are effective in relieving diarrhea but are rarely used for this purpose because of their potentially serious adverse effects. Although paregoric is occasionally useful, other opiates have largely been replaced by the synthetic drugs diphenoxylate and loperamide, which are used only for treatment of diarrhea and do not cause morphinelike adverse effects in recommended doses.

Other nonspecific agents that are sometimes used in diarrhea are anticholinergics (see Chap. 21), psyllium preparations (see Chap. 61), and adsorbent–demulcent products. Anticholinergic drugs, of which atropine is the prototype, are infrequently used because doses large enough to decrease intestinal motility and secretions cause adverse effects. The drugs are occasionally used to decrease abdominal cramping and pain (antispasmodic effects) associated with acute nonspecific diarrhea and chronic diarrhea associated with inflammatory bowel disease. Psyllium preparations (*e.g.*, Metamucil) are most often used as bulk-forming laxatives. They are occasionally used in diarrhea to decrease fluidity of stools. The preparations absorb large amounts of water and produce stools of gelatin-like consistency. Adsorbent–demulcent products include kaolin–pectin preparations. Kaolin is a form of clay that occurs naturally as hydrated aluminum silicate. Pectin is a carbohydrate product obtained from apples and rinds of citrus fruits. Activated attapulgite and bismith salts are other adsorbent–demulcent products used in the treatment of diarrhea. Although widely used, there is no reliable evidence that these agents have therapeutic effects in diarrhea. Furthermore, they may adsorb nutrients and other drugs, including antidiarrheal agents if given concurrently.

Specific drug therapy for diarrhea depends on the cause of the symptom and may include the use of antibacterial, enzymatic, and bile salt-binding drugs. Antibacterial drugs are recommended for use only in carefully selected cases of bacterial enteritis. Although effective in preventing travelers' diarrhea, antibiotics are generally not recommended because their use may promote emergence of drug-resistant microorganisms. Although effective in reducing diarrhea due to *Salmonella* and *E. coli* intestinal infections, antibiotics may induce a prolonged carrier state during which the infection can be transmitted to other people.

Despite the limitations of drug therapy in prevention and treatment of diarrhea, antidiarrheal drugs are generally indicated in the following circumstances:

1. Severe or prolonged diarrhea (more than 2 to 3 days) to prevent severe fluid and electrolyte loss
2. Relatively severe diarrhea in young children and elderly adults. These groups are less able to adapt to fluid and electrolyte losses.
3. In chronic inflammatory diseases of the bowel (ulcerative colitis and Crohn's disease) to allow a more nearly normal lifestyle. Ulcerative colitis is also treated with adrenal corticosteroids and poorly absorbed sulfonamides.
4. In ileostomies or surgical excision of portions of the ileum, to decrease fluidity and volume of stool
5. When specific causes of diarrhea have been determined

Contraindications to use of antidiarrheal agents include diarrhea caused by toxic materials in the gastrointestinal tract. Opiates (morphine, codeine, paregoric) are usually contraindicated in chronic diarrhea because of possible opiate dependence. Diphenoxylate is contraindicated in children under 2 years of age.

Individual antidiarrheal agents are listed in Table 62-1.

Principles of therapy: antidiarrheals

ASSESSMENT GUIDELINES

Assess for acute or chronic diarrhea.

1. Try to determine the duration of diarrhea; number of stools per day; amount, consistency, color, odor, and presence of abnormal components (*e.g.*, undigested food, blood, pus, mucus) in each stool; precipitating factors; accompanying signs and symptoms (*i.e.*, nausea, vomiting, fever, abdominal pain

or cramping); and measures used to relieve diarrhea. When possible, observe stool specimens.

2. Try to determine the cause of the diarrhea. This includes questioning about causes such as chronic inflammatory diseases of the bowel, food intake, possible exposure to contaminated food, living or traveling in areas of poor sanitation, and use of laxatives or other drugs that may cause diarrhea. When available, check laboratory reports on stool specimens (*e.g.*, culture reports).
3. With severe or prolonged diarrhea, especially in young children and elderly adults, assess for dehydration, hypokalemia, and other fluid and electrolyte disorders.

PREVENTIVE NURSING INTERVENTIONS

1. Use measures to prevent diarrhea
   a. Prepare and store food properly and avoid improperly stored foods and those prepared under questionable sanitary conditions. Milk and milk products, cream pies and foods containing mayonnaise (*e.g.*, chicken salad) may cause diarrhea ("food poisoning") if not refrigerated.
   b. Wash hands before handling any foods, after handling raw poultry or meat, and always before eating.
   c. Chew food well.
   d. Do not overuse laxatives (*i.e.*, amount per dose or frequency of use). Many of the commonly used over-the-counter products contain phenolphthalein, a strong stimulant laxative.
2. Whether or not antidiarrheal drugs are used, supportive therapy is required for treatment of diarrhea. Elements of supportive care include the following:
   a. Replacement of fluids and electrolytes. If diarrhea is not severe, fluids such as weak tea, water, bouillon, clear soup, and gelatin may be sufficient. If diarrhea is severe or prolonged, intravenous fluids may be needed (*e.g.*, solutions containing dextrose, sodium chloride, and potassium chloride). Also, oral intake may be restricted to decrease bowel stimulation.
   b. Avoid foods and fluids that may further irritate gastrointestinal mucosa (*e.g.*, highly spiced foods or "laxative" type foods such as raw fruits and vegetables).
   c. Increase frequency and length of rest periods and decrease activity. (Exercise and activity stimulate peristalsis.)
   d. If perianal irritation occurs because of frequent liquid stools, cleanse the area with mild soap and water after each bowel movement. Then apply an emollient such as white petrolatum (Vaseline).

DRUG SELECTION

Choice of antidiarrheal agent depends largely on the cause, severity, and duration of diarrhea.

1. For symptomatic treatment of diarrhea, diphenoxylate with atropine (Lomotil) or loperamide (Imodium) is probably the drug of choice for most people.
2. In bacterial gastroenteritis or diarrhea, choice of antibacterial drug depends on the causative microorganism and susceptibility tests.
3. In ulcerative colitis, sulfonamides and adrenal corticosteroids are the drugs of choice.
4. In diarrhea caused by enzyme deficiency, pancreatic enzymes are given rather than antidiarrheal drugs.
5. In "bile salt" diarrhea, cholestyramine (Questran) is the drug of choice. Colestipol (Colestid), a similar drug, is probably effective also.
6. Although morphine and codeine are contraindicated in chronic diarrhea, they may occasionally be used in the treatment of acute, severe diarrhea. Dosages required for antidiarrheal effects are smaller than those required for analgesia. The following oral drugs and dosages are approximately equivalent in antidiarrheal effectiveness: morphine 4 mg, codeine 30 mg, paregoric 10 ml, diphenoxylate 5 mg, loperamide 2 mg.

USE IN PREGNANCY AND LACTATION

Safety and effectiveness of antidiarrheal agents during pregnancy and lactation have not been established. Diphenoxylate has been used in pregnancy without reported teratogenic or other adverse effects. The drug should not be used during lactation because it is excreted in breast milk. Loperamide has not been studied in relation to pregnancy and lactation.

PEDIATRIC CONSIDERATIONS

In children, diphenoxylate has been used effectively but is contraindicated for children under 2 years of age. Loperamide is also not recommended for use in children under 2 years of age.

TABLE 62-1. ANTIDIARRHEAL DRUGS

Generic name	Trade name	Characteristics	Clinical indications	Routes and dosage ranges	
				Adults	Children
Opiates and related drugs					
Camphorated tincture of opium (paregoric)		1. Contains 0.04% morphine, alcohol, camphor, anise oil, and benzoic acid. 2. Antidiarrheal activity is caused by morphine content. Morphine slows propulsive movements in both small and large intestines. 3. Under Controlled Substances Act, a Schedule III drug when used alone and a Schedule V drug in the small amounts combined with other drugs. 4. Recommended doses and short-term duration of administration do not produce euphoria, analgesia, or dependence.	Symptomatic treatment of acute diarrhea	PO 5–10 ml 1–4 times daily (maximum of 4 doses) until diarrhea is controlled	PO 0.25–0.5 ml/kg 1–4 times daily (maximum of 4 doses) until diarrhea is controlled
Diphenoxylate with atropine sulfate	Lomotil	1. A derivative of meperidine (Demerol) used only for treatment of diarrhea. 2. Most commonly prescribed antidiarrheal drug. Acts to decrease intestinal motility. 3. As effective as paregoric and more convenient to administer. 4. In recommended doses, does not produce euphoria, analgesia, or dependence. In high doses, produces morphine-like effects including euphoria, dependence and respiratory depression. Antidote for overdose is the narcotic antagonist, naloxone (Narcan). 5. Each tablet or 5 ml of liquid contains 2.5 mg of diphenoxylate and 0.025 mg of atropine. The subtherapeutic dose of atropine is added to discourage drug abuse by producing unpleasant, anticholinergic side-effects. 6. Contraindicated in severe liver disease, glaucoma, and children under 2 years of age. Safety during pregnancy and lactation is not established. The drug is excreted in breast milk. 7. A Schedule V drug under the Controlled Substances Act.	Symptomatic treatment of acute or chronic diarrhea	PO 5 mg (2 tablets or 10 ml of liquid) 3–4 times daily. Maximal daily dose, 20 mg	Liquid preparation recommended Ages 8–12 years, PO 10 mg daily in 5 divided doses Ages 5–8 years, PO 8 mg daily in 4 divided doses Ages 2–5 years, PO 6 mg daily in 3 divided doses Under age 2 years, contraindicated
Loperamide	Imodium	1. A derivative of meperidine (Demerol) used only for treatment of diarrhea. 2. Acts to decrease intestinal motility. 3. Compared to diphenoxylate, loperamide is equally effective and may cause fewer adverse reactions in recommended doses. High doses may produce morphine-like effects. 4. Safety has not been established for use in pregnancy, lactation, and in children under 2 years of age. 5. A Schedule V drug under the Controlled Substances Act. 6. Antidote for overdose is the narcotic antagonist, naloxone (Narcan).	Symptomatic treatment of acute or chronic diarrhea	PO 4 mg initially, then 2 mg after each loose stool to a maximal daily dose of 16 mg. For chronic diarrhea, dosage should be reduced to the lowest effective amount	Ages 8–12 years, PO 6 mg daily in 3 divided doses (as liquid or capsule) Ages 5–8 years, PO 4 mg daily in 2 divided doses (as liquid or capsule) Ages 2–5 years, PO 3

TABLE 62-1. ANTIDIARRHEAL DRUGS (*Continued*)

Generic name	Trade name	Characteristics	Clinical indications	Routes and dosage ranges: Adults	Routes and dosage ranges: Children
		7. Each capsule or 10 ml of liquid contains 2 mg of loperamide.		(average 4–8 mg daily)	mg daily in 3 divided doses (as liquid) Under age 2 years, contraindicated
Antibacterial agents					
Ampicillin	Omnipen, Penbriten, others	A broad-spectrum penicillin	1. Bacillary dysentery caused by sensitive strains of *Shigella* 2. Typhoid fever resistant to chloramphenicol 3. Typhoid fever to eliminate the postinfective carrier state	PO, IM, 2–4 g/day, in divided doses, q6h	PO, IM, IV 50–100 mg/kg/day, in divided doses, q6h
Chloramphenicol	Chloromycetin		Typhoid fever (gastroenteritis caused by *Salmonella typhi*)	PO, IV 50 mg/kg/day, in divided doses, q6h	PO 50 mg/kg/day, in divided doses, q6h
Colistin sulfate	Coly-Mycin S		Enteritis caused by susceptible strains of *Escherichia coli* and other gram-negative bacilli resistant to less toxic antibiotics	PO 0.5 g/day in divided doses, q8h	10–15mg/kg/day, in divided doses, q8h
Nalidixic acid	Neg-Gram		Bacillary dysentery caused by strains of *Shigella* that are resistant to other antibiotics but sensitive to nalidixic acid	PO 2–3 g/day, in divided doses, q6h	PO 55 mg/kg/day, in divided doses, q6h
Neomycin			Same as colistin, above	PO 4 g/day, in divided doses q6h	PO 50–100 mg/kg/day, in divided doses, q6h
Tetracycline			1. Cholera 2. Bacillary dysentery caused by sensitive strains of *Shigella*	PO 2 g/day, in divided doses, q6h	PO 40 mg/kg/day, in divided doses, q6h
Trimethoprim-sulfamethoxazole (TMP-SMX)	Bactrim, Septra		1. Bacillary dysentery caused by suscepti-	PO 160 mg of trimethoprim and	PO 8 mg/kg of trimethoprim and

TABLE 62-1. ANTIDIARRHEAL DRUGS (*Continued*)

Generic name	Trade name	Characteristics	Clinical indications	Routes and dosage ranges	
				Adults	*Children*
			ble strains of *Shigella* 2. Typhoid fever resistant to chloramphenicol and ampicillin 3. Enteritis caused by susceptible strains of *E. coli*	800 mg of sulfamethoxazole daily, in divided doses, q12h IV 8–10 mg/kg of trimethoprim and 50 mg/kg sulfamethoxazole daily, in 2–4 divided doses	40 mg/kg of sulfamethoxazole daily, in divided doses, q12h IV 8–10 mg/kg of trimethoprim and 50 mg/kg sulfamethoxazole daily, in 2–4 divided doses
Vancomycin	Vancocin		1. Pseudomembranous colitis due to suppression of normal bacterial flora by antibiotics (primarily clindamycin [Cleocin] or ampicillin) and overgrowth of *Clostridium* organisms 2. Staphylococcal colitis due to broad-spectrum antibiotic therapy, combined with parenteral nafcillin (Unipen)	PO 2 g/day, in divided doses, q6h	PO 44 mg/kg/day, in divided doses, q6h
Miscellaneous drugs					
Cholestyramine	Questran	Binds and inactivates bile salts in the intestine	Diarrhea due to bile salts reaching the colon and causing a cathartic effect. "Bile salt diarrhea" is associated with Crohn's disease or surgical excision of the ileum.	PO 16–32 g/day in 120–180 ml of water, in 2–4 divided doses, before or during meals and at bedtime	
Colestipol	Colestid	Same as cholestyramine, above	Same as colestyramine	PO 15–30 g/day in 120–180 ml of water, in 2–4 divided doses, before or	

TABLE 62-1. ANTIDIARRHEAL DRUGS (*Continued*)

Generic name	Trade name	Characteristics	Clinical indications	Routes and dosage ranges: *Adults*	Routes and dosage ranges: *Children*
				during meals and at bedtime	
Kaolin, pectin, atropine sulfate, hyoscyamine sulfate, hyoscine hydrobromide, alcohol	Donnagel	1. Kaolin and pectin not proved effective in diarrhea; belladonna alkaloids are present in subtherapeutic amounts 2. Not recommended for use			
Above formulation plus paregoric	Donnagel-PG	1. Effectiveness, if any, attributed to paregoric (6 ml paregoric/30 ml of preparation) 2. Schedule V drug under Controlled Substances Act 3. Not recommended for use	Possibly effective for symptomatic treatment of mild, acute diarrhea	PO 30 ml q3h or after each loose stool.	Weight 30 lb or over, PO 5–10 ml q3h or after each loose stool Weight 20–30 lb, PO 5 ml q3h or after each loose stool
Kaolin and pectin mixture	Kaopectate	1. Ingredients not proved effective and mixture not recommended for use 2. Available over the counter			
Kaolin, pectin, and paregoric	Parepectolin	1. Effectiveness, if any, attributed to paregoric (3.7 ml paregoric/30 ml of preparation) 2. Schedule V drug under Controlled Substances Act 3. Not recommended for use	Possibly effective for symptomatic treatment of mild, acute diarrhea	PO 15–30 ml after each loose stool to a maximum of 8 doses/24 hours	PO 2.5–10 ml after each loose stool to a maximum of 8 doses/24 hours
Lactobacillus	Bacid, Lactinex	Not proved effective and not recommended for use			
Pancreatin or pancrelipase	Viokase, Pancrease, Cotazym	Pancreatic enzymes used only for replacement	Diarrhea and malabsorption due to deficiency of pancreatic enzymes	PO 1–3 tablets or capsules or 1–2 packets of powder with meals and snacks	PO 1–3 tablets or capsules or 1–2 packets of powder with each meal
Psyllium preparations	Metamucil, Effersyllium	Absorbs water and decreases fluidity of stools	Possibly effective for symptomatic treatment of diarrhea	PO 6–10 g (1–2 tsp), 2–3 times daily, in a full glass of water or other fluid, mixed immediately before ingestion	
Sulfasalazine	Azulfidine	A poorly absorbed sulfonamide	Ulcerative colitis	PO 2 g/day, in 4 divided doses	Over age 2 months, PO 40–60 mg/kg/day in 3–6 divided doses initially. Maintenance, PO 30 mg/kg/day in 4 divided doses.

NURSING ACTIONS: ANTIDIARRHEALS

Nursing Actions	Rationale/Explanation
1. Administer accurately	
a. With liquid diphenoxylate, use only the calibrated dropper furnished by the manufacturer for measuring dosage.	For accurate measurement
b. Add at least 30 ml of water to each dose of paregoric. The mixture appears milky.	To add sufficient volume for the drug to reach the stomach
c. Do not exceed maximal daily doses of diphenoxylate, loperamide, and paregoric. Also, stop the drugs when diarrhea is controlled.	To decrease risks of adverse reactions, including drug dependence
d. Give cholestyramine and colestipol with at least 120 ml of water. Also, do not give within approximately 4 hours of other drugs.	The drugs may cause obstruction of the gastrointestinal tract if swallowed in a dry state. They may combine with and inactivate other drugs.
2. Observe for therapeutic effects	
a. Decreased number, frequency, and fluidity of stools	Therapeutic effects are usually evident within 24–48 hours.
b. Decreased or absent abdominal cramping pains	
c. Signs of normal fluid and electrolyte balance (adequate hydration, urine output, and skin turgor)	
d. Resumption of usual activities of daily living	
3. Observe for adverse effects	
a. Constipation	Constipation is the most common adverse effect. It can be prevented by using antidiarrheal drugs only as prescribed and stopping the drugs when diarrhea is controlled.
b. Drug dependence	Dependence is unlikely with recommended doses but may occur with long-term use of large doses of paregoric, diphenoxylate, and probably loperamide.
c. With diphenoxylate, anorexia, nausea, vomiting, dizziness, abdominal discomfort, paralytic ileus, toxic megacolon, hypersensitivity (pruritus, urticaria, angioneurotic edema), headache, tachycardia	Although numerous adverse reactions have been reported, their incidence and severity are low when diphenoxylate is used appropriately.
With overdoses of a diphenoxylate–atropine combination, respiratory depression and coma may result from diphenoxylate content and anticholinergic effects (*e.g.,* dry mouth, blurred vision, urinary retention) from atropine content.	Deliberate overdose and abuse are unlikely because of unpleasant anticholinergic effects. Overdose can be prevented by using the drug in recommended doses and only when required. Overdose can be treated with naloxone (Narcan) and supportive therapy.
d. With loperamide, abdominal cramps, dry mouth, dizziness, nausea and vomiting.	Abdominal cramps are the most common adverse effect. No serious adverse effects have been reported with recommended doses of loperamide. Overdose may be treated with naloxone (Narcan), gastric lavage, and administration of activated charcoal.
e. With cholestyramine and colestipol, observe for constipation, nausea, and abdominal distention.	Adverse effects are usually minor and transient because these drugs are not absorbed from the gastrointestinal tract.
4. Observe for drug interactions	Few clinically significant drug interactions have been reported with commonly used antidiarrheal agents.
Drugs that *increase* effects of antidiarrheal agents	
(1) CNS depressants (alcohol, sedative–hypnotics, narcotic analgesics, antianxiety agents, antipsychotic agents)	Additive CNS depression with opiate and related antidiarrheals. Narcotic analgesics have additive constipating effects.

Nursing Actions	Rationale/Explanation
(2) Anticholinergic agents (atropine and synthetic anticholinergic antispasmodics; antihistamines and antidepressants with anticholinergic effects)	Additive anticholinergic adverse effects (dry mouth, blurred vision, urinary retention) with diphenoxylate–atropine (Lomotil)
5. Teach clients	
a. Take antidiarrheal drugs only as prescribed and stop them when diarrhea is controlled.	To avoid adverse effects
b. Report to the physician if diarrhea persists longer than 3 days, if stools contain blood or mucus, and if fever or abdominal pain develops.	These signs and symptoms may indicate more serious disorders for which other treatment measures are needed.
c. Maintain a fluid intake of 2–3 quarts daily.	To avoid dehydration from fluid loss in stools
d. Use measures to prevent diarrhea (*e.g.,* proper handwashing, careful food storage and preparation).	

Selected References

American Medical Association (AMA) Division of Drugs: AMA Drug Evaluations, 5th ed. New York, John Wiley & Sons, 1983

Blaser MJ: Current approach to the management of acute diarrheal illnesses. Drug Ther 13:114–126, February 1983

Facts and Comparisons. St. Louis, J B Lippincott (Updated monthly)

Guyton AC: Textbook of Medical Physiology, 7th ed. Philadelphia, W B Saunders, 1986

Hansten PD: Drug Interactions: Clinical Significance of Drug-Drug Interactions, 5th ed. Philadelphia, Lea & Febiger, 1985

Malseed RT: Pharmacology: Drug Therapy and Nursing Considerations, 2d ed. Philadelphia, J B Lippincott, 1985

63 ANTIEMETICS

Description and uses

Antiemetic drugs are used to prevent or treat nausea and vomiting. Nausea is an unpleasant sensation of abdominal discomfort accompanied by a desire to vomit. Vomiting is the expulsion of stomach contents through the mouth. Nausea may occur without vomiting and vomiting may occur without prior nausea. However, the two symptoms most often occur together.

Nausea and vomiting are common symptoms experienced by virtually everyone at some time or other. These symptoms may accompany almost any illness or stress situation. Causes of nausea and vomiting include the following:

1. Digestive disorders such as gastritis, gastroenteritis, and liver, gallbladder, and pancreatic disease
2. Overeating or ingestion of foods or fluids that irritate the gastrointestinal mucosa
3. Drug therapy. Nausea and vomiting are the most common adverse reactions to drug therapy. Although the symptoms may occur with most drugs, they are especially associated with alcohol, aspirin, anticancer drugs, estrogen preparations, narcotic analgesics, antibiotics, and digitalis preparations.
4. Pain and other noxious stimuli, such as unpleasant sights and odors
5. Emotional disturbances, physical or mental stress
6. Radiation therapy
7. Systemic illness or infection

Vomiting occurs when the vomiting center in the medulla oblongata is stimulated. Stimuli may be relayed to the vomiting center from peripheral (*e.g.*, gastric mucosa, peritoneum, intestines, joints) and central (*e.g.*, cerebral cortex, vestibular apparatus of the ear, neurons in the fourth ventricle, called the *chemoreceptor trigger zone* or CTZ) sites. Although the mechanism is not completely clear, dopamine and acetylcholine apparently play a major role in stimulating the vomiting center. When stimulated, the vomiting center initiates efferent impulses that cause closure of the glottis, contraction of abdominal muscles and the diaphragm, relaxation of the gastroesophageal sphincter, and reverse peristalsis, which moves stomach contents toward the mouth for ejection.

Drugs used in nausea and vomiting belong to several different therapeutic classifications. Most antiemetic agents relieve nausea and vomiting by acting on the vomiting center, CTZ, cerebral cortex, vestibular apparatus, or a combination of these. Antiemetic drugs are generally more effective in prophylaxis than treatment. The three major groups of antiemetic drugs are the phenothiazines, antihistamines, and miscellaneous agents (Table 63-1).

PHENOTHIAZINES

Phenothiazines, of which chlorpromazine (Thorazine) is the prototype, are central nervous system (CNS) depressants used primarily in treatment of psychosis (see Chap. 9). These drugs have widespread effects on the body. Their therapeutic effects in both psychosis and vomiting are attributed to their ability to block dopamine from receptor sites in the brain (antidopaminergic effects). When used as antiemetics, phenothiazines act on the CTZ and the vomiting center. Not all phenothiazines are effective antiemetics.

Phenothiazines are usually effective in preventing or treating nausea and vomiting induced by drugs, radiation therapy, surgery, and most other stimuli. They are generally ineffective in motion sickness.

ANTIHISTAMINES

Antihistamines (*e.g.*, hydroxyzine [Vistaril]) are used primarily to prevent histamine from exerting its widespread effects on body tissues (see Chap. 48). Antihistamines used as antiemetic agents are the "classic" antihistamines or histamine$_1$ receptor blocking agents (as differentiated from cimetidine [Tagamet] and ranitidine [Zantac], which are histamine$_2$ receptor blocking agents). The drugs are thought to relieve nausea and vomiting by blocking the action of acetylcholine in the brain (anticholinergic effects). Antihistamines are especially effective in prevention and treatment of motion sickness. Motion sickness is a disturbance of the vestibular portion of the eighth cranial nerve. Not all antihistamines are effective as antiemetic agents.

MISCELLANEOUS ANTIEMETICS

Miscellaneous antiemetics include several drugs with varied mechanisms of action. *Benzquinamide* (Emete-Con) apparently acts on the CTZ. *Diphenidol* (Vontrol) is thought to act on the vestibular apparatus of the inner ear. *Dronabinol* (Marinol) is a synthetic antiemetic used in the management of nausea and vomiting associated with anticancer drugs and unrelieved by other drugs. The active ingredient is delta-9-tetrahydrocannabinol (THC), a synthetic preparation of the main psychoactive ingredient of marihuana. *Droperidol* (Inapsine) is a butyrophenone related to the antipsychotic drug haloperidol (Haldol). Droperidol produces marked sedation and antiemetic effects, probably resulting from generalized depression of the CNS. It is often used in combination with fentanyl, a narcotic analgesic, for neuroleptanalgesia. The combination product (Innovar) is usually administered by anesthesiologists. However, droperidol may be used alone to prevent nausea and vomiting during surgical or diagnostic procedures. Droperidol may be given preoperatively or during surgery for induction and maintenance of anesthesia.

Metoclopramide (Reglan) has both central and peripheral antiemetic effects. Centrally, metoclopramide antagonizes the action of dopamine, a catecholamine neurotransmitter. Peripherally, metoclopramide stimulates release of acetylcholine, which, in turn, increases the rate of gastric emptying. Metoclopramide is given orally in diabetic gastroparesis and esophageal reflux. Large doses of the drug are given intravenously during chemotherapy with cisplatin (Platinol), an antineoplastic drug that causes severe vomiting in some clients.

Scopolamine, an anticholinergic drug (see Chap. 21), is very effective in relieving nausea and vomiting associated with motion sickness. *Trimethobenzamide* (Tigan) may act on the CTZ but is considered minimally effective. Preparations of *phosphorated carbohydrate solution* (Emetrol, Nausetrol) are hyperosmolar carbohydrate solutions with phosphoric acid. They are thought to exert a direct local action on the wall of the gastrointestinal tract, reducing smooth muscle contraction. These preparations are available over the counter.

INDICATIONS AND CONTRAINDICATIONS

Antiemetic drugs are indicated for prevention and treatment of nausea and vomiting associated with surgery, pain, motion sickness, cancer chemotherapy, radiation therapy, and other causes. Phenothiazines, because of their relatively high incidence and severity of adverse effects, are indicated only when other antiemetic drugs are ineffective or when only a few doses are expected to be required.

Antiemetic drugs are generally contraindicated when their use may prevent or delay diagnosis, when signs and symptoms of drug toxicity may be masked (*e.g.*, during digitalis therapy), and for routine use to prevent postoperative vomiting.

Principles of therapy: antiemetic drugs

ASSESSMENT GUIDELINES

Assess for nausea and vomiting.

1. Identify risk factors (*e.g.*, digestive or other disorders in which nausea and vomiting are symptoms; drugs associated with nausea and vomiting).
2. Interview regarding frequency, duration, and precipitating causes of nausea and vomiting. Also, question the client about accompanying signs and symptoms, characteristics of vomitus (amount, color, odor, presence of abnormal components such as blood), and any measures that relieve nausea and vomiting. When possible, observe and measure the vomitus.

TABLE 63-1. ANTIEMETIC DRUGS

	Generic name	Trade name	Routes and dosage ranges — Adults	Routes and dosage ranges — Children
Phenothiazines	Chlorpromazine	Thorazine	PO 10–25 mg q4–6h IM 25 mg q3–4h until vomiting stops, followed by oral administration if necessary Rectal suppository 25–100 mg q6–8h	PO 0.5 mg/kg q4–6h IM 0.5 mg/kg q6–8h. Maximal daily dose: up to age 5 years or weight 50 lb, 40 mg; age 5–12 years or weight 50–100 lb, 75 mg Rectal suppository 1 mg/kg q6–8h Not recommended for children under 6 months of age
	Perphenazine	Trilafon	PO 8–16 mg daily in divided doses IM 5 mg as a single dose	
	Prochlorperazine	Compazine	PO 5–10 mg 3–4 times daily (sustained-release capsule, 10 mg twice daily) IM 5–10 mg q3–4h to a maximum of 40 mg daily Rectal suppository 25 mg twice daily	Weight over 10 kg: PO 0.4 mg/kg/day, in 3–4 divided doses IM 0.2 mg/kg as a single dose Rectal suppository 0.4 mg/kg/day, in 3–4 divided doses
	Promethazine	Phenergan	PO, IM, rectal suppository 12.5–25 mg q4–6h	Age over 3 months: PO, IM, rectal suppository 0.25–0.5 mg/kg q4–6h
	Thiethylperazine	Torecan	PO, IM, rectal suppository 10–30 mg/day	
	Triflupromazine	Vesprin	PO 20–30 mg/day IM 5–15 mg q4–6h; maximal dose, 60 mg/day IV 1–3 mg as a single dose	Age over 2 years: PO, IM 0.2 mg/kg/day in 3 divided doses. Maximal dose, 10 mg/day.
Antihistamines	Buclizine	Bucladin-S	Motion sickness, PO 50 mg 30 minutes before departure and 4–6 hours later, if needed. Maintenance dose, 50 mg twice daily.	
	Cyclizine	Marezine	Motion sickness, PO 50 mg 30 minutes before departure, then q4–6h as needed, to a maximal daily dose of 300 mg; IM 50 mg 3–4 times daily as needed, rectal suppository 100 mg 3–4 times daily as needed Postoperative vomiting, IM 50 mg preoperatively, 20–30 minutes before surgery is completed or q4–6h as needed	Age 6–10 years: Motion sickness, PO, IM 3 mg/kg/day in 3 divided doses; rectal suppository, 6 mg/kg/day, in 3 divided doses Maximal daily dose, 75 mg
	Dimenhydrinate	Dramamine	PO 50–100 mg q4h IM 50 mg as needed Rectal suppository 100 mg once or twice daily	PO, IM 5 mg/kg/day, in 4 divided doses (maximal daily dose, 150 mg)
	Diphenhydramine	Benadryl	Motion sickness, PO 50 mg 30 minutes before departure and 50 mg before each meal; IM, IV 20–50 mg q2–3h to a maximal daily dose of 400 mg	PO, IM 5 mg/kg/day, in 4 divided doses. Maximal daily dose, 300 mg
	Hydroxyzine	Vistaril, Atarax	PO, IM 25–100 mg, 3–4 times daily	Age over 6 years, PO 50–100 mg daily in 4 divided doses Age under 6 years, PO 50 mg daily in 4 divided doses
	Meclizine	Antivert, Bonine	PO 25–100 mg daily	Dosage not established

TABLE 63-1. ANTIEMETIC DRUGS (*Continued*)

	Generic name	Trade name	Routes and dosage ranges: Adults	Routes and dosage ranges: Children
Miscellaneous agents	Benzquinamide	Emete-Con	IM 0.5–1.0 mg/kg at least 15 minutes before administering antineoplastic drugs or emergence from anesthesia, then q3–4h as needed IV 0.2–0.4 mg/kg as a single dose, injected over 1–3 minutes	
	Diphenidol	Vontrol	PO 25–50 mg 4 times daily IM 20–40 mg 4 times daily IV 20 mg, repeated in 1 hour if necessary. Subsequent doses should be given PO or IM	Age over 6 months or weight over 12 kg, PO 5 mg/kg/day in 4 divided doses; IM 3 mg/kg/day in 4 divided doses
	Dronabinol	Marinol	PO 5 mg/m^2 (square meter of body surface area) 1–3 hours before chemotherapy, then q2–4h for a total of 4–6 doses daily. Dosage can be increased by 2.5 mg/m^2 increments to a maximal dose of 15 mg/m^2, if necessary.	
	Droperidol	Inapsine	Preoperatively, IM 2.5–10 mg 30–60 minutes before procedure	Age 2–12 years, preoperatively, IM 1–1.5 mg/20–25 lb 30–60 minutes before procedure
	Metoclopramide	Reglan	PO 10 mg 30 minutes before meals and at bedtime for 2–8 weeks IV 2 mg/kg 30 minutes before injection of cisplatin and 2 hours after injection of cisplatin, then 1–2 mg/kg q2–3h if needed, up to 4 doses	
	Trimethobenzamide	Tigan	PO 250 mg 3–4 times daily IM, rectal suppository 200 mg 3–4 times daily	PO, rectal suppository 15 mg/kg/day in 3–4 divided doses; IM not recommended
	Scopolamine	Transderm-Scōp	Motion sickness, PO, SC 0.6–1 mg as a single dose Transdermal disc (1.5 mg scopolamine) placed behind the ear every 3 days, if needed	Motion sickness, PO, SC, 0.006 mg/kg as a single dose
	Phosphorated carbohydrate solution	Emetrol	PO 15–30 ml	PO 5–10 ml repeated at 15-minute intervals until vomiting ceases

PREVENTIVE NURSING INTERVENTIONS

Use measures to prevent or minimize nausea and vomiting.

1. Avoid exposure to stimuli when feasible (*e.g.*, unpleasant sights and odors; excessive ingestion of food, alcohol, or aspirin).
2. Because pain may cause nausea and vomiting, administration of analgesics before painful diagnostic tests and dressing changes, or other therapeutic measures, may be helpful.
3. Administer antiemetic drugs before radiation therapy, cancer chemotherapy, or travel.
4. Many oral drugs cause less gastric irritation, nausea, and vomiting if taken with or just after food.

Thus, scheduling and administering drugs may be an important measure in preventing nausea and vomiting. However, food delays or prevents absorption of many drugs and may decrease therapeutic effectiveness. For any drug likely to cause nausea and vomiting, check reference sources to determine whether it can be given with food without altering beneficial effects.

5. When nausea and vomiting occur, assess the client's condition and report to the physician. In some instances, a drug (*e.g.*, digitalis, an antibiotic) may need to be discontinued or reduced in dosage. In other instances (*e.g.*, paralytic ileus, gastrointestinal obstruction), preferred treatment is restriction of oral intake (NPO) and nasogastric intubation.
6. Eating dry crackers before arising may help prevent nausea and vomiting associated with pregnancy.
7. Avoid oral intake of food, fluids, and drugs during acute episodes of nausea and vomiting. Oral intake may increase vomiting and risks of fluid and electrolyte imbalances.
8. Avoid activity during acute episodes of nausea and vomiting. Lying down and resting quietly are often helpful.

DRUG SELECTION

Choice of antiemetic drug depends largely on the client's condition.

1. For ambulatory clients, drugs causing minimal sedation are preferred. However, all antiemetic drugs cause some sedation in usual therapeutic doses.
2. Hydroxyzine (Vistaril) and promethazine (Phenergan) are among the most frequently used antiemetic agents. Hydroxyzine is an antihistamine; promethazine is a phenothiazine with potent antihistaminic effects. Promethazine is most often used clinically for its antihistaminic and antiemetic effects.
3. Although phenothiazines are effective antiemetic agents, they may cause serious adverse effects (*e.g.*, hypotension, sedation, anticholinergic effects, extrapyramidal reactions that simulate signs and symptoms of Parkinson's disease). Consequently, phenothiazines other than promethazine should generally not be used, especially for pregnant, young, elderly, and postoperative clients, unless vomiting is severe and cannot be controlled by other measures.
4. In motion sickness, scopolamine (for 1 to 2 doses) or an antihistamine is the drug of choice.
5. THC, the active ingredient in marihuana, is useful in relieving nausea and vomiting associated with cancer chemotherapy. When given orally or smoked, THC is reportedly as effective as prochlorperazine (Compazine) and oral metoclopramide (Reglan). It may be less effective than parenteral metoclopramide. It may be especially useful when other antiemetic drugs are ineffective. It should be used with caution in clients with hypertension, heart disease, and psychiatric problems that might be aggravated by the drug. Although dronabinol (Marinol) is the only THC preparation currently available for clinical use, other derivatives are undergoing investigation. Dronabinol is a Schedule II drug under the Controlled Substances Act because of the potential for abuse and physical and psychologic dependence. To prevent abuse and dependence, physicians are requested to prescribe only the amount needed for one chemotherapy cycle.
6. Metoclopramide may be the drug of choice when nausea and vomiting are caused by gastric distention or delayed gastric emptying.

DOSAGE AND ADMINISTRATION FACTORS

Dosage and route of administration depend primarily on the reason for use.

1. Doses of phenothiazines are much smaller for antiemetic effects than for antipsychotic effects.
2. Most antiemetic agents are available in oral, parenteral, and rectal dosage forms. As a general rule, oral dosage forms are preferred for prophylactic use, and rectal or parenteral forms are preferred for therapeutic use.
3. Antiemetic drugs are often ordered PRN (as needed). As for any PRN drug, the client's condition should be assessed before drug administration.

USE IN PREGNANCY

During pregnancy, nondrug measures are preferred for controlling nausea and vomiting because of possible drug effects on the fetus. Nausea and vomiting are likely to be most severe during the first trimester, when fetal organs are being formed. No drugs have been proved absolutely safe for use during pregnancy, but teratogenic effects have not been observed with the antihistamines, cyclizine (Marezine) and meclizine (Antivert).

NURSING ACTIONS: ANTIEMETICS

Nursing Actions	*Rationale/Explanation*
1. Administer accurately	
a. For prevention of motion sickness, give antiemetics about 30 minutes before travel and q3–4h, if necessary.	To allow time for drug dissolution and absorption
b. For prevention of vomiting with cancer chemotherapy and radiation therapy, give antiemetic drugs 30–60 minutes before treatment.	Drugs are more effective in preventing than in aborting nausea and vomiting.
c. Inject intramuscular antiemetics deeply into a large muscle mass (*e.g.,* gluteal area).	To decrease tissue irritation
d. As a general rule, do not mix parenteral antiemetics in a syringe with other drugs. An exception is promethazine (Phenergan) which is often mixed with meperidine (Demerol) and atropine sulfate for preanesthetic medication.	To avoid physical incompatibilities
e. Omit antiemetic agents and report to the physician if the client appears excessively drowsy or is hypotensive.	To avoid potentiating adverse effects and CNS depression
2. Observe for therapeutic effects	
a. Verbal reports of decreased nausea	
b. Decreased frequency or absence of vomiting	
3. Observe for adverse effects	
a. Excessive sedation and drowsiness	Excessive sedation may occur with usual therapeutic doses of antiemetics and is more likely to occur with high doses. This may be minimized by avoiding high doses and assessing the client for responsiveness before each dose.
b. Anticholinergic effects—dry mouth, urinary retention	These effects are common to many antiemetic agents and are more likely to occur with large doses.
c. Hypotension, including orthostatic hypotension	May occur with any of the drugs but is most likely with phenothiazines and droperidol.
d. Extrapyramidal reactions—dyskinesia, dystonia, akathisia, parkinsonism	These disorders may occur with phenothiazines and metoclopramide. They are more likely to occur when phenothiazines are used as antipsychotics rather than as antiemetics.
e. With dronabinol, observe for alterations in mood, cognition, and perception of reality, depersonalization, dysphoria, drowsiness, dizziness, anxiety, tachycardia, and conjunctivitis.	According to the manufacturer, these adverse effects are well tolerated. Tachycardia may be prevented with a beta-adrenergic blocking drug such as propranolol (Inderal).
4. Observe for drug interactions	
Drugs that *increase* effects of antiemetic agents	
(1) CNS depressants (alcohol, sedative–hypnotics, antianxiety agents, other antihistamines or antipsychotic agents)	Additive CNS depression
(2) Anticholinergics (*e.g.,* atropine)	Additive anticholinergic effects. Some phenothiazines and antiemetic antihistamines have strong anticholinergic properties.
(3) Antihypertensive agents	Additive hypotension
5. Teach clients	
a. Take the drugs as prescribed.	To avoid adverse effects

Nursing Actions	Rationale/Explanation
b. Do not drive an automobile or operate dangerous machinery if drowsy from antiemetic drugs.	To avoid injury
c. If taking antiemetic drugs regularly, do not take other drugs without the physician's knowledge and consent.	Several drugs interact with antiemetic agents to increase incidence and severity of adverse effects.
d. Report excessive drowsiness or other adverse reactions.	The drug may need to be discontinued or reduced in dose or frequency of administration. Also, a change in drugs may reduce adverse effects in a particular individual.
e. Use nondrug measures to prevent or control nausea and vomiting when feasible.	
f. With dronabinol, teach clients to take the drug only when they can be supervised by a responsible adult.	To increase safety, owing to the mind-altering effects of the drug.

Selected References

Albibi R, McCallum RW: Metoclopramide: Pharmacology and clinical application. Ann Intern Med 98:86–95, January 1983

Anderson PD: Basic Human Anatomy and Physiology: Clinical Implications for the Health Professions. Monterey, CA, Wadsworth, 1984

Facts and Comparisons. St. Louis, J B Lippincott (Updated monthly)

Malseed RT: Pharmacology: Drug Therapy and Nursing Considerations, 2d ed. Philadelphia, J B Lippincott, 1985

Merryman R, Clarke BF: Nausea and vomiting. In Wiener MB, Pepper GA (eds): Clinical Pharmacology and Therapeutics in Nursing, 2d ed, pp 255–264. New York, McGraw-Hill, 1985

Rodman MJ, Karch AM, Boyd EH, Smith DW: Pharmacology and Drug Therapy in Nursing, 3rd ed. Philadelphia, J B Lippincott, 1985

Stoudemire A, Cotanch P, Laszlo J: Recent advances in the pharmacologic and behavioral management of chemotherapy-induced emesis. Arch Intern Med 144:1029–1033, May 1984

X

DRUGS USED IN SPECIAL CONDITIONS

64

ANTINEOPLASTIC DRUGS

Description and uses

Antineoplastic drugs are drugs used in the treatment of cancer. The role of chemotherapy in cancer treatment is increasing in importance. Formerly, chemotherapy was used primarily to treat advanced, metastatic disease, and the goal of treatment was palliation of symptoms. With the advent of newer drugs and newer methods of using older ones, chemotherapy may cure some malignant tumors and is important in the treatment of many others. To participate effectively in cancer chemotherapy, nurses must know the characteristics of both normal and malignant cells and of the drugs used to arrest tumor growth.

CHARACTERISTICS OF NORMAL CELLS

Normal cells undergo an orderly process of replication and retain certain characteristics and functions. Some specific characteristics of normal cells include the following:

1. They reproduce according to a predetermined sequence of events. The normal cell cycle (the interval between the "birth" of a cell and its division into two daughter cells) involves several phases. During the resting phase (G_0), cells are not dividing but are capable of doing so when stimulated. During the first active phase (G_1), ribonucleic acid (RNA) and enzymes required for production of deoxyribonucleic acid (DNA) are developed. During the next phase (S), DNA is synthesized for chromosomes. Then, during G_2, RNA is synthesized and the mitotic spindle is formed. Mitosis occurs in the final phase (M). The resulting two daughter cells may then enter the resting phase (G_0) or proceed through the reproductive cycle.
2. Normal cells reproduce in response to a need (*e.g.*, growth or tissue repair) and stop reproduction when the need has been met.
3. They are well-differentiated in appearance and function. Thus, they can be examined under a microscope and the tissue of origin determined.

CHARACTERISTICS OF MALIGNANT NEOPLASMS

Malignant neoplasms, malignant tumors, and cancer are terms used to describe a group of more than 100 disease processes. Malignant or neoplastic cells differ from normal cells in several ways, including the following:

1. Malignant cells reproduce with the same sequence of events as normal cells, but they may have an accelerated rate of replication, and their growth continues in an uncontrolled fashion.
2. Malignant cells serve no useful purpose in the body. Instead, they occupy space and act as parasites by taking blood and nutrients away from normal tissues.
3. Malignant cells are anaplastic and undifferentiated. *Anaplasia* means loss of structural and func-

tional characteristics of normal cells. *Undifferentiation* indicates that the malignant cells retain few characteristics of the cells from which they originated. Generally, cells that are more anaplastic and undifferentiated are more malignant.

4. Malignant cells can invade normal tissues to cause widespread tissue destruction and eventual death unless treatment measures intervene. Owing to a lack of cohesiveness, increased motility, and possibly production of enzymes that break down normal tissues, malignant cells are able to break away from the primary tumor and spread to other body parts. Malignant cells invade normal tissues primarily by extending into tissues adjacent to the tumor and by traveling through blood and lymph vessels into tissues distant from the tumor site.

ETIOLOGIC FACTORS

Despite extensive study, the cause of cancer is not clear. Since "cancer" is actually many diseases, many etiologic factors are probably involved. Most cancers are thought to be environmental in origin. A number of carcinogens (cancer-causing agents) have been identified, as have a number of risk factors or characteristics that predispose persons to develop cancer. Table 64-1 contains a limited list of known and probable chemical carcinogens. Other carcinogens include radiation (from radioisotopes, ultraviolet light, and sunlight), physical irritation (*e.g.*, of pigmented moles or of the colon from ulcerative colitis), and viruses.

Risk factors cannot predict whether cancer will occur in a person, but they can help to identify people who are more likely to develop cancer. Some risk factors are primarily environmental; others are related to personal characteristics.

Geographic and racial factors

Breast cancer, for example, occurs more often in the United States than in Japan, while the incidence of stomach cancer is higher in Japan. Primary liver cancer is common in some areas of Africa but rare in Europe and North America. These differences have not been fully explained but are probably caused by environmental rather than hereditary or racial factors. Also, people who live in cities are probably more likely to develop cancer because of greater exposure to air pollutants and other carcinogens.

Age and sex

The incidence of cancer increases with age and reaches a peak as a cause of death in the sixth and seventh decades. A smaller peak in cancer mortality occurs during the first 4 years of life. Men are more likely to have leukemia and cancer of the urinary bladder, stomach, lung, and pancreas. Elderly men have a relatively high rate of prostatic cancer. Women are at rather high risk for developing breast cancer; the cervix and endometrium are other common sites. Also, the incidence of lung cancer in women is increasing. Colon cancer occurs about equally in both sexes.

Social customs and lifestyle

The incidence of lung cancer is greatly increased among people who smoke cigarettes. The increased incidence of lung cancer in women is attributed to increased cigarette smoking. Cancers of the mouth, throat, and esophagus are associated with cigarette smoking and alcohol use. There is some evidence that alcohol alone is a carcinogen and, when combined with cigarette smoking, probably acts as a cocarcinogen that increases the cancer-producing effects of cigarette smoking. There is also an increased incidence of liver cancer among alcoholics. Oral cancer is associated with smoking a pipe or chewing tobacco as well as cigarette smoking and alcohol use.

Eating habits also influence the occurrence of cancer. Cancers of the colon, breast, prostate gland, ovary, and endometrium seem to be associated with a high intake of carbohydrate, fat, and animal protein and a low intake of fiber. These eating patterns are more prevalent in affluent, industrialized parts of the world.

Heredity

Hereditary factors are thought to be much less important than environmental factors in cancer development. Most relatives of people with cancer are generally no more likely to develop cancer than the general population. However, some specific types of cancer seem to be related to heredity. For example, close relatives of premenopausal women with breast cancer are more likely to develop breast cancer; close relatives of people with stomach cancer are more likely to develop this disease; and close relatives of people with bronchogenic carcinoma who also smoke cigarettes are much more likely to develop bronchogenic carcinoma. Finally, familial polyposis strongly increases the incidence of colon cancer.

ONCOGENES

Oncogenes (cancer-causing genes) are normal cell structures that have been altered by chromosomal

TABLE 64-1. KNOWN AND PROBABLE CHEMICAL CARCINOGENS

Chemical	Source of Exposure	Location of associated cancer
Aflatoxins	Foods contaminated with aspergillus fungus, such as peanuts, soybeans, corn, wheat, and rice. Contamination is most likely with warm, moist storage conditions.	Liver
Alcohol	Ingestion of alcoholic beverages such as whiskey, beer, or wine	Mouth, pharynx, larynx, esophagus, liver
Alkylating agents (*e.g.*, melphalan [Alkeran], others)	Cytotoxic, immunosuppressive drugs used in the treatment of several types of cancer	Lymphoid tissue (lymphoma, leukemia), bladder (cyclophosphamide [Cytoxan])
Alpha-naphthyline (1 NA) and beta-naphthylamine (2 NA)	Manufacturing, handling, or storing substances containing this chemical. It is used in a wide variety of products, including herbicides, dyes, food colors, color film, paint, plastics, rubber, and petroleum products.	Bladder
Anabolic steroids (Androgens)	Drugs prescribed for debilitated clients to improve nutritional status and promote weight gain	Liver
Arsenic	Manufacturing sodium arsenate, drinking water contaminated by arsenic	Skin and lung
Asbestos	Working in areas where asbestos is used, including shipyards and factories. Several thousand products contain asbestos. These include insulation, floor tiles, and automobile brake linings. Beer, gin, and a number of medicines are filtered through asbestos filters in the manufacturing process. Family members and household contacts of asbestos workers receive considerable exposure from asbestos carried home on clothes.	Bronchi, pleura, peritoneum
Benzene	Working with glues and varnishes	Bone marrow (leukemia)
Benzidine	Working in chemical plants where benzidine is used in the production of aniline dyes, rubber, plastics, printing inks, fireproofing of textiles, various laboratory chemicals. Living in neighborhoods where such plants are located may also result in significant exposure over the years.	Bladder
Bis (chloromethyl) ether (BCME)	Working in chemical plants where BCME is used for water-softening products, to remove impurities such as salt from water or to decolorize or clarify food beverages. BCME is not present in the finished product.	Lung
Dichlorbenzidine (DCB)	Working in chemical plants where DCB is used in the production of pigments for printing inks, textile dyes, plastics, and crayons. DCB is destroyed during the manufacturing process and is not contained in the final products.	Liver, bladder, breasts, skin
Estrogens	Drugs prescribed for menopausal symptoms, menstrual problems. Estrogen is a component of oral contraceptives.	Uterine endometrium, possibly breasts
Hydrocarbons	Cigarette smoke; soot (chimney sweeps may develop cancer of the scrotum); air pollution from industrial wastes, automobile exhausts; coal tar ointments used in treating some skin disorders; gases and particles produced by burning of coal, wood, and oil; foods such as smoked meats, foods burned by charcoal grilling, some vegetables and cereals; food packaging materials; many groups of industrial workers	Lungs, skin
Metallic ores (specific agent unknown)	Workers exposed to chromium in production of chromates and nickel refiners	Lungs
Polyvinyl chloride (PVC)	Workers in chemical plants that use PVC in the production of floor tiles, shoes, phonograph records, automobile upholstery, blood bags, and many other widely used products.	Liver
Tobacco	Cigarette smoking, pipe smoking, chewing tobacco	Lungs, mouth, pharynx, larynx, esophagus, bladder

translocations or mutation. They are introduced into the cell by viruses, where they apparently affect cellular growth factors. The detection of oncogenes in association with specific malignancies (*i.e.,* some leukemias) has great potential for increasing understanding of the malignant process.

CLASSIFICATION OF MALIGNANT NEOPLASMS

Malignant neoplasms are classified in several different ways according to the type of tissue involved, the rate of growth, and other characteristics. With the exception of the acute leukemias, they are considered chronic diseases. These diseases can be broadly categorized as hematologic or solid neoplasms.

Hematologic malignancies

Hematologic malignancies involve the bone marrow and lymphoid tissues; they include leukemias, lymphomas, and multiple myeloma.

Leukemias

Leukemias are cancers of the bone marrow characterized mainly by overproduction of abnormal white blood cells. These cells range from very primitive and immature to nearly normal in morphology. They are unable to function normally as a body defense mechanism against microorganisms and tissue injuries. They also invade the bone marrow and prevent or decrease production of normal red blood cells, white blood cells, and platelets. They eventually infiltrate other organs (liver, spleen, kidneys) and interfere with organ function.

Leukemias are more specifically classified according to the type of abnormal white blood cell. Acute leukemias involve more immature and less functional cells; chronic leukemias involve cells that are more nearly normal and somewhat functional. Granulocytic leukemia indicates abnormal granulocytes, most often neutrophils; myelocytic or myelogenous leukemia indicates that the abnormal cells originate in the bone marrow. Lymphocytic, lymphatic, or lymphogenous leukemia is characterized by abnormal lymphoid tissue.

The four main types of leukemia are (1) acute lymphocytic leukemia, which is more common in children; (2) acute myelogenous leukemia, which occurs in all ages but more often in young adults; (3) chronic lymphocytic leukemia, which is more common in elderly people; and (4) chronic myelogenous leukemia, which is more common in middle age.

Lymphomas

Lymphomas are malignant tumors of lymphoid tissue that are characterized by abnormal proliferation of the white blood cells normally found in lymphoid tissue. Lymphomas usually develop within lymph nodes and may occur anywhere in the body, since virtually all body tissues contain lymphoid structures. They develop as a solid tumor mass without involving peripheral blood. They impair immunity and increase susceptibility to infection. As the disease progresses, there is involvement and functional impairment of the liver, spleen, bone marrow, and other organs. The two main types of malignant lymphomas are known as Hodgkin's disease and non-Hodgkin's lymphoma.

Multiple myeloma

Multiple myeloma is a malignant tumor of the bone marrow in which abnormal plasma cells proliferate. Since normal plasma cells produce antibodies or immunoglobulins and abnormal plasma cells cannot fulfill this function, the body's immune system is handicapped. As the tumor grows, it crowds out normal cells and interferes with other bone marrow functions as well. Although multiple myeloma is a slow-growing tumor, the abnormal plasma cells eventually infiltrate bone and cause extensive destruction. Metastasis eventually occurs in tissues outside bone such as the spleen, liver, and lymph nodes.

Solid neoplasms

Solid tumors are composed of a mass of malignant cells (parenchyma) and a supporting structure of connective tissue, blood vessels, and lymphatics (stroma). The growing tumor develops its own blood supply as new blood vessels grow from preexisting blood vessels of the host. Apparently, neoplastic cells secrete a substance that acts on capillaries to stimulate their growth into the tumor. The two major classifications of solid malignant neoplasms are carcinomas and sarcomas. Each is then subclassified according to the particular kind of body cell involved.

Carcinomas

Carcinomas are derived from epithelial tissues (skin, mucous membrane, linings and coverings of viscera) and are the most common type of malignant tumors. They are further classified by cell type such as adenocarcinoma or basal cell carcinoma.

Sarcomas

Sarcomas are derived from connective tissue (muscle, bone, cartilage, fibrous tissue, fat, blood vessels). They are subclassified by cell type, for example, osteogenic sarcoma, angiosarcoma.

EFFECTS OF CANCER ON THE BODY

Effects of cancer on the host vary according to the extent and location of the disease process. There are few effects initially. As the neoplasm grows, effects occur when the tumor becomes large enough to cause pressure, distortion, or deficient blood supply in surrounding tissues, interfere with organ function, obstruct ducts and organs, and cause malnutrition of normal tissues. More specific effects include anemia, malnutrition, pain, infection, hemorrhagic tendencies, thromboembolic problems, hypercalcemia, cachexia, and occurrence of symptoms related to impaired function of affected organs and tissues.

CHARACTERISTICS OF ANTINEOPLASTIC DRUGS

1. Antineoplastic drugs are cytotoxic. They kill malignant cells by interfering with cell replication. Nutrients and genetic materials are necessary for cell replication. To be effective, the drugs must interfere with the supply and utilization of nutrients (amino acids, purines, pyrimidines) or with the genetic materials in the cell nucleus (DNA or RNA).
2. Some antineoplastic drugs act during specific phases of the cell cycle, such as DNA synthesis or formation of the mitotic spindle. These cell–cycle-specific (CCS) agents include the antimetabolites, the plant alkaloids, and some miscellaneous agents (*e.g.*, asparaginase, hydroxyurea). These drugs are more effective when administered by continuous intravenous infusion because this method prolongs exposure of malignant cells to drug action. Other drugs act during any phase of the cell cycle and are called cell–cycle nonspecific (CCNS). This group includes the alkylating agents, the antibiotic antineoplastics, the nitrosureas, and some miscellaneous agents (*e.g.*, cisplatin, dacarbazine). CCNS agents are more effective when administered in large doses as intermittent boluses.
3. Antineoplastic drugs are most active against rapidly dividing and proliferating cells, although some kill both resting and dividing cells. Since the drugs do not act specifically against malignant cells, normal cells are damaged as well. The normal cells especially endangered are the rapidly proliferating cells of the bone marrow, the lining of the gastrointestinal tract, and the hair follicles. The cytotoxic effects of antineoplastic drugs account for both therapeutic and adverse effects.
4. Each dose of antineoplastic drugs kills some but not all malignant cells. The cell kill effect follows what is called "first-order kinetics." This means that a drug dose kills a specific percentage of cells. If the drug destroys 99% of cells, it reduces one million cells to ten thousand. Succeeding doses would destroy 99% of remaining cells but not all of them. This is important because all malignant cells must be killed to effect a cure. One remaining cell can proliferate and eventually kill the host.
5. Antineoplastic drugs are given mainly by oral and intravenous routes of administration. In some circumstances they may be given intra-arterially or by instillation into a body cavity.
6. Antineoplastic drugs may produce drug resistance. Mechanisms are not clear but may involve killing of sensitive cells while leaving resistant cells, which then proliferate rapidly. Mutant cells may also emerge.
7. Most cytotoxic antineoplastic drugs are potential teratogens.

CLASSIFICATION OF ANTINEOPLASTIC DRUGS

Antineoplastic drugs are classified in several different ways. Some are described in terms of their mechanisms of action (alkylating agents and antimetabolites), others according to their sources (plant alkaloids, antibiotics, enzymes). Another group of drugs used in cancer chemotherapy is the hormones. Hormones are physiologic rather than cytotoxic substances and are useful primarily in certain hormone-dependent cancers. Individual drugs are listed in Table 64-2.

Alkylating agents

Alkylating agents used in cancer chemotherapy include nitrogen mustard and its derivatives (busulfan, chlorambucil, cyclophosphamide, and melphalan). These drugs act by interfering with cell division and structure of DNA during both dividing and resting stages of the malignant cell cycle. Consequently, their spectrum of activity is relatively broad compared to other antineoplastic drugs. They are most effective in hematologic malignancies but are also used in treating breast, lung, and ovarian tumors. All these drugs cause significant bone marrow depression. All except nitrogen mustard may be given orally.

Nitrosureas

The nitrosurea drug group includes carmustine, lomustine, and semustine. These are usually described as

(*Text continues on p. 600.*)

TABLE 64-2. ANTINEOPLASTIC DRUGS

	Generic name	Trade name	Routes and dosage ranges*	Clinical uses	Common or potentially severe adverse reactions
Alkylating drugs					
Nitrogen mustard derivatives	Busulfan	Myleran	PO 4–8 mg daily until white blood cell count decreases by half, then maintenance doses up to 4 mg daily.	Chronic granulocytic leukemia	Bone marrow depression (leukopenia, thrombocytopenia, anemia), pulmonary toxicity
	Chlorambucil	Leukeran	PO 0.1–0.2 mg/kg/day for 3–6 weeks. If maintenance therapy is required, 0.03–0.1 mg/kg/day	Chronic lymphocytic leukemia, non-Hodgkin's lymphomas, carcinomas of breast and ovary	Bone marrow depression, hyperuricemia
	Cyclophosphamide	Cytoxan	Induction of therapy, PO 1–5 mg/kg/day; IV 35–40 mg/kg over several days (20–30 mg/kg for clients with prior chemotherapy or radiation). Oral maintenance therapy, 1.5–2 mg/kg daily.	Hodgkin's disease, non-Hodgkin's lymphomas, neuroblastoma. Often combined with other drugs for acute lymphoblastic leukemia in children; carcinomas of breast, ovary, and lung; multiple myeloma and other malignancies.	Bone marrow depression, anorexia, nausea, vomiting, alopecia, hemorrhagic cystitis
	Mechlorethamine (nitrogen mustard)	Mustargen	IV 0.4 mg/kg in one or two doses. Repeat in 3–6 weeks Intracavitary 0.4 mg/kg instilled into pleural or peritoneal cavities	Hodgkin's disease and non-Hodgkin's lymphomas, lung cancer, pleural and peritoneal malignant effusions	Bone marrow depression, nausea, vomiting. Extravasation may lead to tissue necrosis.
	Melphalan	Alkeran	PO 0.25 mg/kg/day for 7 days, followed by 21 drug-free days, then maintenance dose of 2 mg daily	Multiple myeloma	Bone marrow depression, nausea and vomiting
Nitrosureas	Carmustine (BCNU)		IV 200 mg/m^2 every 6 weeks	Hodgkin's disease, malignant melanoma, multiple myeloma, brain tumors	Bone marrow depression, nausea, vomiting, hepatotoxicity
	Lomustine (CCNU)		PO 130 mg/m^2 every 6 weeks	Hodgkin's disease, brain tumors	Bone marrow depression, nausea, vomiting, hepatotoxicity
	Semustine (Methyl-CCNU)†		PO 200 mg/m^2 every 6 weeks	Hodgkin's disease, non-Hodgkin's lymphomas, brain tumors, malignant melanoma, gastrointestinal malignancies (stomach, colon, pancreas)	Bone marrow depression, nausea, vomiting. Renal toxicity with large total doses

TABLE 64-2. ANTINEOPLASTIC DRUGS (*Continued*)

	Generic name	Trade name	Routes and dosage ranges*	Clinical uses	Common or potentially severe adverse reactions
Antimetabolites	Azathioprine	Imuran	PO, IV 3–5 mg/kg/day, reduced for maintenance and in the presence of impaired renal function	To prevent rejection of renal transplants	Bone marrow depression, nausea
	Cytarabine (ARA-C, cytosine arabinoside)	Cytosar-U	IV 2 mg/kg/day for 10 days	Leukemias of adults and children	Bone marrow depression, nausea, vomiting, stomatitis, diarrhea
	Floxuridine	FUDR	Intra-arterial infusion, 0.1–0.6 mg/kg/day until toxicity occurs	Head and neck tumors, carcinomas of the gastrointestinal tract, liver, pancreas, and biliary tract	Same as cytarabine, above
	Fluorouracil (5-FU)	Adrucil	IV 12 mg/kg/day for 5 days	Carcinomas of the breast, colon, rectum, stomach, and pancreas	Same as cytarabine, above
		Efudex, Fluoroplex	Topical, apply to skin cancer lesion twice daily for several weeks	Solar keratoses, basal cell carcinoma	Pain, pruritus, burning at site of application
	Mercaptopurine	Purinethol	PO 2.5 mg/kg/day	Acute and chronic leukemias	Bone marrow depression, nausea, hyperuricemia
	Methotrexate (MTX, Amethopterin)	Mexate	Induction of remission of acute leukemia in children, PO, IV 3 mg/m^2 day. Maintenance of remission, PO 30 mg/m^2 2 times/week (combined with prednisone for induction and maintenance of remission.) Choriocarcinoma, PO, IM 15 mg/m^2 daily for 5 days	Acute lymphoblastic leukemia in children, lymphocytic lymphoma, choriocarcinoma of the testes, osteogenic carcinoma, and others	Bone marrow depression, nausea, diarrhea, stomatitis
	Thioguanine		PO 2 mg/kg/day	Acute and chronic leukemias	Bone marrow depression, nausea
Antibiotics	Bleomycin	Blenoxane	IV, IM 0.25–0.5 units/kg once or twice weekly	Squamous cell carcinoma, lymphomas, testicular carcinoma, Hodgkin's disease	Pulmonary toxicity, stomatitis, alopecia, hyperpigmentation and ulceration of skin
	Dactinomycin (Actinomycin-D)	Cosmegen	IV 15 μg/kg/day for 5 days and repeated every 2–4 weeks	Rhabdomyosarcoma, Wilms' tumor	Bone marrow depression, anorexia, nausea and vomiting. Extravasation may lead to tissue necrosis.
	Daunorubicin	Cerubidin	IV 60 mg/m^2 daily for 3 days every 3–4 weeks	Acute granulocytic and acute lymphocytic leukemias, lymphomas	Same as doxorubicin, below
	Doxorubicin	Adriamycin	Adults, IV 60–75 mg/m^2 every 21 days	Acute leukemias, lymphomas, carcinomas of	Bone marrow depression, alopecia, stomatitis, gastrointestinal upset,

TABLE 64-2. ANTINEOPLASTIC DRUGS (*Continued*)

	Generic name	Trade name	Routes and dosage ranges*	Clinical uses	Common or potentially severe adverse reactions
			Children, IV 30 mg/m² day for 3 days, repeated every 4 weeks	breast, lung, and ovary	cardiomyopathy. Extravasation may lead to tissue necrosis.
	Mitomycin	Mutamycin	IV 2 mg/m²/day or 50 μg/kg/day for 5 days, repeated after 2 days. This course of therapy may be repeated after recovery of the bone marrow	Carcinomas of stomach, colon, rectum, pancreas, bladder, breast, lung, head and neck, and malignant melanoma	Bone marrow depression, nausea, vomiting, diarrhea, stomatitis. Extravasation may lead to tissue necrosis.
	Plicamycin (formerly known as mithramycin)	Mithracin	IV 25–30 μg/kg/day or every other day for 8–10 doses or until toxicity occurs	Testicular tumors, severe hypercalcemia	Toxicity affecting the bone marrow, liver, and kidneys. Extravasation can cause local tissue inflammation.
Vinca alkaloids	Vinblastine	Velban	IV 0.1 mg/kg weekly, increased gradually by 0.05 mg/kg increments	Metastatic testicular carcinoma. Hodgkin's disease, carcinoma of breast	Bone marrow depression, especially leukopenia, neurotoxicity. Extravasation may lead to tissue necrosis.
	Vincristine	Oncovin	Adults, IV 0.01–0.03 mg/kg weekly Children, IV 0.4–1.4 mg/m² weekly	Hodgkin's disease and other lymphomas, acute leukemia	Neurotoxicity with possible foot drop from muscle weakness, paresthesias, constipation, and other manifestations. Extravasation may lead to tissue necrosis.
Steroid hormones					
Adrenocorticosteroid	Prednisone	Meticorten, others	PO 60–100 mg/m²/day for first few days, then gradual reduction to 20–40 mg/day	Used as adjunct for palliation of symptoms in acute leukemia, Hodgkin's disease, lymphomas, complications of cancer such as thrombocytopenia, hypercalcemia, intracranial metastases	Potentially toxic to almost all body systems. See Chapter 24
Estrogens	Diethylstilbestrol (DES)	Stilbestrol	Breast cancer, PO 1–5 mg 3 times daily Prostate cancer, PO 1–3 mg daily	Carcinoma of prostate gland, carcinoma of breast in postmenopausal women	Feminizing effects in men, anorexia, nausea, vomiting, edema, hypercalcemia, and others. See Chapter 28
	Ethinyl estradiol	Estinyl, others	Breast cancer, PO 0.5 mg/day initially, gradually increased to 3 mg/day in 3 divided doses Prostate cancer, PO 0.15–2 mg daily	Carcinoma of prostate, advanced carcinoma of breast in postmenopausal women	Feminizing effects in men, anorexia, nausea, vomiting, edema, hypercalcemia, and others. See Chapter 28
Progestins	Medroxyprogesterone	Provera, Depo-Provera	IM 400–800 mg twice weekly. PO 200–300 mg/day	Advanced endometrial carcinoma	Usually well tolerated. May cause edema and irritation at injection sites

TABLE 64-2. ANTINEOPLASTIC DRUGS (*Continued*)

	Generic name	Trade name	Routes and dosage ranges*	Clinical uses	Common or potentially severe adverse reactions
	Megestrol	Megace	PO 40–320 mg/day in divided doses	Advanced endometrial carcinoma, breast carcinoma	Usually produces minimal adverse reactions
Androgen	Fluoxymesterone	Halotestin	PO 10 mg, 3 times daily (30 mg/day)	Advanced breast carcinoma in premenopausal women	Masculinizing effects, hypercalcemia
Hormone inhibitors					
Adrenocorticosteroid inhibitor	Aminoglutethimide	Cytadren	PO 250 mg 4 times daily	Advanced breast carcinoma	Adrenal insufficiency
Antiestrogen	Tamoxifen	Nolvadex	PO 20–40 mg/day in 2 divided doses	Advanced breast cancer in postmenopausal women	Hot flashes, nausea, and vomiting, ocular toxicity
Miscellaneous antineoplastic agents	Asparaginase	Elspar	IV 1000 IU/kg/day for 10 days	Acute lymphocytic leukemia refractory to other drugs. Usually used in conjunction with other agents	Abnormal functioning of the liver, kidneys, pancreas, central nervous system, and the blood-clotting mechanism; hypersensitivity reactions
	Cisplatin	Platinol	IV 100 mg/m² once every 4 weeks	Carcinomas of testes, bladder, ovary, head and neck, and endometrium	Renal toxicity and ototoxicity
	Dacarbazine	DTIC-Dome	IV 3.5 mg/kg/day for 10 days, repeated every 28 days	Malignant melanoma, Hodgkin's disease, sarcoma	Bone marrow depression, nausea, and vomiting; increased blood urea nitrogen, serum glutaminic-oxalic transaminase, and serum glutaminic-pyruvic transaminase. Extravasation may cause severe pain and tissue damage.
	Etoposide	VePesid	IV 50–100 mg/m²/day on days 1–5, or 100 mg/m²/day on days 1, 3, and 5, every 3–4 weeks	Testicular cancer, acute leukemias, lymphomas, small-cell lung cancer	Bone marrow depression, anaphylaxis, nausea, vomiting, alopecia
	Hydroxyurea	Hydrea	PO 80 mg/kg as single dose every third day or 20–30 mg/kg as a single dose daily	Chronic granulocytic leukemia, malignant melanoma	Bone marrow depression, gastrointestinal upset
	Mitotane	Lysodren	PO 8–10 g daily in 3–4 divided doses. Maximal daily dose, 19 g	Inoperable carcinoma of the adrenal cortex	Anorexia, nausea, damage to adrenal cortex
	Procarbazine	Matulane	PO 100–200 mg/day for 1 week, then 300 mg/day until maximal response or toxicity occurs	Hodgkin's disease	Bone marrow depression, nausea, and vomiting

* Dosages change frequently according to use in different types of cancer and in combination with other antineoplastic drugs.
† Investigational drug available from the National Cancer Institute.

alkylating agents. However, their mechanism of action is relatively complex, and other factors may be involved. These drugs have been used in clients with gastrointestinal and lung tumors. These drugs have two unique features. First, they are highly lipid soluble and cross the blood–brain barrier to enter the brain and cerebrospinal fluid. Second, they cause delayed bone marrow depression, with maximum leukopenia and thrombocytopenia occurring about 5 to 6 weeks after drug administration.

Antimetabolites

Antimetabolites include a folic acid antagonist (methotrexate), purine antagonists (mercaptopurine and thioguanine), pyrimidine antagonists (fluorouracil and floxuridine), and an inhibitor of DNA polymerase (cytarabine). The drugs are similar to nutrients needed by the cells for reproduction and are allowed to enter the cells. Once inside the cell, the drugs deprive the cell of necessary substances or cause formation of abnormal DNA. Either action kills the cell.

The antimetabolites have been used to treat the entire spectrum of cancers. Effectiveness of individual drugs varies with different kinds of cancer. Toxic effects mainly involve the bone marrow, epithelial lining of the gastrointestinal tract, and hair follicles.

Some antimetabolites can be given both orally and parenterally; others are given only by one route. The effectiveness of these drugs depends greatly on the schedule of administration. They exert their cytotoxic effects only during one phase of the reproductive cycle of the cell, that is, when DNA is being synthesized. Although there is no way a chemotherapist can determine exactly when a drug is most likely to be effective (*i.e.,* kill the largest number of malignant cells), information has been accumulated empirically through extensive clinical trials. Thus, recommendations regarding dosage schedules should be followed as precisely as possible.

Alkaloids

Plant alkaloids, vinblastine and vincristine, are derived from the periwinkle plant. They exert their cytotoxic effects by inhibiting cell division. Despite structural similarities, these two drugs have different ranges of antineoplastic activity. Either may be effective in treating Hodgkin's disease and choriocarcinoma. Vinblastine is also useful in testicular carcinoma, and vincristine is used in acute lymphoblastic leukemia, non-Hodgkin's lymphomas, oat-cell carcinoma of the lung, and Wilms' tumor. These drugs differ in toxic effects. Vinblastine is more likely to cause bone marrow depression, and vincristine is more likely to cause peripheral nerve toxicity. Vindesine is an investigational plant alkaloid.

Antibiotics

Antibiotics include bleomycin, dactinomycin, daunorubicin, doxorubicin, mithramycin, and mitomycin. These drugs differ in activity and toxicities. They have some anti-infective activity, but they are too toxic for this use. The major toxicity is bone marrow depression. The anthracycline drugs, daunorubicin and doxorubicin, also cause cardiotoxicity. Bleomycin may cause significant pulmonary toxicity. All these drugs, except bleomycin, must be given intravenously because they are extremely irritating to tissues and cause tissue necrosis if extravasation occurs.

Hormones

Hormones used in cancer chemotherapy exert beneficial effects by altering the hormonal environment that promotes cancer growth. The sex hormones (estrogens, progestins, androgens) are useful in cancers of the sex organs, including the breast and prostate gland. The adrenal corticosteroids suppress formation and function of lymphocytes and are therefore most useful in the treatment of acute leukemia in children and of malignant lymphoma. They may also be used in treating complications of cancer such as intracranial metastases and hypercalcemia. Related agents include tamoxifen (Nolvadex), an antiestrogen that competes with estrogen for binding sites in breast tissue, and aminoglutethimide (Cytadren), an adrenocorticosteroid-inhibiting agent that produces a "medical adrenalectomy."

Radioactive iodine

Radioactive iodine (^{131}I) is used only for treatment of thyroid cancer. Radioactive gold and phosphorus have been used to treat malignant effusions but are now considered obsolete.

Miscellaneous agents

Miscellaneous antineoplastic agents generally have a limited spectrum of antineoplastic activity and high toxicity.

INDICATIONS

Cytotoxic antineoplastic drugs are clearly indicated only in the treatment of malignant neoplasms. Goals of chemotherapy vary according to the clinical situation. In some cases, chemotherapy is curative. In others, it is palliative. In still others, it is employed to induce or maintain remissions (symptom-free periods that last for varying lengths of time).

Chemotherapy is the primary treatment of choice for a few types of cancer, including Burkitt's lymphoma, choriocarcinoma, Hodgkin's disease, acute leukemia, carcinoma of the testes, Wilms' tumor, Ewing's sarcoma, and retinoblastoma. Most of these malignant tumors are relatively rare. Chemotherapy is relatively ineffective in the most common cancers in the United States. These include cancers of the lung, rectum, pancreas, colon, and prostate gland.

In hematologic neoplasms, drug therapy is the primary treatment of choice because the systemic distribution of the disease precludes use of the other two treatments for cancer (surgery and radiation). In solid tumors, drug therapy is often used to kill malignant cells remaining after surgery or radiation therapy. Chemotherapy is more effective when the tumor mass has been removed or reduced. Chemotherapy used in conjunction with surgery or irradiation is called *adjuvant chemotherapy*. Adjuvant chemotherapy is being increasingly used to destroy malignant cells in breast and other cancers. Drug therapy is also used in advanced malignant disease for palliation of symptoms. Once metastasized, solid tumors become systemic diseases and are no longer readily accessible to surgical excision or radiation therapy.

Antineoplastic drugs are sometimes used in the treatment of nonmalignant conditions. One of these is polycythemia vera, an uncommon condition characterized by abnormal proliferation of blood cells. Another use is in organ transplantation, in which the drugs are given to suppress the recipient's immune system and thereby prevent rejection of the transplanted organ. This regimen has been very successful in renal transplants but less successful in other organ transplants. The main drug used for this purpose is azathioprine (Imuran). It is a derivative of mercaptopurine and has similar cytotoxic effects and adverse reactions.

Principles of therapy: antineoplastic drugs

ASSESSMENT GUIDELINES

Assess the client's condition before drug therapy is started and frequently throughout the course of treatment. Knowledge about the type of malignancy the client has is necessary for adequate assessment. Useful information includes the main organs affected, whether the tumor grows slowly or rapidly, and usual patterns of metastasis. Specific assessment data include the following:

1. *Grade* of the malignancy. Tumor grading is an attempt to determine the degree of malignancy. It is done by biopsy and histologic examination. Grade 1 and 2 tumors show cellular differentiation and are similar to the normal tissue of origin. Grade 3 and 4 tumors are less differentiated, bear little resemblance to the normal tissue of origin, and are more malignant. Generally, the higher the tumor grade, the poorer the prognosis. Criteria for each grade vary with the type of cancer.
2. *Stage* of the malignancy. Staging is a way to determine the extent of the malignant process, that is, whether the tumor is localized or has spread. It also determines which organs are involved in the malignant process. One system of staging is the TNM system. T stands for the primary tumor; subcategories (T_1, T_2, T_3) indicate increasing size. N indicates involvement of regional lymph nodes; N_0 means no involvement, and N_1 and N_2 indicate increasing nodal disease. M stands for metastasis; M_0 indicates absence of metastasis and M_1 indicates metastatic spread.

   Staging is done by the physician on the basis of a history and physical examination and diagnostic tests such as x-ray studies, radioisotope scans, tissue biopsies, cytologic examination of various body secretions, endoscopies, liver and other organ function studies, and, sometimes, exploratory laparotomy or thoracotomy.
3. Laboratory test results. Several laboratory tests are useful in cancer chemotherapy. These are usually done before the beginning of drug therapy, to establish baseline data for later comparison, and during drug therapy, to monitor drug effects.
   a. One test is a blood test for carcinoembryonic antigen (CEA). This is a substance secreted by several types of malignant cells, especially by cells originating in the gastrointestinal tract. It is not a good screening test because a number of false-positive and false-negative results occur. It can be useful in selected circumstances, however. For example, a rising CEA level may indicate progression of malignant disease and a need for evaluation or treatment. If CEA levels are elevated before surgery and disappear after surgery, this is a good indication of adequate tumor excision. If a rise in CEA levels occurs later, it probably indicates recurrence of the tumor. In chemotherapy, falling CEA levels indicate drug effectiveness.
   b. Another common laboratory test is the complete blood count (CBC), done to check for

anemia and other abnormalities. Of special interest are the leukocyte and platelet counts, since most antineoplastic drugs cause bone marrow depression manifested mainly by leukopenia and thrombocytopenia. A CBC and white blood cell differential are done before each cycle of chemotherapy. The tests are used to determine dosage and frequency of drug administration, to monitor bone marrow function so that fatal bone marrow depression does not occur, and to assist the nurse in planning care. For example, the person is very susceptible to infection when the leukocyte count is low, and bleeding is likely when the platelet count is low. Nursing measures can be taken to prevent or minimize both of these complications of chemotherapy.

c. Other tests often ordered include serum calcium, uric acid, and others, depending on the particular organs affected by the malignant disease.

4. Clinical manifestations of the malignancy. Common signs and symptoms include anemia, malnutrition, weight loss, pain, and infection; other symptoms depend on the particular organs affected.
5. Whether other disease conditions are present and, if the client has had previous cancer treatment, the response obtained.
6. Emotional and mental status. Anxiety and depression are common features at any point in cancer diagnosis and treatment. Other aspects of nursing assessment include the client's coping mechanisms, family relationships, and financial resources.

PLANNING WITH CLIENT AND FAMILY

Once the diagnosis of cancer is made, the tumor is graded and staged, the client's physical and mental status is assessed, and the physician decides that the anticipated benefits of chemotherapy outweigh the disadvantages, additional factors must be discussed with the client and family.

1. What is the goal of chemotherapy? It may be to cure the malignant disease, decrease tumor size, relieve symptoms, kill metastatic cells left by surgery or radiation therapy, or prolong life. When the goal is cure or induction of remission, adverse reactions and other disadvantages of chemotherapy may be acceptable. When expected benefit is minimal, even moderate morbidity due to drug therapy may not be acceptable.
2. What adverse reactions are likely to occur? Which should be reported to the physician? How will they be managed if they occur? Even if the realities of chemotherapy are quite unpleasant, it is usually better for the client to know what they are than to fear the unknown. Some specific effects that should be discussed, depending on the drugs to be used, include alopecia, amenorrhea, oligospermia, and possibly permanent sterility. Since most of these drugs are teratogenic, clients in the reproductive years are advised to avoid pregnancy during treatment.
3. Who will administer the drugs, where, and for how long? Cancer chemotherapy is highly specialized. Because the drugs are highly toxic to normal body cells as well as to malignant ones and require meticulous techniques of administration, they are preferably given at a cancer treatment center or by a physician–oncologist experienced in their use. There are also nurse–oncologists who are qualified to administer the drugs and monitor their effects. Some clients undergo chemotherapy at a cancer center far from home; others undergo treatment at a nearby hospital, clinic, physician's office, or even at home. The duration of treatment may be short or long term, depending largely on the type of tumor and response to drug therapy. Thus, estimates of weeks, months, or years of drug therapy must be discussed. The time required for one drug treatment should be described as well, so that the client can schedule other activities. Usual practice requires that blood be drawn for CBC and perhaps other tests. The results of these tests must be reported before antineoplastic drugs are given. If excessive leukopenia or thrombocytopenia is reported, drug therapy may be discontinued or postponed. Clients should be informed about the frequent venipunctures required for blood tests and drug administration.
4. How can the client help to maximize therapeutic benefits of chemotherapy and minimize adverse effects? One self-help measure is to eat a well-balanced diet. This may require great effort in the presence of anorexia, nausea, vomiting, diarrhea, or stomatitis. Another self-help measure is frequent and thorough oral hygiene. A third measure is to keep all appointments for drug administration and blood tests.

DRUG SELECTION

Choice of drug or combination of drugs depends largely on which drugs have been effective in similar types of cancer. Other factors to be considered include primary tumor sites, presence and extent of metastases, physical status of the client, and other disease conditions that affect chemotherapy, such as liver or kidney disease.

COMBINATION DRUG THERAPY

Combinations of several drugs are being increasingly used in the continuing effort to increase therapeutic effects without increasing toxic effects. The effectiveness of various combinations is determined by clinical testing and is usually expressed as a percentage of the clients who respond favorably. Combinations may also prevent or delay the development of drug resistance. Combinations are based on knowledge of tumor cell kinetics and drug actions. Some general characteristics of effective drug combinations include the following:

1. Each drug should exert antineoplastic activity when used alone.
2. Each drug should act by a different mechanism. They can be combined to produce either sequential inhibition or concurrent inhibition. For example, one drug can be chosen to damage the DNA, RNA, or proteins of the malignant cell, and another drug can be chosen to prevent their repair or synthesis.
3. Drugs should act at different times in the reproductive cycle of the malignant cell. For example, more malignant cells are likely to be destroyed by combining CCS and CCNS drugs. The first group kills only dividing cells; the second groups kills cells during any part of the life cycle, including the resting or nondividing phase.
4. Consecutive doses kill a percentage of the tumor cells remaining after earlier doses and further decrease the tumor burden.
5. Toxic reactions of the various drugs should not overlap so that maximal tolerated doses may be given. It is preferable to use drugs that are not toxic to the same organ system (*e.g.*, bone marrow, kidney) and to use drugs that do not exert their toxic effects at the same time. However, adverse reactions to drug combinations may differ considerably from those of each drug when given alone.
6. Combinations usually require different dosages and schedules than single-agent drug therapy.
7. Most drug combinations are designated by letters that indicate individual components. An exception is the COOPER combination, which is named after the physician who developed it. Commonly used drug combinations include the following:
   a. In breast cancer, several combinations may be used. One regimen combines cyclophosphamide, methotrexate, and fluorouracil (CMF). Another uses cyclophosphamide, methotrexate, fluorouracil, vincristine, and prednisone (COOPER; also designated CMFVP). A third uses cyclophosphamide, doxorubicin (Adriamycin) and fluorouracil (CAF). A fourth combines cyclophosphamide, methotrexate, fluorouracil, and prednisone (CMFP).
   b. In leukemia, a combination of cyclophosphamide, vincristine (Oncovin), cytarabine, and prednisone (COAP) may be used.
   c. In Hodgkin's disease, the preferred regimen is mechlorethamine, vincristine (Oncovin), procarbazine, and prednisone, the MOPP regimen. In non-Hodgkin's lymphomas, cyclophosphamide, vincristine, and prednisone (CVP) may be used.

DOSAGE AND ADMINISTRATION FACTORS

Antineoplastic drugs are usually given in relatively high doses, on an intermittent or cyclic schedule. This regimen seems to be more effective than low doses given continuously or massive doses given once. It also produces less immunosuppression and provides drug-free periods during which normal tissues can repair themselves of damage inflicted by the drugs. Fortunately, normal cells repair themselves faster than malignant cells. Succeeding doses are given as soon as tissue repair becomes evident, usually when leukocyte and platelet counts return to normal or acceptable levels. At present, it is unknown whether the peak blood concentration of a drug, its duration, or both determine drug effects in clients.

Each antineoplastic drug must be used in the schedule, route, and dose judged to be most effective for a particular type of neoplastic disease. With combinations of drugs, the recommended schedule should be followed precisely because both safety and effectiveness may be schedule dependent. When chemotherapy is used as an adjuvant to surgery, it usually should be started as soon as possible after surgery, given in maximal tolerated doses just as if advanced disease were present, and continued for several months (usually a year for breast cancer).

Dosage of antineoplastic drugs must be calculated and regulated very carefully to avoid unnecessary toxicity. The age, nutritional status, blood count, kidney and liver function, and previous chemotherapy or radiation therapy must all be considered when determining dosage for a client. Additional factors that influence dosage are as follows:

1. Dosage is usually based on the recipient's body weight (mg/kg) or surface area (mg/m^2).

2. The usual dosages listed for individual drugs apply only when the drug is used as a single agent. In drug combinations, the amount of each agent must be determined by clinical investigations.
3. Dosage may be reduced on the basis of bone marrow depression (as indicated by leukopenia or thrombocytopenia), liver disease, or kidney disease.
4. Sex hormones used in cancer chemotherapy must be given in larger amounts (pharmacologic doses) than when they are used in hormone replacement therapy (physiologic doses). Consequently, adverse reactions are likely to be increased in both incidence and severity.

NURSING INTERVENTIONS IN PREVENTION AND TREATMENT OF ADVERSE REACTIONS

Since all antineoplastic drugs may cause adverse reactions ranging from relatively minor to life threatening, measures are needed to prevent or minimize incidence and intensity of adverse reactions. If they cannot be prevented, they must be detected as early as possible so that treatment may be started and damaging effects may be decreased.

1. *Nausea and vomiting* are common with most antineoplastic drugs. They usually occur within 1 or 2 hours of drug administration and may last for several hours. Various measures to prevent or treat nausea and vomiting have met with varying amounts of success.
   a. Giving antineoplastic drugs at bedtime, often with a sedative type of drug as well, may allow the client to sleep through the hours when nausea and vomiting are likely to be more severe.
   b. Antiemetic drugs may be given before or after administration of antineoplastic drugs. Although they may not completely control nausea and vomiting, they may exert a sedative effect and psychologic benefits. Some clients may experience nausea and vomiting for 2 to 3 days after chemotherapy. In these people, administration of antiemetics on a regular schedule may be beneficial.
   c. Reducing food intake before drug administration apparently makes little difference in the degree of nausea and vomiting.
   d. Oral intake after drug administration is probably best determined by the client through trial and error. Some clients feel better if they avoid oral intake for a few hours; others tolerate small amounts of liquid and dry carbohydrates such as crackers. As soon as nausea and vomiting are relieved, a normal diet can be resumed.
   e. Anorexia and altered taste perception are related problems that interfere with nutrition. Well-balanced meals, consisting of foods the client is able and willing to eat, are very important. There are also nutritional supplements that can be used to increase intake of protein and calories.
2. *Alopecia* occurs with several of the more frequently used antineoplastic drugs such as cyclophosphamide, doxorubicin, methotrexate, and vincristine. Complete hair loss can be psychologically devastating, especially for women. Measures to help decrease the impact of alopecia include the following:
   a. Warn clients before drug therapy is started. Reassure them that alopecia is usually temporary and reversible when drug therapy is stopped. Sometimes, hair growth returns even while drug therapy continues. Hair may grow back with a different color and texture.
   b. Suggest the purchase of wigs, hats, and scarves. This should be done before hair loss is expected to occur.
   c. Suggest the avoidance of permanent waves, hair coloring, or other hair treatments that damage the hair and may affect the degree of hair loss.
   d. Allow the client to express feelings about his altered body image.
   e. Two investigational techniques to prevent alopecia have been tried, with varying success. The rationale for both techniques is to decrease blood flow to the scalp and hair follicles during the intravenous administration of antineoplastic drugs and for a few minutes afterward. This presumably decreases drug effect on the hair follicles. These techniques are probably contraindicated in leukemia and other disorders that metastasize to or originate in the scalp, since they may prevent drugs from reaching malignant cells in the scalp.
      (1) One technique is the scalp tourniquet, which is left in place about 20 minutes. This procedure has probably been used most extensively with vincristine, which is rapidly cleared from the blood after intravenous injection.
      (2) In the other technique, called scalp hypothermia, ice bags are applied to the scalp for about 45 minutes, starting about 10 minutes before drug administration.
3. *Stomatitis* occurs often with the antimetabolites, an-

tibiotics, and plant alkaloids used in cancer chemotherapy. It is likely to interfere with nutrition, lead to oral infections and bleeding, and cause considerable discomfort. Some guidelines for minimizing or treating stomatitis are listed as follows. Most of these can be done by the client after their purpose has been explained by the nurse. Others must be done by or with the assistance of the nurse.

a. Brush the teeth at last twice daily with a soft-bristled toothbrush. Stop brushing teeth if the platelet count drops below 20,000/mm^3 because gingival bleeding is likely. Teeth may then be cleaned with gauze or cotton-tipped applicators dipped in a dilute hydrogen peroxide solution.
b. Floss teeth daily with unwaxed floss. Stop if the platelet count drops below 20,000/mm^3 to prevent gingival bleeding.
c. Rinse the mouth several times daily. Various solutions may be used, such as equal parts of hydrogen peroxide, water, and Cepacol mouthwash; hydrogen peroxide diluted with water in a 1:4 ratio; normal saline; or water. Any of these solutions serves a useful purpose in removing debris from the mouth. The solutions containing hydrogen peroxide are probably more effective in mechanically removing food particles and other debris. Undiluted hydrogen peroxide and commercial mouthwashes are not recommended because they are likely to cause further irritation of oral mucosa. If stomatitis becomes severe, the mouth may need to be rinsed every 2 to 4 hours. Rinsing before meals may decrease unpleasant taste and increase appetite. Rinsing immediately after meals is needed to remove food particles, which promote growth of microorganisms.
d. Do not use lemon–glycerin swabs for oral care. They are ineffective as cleansing agents. In addition, lemon is acidic and may decalcify tooth enamel; glycerin is drying and irritating to oral mucosa.
e. Encourage oral fluids. Systemic dehydration and local dryness of the oral mucosa contribute to the development and progression of stomatitis. Pain and soreness contribute to dehydration. Fluids usually tolerated by the person with stomatitis include tea, carbonated beverages, and ices such as Popsicles. Gelatin desserts are also usually well tolerated and add to fluid intake. Fruit juices are not usually recommended, especially citrus juices such as orange and grapefruit, because they may produce pain, burning, and further tissue irritation. They may be tolerated if diluted with water or carbonated beverages such as Sprite or Seven-Up. Drinking fluids through a straw may be more comfortable, since this decreases contact of fluids with painful ulcerations.
f. Encourage soft, bland, cold, nonacidic foods. Although individual tolerances vary, it is usually better to avoid highly spiced or rough foods.
g. Remove dentures entirely or at least 8 hours daily, since they may irritate oral mucosa.
h. Inspect the mouth daily for signs of inflammation and lesions.
i. Give medications for pain. Local anesthetic solutions such as viscous lidocaine can be used about 15 minutes before meals to make eating more comfortable. Because the mouth and throat are anesthetized, there may be difficulty in swallowing and detecting the temperature of hot foods. Aspiration or burns may occur. Doses should not exceed 15 ml every 3 hours or 120 ml in 24 hours. If systemic analgesics are used, they should be given about 30 to 60 minutes before eating.
j. In oral infections resulting from stomatitis, local or systemic anti-infective drugs are used. Fungal infections with *Candida albicans,* which are common, can be treated with mycostatin (Nystatin) oral tablets, oral suspension, or vaginal tablets used as lozenges and allowed to dissolve in the mouth. Severe infections may require systemic antibiotics, depending on the causative organism as identified by cultures of mouth lesions.

4. *Infection* is common because both the disease and its treatment lower host resistance to infection. Measures to prevent infection are aimed toward increasing host resistance and decreasing exposure to pathogenic microorganisms. Measures to minimize infection are aimed toward early detection and treatment.
   a. Assist in maintaining a well-balanced diet. Oral hygiene before meals and analgesics when appropriate may increase food intake. High-protein, high-calorie foods and fluids can be given between meals. Several types of nutritional supplements are available commercially and can be taken with or between meals. Provide fluids with high nutritional value, such as milkshakes and eggnog, rather than coffee, tea, or carbonated beverages if the client is able to tolerate them and has an adequate intake of water and other fluids.

b. Frequent and thorough handwashing by the client and everyone involved in care is probably the single best way to reduce exposure to pathogenic microorganisms.
c. Teach the client to practice meticulous personal hygiene and to avoid contact with people who have infections, when possible.
d. Avoid in-dwelling venous and urinary catheters when possible. If they are necessary, take particular care to prevent them from becoming sources of infection. For venous lines, change the dressing every 24 or 48 hours, using sterile technique; cleanse the venipuncture site with povidone-iodine (Betadine) and inspect the area for any signs of inflammation. The site must be changed regularly, every 2 or 3 days or if signs of phlebitis occur. For urinary catheters, cleansing the perineal area with soap and water at least once daily is recommended.
e. Signs and symptoms of infection may not be very obvious in the person whose defenses against infection are compromised. Fever is probably the most consistent symptom. If it occurs, it is presumed to be caused by infection, and it should be investigated to determine the source. Rectal temperature measurements are usually avoided because of the risk of mucosal trauma and subsequent infection.
f. When infection is suspected, possible sources are cultured and antibiotics initiated without waiting for culture reports.
g. If severe leukopenia develops, some physicians order protective or reverse isolation to decrease exposure to pathogens. Others, however, do not think isolation is very helpful, since most infections are caused by microorganisms from the patient's own body rather than exogenous sources. Transfusions of white blood cells may be given in some circumstances.

5. *Bleeding* may be caused by thrombocytopenia, and precautions should be instituted if the platelet count drops to 50,000/mm^3 or below. Bleeding may occur with seemingly minor trauma or spontaneously. Measures to avoid bleeding include:
   a. Avoid trauma, including venipuncture, injections, and rectal temperatures when possible.
   b. Use an electric razor for shaving.
   c. Check skin, urine, and stool for blood.
   d. For platelet counts under 20,000/mm^3, stop brushing the teeth. Platelet transfusions may be given.
6. *Extravasation* is the leakage of drug into subcutaneous tissues around an intravenous injection site. Many of the cytotoxic antineoplastic drugs cause severe inflammation, pain, and even tissue necrosis if extravasation occurs. Thus, efforts are needed to prevent extravasation if possible or to minimize tissue damage if it occurs.
   a. Start an intravenous infusion. Avoid veins that are small, located in an edematous extremity, or located near a joint.
   b. With the intravenous infusion running rapidly, inject the drug into the intravenous tubing with a small gauge needle. This provides for relatively slow administration and rapid dilution of the drug. In addition, if extravasation should occur, it can be detected quickly and stopped when only small amounts of drug have been injected into subcutaneous tissues.
   c. After the drug has been injected, continue the rapid flow rate of the intravenous fluid for 2 to 5 minutes to thoroughly flush the vein.
   d. If extravasation occurs, various techniques have been suggested to decrease tissue damage. These include injection of hydrocortisone through the intravenous line before it is removed, subcutaneous infiltration of hydrocortisone around the extravasated area, and application of ice bags or cold compresses. Nurses involved in cancer chemotherapy must know the procedure to be followed in their facility if extravasation occurs so that it can be instituted immediately.
7. *Hyperuricemia* results from rapid breakdown or destruction of malignant cells whether it occurs spontaneously or as a result of antineoplastic drugs. Uric acid crystals can cause kidney damage. Uric acid nephropathy is the main danger to the client. The following measures minimize these effects:
   a. Maintaining a high fluid intake, with intravenous fluids if necessary, and a high urine output.
   b. Alkalinizing the urine with sodium bicarbonate or other agents.
   c. Administering allopurinol to inhibit uric acid formation.

GUIDELINES FOR HANDLING ANTINEOPLASTIC DRUGS

Antineoplastic drugs exert adverse effects on nurses and other people who prepare and administer the drugs. These effects include contact dermatitis and mutagenic cells in the urine. The extent and long-term consequences of the mutagenic cells are not yet known. Guidelines for handling the drugs to avoid adverse effects include the following:

1. Avoid contact with solutions for injection by wearing disposable gloves, eye protectors, and protective clothing (*e.g.*, long-sleeved garments).
2. If handling a powder form of a drug, wear a mask to avoid inhaling the powder.
3. Prepare the drugs on disposable trays or towels so that spills can be contained.
4. Dispose of contaminated materials in specific chemotherapy waste containers. The containers should be incinerated at temperatures of 1800°F to 2000°F.

NURSING ACTIONS: ANTINEOPLASTIC DRUGS

Nursing Actions	*Rationale/Explanation*
1. Administer accurately	
a. If not used to giving cytotoxic antineoplastic drugs regularly, read package inserts or other recent drug references regarding administration of individual drugs.	Obtaining current information is necessary for several reasons, including the relatively large number and varied characteristics of the drugs, differences in administration according to the type of neoplasm being treated and other client characteristics, continuing development of new dosages, routes and schedules of administration through clinical research, and continuing development of new or altered drug combination regimens.
b. For drugs to be given parenterally,	
(1) Prepare the drug solution immediately before use when possible.	Many of the drugs are available in a powder form, which must be reconstituted before administration. Increasingly, preparation is done in the pharmacy under a vertical laminar flow hood. This is the preferred method, because it prevents contamination of the solution and dissemination of drug particles into the environment. Several drugs are unstable in solution and therefore need to be given soon after mixing. Others may be stable for varying lengths of time.
(2) If necessary to use a prepared drug solution at a later time, label it with an expiration time and store it correctly, usually under refrigeration.	Expiration times vary with individual drugs and the method of storage. Most drug solutions last longer when refrigerated.
(3) Wear gloves when mixing the drugs (cyclophosphamide, dacarbazine, dactinomycin, doxorubicin, mechlorethamide, vinblastine, and vincristine)	To avoid chemical burns, since a number of the drugs are very irritating to the skin. Safety glasses are also recommended for those who wear contact lenses. If some drug solution gets on the skin despite precautions, wash the area with large amounts of water as with any chemical burn.
(4) Give intravenous drugs through a small needle (23 to 25 gauge) over a period of 2 to 3 minutes or inject into the tubing of a rapidly flowing intravenous infusion.	To decrease tissue irritation. The second method is recommended for the more irritating drugs such as doxorubicin so that extravasation into subcutaneous tissues becomes immediately apparent if it occurs.
c. For drugs to be given orally, the total dose of most drugs can be given at one time. An exception is mitotane, which is given in 3 to 4 divided doses.	
2. Observe for therapeutic effects	Therapeutic effects depend to a large extent on the particular type of malignancy being treated. They may not become evident for several weeks after chemotherapy is begun. Some
a. Increased appetite	

Nursing Actions	Rationale/Explanation
b. Increased sense of well being **c.** Improved mobility **d.** Decreased pain	clients experience anorexia, nausea, and vomiting for 2–3 weeks after each cycle of drug therapy.
e. With busulfan, given for chronic myelogenous leukemia, also observe for decreased white blood cell count and decreased size of the spleen.	Decreased white blood cell count and splenomegaly usually become evident about the second or third week of drug therapy.
f. With melphalan, given for multiple myeloma, also observe for decreased amounts of abnormal proteins in urine and blood, decreased levels of serum calcium, and increased hemoglobin.	
3. Observe for adverse effects	Because they are toxic to normal cells as well as malignant ones, cytotoxic antineoplastic drugs may have adverse effects on almost any body tissue. These adverse effects range from common to rare, from relatively mild to life threatening. Some are expected, such as bone marrow depression, and this is used to guide drug therapy. Most of the adverse effects occur with usual dosage ranges and are likely to be increased in incidence and severity with larger doses.
a. Hematologic effects (1) Bone marrow depression with leukopenia (decreased white blood cell count), thrombocytopenia (decreased platelets), and anemia (decreased red blood cell count, hemoglobin, and hematocrit)	For most of these drugs, white blood cell count and platelet counts reach their lowest points about 7 to 14 days after drug administration and return toward normal after about 21 days. Normal leukocyte and platelet counts signify recovery of bone marrow function. Anemia may occur later because the red blood cell is longer lived than white cells and platelets.
(2) Decreased antibodies and lymphocytes	Most of these drugs have immunosuppressant effects, which impair body defenses against infection.
b. Gastrointestinal effects—anorexia, nausea, vomiting, diarrhea, constipation, stomatitis and other mucosal ulcerations, oral candidiasis	Anorexia, nausea, and vomiting are very common. They usually occur within a few hours of drug administration. Nausea and vomiting often subside within approximately 12 to 24 hours, but anorexia may persist. Constipation is most likely to occur with vincristine. Mucosal ulcerations may occur anywhere in the gastrointestinal tract and can lead to serious complications (infection, hemorrhage, perforation). Their occurrence is usually an indication to stop drug therapy, at least temporarily. Fungal and bacterial infections may interfere with nutrition. They may be relatively mild or severe.
c. Integumentary effects—alopecia, dermatitis, tissue irritation at injection sites	Complete hair loss may take several weeks to occur. Alopecia is most significant in terms of altered body image, possible mental depression, and other psychologic effects. Several drugs may cause phlebitis and sclerosis of veins used for injections as well as pain and tissue necrosis if allowed to leak into subcutaneous tissues around the injection site.
d. Renal effects (1) Hyperuricemia and uric acid nephropathy	When malignant cells are destroyed by drug therapy, they release uric acid into the bloodstream. Uric acid crystals may precipitate in the kidneys and cause impaired function or even renal failure. Adverse effects on the kidneys are especially associated with methotrexate and cisplatin. Hyperuricemia can be decreased by an ample fluid intake or by administration of allopurinol.

Nursing Actions	**Rationale/Explanation**
(2) With cyclophosphamide, hemorrhagic cystitis (blood in urine, dysuria, burning on urination)	Hemorrhagic cystitis is thought to occur in about 10% of the clients who receive cyclophosphamide and to result from irritating effects of drug metabolites on the bladder mucosa. The drug is stopped if this occurs. Cystitis can be decreased by an ample fluid intake.
e. Pulmonary effects—cough, dyspnea, chest x-ray changes	Adverse reactions affecting the lungs are associated mainly with bleomycin, busulfan, and methotrexate. With bleomycin particularly, pulmonary toxicity may be severe and progress to pulmonary fibrosis.
f. Cardiovascular effects—congestive heart failure (dyspnea, edema, fatigue), arrhythmias, electrocardiographic changes	Cardiomyopathy is associated primarily with daunorubicin and doxorubicin. This is a life-threatening adverse reaction. The heart failure may be unresponsive to digitalis preparations.
g. Nervous system effects—peripheral neuropathy with vincristine, manifested by muscle weakness, numbness and tingling of extremities, foot drop and decreased ability to walk.	This is a fairly common effect of vincristine, which may worsen for several weeks after drug administration. There is usually some recovery of function eventually.
h. Endocrine effects—menstrual irregularities, sterility in both males and females	
4. Observe for drug interactions	
a. Drugs that *increase* effects of cytotoxic antineoplastic drugs	
(1) Allopurinol	Allopurinol is usually given to prevent or treat hyperuricemia, which may occur with cancer chemotherapy. When given with mercaptopurine, allopurinol facilitates the formation of the active metabolite. Consequently, doses of mercaptopurine must be reduced to one third to one fourth of the usual dose.
(2) Anticoagulants, oral	Increased risk of bleeding
(3) Bone marrow depressants	Increased bone marrow depression
(4) Other antineoplastic drugs	Additive cytotoxic effects, both therapeutic and adverse
b. Drugs that *increase* effects of cyclophosphamide	
(1) Anesthetics, inhalation	Lethal combination. Discontinue cyclophosphamide at least 12 hours before general inhalation anesthesia is to be given.
(2) Barbiturates	Potentiate cyclphosphamide by induction of liver enzymes, which accelerate transformation of the drug into its active metabolites
(3) Other alkylating antineoplastic drugs	Increased bone marrow depression
c. Drugs that *increase* effects of methotrexate	
(1) Alcohol	Additive liver toxicity. Avoid concomitant use.
(2) Aspirin; analgesics and antipyretics containing aspirin or other salicylates; barbiturates; phenytoin; sulfonamides	Potentiate methotrexate by displacing it from protein-binding sites in plasma. Salicylates also block renal excretion of methotrexate. This may cause pancytopenia and liver toxicity. Salicylates are present in many prescription and nonprescription drugs such as headache remedies, pain relievers, and cold remedies.
(3) Other hepatotoxic drugs	Additive liver toxicity
(4) Other antineoplastic drugs	Additive cytotoxic effects, both therapeutic and adverse. Methotrexate is one component of several drug combinations used to treat breast cancer.
d. Drugs that *decrease* effects of methotrexate	
Leucovorin (citrovorum factor, folinic acid)	Leucovorin antagonizes the toxic effects of methotrexate and is used as an antidote for high-dose methotrexate regimens or

Nursing Actions	Rationale/Explanation
	for overdose. It must be given exactly at the specified time, before affected cells become too damaged to respond.
5. Teach clients	
a. Keep all appointments for drug therapy and blood tests.	Drugs must be given on schedule for maximal therapeutic effects. Regular blood tests are necessary to avoid excessive adverse reactions to drug therapy.
b. Try to maintain the best possible nutritional status.	Drug therapy seems to be better tolerated by well-nourished clients.
c. Maintain a fluid intake of 3 to 4 quarts each day if not contraindicated by heart or kidney disease.	To decrease kidney damage
d. Use wigs, scarves, and hats to minimize the impact of alopecia, if expected with the planned drug therapy. These should be purchased before the start of chemotherapy.	To maintain a positive body image as much as possible and promote mental health
e. Avoid people with infections. Wash hands frequently and thoroughly.	Clients taking anticancer drugs pick up infections easily. Avoiding exposure to potential infections is desirable. Many infections are caused by fungi and bacteria in one's own body. Handwashing helps to decrease infection from sources both inside and outside the body.
f. Shave with an electric razor, avoid injections if possible, and avoid aspirin-containing preparations such as some pain medications and cold remedies.	To decrease risk of bleeding. Antineoplastic drugs cause thrombocytopenia (decreased platelets), which, in turn, increases the risk of spontaneous bleeding and of bleeding from trauma. Aspirin increases the risk of bleeding by interfering with platelet aggregation, an essential step in blood coagulation.
g. Report symptoms	
(1) Mouth soreness or ulcerations	May indicate infection, need for special oral care, or need to stop drug therapy.
(2) Any evidence of bleeding, such as excessive bruising of skin, bleeding from the gums or nose, seeing blood in urine or feces	May indicate a need to stop drug therapy and, if severe, to start treatment measures to control bleeding
(3) Fever	Fever may indicate infection and need for prompt treatment.
h. If necessary to go to another physician or a dentist, inform about cancer chemotherapy *before* any diagnostic test or treatment is begun.	Some diagnostic tests and treatment measures may be contraindicated or require special precautions in an individual taking antineoplastic drugs.
i. With vincristine, eat high-fiber foods such as raw fruits and vegetables and whole cereal grains, if able. Also try to maintain a high-fluid intake. A stool softener or bulk laxative may also be prescribed on a daily basis.	To prevent the constipation that may occur during vincristine therapy.
j. With cyclophosphamide, drink 2 to 3 quarts of fluid daily, if possible, and urinate often, especially at bedtime. If blood is seen in the urine or signs of cystitis occur despite precautions, report this immediately.	Products of cyclophosphamide breakdown are irritating to the bladder lining and may cause bleeding, burning on urination, and other signs of cystitis. High fluid intake and frequent emptying of the bladder help to decrease bladder damage. If blood appears in the urine or if cystitis occurs, the drug should be discontinued.
k. With doxorubicin, inform the client that the urine may turn red for 1 to 2 days after drug administration.	To decrease the anxiety that may occur if the client thinks the red urine is from bleeding. The discoloration is harmless.
l. Also with doxorubicin, tell the client to report edema, shortness of breath, and excessive fatigue.	These are signs of heart failure and require that drug therapy be stopped.

Selected References

Anderson PD: Basic Human Anatomy and Physiology: Clinical Implications for the Health Professions. Monterey, CA, Wadsworth, 1984

Bourke GJ (ed): The Epidemiology of Cancer. Philadelphia, Charles Press, 1983

Brinton LA: The relationship of exogenous estrogens to cancer risk. Cancer Detect Prevent 7:159–171, 1984

Calabresi P, Parks RE Jr: Antiproliferative agents and drugs used for immunosuppression. In Gilman AG, Goodman LS, Rall TW, Murad F (eds): The Pharmacological Basis of Therapeutics, 7th ed, pp 1247–1306. New York, Macmillan, 1985

Calabresi P, Schein PS, Rosenberg SA (eds): Medical Oncology. New York, Macmillan, 1985

Cancer chemotherapy. Med Lett Drugs Ther 27:13–20, February 1985

Creasey WA: Diet and Cancer. Philadelphia, Lea & Febiger, 1985

DeVita VT, Hellman S, Rosenberg SA (eds): Cancer: Principles and Practices of Oncology. Philadelphia, J B Lippincott, 1985

Donovan M: Cancer pain: You can help! Nurs Clin North Am 17:713–728, December 1982

Etoposide (VP 16-213: VePesid). Med Lett Drugs Ther 26:48–49, May 1984

Facts and Comparisons. St. Louis, J B Lippincott (Updated monthly)

Gordon H: Oncogenes. Mayo Clin Proc 60:697–713, October 1985

Griffiths MJ, Murray KH, Russo PC: Oncology Nursing: Pathophysiology, Assessment, and Intervention. New York, Macmillan, 1985

Hughes CB: Giving cancer drugs: Some guidelines. Am J Nurs 86:34–38, January 1986

Mattia MA, Blake SL: Hospital hazards: Cancer drugs. Am J Nurs 83:758–762, May 1983

Petton S: Easing the complications of chemotherapy—a matter of little victories. Nursing 14:58–63, February 1984

Stoudemire A, Cotanch P, Laszlo J: Recent advances in the pharmacologic and behavioral management of chemotherapy-induced emesis. Arch Intern Med 144:1029–1033, May 1984

Veronesi U: Breast cancer—1985: Changing management strategies. Drug Ther 15:26–42, August 1985

Walter J: Care of the patient receiving antineoplastic drugs. Nurs Clin North Am 17:607–629, December 1982

Wissing VS: Breast cancer: The hormone factor. Am J Nurs 84:1117–1118, September 1984

65

DRUGS USED IN OPHTHALMIC CONDITIONS

Description and uses

STRUCTURES OF THE EYE

The eye is the major sensory organ through which the person receives information about the external environment. An in-depth discussion of vision and ocular anatomy is beyond the scope of this chapter. A limited number of characteristics and functions are described to facilitate understanding of ocular drug therapy. These include the following:

1. The eyelids and lacrimal system function to protect the eye. The *eyelid* is a covering that acts as a barrier to the entry of foreign bodies, strong light, dust, and other potential irritants. The *conjunctiva* is the mucous membrane lining of the eyelids. The *canthi* (singular, canthus) are the angles or corners where upper and lower eyelids meet. The *lacrimal system* produces a fluid that constantly moistens and cleanses the anterior surface of the eyeball. The fluid drains through two small openings in the inner canthus and flows through the nasolacrimal duct into the nasal cavity. When the conjunctiva is irritated or certain emotions are experienced (*e.g.*, sadness), the lacrimal gland produces more fluid than the drainage system can accommodate. The excess fluid overflows the eyelids and becomes *tears*.
2. The eyeball is a spherical structure composed of the sclera, cornea, choroid, and retina, plus special refractory tissues. The *sclera* is a white, opaque fibrous tissue that covers the posterior five sixths of the eyeball. The *cornea* is a transparent, special connective tissue that covers the anterior one sixth of the eyeball. The cornea contains no blood vessels. The *choroid* is composed of blood vessels and connective tissue. It continues forward to form the iris. The *iris* is composed of pigmented cells, the opening called the *pupil,* and muscles that control the size of the pupil by contracting or dilating in response to stimuli. The *retina* is the innermost layer of the eyeball. For vision to occur, light rays must enter the eye through the cornea, travel through the pupil, lens, and vitreous body (see below), and be focused on the retina. Light rays do not travel directly to the retina. Instead, they are deflected in various directions according to the density of the ocular structures through which they pass. This process, called *refraction,* is controlled by the aqueous humor, lens, and vitreous body. The *optic disk* is the area of the retina where ophthalmic blood vessels and the optic nerve enter the eyeball.
3. Structure and function of the eyeball are further influenced by the lens, aqueous humor, and vitreous body. The *lens* is an elastic, transparent structure whose function is to focus light rays to form

images on the retina. It is located behind the iris and held in place by suspensory ligaments attached to the ciliary body. The *aqueous humor* is a clear fluid produced by capillaries in the ciliary body. Most of the fluid flows through the pupil into the anterior chamber (between the cornea and the lens and anterior to the iris). A small amount flows into a passage called the canal of Schlemm, from which it enters the venous circulation. Under normal circumstances, production and drainage of aqueous humor are approximately equal, and a normal intraocular pressure (about 15 to 25 mm Hg) is maintained. Impaired drainage of aqueous humor causes increased intraocular pressure. The *vitreous body* is a transparent, jellylike mass located in the posterior portion of the eyeball. It functions to refract light rays and maintain normal shape of the eyeball.

DISORDERS OF THE EYE

The eye is subject to the development of many disorders that threaten structure, function, or both. Some disorders in which ophthalmic drugs play a prominent role, either alone or in conjunction with other therapeutic modalities, include the following:

Refractive errors

Refractive errors include myopia (nearsightedness), hyperopia (farsightedness), presbyopia, and astigmatism. These conditions impair vision by interfering with the ability of the eye to focus light rays on the retina. Ophthalmic drugs are used only in diagnosis of the conditions; treatment involves prescription of eyeglasses or contact lenses.

Glaucoma

Glaucoma is a common *preventable* cause of blindness. It occurs when the inflow of aqueous humor into the anterior chamber is greater than the outflow. As a result, intraocular pressure is increased, blood vessels and the optic nerve are compressed, ocular tissues are damaged, and blindness occurs if the condition is not treated effectively.

The most common type of glaucoma is called primary open-angle glaucoma. It is a chronic disorder of unknown cause. A less common but more dramatic type is called narrow-angle glaucoma. Acute glaucoma results from a sudden, severe increase in intraocular pressure and is characterized by progressive ocular damage and loss of vision. Acute glaucoma occurs in people with narrow-angle glaucoma when pupils are dilated and outflow of aqueous humor is blocked. Darkness and numerous drugs (*e.g.*, anticholinergics, antihistamines, antipsychotics, and antidepressants) may precipitate acute glaucoma. Secondary glaucoma may follow traumatic or inflammatory conditions of the eye.

Inflammatory or infectious conditions

Inflammation may be caused by bacteria, viruses, allergic reactions, or irritating chemicals. Infections may result from foreign bodies, contaminated hands, contaminated equipment or solutions used in treatment, or infections in contiguous structures (*e.g.*, nose, face, sinuses). Common inflammatory and infectious disorders include the following:

1. Conjunctivitis is often caused by allergic reactions that are characterized by a watery discharge and pruritus. A highly contagious form of conjunctivitis ("pinkeye") commonly occurs in children. Chronic conjunctivitis is usually caused by *Staphylococcus aureus, Streptococcus viridans,* or *Diplococcus pneumoniae* and is characterized by mucoid or mucopurulent discharge and red, edematous conjunctiva. Conjunctivitis with a purulent discharge is most often caused by the gonococcus; corneal ulcers and scarring may result.
2. Blepharitis is a chronic infection of glands and lash follicles on the margins of the eyelids. A hordeolum (commonly called a "sty") is often associated with blepharitis. The most common causes are seborrhea and staphylococcal infections.
3. Keratitis (inflammation of the cornea) may be caused by microorganisms, trauma, allergy, ischemia, and drying of the cornea (*e.g.*, from inadequate lacrimation or inability to close the eyelid). The major symptom is pain, which ranges from mild to severe. Vision may not be affected initially. However, if not treated effectively, corneal ulceration, scarring, and impaired vision may result.
4. Bacterial corneal ulcers are most often caused by pneumococci and staphylococci. Pseudomonal ulcers are less common but may rapidly progress to perforation. Fungal ulcers may follow topical corticosteroid therapy or injury with vegetable matter such as a tree branch. Viral ulcers are usually caused by the herpes virus.

OPHTHALMIC DRUGS

Drugs used to diagnose or treat ophthalmic disorders represent numerous therapeutic classifications, most of which are discussed in other chapters. Some drugs are used exclusively or primarily by ophthalmologists. Major classes of drugs used in ophthalmology include the following:

1. Anti-infective drugs are used to treat bacterial, viral, and fungal infections (see Chaps. 33 through 43). They are usually applied topically but may be injected subconjunctivally or intravenously (IV) in severe infections.
2. Autonomic drugs are used extensively in ophthalmology for both diagnostic and therapeutic purposes (see Chaps. 17 through 21). Some are used to dilate the pupil before ophthalmologic examinations or surgical procedures; some are used to constrict the pupil and decrease intraocular pressure in glaucoma. Autonomic drugs indicated in one disorder may be contraindicated in another. For example, anticholinergic drugs are usually contraindicated in glaucoma. Adrenergic mydriatics (*e.g.,* epinephrine, phenylephrine) should be used cautiously in clients with hypertension, cardiac arrhythmias, arteriosclerotic heart disease, and hyperthyroidism.
3. Corticosteroids (see Chap. 24) are frequently used to treat inflammatory conditions of the eye, thereby reducing scarring and preventing loss of vision. Corticosteroids are generally more effective in acute than chronic inflammatory conditions. These drugs are potentially toxic. Therefore, they should not be used to treat minor disorders or disorders that can be effectively treated with safer drugs. When used, corticosteroids should be administered in the lowest effective dose and for the shortest effective time. Long-term use should be avoided when possible. When used in ophthalmologic conditions, corticosteroids may be administered topically, systemically, or both. Corticosteroids are contraindicated in eye infections caused by the herpes virus because the drugs increase the severity of the infection.
4. Carbonic anhydrase inhibitors and osmotic diuretics are given to decrease intraocular pressure in glaucoma and before certain surgical procedures. Carbonic anhydrase inhibitors were initially used as diuretics, but their effectiveness in lowering intraocular pressure (by decreasing production of aqueous humor) does not depend on diuretic effects.
5. Miscellaneous drugs used by the ophthalmologist include a chelating agent, dyes, and an enzyme, as follows:
    a. A chelating agent, disodium edetate (Endrate), is used to remove calcium deposits in the cornea, which cause pain or impair vision. The drugs may also be used for emergency treatment of calcium hydroxide burns of the eye. There is no ophthalmic preparation available. The IV preparation is diluted with sterile normal saline to a concentration of 0.35% to 1.85%. The dilute solution is used to irrigate the eye for about 15 minutes.
    b. Fluorescein (Ful-Glo) is the most commonly used dye. This agent is useful in diagnosing lesions or foreign bodies in the cornea, fitting contact lenses, and studying the lacrimal system and flow of aqueous humor. Rose bengal is another dye that may be used.
    c. Alpha chymotrypsin (Catarase) is an enzyme that may be used to facilitate intracapsular cataract extraction.

Drug therapy of ophthalmic conditions is unique because of the location, structure, and function of the eye. Many systemic drugs are unable to cross the blood–eye barrier and achieve therapeutic concentrations in ocular structures. Some drugs penetrate the eye better than others, however, depending on the serum drug concentration, size of drug molecules, solubility of the drug in fat, extent of drug protein binding, and whether inflammation is present in the eye. Generally, penetration is greater if the drug achieves a high concentration in the blood, has small molecules, is fat soluble, and is poorly bound to serum proteins and if inflammation is present.

Because of the difficulties associated with systemic therapy, various methods of administering drugs locally have been developed. The most common method of drug administration in ocular therapeutics is topical application of ophthalmic solutions (eye drops) to the conjunctiva. Drugs are distributed through the tear film covering the eye and may be used for superficial disorders (*e.g.,* conjunctivitis) or for relatively deep ocular disorders (*e.g.,* when epinephrine is given for glaucoma, the drug must penetrate the cornea, anterior chamber, and ciliary processes to exert therapeutic effects). Other topical dosage forms include ophthalmic ointments and a specialized method of administering pilocarpine so that the drug is slowly released over a 1-week period (Ocusert). Ocusert is a small plastic device inserted into the conjunctival area and replaced weekly by the client. It is used for long-term management of glaucoma.

Other methods of local administration of drugs involve special injection techniques used by ophthalmologists. These include injections through the conjunctiva to subconjunctival tissues or under the fibrous capsule beneath the conjunctiva (sub-Tenon's injection). These injections are painful, and topical anesthetic solutions should be applied before the procedure. Antibiotics and corticosteroids are the drugs most likely to be administered by subconjunctival or sub-

Tenon's injection. A third type of injection, called retrobulbar injection, involves injection of a drug behind the globe of the eyeball. Corticosteroids and preoperative local anesthetics may be administered this way.

Individual drugs are listed in Tables 65-1 and 65-2.

Principles of therapy: ophthalmic drugs

ASSESSMENT GUIDELINES

Assess the client's condition in relation to ophthalmic disorders.

1. Determine whether the client has impaired vision and, if so, the extent or severity of the impairment. Minimal assessment of the vision-impaired client includes ability to participate in activities of daily living, including safe ambulation. Maximal assessment depends on the nurse's ability and working situation. Some nurses do complete vision testing and ophthalmoscopic examinations.
2. Identify risk factors for eye disorders. These include trauma, allergies, infection in one eye (a risk factor for infection in the other eye), hard contact lenses, infections of facial structures or skin, and occupational exposure to chemical irritants or foreign bodies.
3. Signs and symptoms vary with particular disorders.
   a. Pain is usually associated with corneal abrasions or inflammation. Sudden, severe pain may indicate acute angle-closure glaucoma. Acute glaucoma requires immediate treatment to lower intraocular pressure and minimize damage to the eye.
   b. Signs of inflammation (redness, edema, heat, tenderness) are especially evident with infection or inflammation of external ocular structures such as the eyelids and conjunctiva. A mucoid or purulent discharge often occurs also.
   c. Pruritus is most often associated with allergic conjunctivitis.
   d. Photosensitivity commonly occurs with keratitis.

PREVENTIVE NURSING INTERVENTIONS

Use measures to prevent or minimize ocular disorders.

1. Treat eye injuries appropriately.
   a. For chemical burns, irrigate the eyes with copious amounts of water as soon as possible (*i.e.*, near the area where injury occurred; do not wait for transport to a first-aid station, hospital, or other health care facility). Damage continues as long as the chemical is in contact with the eye.
   b. For thermal burns, apply cold compresses to the area.
   c. Superficial foreign bodies may be removed by irrigation with water. Foreign bodies embedded in ocular structures must be removed by a physician.
2. Teach clients to observe the following precautions:
   a. Wear safety goggles when working in high-risk areas. These are often provided by employers.
   b. Avoid overwearing of hard contact lenses. This is a common cause of corneal abrasion and may cause corneal ulceration. The lens wearer should consult a physician when eye pain occurs. Antibiotics are often prescribed for corneal abrasions to prevent development of ulcers.
   c. Avoid regular use of nonprescription eye drops (*e.g.*, Murine, Clear & Brite, Visine). Persistent eye irritation and redness should be reported to a physician.
   d. Avoid eyestrain by using appropriate lighting for reading and handwork. Also, limit periods of reading, watching television, and other visual activities.
   e. Minimize exposure to dust, smog, cigarette smoke, and other eye irritants when possible.
   f. Have regular eye examinations and testing for glaucoma after 40 years of age.
   g. Avoid straining at stool (use laxatives or stool softeners if necessary), heavy lifting, bending over, coughing, and vomiting when possible. These activities increase intraocular pressure which may cause ocular damage in glaucoma and after intraocular surgery.
3. Warm wet compresses are often useful in ophthalmic inflammation or infections. They relieve pain and promote healing by increasing blood supply to the affected area.

THERAPEUTIC GUIDELINES

Ocular infections

For drug therapy of ocular infections, guidelines for choice of drug, dosage, and route of administration include the following:

1. Drug therapy is usually initiated as soon as culture material (eye secretions) has been obtained, often with a broad-spectrum antibacterial agent or a combination of two or more antibiotics.
2. Topical administration is used most often, and recommended drugs include bacitracin, colistimethate sodium, chloramphenicol, polymyxin B, and

(*Text continues on p. 619.*)

TABLE 65-1. DRUGS USED IN OCULAR DISORDERS*

Ocular effects	Clinical indications	Generic name	Trade name	Routes and dosage ranges: Adults	Routes and dosage ranges: Children
Autonomic drugs					
Adrenergics					
1. Decreased production of aqueous humor 2. Mydriasis 3. Decreased intraocular pressure 4. Vasoconstriction 5. Photophobia	1. Glaucoma 2. Ophthalmoscopic examination 3. Reduction of adhesion formation with uveitis 4. Preoperative and postoperative mydriasis 5. Local hemostasis	Dipivefrin (0.1% solution)	Propine	Topically, 1 drop in affected eye(s) twice daily q12h	
		Epinephrine bitartrate (1% solution)	Epitrate	Topically, 1 drop in each eye once or twice daily	Same as adults
		Epinephrine hydrochloride (0.25%, 0.5%, 1%, and 2% solutions)	Epifrin, Glaucon	Topically, 1 drop in each eye once or twice daily	Same as adults
		Hydroxyamphetamine (1% solution)	Paredrine	Prior to ophthalmoscopy, topically, 1 drop in each eye	
		Phenylephrine (2.5% and 10% solutions)	Neo-Synephrine	Before ophthalmoscopy or refraction, topically, 1 drop of 2.5% or 10% solution Preoperatively, topically, 1 drop of 2.5% or 10% solution 30–60 minutes before surgery Postoperatively, topically, 1 drop of 10% solution once or twice daily	Refraction, topically, 1 drop of 2.5% solution
Antiadrenergic (beta-blocking) drugs					
1. Decreased production and increased outflow of aqueous humor 2. Reduced intraocular pressure	Glaucoma	Timolol maleate	Timoptic	Topically, 1 drop of 0.25% or 0.5% solution in each eye twice daily (q12h)	
		Betaxolol	Betoptic	Topically to each eye, 1 drop ql2h	
		Levobunolol	Betagan	Topically to the affected eye, 1 drop once or twice daily	
Cholinergics					
1. Increased outflow of aqueous humor 2. Miosis	Glaucoma	Pilocarpine (0.25%–10% solutions)	Almocarpine, Isopto Carpine, Pilocar, Pilocel, Pilomiotin	Chronic glaucoma, topically, 1 drop of 1% or 2% solution instilled in each eye q6–8h initially. Then, drug concentration and frequency of administration are adjusted to maintain intraocular pressure in the desired range. Drops are usually instilled 4 times daily.	
		Pilocarpine ocular therapeutic system	Ocusert Pilo-20, Ocusert Pilo-40	One system placed into conjunctival sac per week, according to package directions. Each system releases 20 or 40 μg pilocarpine per hour for 1 week.	
		Carbachol	Carbacel, Isopto Carbachol	Topically, 1 drop of 0.75%–3% solution instilled in each eye initially. Then	

TABLE 65-1. DRUGS USED IN OCULAR DISORDERS* (*Continued*)

Ocular effects	Clinical indications	Generic name	Trade name	Routes and dosage ranges: *Adults*	*Children*
				drug concentration and frequency of administration are adjusted to maintain intraocular pressure in the desired range.	
Anticholinesterase agents					
1. Increased outflow of aqueous humor 2. Miosis	Glaucoma	Demecarium bromide	Humorsol	Topically, 1 drop of 0.125%–0.25% solution in each eye twice a day to twice a week, depending on condition	
		Echothiophate iodide	Phospholine iodide	Topically, 1 drop of solution (0.03%, 0.06%, 0.125%, or 0.25%) in each eye q12–48h	
		Isoflurophate	Floropryl	Topically, $\frac{1}{4}$-inch strip of ointment in the lower conjunctival sac of each eye q12–72h	
		Physostigmine sulfate	Eserine sulfate	Topically, 0.25% ointment 3–4 times daily	
		Physostigmine salicylate	Isopto Eserine	Topically, 1–2 drops of 0.25%–0.5% solution in each eye up to 4 times daily	
Anticholinergics					
1. Mydriasis 2. Cycloplegia 3. Photophobia	1. Mydriasis for refraction and other diagnostic purposes 2. Pre- and postoperatively in intraocular surgery 3. Treatment of uveitis 4. Treatment of some secondary glaucoma	Atropine sulfate (0.5%–3% solutions)		Before intraocular surgery, topically, 1 drop of solution Following intraocular surgery, topically, 1 drop of solution once daily	
		Cyclopentolate hydrochloride	Cyclogyl	For refraction, topically, 1 drop of 0.5%, or 2% solution instilled once Before ophthalmoscopy, 1 drop of 0.5% solution	For refraction, topically, 1 drop of 0.5%, 1% or 2% solution, repeated in 10 minutes
		Homatropine hydrobromide (2% and 5% solutions)	Isopto Homatropine	Refraction, topically, 1 drop of 5% solution every 5 minutes for 2–3 doses or 1–2 drops of 2% solution every 10–15 minutes for 5 doses Uveitis, topically, 1 drop of 2% or 5% solution 2–3 times daily	
		Scopolamine hydrobromide (0.25% solution)	Isopto Hyoscine	Refraction, topically, 1–2 drops in affected eye(s) 1 hour before examination	
		Tropicamide (0.5% and 1% solutions)	Mydriacyl	Before refraction or ophthalmoscopy, topically, 1 drop of 0.5% or 1% solution, repeated in 5 minutes, then every 20–30 minutes as needed to maintain mydriasis	

TABLE 65-1. DRUGS USED IN OCULAR DISORDERS* (*Continued*)

Ocular effects	Clinical indications	Generic name	Trade name	Routes and dosage ranges: Adults	Routes and dosage ranges: Children
Diuretics					
Carbonic anhydrase inhibitors					
1. Decreased production of aqueous humor 2. Decreased intraocular pressure	1. Glaucoma 2. Preoperatively in intraocular surgery	Acetazolamide	Diamox	PO 250 mg q6h Sustained-release capsules (Diamox Sequels), PO 500 mg, q12h	PO 10–15 mg/kg/day in divided doses
				IV, IM 500 mg initially, repeated in 2–4 hours if necessary	IV, IM 5–10 mg/kg/day in divided doses, q6h
		Dichlorphenamide	Daranide	PO 50–200 mg q6–8h. Maintenance dosage, 25–50 mg 1–3 times daily	
		Methazolamide	Neptazane	PO 50–100 mg q8h	
Osmotic agents					
1. Reduced volume of vitreous humor 2. Decreased intraocular pressure	1. Preoperatively in intraocular surgery 2. Treatment of acute glaucoma	Glycerin	Osmoglyn	PO 1–1.5 g/kg, usually given as a 50% or 75% solution 1–1½ hours before surgery	Same as adults
		Isosorbide	Ismotic	Emergency reduction of intraocular pressure (*e.g.,* acute angle-closure glaucoma), PO 1.5 g/kg up to 4 times daily if necessary	
		Mannitol	Osmitrol	IV 1.5–2 g/kg given as a 20% solution over 30–60 minutes	Same as adults
Miscellaneous agents					
Anesthetics, local					
Surface anesthesia of conjunctiva and cornea	1. Tonometry 2. Subconjunctival injections 3. Removal of foreign bodies 4. Removal of sutures	Benoxinate hydrochloride	Dorsacaine	Before tonometry and other minor procedures, topically, 1–2 drops of 0.4% solution	
				Deeper anesthesia, topically, 2 drops of 0.4% solution every 90 seconds for 3 doses	
		Proparacaine hydrochloride	Alcaine, Ophthaine	Minor procedures, topically, 1–2 drops of 0.5% solution; instillation may be repeated for deeper anesthesia	
		Tetracaine hydrochloride	Pontocaine	Minor procedures, topically, 1–2 drops of 0.5% solution; 2–4 instillations are required for deeper anesthesia	
Antiallergic agent					
	Allergic keratitis or conjunctivitis	Cromolyn sodium	Opticrom	1–2 drops in each eye 4–6 times daily at regular intervals	Same as adults
Antiseptic					
	Prophylaxis of gonorrheal	Silver nitrate ophthalmic			Newborns, topically, 2 drops

TABLE 65-1. DRUGS USED IN OCULAR DISORDERS* (*Continued*)

Ocular effects	Clinical indications	Generic name	Trade name	Routes and dosage ranges: *Adults*	Routes and dosage ranges: *Children*
	ophthalmia neonatorum				of 1% solution in each eye
Lubricants					
Serve as "artificial tears"	1. Prevent damage to the cornea in clients with keratitis 2. Protect the cornea during gonioscopy and other procedures 3. Moisten hard contact lenses 4. Lubricate artificial eyes	Methylcellulose	Methulose, Visculose, others	Topically, 1–2 drops as needed	
		Polyvinyl alcohol	Liquifilm, others	Topically, 1–2 drops as needed	

* Anti-infective and anti-inflammatory agents are listed in Table 65-2.

sulfacetamide sodium. These agents are rarely given systemically. They do not cause sensitization to commonly used systemic antibiotics and do not promote growth of drug-resistant microorganisms.

3. In severe infections, antibacterial drugs may be given both topically and systemically. Because systemic antibiotics penetrate the eye poorly, large doses are required to attain therapeutic drug concentrations in ocular structures. Drugs that reach therapeutic levels in the eye, when given in proper dosage, include ampicillin, cephalothin, dicloxacillin, and methicillin. Gentamicin and other antibiotics penetrate the eye when inflammation is present.
4. Combination products containing two or more antibacterials are available for topical treatment of external ocular infections. These products are most useful when therapy must be initiated before the infecting microorganism is identified. Mixtures provide a broader spectrum of antibacterial activity than a single drug. Most of the available combination products contain various amounts of polymyxin B, neomycin, and bacitracin (*e.g.*, Mycitracin, Neo-Polycin, Neosporin).
5. Fixed-dose combinations of an antibacterial agent and corticosteroid are available for topical use in selected conditions (*e.g.*, staphylococcal keratitis, blepharoconjunctivitis, allergic conjunctivitis, and some postoperative inflammatory reactions). *Chloramphenicol* and corticosteroid mixtures include Chloromycetin-hydrocortisone and Chloroptic-P. A combination of *chloramphenicol, polymyxin B,* and corticosteroid is available as Ophthocort. *Neomycin* and corticosteroid mixtures include Cor-Oticin, Neo-Cortef, NeoDecadron, Neo-Delta-Cortef, Neo-Hydeltrasol, and Neo-Medrol. *Neomycin, polymyxin B,* and corticosteroid mixtures include Poly-Pred and Maxitrol. *Neomycin, polymyxin B, bacitracin,* and corticosteroid mixtures include Cortisporin and Coracin. *Sulfacetamide sodium* and corticosteroid mixtures include Blephamide, Cetapred, Metimyd, Optimyd, Sulfapred, and Vasocidin.
6. Trifluridine (Viroptic) is probably the drug of choice in eye infections caused by the herpes simplex virus.
7. In fungal infections, natamycin (Natacyn) may be preferred because it has a broad spectrum of antifungal activity and is nonirritating and nontoxic.

Glaucoma

For drug therapy of chronic, primary open-angle glaucoma, pilocarpine has long been the drug of choice.

TABLE 65-2. OPHTHALMIC ANTI-INFECTIVE AND ANTI-INFLAMMATORY AGENTS

	Generic name	Trade name	Routes and dosage ranges	
			Adults	*Children*
Antibacterial agents	Bacitracin	Baciguent	Ophthalmic ointment, topically, instill in infected eye 1–3 times daily	
	Chloramphenicol	Chloromycetin Ophthochlor (0.5% solution) Antibiopto (0.5% solution) Chloroptic (0.5% solution, 1% ointment) Econochlor (0.5% solution, 1% ointment)	Mild conjunctivitis: topically, 1 drop of 0.5% ophthalmic solution q1–2h or ointment instilled 3–4 times daily Severe conjunctivitis, corneal ulcers: topically, 1 drop of 0.5% solution every 30 minutes	Topically, same as adults
	Erythromycin	Ilotycin ophthalmic (0.5% ointment)		Prevention of gonorrheal ophthalmia neonatorum: topically 0.5–1 cm in each eye
	Gentamicin sulfate	Garamycin	Topically, ophthalmic solution (0.3%) 1 drop q1–4h; ophthalmic ointment (0.3%), instill 2–3 times daily	Topically, same as adults
	Polymyxin B sulfate		Corneal ulcers due to *Pseudomonas aeruginosa:* topically, 1 drop of a freshly prepared solution (20,000 units/ml), instilled 2–10 times hourly	
	Sulfacetamide sodium	Bleph-10 Liquifilm (10% solution or ointment) Isopto-Cetamide (15% solution) Sulfacel-15 (15% solution) Cetamide (10% ointment) Sodium Sulamyd (10% and 30% solution, 10% ointment) Also available generically as 10% and 30% solutions	Acute catarrhal conjunctivitis caused by *Staphylococcus aureus, Diplococcus pneumoniae, Hemophilus influenzae, Neisseria catarrhalis:* topically, 1 drop of 10% or 15% solution every 10–30 minutes Chronic conjunctivitis due to *Proteus* organisms: topically, 10% ointment instilled 3–4 times daily Chronic blepharoconjunctivitis due to *S. aureus:* topically, 1 drop of 30% solution 3–4 times daily Corneal ulcers due to *E. coli* or *Klebsiella pneumoniae:* 1 drop of 10% solution every 30 minutes or 10% ointment instilled 3–4 times daily	

TABLE 65-2. OPHTHALMIC ANTI-INFECTIVE AND ANTI-INFLAMMATORY AGENTS (*Continued*)

	Generic name	Trade name	Routes and dosage ranges	
			Adults	***Children***
	Sulfisoxazole diolamine	Gantrisin (4% solution and ointment)	Topically, solution, 2–3 drops in affected eye 3 or more times daily; ointment, instill in affected eye 4 times daily	
	Tetracycline	Achromycin	Inclusion conjunctivitis: topically, 1% solution or ointment instilled 3–4 times daily for 30 days	Topically, same as adults
	Tobramycin	Tobrex (0.3% solution and ointment)	Topically, 1–2 drops 2–6 times daily or ointment 2–3 times daily	
Antiviral agents	Idoxuridine	Stoxil	Herpes simplex infection of eyelids, conjunctiva, and cornea: topically, 1 drop of 0.1% solution q1h during daytime hours and q2h at night, or 0.5% ointment instilled 4–5 times daily. Treatment should be continued for at least 2 weeks.	
	Trifluridine	Viroptic	Keratoconjunctivitis or corneal ulcers caused by herpes simplex virus: topically, 1 drop of 1% solution q2h while awake (maximal daily dose, 9 drops) until corneal ulcer heals, then 1 drop q4h (minimal dose, 5 drops daily for 7 days)	
	Vidarabine	Vira-A	Keratoconjunctivitis caused by herpes simplex virus: topically, 3% ointment instilled q3h	
Antifungal agent	Natamycin	Natacyn	Topically, 1 drop of 5% suspension q1–2h	
Corticosteroids	Dexamethasone	Decadron Phosphate Ophthalmic (0.1% solution, 0.05% ointment) Maxidex (0.1% solution. 0.05% ointment)	Topically, 1 drop of solution q1–2h until response is obtained, then less frequently; ointment, apply 3–4 times daily	
	Fluorometholone	FML Liquifilm (0.1% suspension)	Topically, 1 drop q1–2h until response is obtained, then less frequently	
	Hydrocortisone	Hydrocortone (1.5% ointment)	Topically, 1 drop of 0.2% or 0.5% sus-	

TABLE 65-2. OPHTHALMIC ANTI-INFECTIVE AND ANTI-INFLAMMATORY AGENTS (*Continued*)

Generic name	Trade name	Routes and dosage ranges: Adults	Routes and dosage ranges: Children
		pension q1–2h until response is obtained, then less frequently; ointment, apply 3–4 times daily	
Medrysone	HMS Liquifilm (1% suspension)	Topically, 1 drop q1–2h until response is obtained, then less frequently	
Prednisolone acetate	Econopred (0.125% or 1% suspension)	Topically, 1 drop q1–2h until response is obtained, then less frequently	
Prednisolone sodium phosphate	Inflamase (0.125% and 1% solution) Metreton (0.5% solution)	Topically, 1 drop q1–2h until response is obtained, then less frequently; ointment, apply 3–4 times daily	

Timolol (Timoptic) has recently become the preferred drug in many cases. Timolol is effective in lowering intraocular pressure, does not cause miosis as pilocarpine does, and is administered only twice daily (every 12 hours). The long-acting anticholinesterase agents (*e.g.*, demecarium [Humorsol]) are used only in severe glaucoma that is resistant to other drugs. These drugs cause a higher incidence of cholinergic systemic side-effects and development of cataracts with long-term use.

Use of ophthalmic ointments

Many ophthalmic drugs are available as eye drops (solutions or suspensions) and ointments. Ointments require less frequent administration and often produce higher concentrations of drug in target tissues. However, ointments also cause blurred vision, which limits their daytime use, at least for ambulatory clients. In some situations, drops may be used during waking hours and ointments at bedtime. However, the two formulations are *not* interchangeable.

PEDIATRIC CONSIDERATIONS

Topical ophthalmic drug therapy in children differs little from that in adults. Few studies of ophthalmic drug therapy in children have been reported, and many conditions for which adults need therapy (*e.g.*, cataract, glaucoma) rarely occur in children. A major use of topical ophthalmic drugs in children is to dilate the pupil and paralyze accommodation for ophthalmoscopic examination. As a general rule, the short-acting mydriatics and cycloplegics (*e.g.*, cyclopentolate, tropicamide) are preferred because they cause fewer systemic adverse effects than atropine and scopolamine. In addition, lower drug concentrations are usually given empirically because of the smaller size of children and the potential risk of systemic adverse effects.

NURSING ACTIONS: OPHTHALMIC DRUGS

Nursing Actions	*Rationale/Explanation*
1. Administer accurately	
a. Read labels of ophthalmic medications carefully.	To avoid error. For example, many drugs are available in several concentrations. The correct concentration must be given as well as the correct drug.

Nursing Actions	***Rationale/Explanation***
b. Read medication orders carefully and accurately.	To avoid error. Abbreviations (*e.g.,* O.S., O.D., O.U.) are often used in physicians' orders and must be interpreted accurately.
c. For hospitalized clients, keep eye medications at the bedside when possible.	Eye medications should be ordered for and used by one person only. They are dispensed in small amounts for this purpose. This minimizes cross contamination and risk of infection.
d. Wash hands before approaching the client for instillation of eye medications.	To reduce risks of infection.
e. To administer eye drops, have the client lie down or tilt the head backward and look upward. Then, pull down the lower lid to expose the conjunctival sac and drop the medication into the sac. Alternate method: gently grasp the lower lid and pull it outward to form a pouch into which medication is instilled. After instillation, have the client close the eyes gently and apply pressure to the inner canthus briefly (nurse or client).	Absorption of the drug and its concentration in ocular tissues depend partly on the length of time the medication is in contact with ocular tissues. Contact time is increased by the "pouch" method of administration, closing the eyes (delays outflow into the nasolacrimal duct), and by pressure on the inner canthus (delays outflow and decreases side-effects resulting from systemic absorption).
f. When instilling ophthalmic ointments, position the client as above, and apply a one-quarter- to one-half-inch strip of ointment to the conjunctiva.	
g. Do not touch the dropper tip or ointment tip to the eye or anything else.	To avoid contamination of the medication and infection
h. When crusts or secretions are present, cleanse the eye prior to administering medication.	If the eye is not cleansed, the drug may not be absorbed.
i. When two or more eye drops are scheduled for the same time, they should be instilled about 5 minutes apart.	To avoid drug loss by dilution and outflow into the nasolacrimal duct
2. Observe for therapeutic effects	Therapeutic effects depend on the reason for use.
a. With mydriatics, observe for dilation of the pupil.	Mydriasis begins within 5 to 15 minutes after instillation.
b. With miotics, observe for constriction of the pupil.	
c. With anti-infective drugs, observe for decreased redness, edema, and drainage.	
d. With osmotic agents, observe for decreased intraocular pressure.	With oral glycerin, maximal decrease in intraocular pressure occurs approximately 1 hour after administration, and effects persist for about 5 hours. With intravenous mannitol, maximal decrease in intraocular pressure occurs within 30 to 60 minutes, and effects last 6 to 8 hours.
3. Observe for adverse effects	
a. Local effects	
(1) Irritation and discomfort, lacrimation, contact dermatitis of eyelids, allergic conjunctivitis	These effects may occur with any topical ophthalmic agents, from the drug itself, or from the preservatives in the formulation.
(2) With antibacterial agents—superinfection or sensitization	Superinfection caused by drug-resistant organisms may occur. Sensitization means that topical application induces antibody formation. Therefore, if the same or a related drug is subsequently administered systemically, an allergic reaction may occur. The allergic reaction most often involves dermatitis; occasionally urticaria or anaphylaxis occurs. Penicillin is the most frequently involved drug. Other drugs include strep-

Nursing Actions	Rationale/Explanation
	tomycin, neomycin, gentamicin, and sulfonamides (with the exception of sulfacetamide sodium). Sensitization can be prevented or minimized by avoiding topical administration of antibacterial agents that are commonly given systemically.
(3) With anticholinergics, adrenergics, topical corticosteroids—glaucoma	Mydriatic drugs (anticholinergics and adrenergics) may cause an acute attack of angle-closure glaucoma in clients with narrow angles by blocking outflow of aqueous humor. Topical corticosteroids raise intraocular pressure in some clients. The "glaucomatous" response occurs most often in clients with chronic, primary open-angle glaucoma and their relatives. It may also occur in clients with myopia or diabetes mellitus. The magnitude of increased intraocular pressure depends on the concentration, frequency of administration, duration of therapy, and anti-inflammatory potency of the corticosteroid. Increased intraocular pressure has been reported most often with 0.1% dexamethasone (Decadron). This adverse effect can be minimized by checking intraocular pressure every 2 months in clients receiving long-term therapy with topical corticosteroids.
(4) Cataract formation	This is most likely to occur with long-term use of anticholinesterase agents.
(5) With miotic drugs—decreased vision in dim light	These agents prevent pupil dilation, which normally occurs in dim light or darkness.
b. Systemic effects	Systemic absorption and adverse effects of eye drops can be prevented or minimized by applying pressure to the inner canthus during and after instillation of the medications. Pressure may be applied by the nurse or the client.
(1) With miotics—sweating, nausea, vomiting, diarrhea, abdominal pain, bradycardia, hypotension, bronchoconstriction. Toxic doses produce ataxia, confusion, convulsions, coma, respiratory failure, and death.	These cholinergic or parasympathomimetic effects occur rarely with pilocarpine or carbachol. They are more likely to occur with the long-acting anticholinesterase agents, especially echothiophate (Phospholine iodide). Acute toxicity may be reversed by an anticholinergic agent, atropine, given IV.
(2) With anticholinergic mydriatics—dryness of the mouth and skin, fever, rash, tachycardia, confusion, hallucinations, delirium	These effects are most likely to occur with atropine and in children and elderly clients. Tropicamide (Mydriacyl) rarely causes systemic reactions
(3) With adrenergic mydriatics—tachycardia, hypertension, premature ventricular contractions, tremors, headache	Systemic effects are uncommon. They are more likely to occur with repeated instillations of high drug concentrations (*e.g.,* epinephrine 2%, phenylephrine [Neo-Synephrine] 10%).
(4) With carbonic anhydrase inhibitors—anorexia, nausea, vomiting, diarrhea, paresthesias, weakness, lethargy	Nausea, malaise, and paresthesias (numbness and tingling of extremities) commonly occur.
(5) With osmotic diuretics—dehydration, nausea, vomiting, headache. Hyperglycemia and glycosuria with glycerin (Osmoglyn)	These agents may produce profound diuresis and dehydration. Oral agents (*e.g.,* glycerin) are less likely to cause severe systemic effects than intravenous agents (*e.g.,* mannitol). These agents are usually given in a single dose, which decreases the risks of serious adverse reactions unless large doses are given.
(6) With corticosteroids, see Chapter 24.	Serious adverse effects may occur with long-term use of corticosteroids.
(7) With antibacterial agents, see Chapter 33 and the chapter on the individual drug group.	Adverse effects may occur with all antibacterial agents.
4. Observe for drug interactions	
a. Drugs that *increase* effects of adrenergic (sympathomimetic) ophthalmic drugs	

Nursing Actions	***Rationale/Explanation***
(1) Anticholinergic ophthalmic drugs	The combination (*e.g.*, atropine and phenylephrine) produces additive mydriasis.
(2) Systemic adrenergic drugs	Additive risks of adverse effects (*e.g.*, tachycardia, cardiac arrhythmias, hypertension)
b. Drugs that *decrease* effects of adrenergic ophthalmic preparations Cholinergic and anticholinesterase ophthalmic drugs	Antagonize mydriatic effects of adrenergic drugs.
c. Drugs that *increase* effects of antiadrenergic ophthalmic preparations Systemic antiadrenergics (*e.g.*, propranolol, atenolol, metoprolol, nadolol, timolol)	When the client is receiving a topical beta blocker in ocular disorders, administration of systemic beta-blocking agents in cardiovascular disorders may cause additive systemic toxicity.
d. Drugs that *increase* effects of anticholinergic ophthalmic agents (1) Adrenergic ophthalmic agents	Additive mydriasis
(2) Systemic anticholinergic drugs (*e.g.*, atropine) and other drugs with anticholinergic effects (*e.g.*, some antihistamines, antipyschotic agents, and tricyclic antidepressants)	Additive anticholinergic effects (mydriasis, blurred vision, tachycardia). These drugs are hazardous in glaucoma.
e. Drugs that *decrease* effects of cholinergic and anticholinesterase ophthalmic drugs (1) Anticholinergics and drugs with anticholinergic effects (*e.g.*, atropine, antipsychotic agents, tricyclic antidepressants, some antihistamines)	Antagonize antiglaucoma (miotic) effects of cholinergic and anticholinesterase drugs
(2) Corticosteroids	Long-term use of corticosteroids, topically or systemically, raises intraocular pressure and may cause glaucoma. Therefore, corticosteroids decrease effects of all drugs used for glaucoma.
(3) Sympathomimetic drugs	Antagonize miotic (antiglaucoma) effects
5. Teach clients **a.** The correct procedure for administering eye medications (including maintenance of sterility)	If the client is unable to administer the drugs, a family member may be taught the procedure. Written instructions are preferred to verbal ones.
b. To discard cloudy or discolored solutions	These changes indicate deterioration. Phenylephrine (Neo-Synephrine) solutions become cloudy, epinephrine solutions turn brown, and physostigmine becomes pink or red.
c. With glaucoma (1) Do not take any drugs without the physician's knowledge and consent.	Many drugs given for purposes other than eye disorders may cause or aggravate glaucoma.
(2) Wear a Medic-Alert bracelet or carry identification that states that the person has glaucoma.	To avoid administration of drugs that aggravate glaucoma or to maintain treatment of glaucoma (*e.g.*, in emergencies)
d. With eye infections (1) Avoid touching the unaffected eye. (2) Wash hands before and after contact with the infected eye. (3) Use a separate towel.	These measures are indicated to avoid spreading the infection to the unaffected eye or to other people.

Selected References

Anderson PD: Basic Human Anatomy and Physiology: Clinical Implications for the Health Professions. Monterey, CA, Wadsworth, 1984

Cromolyn sodium for allergic conjunctivitis. Med Lett Drugs Ther 27:7–8, January 1985

Facts and Comparisons. St. Louis, J B Lippincott (Updated monthly)

Hansten PD: Drug Interactions: Clinical Significance of Drug–Drug Interactions, 5th ed. Philadelphia, Lea & Febiger, 1985

Malseed RT: Pharmacology: Drug Therapy and Nursing Considerations, 2d ed. Philadelphia, J B Lippincott, 1985

Resler MM, Tumulty G: Glaucoma update. Am J Nurs 83:752–756, May 1983

Sagaties MJ, Constantine JB: Ophthalmologic disorders. In Wiener MB, Pepper GA (eds): Clinical Pharmacology and Therapeutics in Nursing, 2d ed, pp 776–795. New York, McGraw-Hill, 1985

Sasso SC: Erythromycin for eye prophylaxis. Am J Maternal–Child Nurs 9:417, November–December 1984

66

DRUGS USED IN DERMATOLOGIC CONDITIONS

Description and uses

FUNCTIONS OF THE SKIN

The skin, the largest organ of the body, is the interface between the body's internal and external environments. The skin is composed of the epidermis and dermis. Epidermal or epithelial cells begin in the basal layer of the epidermis and migrate outward, undergoing degenerative changes in each layer. The outer layer, called the *stratum corneum,* is composed of dead cells and keratin. The dead cells are constantly being shedded (desquamated) and replaced by newer cells. Normally, about 1 month is required for cell formation, migration, and desquamation. When dead cells are discarded, keratin remains on the skin. Keratin is a tough protein substance that is insoluble in water, weak acids, and weak bases. Hair and nails, which are composed of keratin, are referred to as appendages of the skin.

Melanocytes are pigment-producing cells located at the junction of the epidermis and the dermis. These cells produce yellow, brown, or black skin coloring in response to genetic influences, melanocyte-stimulating hormone released from the anterior pituitary gland, and exposure to ultraviolet light (*e.g.,* sunlight).

The dermis is composed of elastic and fibrous connective tissue. Dermal structures include blood vessels, lymphatic channels, nerves and nerve endings, sweat glands, sebaceous glands, and hair follicles. The dermis is supported underneath by subcutaneous tissue, which is composed primarily of fat cells.

The skin has numerous functions, most of which are protective. Functions include the following:

1. Serves as a physical barrier against loss of fluids and electrolytes and against entry of potentially harmful substances (*e.g.,* microorganisms and other foreign bodies)
2. Detects sensations of pain, pressure, touch, and temperature through sensory nerve endings
3. Assists in regulating body temperature through production and elimination of sweat
4. Serves as a source of vitamin D when exposed to sunlight or other sources of ultraviolet light. Skin contains a precursor for vitamin D.
5. Serves as an excretory organ. Water, sodium, chloride, lactate, and urea are excreted in sweat.
6. Inhibits growth of many microorganisms by its acid *p*H (approximately 4.5 to 6.5).

Mucous membrane is composed of a surface layer of epithelial cells, a basement membrane, and a layer of connective tissue. Mucous membranes line body cavities that communicate with the external environment (*i.e.*, mouth, vagina, anus). They receive an abundant blood supply. Capillaries lie just beneath the epithelial cells.

Dermatologic disorders may be primary (*i.e.*, originate in the skin or mucous membranes) or secondary (*i.e.*, result from a systemic condition such as measles, lupus erythematosus, or adverse drug reactions). This chapter focuses on primary skin disorders and the topical medications used to prevent or treat them.

DISORDERS OF THE SKIN

Because the skin is constantly exposed to the external environment, it is susceptible to numerous disorders. Dermatologic disorders of concern to the nurse include the following:

Inflammatory disorders

Dermatitis

Dermatitis is a general term denoting an inflammatory response of the skin to various injuries from irritants, allergens, or trauma. *Eczema* is often used as a synonym for dermatitis. Whatever the cause, dermatitis is usually characterized by erythema, pruritus, and skin lesions. Dermatitis may be acute or chronic.

1. Atopic dermatitis is a chronic disorder characterized primarily by pruritus. Its cause is uncertain but may involve allergic, hereditary, or psychologic elements.
2. Contact dermatitis results from irritants (*e.g.*, strong soaps, detergents, acids, alkalis) or allergens (*e.g.*, clothing materials or dyes, jewelry, cosmetics, hair dyes). Irritants cause dermatitis in any person with sufficient contact or exposure. Allergens cause dermatitis only in sensitized or hypersensitive persons. The location of the dermatitis may indicate the cause (*e.g.*, facial dermatitis may indicate an allergy to cosmetics).
3. Seborrheic dermatitis is a disease of the sebaceous glands characterized by excessive production of sebum. A simple form of seborrheic dermatitis involving the scalp is dandruff, which is characterized by flaking and itching of the skin. More severe forms of seborrheic dermatitis are characterized by greasy, yellow scales or crusts with variable amounts of erythema and itching. Seborrheic dermatitis may occur on the scalp, face, or trunk.
4. Urticaria ("hives") is an allergic reaction to external agents (*e.g.*, insect bites) or to internal allergens that reach the skin through the bloodstream (*e.g.*, from foods or drugs). The characteristic skin lesion of urticaria is the wheal, a raised edematous area with a pallid center and erythematous border, which itches severely. Topical medications may be applied to relieve itching, but systemic drug therapy with antihistamines and perhaps epinephrine is the major element of drug therapy.

Psoriasis

Psoriasis is a chronic skin disorder characterized by erythematous, dry, scaling lesions. The lesions may occur anywhere on the body but commonly involve the skin covering bony prominences, such as the elbows and knees. The disease is characterized by remissions and exacerbations. It is not contagious.

The cause of psoriasis is unknown. The pathophysiology involves excessively rapid turnover of epidermal cells. Instead of approximately 30 days from formation to elimination of normal epidermal cells, epidermal cells involved in psoriasis are abnormal in structure and have a life span of only 3 to 4 days.

Skin lesions may be tender, but they do not usually cause severe pain or itching. However, the lesions are unsightly and usually cause embarrassment and mental distress.

Dermatologic infections

Bacterial infections

Bacterial infections of the skin are common; they are most often caused by streptococci or staphylococci.

1. Cellulitis is characterized by erythema, tenderness, and edema, which may spread to subcutaneous tissue. Erysipelas is a form of cellulitis. Generalized malaise, chills, and fever may occur.
2. Folliculitis is an infection of the hair follicles that most often occurs on the scalp or bearded areas of the face.
3. Furuncles and carbuncles are infections usually caused by staphylococci. Furuncles (boils) may result from folliculitis. They usually occur in the neck, face, axillae, buttocks, thighs, and perineum. Furuncles tend to recur. Carbuncles involve many hair follicles and include multiple pustules. Carbuncles may cause fever, malaise, leukocytosis, and bacteremia. Healing of carbuncles often produces scar tissue.
4. Impetigo is a superficial skin infection caused by streptococci or staphylococci. An especially contagious form is caused by Group A beta-hemolytic streptococci. This form occurs most often in children.

Fungal infections

Fungal infections of the skin and mucous membranes are most often caused by *Candida albicans*.

1. Oral candidiasis (thrush) involves mucous membranes of the mouth. It often occurs as a superinfection following the use of broad-spectrum systemic antibiotics.
2. Candidiasis of the vagina and vulva occurs with systemic antibiotic therapy and in women with diabetes mellitus.
3. Intertrigo involves skin folds or areas where two skin surfaces are in contact (*e.g.*, groin, pendulous breasts).
4. Tinea infections (ringworm) are caused by fungi (dermatophytes). These infections may involve the scalp (tinea capitis), the body (tinea corporis), the foot (tinea pedis), and other areas of the body. Tinea pedis, commonly called "athlete's foot," is the most common type of ringworm infection.

Viral infections

Viral infections of the skin include veruccal (warts) and herpes infections. There are two types of herpes simplex infections. Type 1 infections usually involve the face or neck (*e.g.*, fever blisters or cold sores on the lips), and type 2 infections involve the genital organs. Other herpes infections include herpes zoster (shingles) and varicella (chickenpox).

Trauma

Trauma refers to a physical injury that disrupts the skin. When the skin is broken, it may not be able to function properly. The major problem associated with skin wounds is infection. Common wounds include the following:

1. Lacerations (cuts or tears), abrasions (shearing or scraping of the skin), and puncture wounds
2. Surgical incisions
3. Burn wounds

Ulcerations

Cutaneous ulcerations are usually caused by trauma and impaired circulation. They may become inflamed or infected.

1. Pressure sores (decubitus ulcers) may occur anywhere on the body where external pressure decreases blood flow. Common sites include the sacrum, trochanters, ankles, and heels. Cutaneous ulcers may also result from improper moving and lifting techniques. For example, when a person is pulled across bed linens rather than lifted, friction and shearing force may cause skin abrasions. Abraded skin is susceptible to infection and ulcer formation.

   Decubitus ulcers are most likely to develop in clients who are immobilized, incontinent, malnourished, and debilitated.
2. Venous stasis ulcers are commonly located on the lower extremities.

Acne

Acne is a common disorder characterized by excessive production of sebum and obstruction of hair follicles, which normally carry sebum to the skin surface. As a result, hair follicles expand and form comedones (blackheads and whiteheads). The most severe form of acne is acne vulgaris, in which follicles become infected and irritating secretions leak into surrounding tissues to form pustules, cysts, and abscesses.

Acne occurs most often on the face, upper back, and chest because large numbers of sebaceous glands are located in these areas. Etiologic factors include increased secretion of male hormones (which occurs at puberty in both males and females); bacteria, which cause sebum to break down into irritating fatty acids; oil-based cosmetics, which plug hair follicles; and certain medications (*e.g.*, phenytoin [Dilantin], corticosteroids, and iodides). There is no evidence that certain foods and emotional stress cause acne.

External otitis

External otitis is a general term for inflammatory processes involving the external ear. The external ear, including the meatus, canal, and tympanic membrane (ear drum), is lined with epidermal tissue. The epidermal tissue is susceptible to the same skin disorders that affect other parts of the body. External otitis may be acute or chronic, and it may be treated with topical medications.

Anorectal disorders

Hemorrhoids and anal fissures are common anorectal disorders characterized by pruritus, bleeding, and pain. Inflammation and infection may occur.

TYPES OF DERMATOLOGIC DRUGS

Many different agents are used to prevent or treat dermatologic disorders (Tables 66-1 to 66-3). Most agents fit into one or more of the following categories:

(*Text continues on p. 635.*)

TABLE 66-1. ANTISEPTICS

	Generic name	Trade name	Characteristics	Clinical indications
Alcohols	Ethanol (ethyl alcohol) Isopropyl alcohol	Rubbing Alcohol U.S.P. (70% ethanol) Isopropyl Alcohol (99% solution), Isopropyl Rubbing Alcohol (70% solution)	1. Bactericidal to common bacteria. When applied to skin, kills approximately 90% of bacteria within 2 minutes if the area is kept moist for that period. When applied in a single wipe and left to evaporate (*e.g.,* before injections), approximately 75% of bacteria are killed. 2. Erratic against viruses and fungi; ineffective against spores. 3. Irritating to intact skin with prolonged contact. Irritating to denuded skin areas or open wounds; causes burning type of pain, increases tissue injury, and coagulates protein to form a mass under which bacteria may proliferate. 4. Isopropyl alcohol is slightly more antiseptic than ethyl alcohol. It has the same indications for use.	Cleansing of intact skin before injections or surgical incisions
Biguanide	Chlorhexidine gluconate	Hibiclens (4% Aqueous Emulsion) Hibitane (1% Aqueous Solution)	1. Effective against both gram-positive and gram-negative bacteria. 2. Some studies indicate chlorhexidine (4%) is more effective than 3% hexachlorophene (pHisoHex) or povidone–iodine (Betadine) for handwashing and surgical scrubs. 3. Little, if any, absorption occurs through the skin of adults. Absorption from the skin of neonates is unknown but probably slight. 4. Some gram-negative organisms are resistant to the drug, and infection may occur.	1. Handwashing 2. Preoperative skin cleansing for client and health care personnel (surgical scrub) 3. Treatment of superficial cutaneous infections 4. Wound cleansing 5. Neonatal skin cleansing to reduce incidence of staphylococcal and streptococcal infections 6. Treatment of oral ulcers (as an ingredient in mouthwashes) 7. Prevention of dental caries.
Iodine preparations	Iodine tincture, U.S.P. (2% iodine and 2.4% sodium iodide diluted in 50% ethanol) Iodine topical solution, U.S.P. (2% iodine and 2.4% sodium iodide in water) Povidone–iodine (a 10% solution contains 1% available iodine) Poloxamer-Iodine	 Betadine, Isodine, others Prepodyne	1. Iodine preparations kill most microorganisms (bacteria, fungi, viruses). When applied to the skin, a 1% solution kills approximately 90% of bacteria within 90 seconds. 2. Antiseptic activity depends on the concentration of iodine. Sodium iodide increases solubility; polyvinylpyrrolidone (povidone) is a carrier substance that increases solubility of iodine and releases iodine slowly, for a sustained action; poloxamer functions as a carrier substance. 3. Betadine, a commonly used iodine preparation, is available in numerous concentrations and dosage forms.	1. Prevention or treatment of infections of the skin, scalp, and mucous membranes of the mouth and vagina 2. Preoperative cleansing of the skin 3. Treatment of wounds and abrasions

TABLE 66-1. ANTISEPTICS (*Continued*)

	Generic name	Trade name	Characteristics	Clinical indications
			These include the following (concentrations expressed in terms of available iodine): aerosol spray 0.5%; ointment 1%; shampoo 0.75%; skin cleanser 0.75%; solution 1%; surgical scrub 0.75%; vaginal douche solution and vaginal gel 1%. 4. Iodine topical solution should not be confused with strong iodine solution (Lugol's solution) used for the treatment of hyperthyroidism.	
Chlorine preparations	Sodium hypochlorite solution, diluted	Modified Dakin's solution	1. Exerts bactericidal action by releasing hypochlorous acid 2. Irritating to tissues 3. Dissolves necrotic materials 4. Dissolves blood clots and delays clotting 5. Undiluted solutions are too strong for use as antiseptics.	Infected wounds when other methods or agents are not available
	Sodium oxychlorosene	Clorpactin sodium	A mixture of sodium hypochlorite solution and alkylbenzene sulfonates. The alkylbenzene sulfonates have surfactant properties that increase penetration and antibacterial effects.	Treatment of infected wounds
Metallic antiseptics	Silver nitrate		Silver nitrate is available in solid form (Toughened silver nitrate, U.S.P.) for use as a caustic in removing warts and cauterizing wounds; an ophthalmic solution for use in newborn infants; and a solution (0.5%) for use in treatment of burn wounds. It is infrequently used in burn treatment because it stains the skin black and causes hypochloremia.	1. Cauterizing warts or wounds 2. Prophylaxis of ophthalmia neonatorum in newborns 3. Treatment of burn wounds
	Silver sulfadiazine	Silvadene	1. Silver sulfadiazine is widely used in treatment of burn wounds. 2. Exerts antibacterial action against *Pseudomonas* and many other organisms that infect burn wounds. The drug penetrates eschar. 3. Does not stain the skin or cause pain at application sites.	Prevention of infection in burn wounds
	Zinc oxide	Zinc Oxide Ointment (20% zinc oxide) Calamine Lotion, U.S.P. (8% calamine and 8% zinc oxide)	1. Available in many preparations and dosage forms (powders, ointments, pastes, lotions) 2. Also has astringent properties	1. Eczema 2. Impetigo 3. Tinea infections (ringworm) 4. Venous stasis ulcers 5. Pruritus 6. Psoriasis
	Zinc pyrithione	Zincon, others	1. Used in concentrations of 0.1%–2% 2. A common ingredient in over-the-counter dandruff shampoos.	1. Seborrhea 2. Dandruff

TABLE 66-1. ANTISEPTICS (*Continued*)

	Generic name	Trade name	Characteristics	Clinical indications
	Zinc sulfate		1. For topical application to the skin, zinc sulfate is used in a concentration of 4%. In vaginal deodorants, concentrations of 0.25%–4% are used. 2. Zinc sulfate may also be given orally in cases of zinc deficiency. 3. In addition to antiseptic properties, zinc sulfate also has astringent, antiperspirant, and caustic activity.	1. Acne 2. Lupus erythematosus 3. Impetigo 4. Ivy poisoning 5. Leg ulcers, in people with low serum levels of zinc
Oxidizing agents	Hydrogen peroxide topical solution, U.S.P. (3% hydrogen peroxide in water)		1. Hydrogen peroxide is probably more effective as a debriding and cleansing agent than as an antiseptic. It is of doubtful value on intact skin. However, when it comes in contact with wounds or blood, it rapidly decomposes into oxygen and water. The liberated oxygen exerts a brief antibacterial effect and loosens infected material. 2. Prolonged use of hydrogen peroxide as a mouthwash, even half strength, may cause hypertrophy of filiform papillae of the tongue ("hairy tongue"). This condition is reversible when hydrogen peroxide is discontinued.	1. Wound cleansing 2. Mouthwash (diluted in equal parts with water or normal saline and a commercial mouthwash such as Cepacol) 3. To remove cerumen from the external ear. 4. Cleansing of tracheostomy tubes (inner cannulae)
	Benzoyl peroxide	Benzoyl peroxide lotion, U.S.P. (5% or 10% hydrous benzoyl peroxide)	1. Benzoyl peroxide slowly releases oxygen and is bactericidal for anaerobic bacteria (*e.g., Corynebacterium*). 2. This agent also has irritant, keratolytic, and antiseborrheic properties.	Acne
Phenol derivatives	Hexachlorophene and entsufon sodium emulsion	pHisoHex	1. pHisoHex is a commonly used preparation of hexachlorophene. It contains 3% hexachlorophene and entsufon sodium, a detergent. 2. Bacteriostatic against gram-positive bacteria, including staphylococci. Relatively ineffective against gram-negative organisms and fungi. Gram-negative bacterial and fungal infections may increase in incidence during chronic use of hexachlorophene preparations. 3. A single washing with a hexachlorophene substance is no more effective than soap in reducing the number of microorganisms on the skin. Repeated wash-	1. Handwashing, especially for health care personnel and food handlers 2. Preoperative skin cleansing

TABLE 66-1. ANTISEPTICS (*Continued*)

	Generic name	Trade name	Characteristics	Clinical indications
			ings leave a residual film on the skin that produces a steady reduction in bacterial flora. Cleansing with alcohol or washing with soap removes the antibacterial residual film. 4. Hexachlorophene is absorbed systemically from intact skin, especially after repeated applications. Systemic absorption is increased if the skin is broken; thus hexachlorophene should *not* be applied to open wounds. 5. Short-term use for daily bathing in newborn nurseries is probably effective in preventing infection. 6. Use on the skin in any age group should be followed by thorough rinsing.	
	Resorcinol		1. Bactericidal and fungicidal 2. Also has mild irritant and keratolytic characteristics 3. Usually applied as a 10% ointment or lotion	1. Acne 2. Ringworm (tinea) infections 3. Dermatitis 4. Psoriasis 5. Other cutaneous lesions
Miscellaneous antiseptics	Acetic acid		1. Bactericidal to many microorganisms, including *Pseudomonas aeruginosa,* in a 5% concentration 2. Bacteriostatic in concentrations lower than 5%	1. Irrigations and dressings of surgical wounds (1% solution), bladder irrigations (0.25% solution) 2. Vaginal infections due to *Trichomonas, Candida,* or *Hemophilus* organisms. Administered as a vaginal douche. 3. External otitis (5% solution, instilled in the auditory canal)
	Gentian violet, U.S.P.	Gentian Violet Topical Solution, U.S.P. (1% gentian violet in 10% ethanol) Gentian Violet Cream (1.35% gentian violet in an absorbable base) Genapax tampons Hyva vaginal tablets	1. Effective against gram-positive bacteria (bacteriostatic and bactericidal) and many fungi; ineffective against gram-negative and acid-fast (*e.g.,* tuberculosis) bacteria 2. Stains granulation tissue; should not be applied to ulcerative facial lesions	1. Oral and vaginal fungal infections 2. Infected wounds and mucous membranes
	Sulfur		1. Has fungicidal and keratolytic properties 2. May be used alone or in combination with other keratolytic agents (*e.g.,* coal tar, resorcinol, 2% salicylic acid). 3. Widely used in dermatology	1. Psoriasis 2. Seborrhea 3. Dermatitis

TABLE 66-2. DERMATOLOGIC ANTI-INFECTIVE AND ANTI-INFLAMMATORY AGENTS

	Generic name	Trade name	Routes and dosage ranges (adults and children)
Antibacterial agents	Bacitracin	Baciguent ointment	Topically to skin lesions once or twice daily
	Neomycin sulfate	Myciguent ointment	Topically to skin once or twice daily
Combination agents	Bacitracin and polymyxin B	Polysporin ointment	Topically to skin 2–5 times daily
	Polymyxin B sulfate, neomycin sulfate, and bacitracin	Neosporin ointment, Mycitracin ointment, Neo-Polycin ointment	Topically to skin 2–5 times daily
Antifungal agents	Acrisorcin	Akrinol	Tinea versicolor: topically to skin, morning and night
	Amphotericin B	Fungizone	Cutaneous candidiasis: topically to skin 2–4 times daily
	Clotrimazole	Lotrimin, Mycelex	Cutaneous dermatophytosis, cutaneous and vaginal candidiasis: topically to skin or vaginal mucosa once daily
	Ciclopirox	Loprox	Same as econazole
	Econazole	Spectazole	Tinea infections, cutaneous candidiasis: topically to skin twice daily for 2–4 weeks
	Haloprogin	Halotex	Tinea pedis (athlete's foot), cutaneous candidiasis: topically to skin twice daily for 2–4 weeks
	Iodochlorhydroxyquin	Vioform	Localized dermatophytosis: topically to skin several times daily
	Miconazole	MicaTin	Dermatophytosis, cutaneous candidiasis: topically to skin once or twice daily for 4 weeks
	Nystatin	Mycostatin	Candidiasis of skin and oral mucous membranes, topically to lesions 2–3 times daily Vaginal candidiasis: topically to vaginal mucosa once or twice daily for 14 days
	Tolnaftate	Tinactin	Dermatophytosis: topically to skin twice daily
	Undecylenic acid	Desenex, others	Dermatophytosis, especially tinea pedis (athlete's foot): topically to skin or mucous membranes. Dosage recommendations vary among manufacturers.
Antiviral agent	Acyclovir	Zovirax	Herpes genitalis (initial lesions) and herpes labialis in immunosuppressed clients: topically to lesions q3h or at least 6 times daily for 7 days
Corticosteroids	Amcinonide	Cyclocort	Topically to skin 2–3 times daily
	Betamethasone benzoate	Benisone, Uticort	Topically to skin 1–4 times daily
	Betamethasone dipropionate	Diprosone	Topically to skin 1–4 times daily
	Betamethasone valerate	Valisone	Topically to skin 1–4 times daily
	Clocortolone	Cloderm	Topically to skin 1–3 times daily
	Desonide	Tridesilon	Topically to skin 2–3 times daily
	Desoximetasone	Topicort	Topically to skin 1–2 times daily
	Dexamethasone	Decaspray, Decaderm	Topically to skin 2–3 times daily
	Dexamethasone sodium phosphate	Decadron	Topically to skin 2–3 times daily
	Diflorasone	Florone, Maxiflor	Topically to skin 2–3 times daily
	Fluocinolone acetonide	Synalar, others	Topically to skin 3–4 times daily
	Fluocinonide	Lidex	Topically to skin 3–4 times daily
	Flurandrenolide	Cordran	Topically to skin 2–3 times daily

TABLE 66-2. DERMATOLOGIC ANTI-INFECTIVE AND ANTI–INFLAMMATORY AGENTS (*Continued*)

Generic name	Trade name	Routes and dosage ranges (adults and children)
Halcinonide	Halog	Topically to skin 2–3 times daily
Hydrocortisone	Cortril, others	Topically to skin 3–4 times daily
Hydrocortisone acetate	Hydrocortone, others	Topically to skin 3–4 times daily
Methylprednisolone acetate	Medrol acetate	Topically to skin 1–4 times daily, then reduced when disease process is controlled
Triamcinolone acetonide	Aristocort, Kenalog, others	Topically to skin 3–4 times daily

1. *Antiseptics* kill or inhibit the growth of bacteria, viruses, or fungi. They are used primarily to prevent infection. They are occasionally used in the treatment of dermatologic infections. Soaps and detergents are not antiseptics because they do not kill or inhibit growth of microorganisms. However, soaps and detergents facilitate mechanical cleansing of the skin, especially when applied with friction. Skin surfaces should generally be clean before application of antiseptics. Antiseptics are sometimes called "skin disinfectants." Generally, however, the term *disinfectant* refers to agents used for sterilizing inanimate objects (*e.g.*, instruments). Disinfectants are usually too strong for application to the skin and mucous membranes.
2. *Anti-infective agents* are used to treat infections caused by bacteria, fungi, and viruses. (These drugs are extensively discussed in Chaps. 33 through 43). When used in dermatologic infections, antiinfective drugs may be administered locally (topically) or systemically (orally or parenterally). In many bacterial infections (*e.g.*, furuncles), systemic antibiotics are preferred. Generally, topical antibiotics have limited clinical utility in bacterial infections. However, topical therapy of fungal infections is very effective. Topical antiviral therapy is available for treatment of ophthalmic viral infections (see Chap. 65); herpes genitalis, an infectious viral disease transmitted primarily by sexual contact; and herpes labialis ("fever blisters") in immunosuppressed clients (see Chap. 42).
3. *Anti-inflammatory* agents are used to treat the inflammation that is present in many dermatologic conditions. The major anti-inflammatory agents are the adrenal corticosteroids (see Chap. 24). When used in dermatologic conditions, corticosteroids are most often applied topically. However, they may also be administered orally and parenterally in severe dermatologic disorders.
4. *Astringents* (*e.g.*, dilute solutions of aluminum or zinc salts) are used for drying effects on exudative lesions.
5. *Emollients* or lubricants (*e.g.*, mineral oil, lanolin, petrolatum) are used to relieve pruritus and dryness of the skin.
6. *Enzymes* are used to debride burn wounds, decubitus ulcers, and venous stasis ulcers. They promote healing by removing necrotic tissue.
7. *Keratolytic* agents (*e.g.*, salicylic acid) are used to remove warts, corns, calluses, and other keratin-containing skin lesions.
8. *Sunscreens* are used to protect the skin from excessive exposure to sunlight, thereby preventing sunburn and possibly preventing skin cancer. The most effective screening agent is para-aminobenzoic acid (PABA) in 55% to 70% alcohol.

   Sunscreening preparations are labeled in terms of "sun-protection factor" (SPF), with an SPF of 15 being the most protective. Agents with high SPF values are recommended for people with fair skin who sunburn easily, people who are allergic to sunlight, and people who are using topical or systemic medications with photosensitizing or phototoxic characteristics (*e.g.*, tetracycline). Agents with low SPF values may be used by people who wish to tan the skin without experiencing sunburn.
9. Agents affecting skin pigmentation may be used, with variable degrees of effectiveness, to increase or decrease pigmentation. *Melanizing agents* (*e.g.*, trioxsalen, methoxsalen) may be used to increase skin pigmentation in vitiligo. Vitiligo is a disorder characterized by white patches of skin surrounded by normally pigmented skin. *Demelanizing agents* (*e.g.*, hydroquinone, monobenzone) are occasionally used for hyperpigmented areas of the skin such as freckles or chronic inflammatory lesions.

Most dermatologic medications are applied topically. To be effective, topical agents must be in contact with the underlying skin or mucous membrane. Nu-

TABLE 66-3. MISCELLANEOUS DERMATOLOGIC AGENTS

	Generic name	Trade name	Dermatologic effects	Clinical indications	Method of administration
Demelanizing agents	Hydroquinone	Eldoquin	Decreases skin pigmentation	1. Freckles 2. Melasma	Topically to hyperpigmented areas of the skin 1–2 times daily
	Monobenzone	Benoquin	Decreases skin pigmentation	Vitiligo—for permanent depigmentation of areas containing normal pigmentation (*i.e.,* to relieve "spotted" appearance)	Topically, to pigmented areas only, 2–3 times daily
Melanizing agents	Methoxsalen	Oxsoralen	Increases skin pigmentation	Vitiligo	Topically to small lesions, followed by sunlight or ultraviolet light
	Trioxsalen	Trisoralen	Increases skin pigmentation	1. Vitiligo 2. Increase tolerance to sunlight	Vitiligo: PO 10 mg daily, followed in 2 hours by exposure to sunlight To increase tolerance to sunlight: PO 10 mg daily for no longer than 14 days
Enzymes	Collagenase	Santyl	Debriding effects	Enzymatic debridement of infected wounds (*e.g.,* burn wounds, decubitus ulcers)	Topically once daily until the wound is cleansed of necrotic material
	Fibrinolysin-deoxyribonuclease	Elase	See collagenase, above	See collagenase, above	See collagenase, above
	Papain	Panafil	Debriding effects	Debridement of surface lesions	Topically 1–2 times daily
	Sutilains	Travase	Debriding effects	Debridement of wounds	Topically to wound 3–4 times daily
	Trypsin	Granulex	Debriding effects	Debridement of infected wounds (*e.g.,* decubitus and varicose ulcers)	Topically by spray twice daily
Other agents	Aluminum acetate solution (Burow's solution)		Astringent, antipruritic, anti-inflammatory	1. Weeping or "wet" skin lesions due to infection or inflammation 2. External otitis	Topically to skin, as wet dressings Topically to external ear, as irrigating solution to remove debris
	Coal tar	Balnetar, Zetar, others	Irritant	1. Psoriasis 2. Dermatitis	Topically to skin, in various concentrations and preparations (*e.g.,* creams, lotions, shampoos, bath emulsion). Also available in combination with hydrocortisone and other substances
	Colloidal oatmeal	Aveeno	Antipruritic	Pruritus	Topically as a bath solution (1 cup in bathtub of water)
	Fluorouracil	Efudex	Antineoplastic	1. Actinic keratoses 2. Superficial basal cell carcinomas	Topically to skin lesions twice daily for 2–6 weeks
	Isotretinoin	Accutane	Inhibits sebum production and keratinization	1. Severe cystic acne 2. Disorders characterized by excessive	PO 1–2 mg/kg/day, in 2 divided doses, for 15–20 weeks

TABLE 66-3. MISCELLANEOUS DERMATOLOGIC AGENTS (*Continued*)

Generic name	Trade name	Dermatologic effects	Clinical indications	Method of administration
			keratinization (*e.g.*, pityriasis, ichthyosis) 3. *Mycosis fungoides*	
Salicylic acid		Keratolytic, antifungal	1. Removal of warts, corns, calluses 2. Superficial fungal infections 3. Seborrheic dermatitis 4. Acne 5. Psoriasis	Topically to lesions
Selenium sulfide	Selsun	Antifungal, antidandruff	1. Dandruff 2. Tinea versicolor	Topically to scalp as shampoo once or twice weekly
Tretinoin	Retin-A	Irritant	Acne vulgaris	Topically to skin lesions once daily

merous dosage forms have been developed for topical application of drugs to various parts of the body and for various therapeutic purposes. Basic components of topical agents are one or more active ingredients and a usually inactive vehicle. The vehicle is a major determinant of the drug's ability to reach affected skin and mucous membrane. Many topical preparations contain other additives (*e.g.*, preservatives, emulsifiers, emollients, dispersing agents) that further facilitate application to skin and mucous membranes. Commonly used vehicles and dosage forms include ointments, creams, lotions, powders, sprays, aerosols, gels, otic solutions, and vaginal and rectal suppositories. Many topical drug preparations are available in several dosage forms.

Topical medications are used primarily for local effects when systemic absorption is undesirable. Factors that influence percutaneous absorption of topical agents include the following:

1. *Degree of skin hydration.* Drug penetration and percutaneous absorption are increased when keratin in the outermost layer of the epidermis is well hydrated.
2. *Drug concentration.* Since percutaneous absorption occurs by passive diffusion, higher concentrations increase the amount of drug absorbed.
3. *Skin condition.* Absorption from abraded or damaged skin is much greater than from intact skin.
4. *Length of contact time.* Absorption is increased when drugs are left in place for prolonged periods.
5. *Size of area.* Absorption is increased when topical medications are applied to large areas of the body.
6. *Location of area.* Absorption from mucous membranes and facial skin is comparatively rapid. Absorption from thick-skinned areas (*e.g.*, palms of hands and soles of feet) is comparatively slow.

Principles of therapy: dermatologic drugs

ASSESSMENT GUIDELINES

Assess the client's skin for any characteristics or lesions that may indicate current or potential dermatologic disorders.

1. When a skin rash is present, interview the client and inspect the area to determine the following:
   a. Appearance of individual lesions. Lesions should be described as specifically as possible so that changes can be identified. Terms commonly used in dermatology include *macule* (flat spot), *papule* (raised spot), *nodule* (small solid swelling), *vesicle* (blister), *pustule* (pus-containing lesion), *petechia* (flat, round, purplish red spot the size of a pinpoint, caused by intradermal or submucosal bleeding), and *erythema* (redness). Lesions may also be described as weeping or dry, scaly and crusty.
   b. Location or distribution. Some skin rashes occur exclusively or primarily on certain parts of the body (*e.g.*, face, extremities, trunk), and distribution may indicate the cause.
   c. Accompanying symptoms. Pruritus occurs with most dermatologic conditions. Fever, malaise, and other symptoms may occur as well.

d. Historical development. Appropriate questions include:
   (1) When and where did the skin rash appear?
   (2) How long has it been present?
   (3) Has it changed in appearance or location?
   (4) Has it occurred previously?
e. Etiologic factors. In many instances, appropriate treatment is determined by cause. Some etiologic factors include the following:
   (1) *Drug therapy.* Many commonly used drugs may cause skin lesions. These drugs include antibiotics (*e.g.*, penicillins, sulfonamides, tetracyclines), barbiturates, narcotic analgesics, phenothiazine antipsychotic agents, (*e.g.*, chlorpromazine [Thorazine]), and thiazide diuretics. Skin rashes due to drug therapy are usually generalized and appear abruptly.
   (2) *Irritants or allergens* may cause contact dermatitis. For example, dermatitis involving the hands may be caused by soaps, detergents, or various other cleansing agents. Dermatitis involving the trunk may result from allergic reactions to clothing.
   (3) *Communicable diseases* (*i.e.*, measles, scarlatina, chickenpox) cause characteristic skin rashes and systemic signs and symptoms.

2. When skin lesions other than rashes are present, assess appearance, size or extent, amount and character of any drainage, and whether the lesion appears infected or contains necrotic material. Bleeding into the skin is usually described as *petechiae* (pinpoint hemmorhages) or *ecchymoses* (bruises). Burn wounds are usually described in terms of depth (partial or full thickness of skin) and percentage of body surface area. Burn wounds with extensive skin damage are rapidly colonized with potentially pathogenic microorganisms. Venous stasis, decubitus, and other cutaneous ulcers are usually described in terms of diameter and depth.
3. When assessing the skin, consider the age of the client. Infants are likely to have "diaper" dermatitis, miliaria (heat rash), and tinea capitis (ringworm infection of the scalp). School-age children have a relatively high incidence of measles, chickenpox, and tinea infections. Adolescents commonly have acne. Elderly adults are more likely to have dry skin, actinic keratoses, and skin neoplasms.
4. Assess for skin neoplasms. *Basal cell carcinoma* is the most common type of skin cancer. It may initially appear as a pale nodule, most often on the head and neck. *Squamous cell carcinomas* may appear as ulcerated areas. These lesions may occur anywhere on the body but are more common on sun-exposed parts such as the face and hands. *Malignant melanoma* is the most serious skin cancer. It involves melanocytes, the pigment-producing cells of the skin. Malignant melanoma may occur in pigmented nevi (moles) or previously normal skin. In nevi, malignant melanoma may be manifested by enlargement and ulceration. In previously normal skin, lesions appear as irregularly shaped pigmented areas. Although it can occur in almost any area, malignant melanoma is most likely to be located on the back in whites and in toe webs and soles of the feet in blacks and Orientals.
5. When assessing dark-skinned persons, color changes and skin rashes are more difficult to detect. Some guidelines include the following:
   a. Adequate lighting is required. Nonglare daylight is best. The illumination provided by overbed lights or flashlights is inadequate for most purposes.
   b. Some skin rashes may be visible on oral mucous membranes.
   c. Petechiae are not visible on dark brown or black skin. However, they may be visible on oral mucous membranes or the conjunctiva.
6. When skin disorders are present, assess the client's psychologic response to the condition. Many clients, especially those with chronic disorders, feel self-conscious and depressed.

PREVENTIVE NURSING INTERVENTIONS

Use measures to prevent or minimize skin disorders.

1. Avoid known irritants or allergens. Have the client substitute nonirritating soaps or cleaning supplies for irritating ones; use hypoallergenic jewelry and cosmetics, if indicated; wear cotton clothing, if indicated.
2. Use general measures to promote health and increase resistance to disease (*i.e.*, maintain nutrition, rest, and exercise). In addition, practice safety measures to avoid injury to the skin. Any injury, especially those that disrupt the integrity of the skin (*e.g.*, lacerations, puncture wounds, scratching of skin lesions), increases the likelihood of skin infections.
3. Use measures to relieve dry skin and pruritus. Dry skin causes itching, and itching promotes scratching. Scratching relieves itching only if it is strong enough to damage the skin and serve as a counterirritant. Skin damaged or disrupted by scratching is susceptible to invasion by pathogenic microorganisms. Thus, dry skin may lead to serious skin disorders. Older adults are especially likely to have dry, flaky skin. Measures to decrease skin dryness include the following:

a. Alternating complete and partial baths. For example, a person may take a complete shower or tub bath and a sponge bath (of face, hands, underarms, and perineal areas) on alternate days. Warm water, mild soaps, and patting dry are recommended because hot water, harsh soaps, and rubbing with a towel have drying effects on the skin.
b. Liberal use of lubricating creams, lotions, and oils. Bath oils, which usually contain mineral oil or lanolin oil and a perfume, are widely available. If bath oils are used, precautions against falls are necessary, since the oils make bathtubs and shower floors slippery. Creams and lotions may be applied several times daily.

4. Prevent decubitus ulcers by avoiding trauma to the skin and prolonged pressure on any part of the body. In clients at high risk for developing decubitus ulcers, major preventive measures include frequent changes of position and correct lifting techniques. Various pressure-relieving devices are also useful. These include water beds, air or foam rubber mattresses, and chair pads. Daily inspection of the skin is needed for early detection and treatment of beginning decubitus ulcers.
5. Avoid excessive exposure to sunlight and other sources of ultraviolet light. Although controlled amounts of ultraviolet light are beneficial in some dermatologic disorders (*i.e.*, acne, psoriasis), excessive amounts cause wrinkling, dryness, and malignancies. If prolonged exposure is necessary, the use of sunscreening lotions decreases skin damage.
6. When skin rashes are present, cool, wet compresses or baths are often effective in relieving pruritus. Water or normal saline may be used alone or with additives such as aluminum acetate solution (Burow's solution), colloidal oatmeal (Aveeno), or baking soda. A cool environment also tends to decrease pruritus. The client's fingernails should be cut short and kept clean to avoid skin damage and infection from scratching.

DRUG SELECTION IN VARIOUS SKIN CONDITIONS

Choice of dermatologic agents depends primarily on the reason for use and client response. Some guidelines include the following:

1. For routine handwashing of health care personnel and preoperative skin cleansing of surgical staff and clients, chlorhexidene (Hibiclens) and the iodophors (Betadine, Prepodyne) are the antiseptics of first choice. Alcohol is effective but too drying for routine use. pHisoHex is not effective against gram-negative bacteria and is absorbed systemically from intact skin.
2. Topical medications for inflammatory and noninflammatory skin disorders vary greatly. Generally, though, astringents and lotions are used as drying agents for "wet," oozing lesions, and ointments and creams are used as "wetting" agents for dry, scaling lesions. Topical corticosteroids are available in several dosage forms for use in both acute and chronic inflammatory disorders. Hydrocortisone is the topical corticosteroid of choice for use on the face or other cosmetically important areas. It is available over the counter in a 0.5% concentration. The fluorinated corticosteroids may cause skin eruptions, dermatitis, and acne; therefore, these compounds are generally used on areas other than the face.
3. For topical antibiotic therapy, bacitracin, neomycin, and polymyxin are usually preferred. These drugs are often used in combination, and various preparations are available (*e.g.*, Neosporin). Although other antibiotics are available in dosage forms for topical use (*e.g.*, gentamicin, chloramphenicol, tetracyclines), these drugs should generally not be used. These drugs may cause sensitization when used topically. If a sensitized client receives the drug systemically at a later time, serious allergic reactions may occur.
4. In acne, benzoyl peroxide, 5% or 10%, is one of the most effective topical agents. Systemic tetracycline in low doses may be used for long-term treatment of acne. Because of potentially severe adverse effects, isotretinoin is recommended for use only in severe cystic acne that is resistant to other treatments. Because of teratogenic effects, it is contraindicated during pregnancy. Women of childbearing potential should use an effective method of contraception during and for at least 1 month after isotretinoin therapy.
5. In external otitis, otic preparations of various dermatologic medications are used. Polymyxin B (Cortisporin Otic Solution) and neomycin (Otobiotic Otic Solution) are the most commonly used antibiotics, although others (*e.g.*, tetracyclines, sulfonamides, gentamicin) are available. Acetic acid solution 5% may also be administered as an otic anti-infective agent. Acetic acid is effective against *Pseudomonas* and many other organisms that cause external ear disease. It establishes an acidic environment, which prevents growth of the organisms and does not produce resistant organisms. Hydrocortisone is the corticosteroid most often included in topical otic preparations. It relieves pruritus and inflammation in chronic external otitis. Local anesthetics, usually benzocaine, are included in some otic formulations. However, local anesthetics are

not well absorbed from the ear and are generally ineffective in relieving severe pain associated with acute external otitis or otitis media. Systemic analgesics are usually required.

6. In decubitus ulcers, the only clear-cut guideline for treatment is avoiding further pressure on the affected area. Many topical agents are used, most often with specific procedures for dressing changes, skin cleansing, and so on. No one agent or procedure seems clearly superior. Consistent implementation of a decubitus care protocol (*i.e.*, position changes, inspection of current or potential pressure areas, dressing changes, use of an air mattress) may be more effective than drug therapy.
7. In anorectal disorders, most preparations contain a local anesthetic, emollients, and perhaps a corticosteroid. These preparations relieve pruritus and pain but do not cure the underlying condition. Some preparations contain ingredients of questionable value, such as vasoconstrictors, astringents, and weak antiseptics. No particular mixture is clearly superior.

DOSAGE FORMS

Choice of dosage form for topical drug therapy depends largely on the reason for use. Guidelines include the following:

1. *Ointments* are oil-based substances that usually contain a medication in an emollient vehicle such as petrolatum or lanolin. Ointments occlude the skin and promote retention of moisture. Thus, they are especially useful in chronic skin disorders characterized by dry lesions. Ointments should generally be avoided in hairy, moist, and intertriginous areas of the body because of potential maceration, irritation, and secondary infection.
2. *Creams* (emulsions of oil in water, which may be greasy or nongreasy) and *gels* (transparent colloids, which dry and leave a film over the area) retain moisture in the skin but are less occlusive than ointments. These preparations are cosmetically acceptable for use on the face and other visible areas of the body. They may also be used in hairy, moist, intertriginous areas. Creams and gels are especially useful in subacute dermatologic disorders.
3. *Lotions* are suspensions of insoluble substances in water. They cool and dry and protect the skin. They are most useful in subacute dermatologic disorders. *Sprays* and *aerosols* are similar to lotions.
4. *Powders* have absorbent, cooling, and protective effects. Generally, powders should not be applied in acute, exudative disorders or on denuded areas because they tend to cake, occlude the lesions, and retard healing. Also, some powders (*e.g.*, cornstarch) may lead to secondary infections by promoting growth of bacteria and fungi.
5. *Pastes* are semisolid preparations composed primarily of powder. Pastes adhere strongly to the area of application and are difficult to remove. They are generally less macerating, penetrating, and occlusive than ointments. Pastes should not be used on hairy areas of the body.
6. Topical otic medications are usually delivered in a liquid vehicle. However, creams or ointments may be used for dry, crusted lesions, and powders may be used for drying effects.
7. Topical vaginal medications may be applied as douche solutions, vaginal tablets, or vaginal creams used with an applicator.
8. Dosage of corticosteroids applied topically to skin depends on the potency of the preparation (percentage of drug contained in the ointment, lotion, or other vehicle), the area of application, and the method of application. The skin covering the face, scalp, scrotum, and axillae is more permeable to corticosteroids than other skin surfaces, and these areas can usually be treated with smaller amounts or less frequent application. In addition, drug absorption is increased by applying an occlusive dressing over the affected area. Systemic toxicity may occur. For this reason, drug application is usually done less frequently when occlusive dressings are used.
9. Anorectal medications may be applied as ointments, creams, foams, and rectal suppositories.

NURSING ACTIONS: DERMATOLOGIC DRUGS

Nursing Actions	*Rationale/Explanation*
1. Administer accurately	
a. Use the correct preparation for the intended use (*i.e.*, dermatologic, otic, vaginal, anorectal).	Preparations may differ in drug contents and concentrations.

Nursing Actions	*Rationale/Explanation*
b. For topical application to skin lesions	
(1) Wash the skin and pat it dry.	To cleanse the skin and remove previously applied medication. This facilitates drug contact with the affected area of the skin.
(2) Apply a small amount of the drug preparation and rub it in well.	A thin layer of medication is effective and decreases the incidence and severity of adverse effects.
(3) For burn wounds, broken skin, or open lesions, apply the drug with sterile gloves or sterile cotton-tipped applicators.	To prevent infection
(4) Use the drug only for the individual client (*i.e.,* do not use the same tube for more than one client).	To avoid bacterial cross contamination between clients
(5) Wash hands before and after application.	Wash hands before to avoid exposing the client to infection; wash hands afterward to avoid transferring the drug to your own face or eyes and causing adverse reactions.
2. Observe for therapeutic effects	Therapeutic effects depend on the medication being used and the disorder being treated.
a. With dermatologic conditions, observe for healing of skin lesions.	
b. With external otitis, observe for decreased pain and pruritus.	
c. With vaginal disorders, observe for decreased vaginal discharge and pruritus.	
d. With anorectal disorders, observe for decreased pain and pruritus.	
3. Observe for adverse effects	Incidence of adverse effects is low with topical agents.
a. Local irritation or inflammation—erythema, skin rash, pruritus	Local adverse effects may occur with antiseptics (*e.g.,* iodine preparations), local anesthetics (*e.g.,* in anorectal preparations), and antibiotics. When topical antibiotics are applied to the external ear, the drugs may cause a cutaneous reaction that resembles the disorder being treated.
b. With topical corticosteroids, observe for acneiform facial lesions and other skin changes (atrophy, thinning, development of striae).	Facial lesions occur with chronic use of fluorinated corticosteroids. They can be avoided by using hydrocortisone on facial lesions. Other skin changes occur with prolonged use of topical corticosteroids.
c. With topical antibiotics, superinfection and sensitization may occur.	Superinfection with drug-resistant organisms may occur with any antibacterial agent. It is less likely to occur with mixtures that have a broad spectrum of antibacterial activity. Sensitization may cause serious allergic reactions if the same drug is given systemically at a later time.
d. With isotretinoin, observe for hypervitaminosis A (nausea, vomiting, headache, blurred vision, eye irritation, conjunctivitis, skin disorders, abnormal liver function, musculoskeletal pain, increased plasma triglycerides, others).	Adverse effects commonly occur with usual doses but are more severe with higher doses.
4. Observe for drug interactions	Clinically significant drug interactions rarely occur with topical agents.
5. Teach clients	
a. Promote healthy skin by personal hygiene measures, avoiding excessive exposure to sunlight, avoiding skin injuries, and lubricating dry skin.	Healthy skin is less susceptible to inflammation, infections and other disorders. It also heals more rapidly if disorders or injuries occur.

Nursing Actions	Rationale/Explanation
b. When skin lesions are present, try to avoid scratching, squeezing, or rubbing the affected area.	To avoid additional skin damage and infection
c. Use topical medications only as prescribed or according to the manufacturer's instructions (for over-the-counter products).	Most topical agents are quite safe if used properly but may cause adverse effects if used improperly.
d. For minor wounds and abrasions, cleansing with soap and water is usually adequate. If an antiseptic is used, an iodine preparation (*e.g.,* aqueous iodine solution 1%) is preferred.	Iodine preparations are effective in preventing infection. Alcohol should not be applied to open wounds. Hydrogen peroxide may facilitate mechanical cleansing, but it is a weak antiseptic. Common household agents, for instance, merbromin (Mercurochrome) and thimerosal (Merthiolate), are weak antiseptics. These mercury compounds are generally not recommended for use.
e. With isotretinoin, avoid vitamin supplements containing vitamin A and excessive exposure to sunlight	To decrease risks of excessive vitamin A intake and photosensitivity

Selected References

Adverse effects with isotretinoin. FDA Drug Bull 13:21–22, November 1983

Anders JE, Leach EE: Sun versus skin. Am J Nurs 83:1015–1020, July 1983

Arnell I: Treating decubitus ulcers: Two methods that work. Nursing 13:50–55, June 1983

Burkhart CG: Scabies: An epidemiologic reassessment. Ann Intern Med 98:498–503, April 1983

Carey K (ed): Drug Interactions. Springhouse, PA, Springhouse Corp, 1984

Facts and Comparisons. St. Louis, J B Lippincott (Updated monthly)

Harvey SC: Antiseptics and disinfectants; fungicides; ectoparasiticides. In Gilman AG, Goodman LS, Rall TW, Murad F (eds): The Pharmacological Basis of Therapeutics, 7th ed, pp 959–979. New York, Macmillan, 1985

Lesher JL, Smith JG: Athlete's foot: A logical approach to treatment. Drug Ther 14:113–120, September 1984

Malseed RT: Pharmacology: Drug Therapy and Nursing Considerations, 2d ed. Philadelphia, J B Lippincott, 1985

Neuberger GB, Reckling JB: A new look at wound care. Nursing 15:34–41, February 1985

Shannon ML: Five famous fallacies about pressure sores. Nursing 14:34–41, October 1984

Sunscreens. Med Lett Drugs Ther 26:56–58, June 8, 1984

Susong CR, Nordlund JJ: Vitiligo: Guidelines for successful therapy. Drug Ther 15:133–139, February 1985

Swinyard EA, Pathak MA: Surface-acting drugs. In Gilman AG, Goodman LS, Rall TW, Murad F (eds): The Pharmacological Basis of Therapeutics, 7th ed, pp 946–958. New York, Macmillan, 1985

Update on birth defects with isotretinoin. FDA Drug Bull 14:15–16, August 1984

Witkowski JA, Parish LC: Poison ivy, poison oak, poison sumac. Drug Ther 14:81–88, June 1984

67

DRUGS AFFECTING UTERINE MOTILITY

Description and uses

The uterus is the small, hollow organ in which the fetus develops during pregnancy. It is composed of the myometrium and the endometrium. The *myometrium* is a thick, muscular layer. The *fundus* is the upper portion and the *cervix* is the lower portion of the myometrium. The cervix extends into the vagina. The *endometrium* is the secretory mucous membrane that forms the inner lining of the uterus. Cyclical changes in response to estrogens and progesterone result in the shedding of the endometrium (menstruation) or, if conception occurs, further proliferation to nourish a developing embryo (see Chap. 28). In this chapter, drugs that cause contraction or relaxation of the myometrium are discussed.

Changes in uterine motility may be physiologic or pathologic. Motility of the nonpregnant uterus is limited. However, motility increases during menstruation and may cause pain or discomfort (*i.e.,* menstrual cramps or dysmenorrhea). During pregnancy, the myometrium becomes more responsive to stimuli. Beginning in early pregnancy, the uterus undergoes intermittent, painless periods of contraction and relaxation called Braxton–Hicks contractions. At the end of the gestational period, uterine contractions occur regularly and increase in duration and intensity. The strong muscular contractions help to expel the fetus from the uterine cavity, and birth occurs. After birth of the infant, additional contractions aid expulsion of the placenta and control uterine bleeding. Uterine contractions occurring before the end of gestation may cause abortion or premature birth. Abnormal contractions may occur spontaneously, without known cause, or be induced by abortifacients (agents that cause abortion).

Drugs may be given to increase or decrease uterine motility. Drugs used to increase motility are the oxytocic agents, which stimulate contraction by increasing the tone and motility of uterine smooth muscle. Drugs used to decrease motility are $beta_2$-adrenergic agents, central nervous system (CNS) depressants (*e.g.,* intravenous alcohol solutions, sedative–hypnotic drugs), and relatively large doses of magnesium sulfate.

OXYTOCIC AGENTS

Oxytocin is a hormone that is produced in the hypothalamus and stored and released by the posterior pituitary gland (see Chap. 23). Oxytocin functions in childbirth by stimulating uterine contractions and in lactation by promoting milk "let-down" (movement of breast milk from the glands to the nipples). A synthetic form of oxytocin is used in obstetrics, primarily for its uterine effects.

Ergot alkaloids are oxytocic agents obtained from a parasitic fungus that grows on cereal grains, especially rye. Ergot alkaloids markedly increase the force and frequency of uterine contractions. Small doses produce contractions followed by relaxation; larger doses produce more forceful and prolonged contractions with little uterine relaxation between contractions. These agents stimulate contraction in both the pregnant and nonpregnant uterus. However, the uterus is most responsive during pregnancy and immediately after delivery. Ergonovine and methylergonovine are the two ergot alkaloids used clinically for their oxytocic effects. Another ergot alkaloid, ergotamine, is used only for the relief of migraine (see Chap. 6).

Prostaglandins are very active biologic substances synthesized in the body from fatty acids and found in almost every body tissue and fluid. In the female reproductive system, prostaglandins of the E and F types are found in the ovaries, myometrium, and menstrual fluid. The cervix is exposed to additional prostaglandins after coitus because high concentrations are found in the seminal fluid. Prostaglandins stimulate contraction of smooth muscle in the uterus. The PGF series of prostaglandins stimulates contraction of the pregnant or nonpregnant uterus; the PGE_2 series of prostaglandins stimulates contraction of the pregnant uterus, especially during the second and third trimesters of pregnancy. Prostaglandins are probably important in initiating and maintaining the normal birth process. However, prostaglandins are capable of inducing labor if administered at any time during pregnancy.

UTERINE RELAXANT AGENTS

Uterine relaxants are drugs used for prevention or treatment of premature labor. Numerous agents have been tried with varying levels of success. At present, $beta_2$-adrenergic agents are the drugs of choice. Ritodrine (Yutopar) is the only one approved for use in the United States. Terbutaline (Brethine), commonly used as a bronchodilator in respiratory disorders, is also used to relax uterine muscles, but such usage is considered investigational. Other $beta_2$-adrenergic drugs and calcium channel blocking agents are being investigated for possible use.

Individual agents

OXYTOCIN

Oxytocin (Pitocin, Syntocinon) is a synthetic drug that is identical to the endogenous hormone released from the posterior pituitary gland. It is used to induce labor at or near full-term gestation and to stimulate labor when uterine contractions are weak and ineffective. it is occasionally used to prevent or control uterine bleeding after delivery, to complete an incomplete abortion, and to promote milk ejection during lactation. When given intravenously, oxytocin causes uterine contractions in approximately 1 minute. Duration of action is short. When given intramuscularly, oxytocin acts within 3 to 7 minutes and effects last 30 to 60 minutes. Oxytocin is occasionally used as a nasal spray to promote milk ejection.

Oxytocin is contraindicated for antepartal use in the presence of fetal distress, cephalopelvic disproportion, prematurity, placenta previa, previous uterine surgery, and severe toxemia.

Routes and dosage ranges

Adults: During labor and delivery, IV 2 milliunits/minute, gradually increased to 20 milliunits/minute, if necessary, to produce 3–4 contractions within 10-minute periods. Prepare solution by adding 10 units (1 ml) of oxytocin to 1000 ml of 0.9% sodium chloride or 5% dextrose in 0.45% sodium chloride

To control postpartal hemorrhage, IV 10–40 units added, as above, to 1000 ml of 0.9% sodium chloride, infused at a rate to control bleeding

To prevent postpartal bleeding, IM 3–10 units (0.3–1 ml) as a single dose

To promote milk ejection, topically, 1 spray of nasal solution to one or both of the nostrils 2–3 minutes before nursing the infant

ERGOT ALKALOIDS

Ergonovine maleate (Ergotrate) is a naturally occuring ergot alkaloid. **Methylergonovine maleate** (Methergine) is a semisynthetic derivative of ergonovine. These oxytocic agents have the same indications for use, adverse effects, and contraindications. They are occasionally used to stimulate uterine contraction and control bleeding after delivery of the placenta. They are also used to control uterine bleeding after abortion. Ergonovine and methylergonovine have a rapid onset and prolonged duration (3 hours or more) of action. Both drugs are available in tablets or 1-ml ampules containing 0.2 mg.

Ergonovine and methylergonovine are contraindicated in severe hypertension or toxemia and before delivery of the placenta.

Routes and dosage ranges

Adults: After delivery of the placenta, IM 0.2 mg, repeated in 2–4 hours if bleeding is severe

Severe uterine bleeding, IV 0.2 mg

To prevent excessive postpartal bleeding, PO 0.2 mg 2–4 times daily for 2–7 days if necessary

PROSTAGLANDINS

Dinoprost tromethamine (prostin F_2 alpha) and **dinoprostone** (prostin E_2) are prostaglandins used to induce abortion during the second trimester of pregnancy. Dinoprost is injected transabdominally into the amniotic sac by the physician. The drug promotes cervical dilatation and uterine contraction. Abortion usually occurs within 8 to 24 hours. Dinoprostone is administered as a vaginal suppository. Uterine contractions start within 30 minutes, and abortion usually occurs within 24 to 48 hours. Dinoprostone may also be used to evacuate the uterus in cases of missed abortion or fetal death up to 28 weeks of gestation and in the management of hydatidiform mole (benign gestational trophoblastic disease).

Prostaglandins are contraindicated in the presence of pelvic inflammatory disease.

Routes and dosage ranges

Dinoprost

Adults: Intra-amniotically 40 mg, followed by an additional dose of 10–40 mg after 2–4 hours if abortion is not established or complete

Dinoprostone

Adults: Intravaginally 20 mg, repeated every 3–5 hours until abortion occurs

UTERINE RELAXANT AGENT

Ritodrine hydrochloride (Yutopar) is a β_2-adrenergic receptor agonist that inhibits uterine contractility. Ritodrine is used in the management of premature labor occurring after 20 weeks of gestation.

Ritodrine is contraindicated before 20 weeks of gestation and in the presence of fetal death, antepartal hemorrhage, or severe maternal diseases (*i.e.*, cardiovascular disorders such as congestive heart failure, arrhythmias or hypertension, pheochromocytoma, uncontrolled diabetes mellitus, bronchial asthma, and hyperthyroidism).

Routes and dosage ranges

Adults: IV infusion 0.1 mg/minute initially, increased by 50 μg/minute every 10 minutes to a maximal dose of 350 μg/minute if necessary to stop labor. The infusion should be continued for 12 hours after uterine contractions cease. Prepare the solution by adding 150 mg of ritodrine to 500 ml of intravenous fluid for a concentration of 0.3 mg/ml.

PO 10 mg 30 minutes before discontinuing the intravenous infusion, then 10 mg q2h for 24 hours, then 10–20 mg q4–6h as long as necessary to maintain the pregnancy. Maximal oral dose, 120 mg daily

Principles of therapy: drugs affecting uterine motility

1. Assess the client's status in relation to pregnancy and purpose of drug therapy.
   a. When spontaneous labor occurs in normal, full-term pregnancy, assess frequency and quality of uterine contractions, amount of cervical dilatation, fetal heart rate and quality, and maternal blood pressure. In this situation, drugs affecting uterine motility are used only after delivery of the infant and the placenta.
   b. With threatened abortion or premature labor, determine the length of gestation, the frequency and quality of uterine contractions if possible, the amount of vaginal bleeding, and the length of labor. Also determine whether any tissue has been expelled from the vagina. When abortion is inevitable, oxytocic agents may be given to facilitate termination of the pregnancy. When attempts to stop labor and maintain the pregnancy are desired, a uterine relaxant may be given.
2. For induction or augmentation of labor, oxytocin is the drug of choice because physiologic doses produce a rhythmic uterine contraction–relaxation pattern that approximates the normal labor process.
3. For prevention or control of postpartal uterine bleeding, oxytocin is also the drug of choice because it is less likely to cause hypertension than ergonovine and methylergonovine.
4. For induction of elective abortion, various methods are used, depending primarily on the length of gestation. The role of the nurse varies according to state laws and agency policies. General guidelines include the following:
   a. All candidates for abortion should receive preabortion counseling regarding methods and expected outcomes. Postabortion counseling may also be needed for instruction in contraceptive techniques.
   b. For first trimester abortions, suction curettage is a commonly used, safe, and effective method.
   c. For second trimester abortions, several methods have been used. One method involves intra-amniotic instillation of hypertonic (20%) sodium chloride solution. Intra-amniotic instillation involves insertion of a spinal-length needle through the abdominal

and uterine walls into the amniotic sac, withdrawal of amniotic fluid, and instillation of sodium chloride solution. This method has largely been replaced by prostaglandin administration. A third method involves dilatation of the cervix and curettage of the endometrium to mechanically remove products of conception. Except for intravaginal or intramuscular administration of prostaglandins, abortions are performed by the physician. The role of the nurse involves assisting the client and the physician as well as observing client responses before, during, and after the procedure.

NURSING ACTIONS: DRUGS AFFECTING UTERINE MOTILITY

Nursing Actions	*Rationale/Explanation*
1. Administer accurately	
a. For intravenous infusion of oxytocin, mix the drug in an intravenous solution containing sodium chloride and "piggyback" the solution into a primary intravenous line. Use an infusion pump to administer.	Oxytocin has an antidiuretic effect and may cause water intoxication. This is less likely to occur if the drug is given in a saline solution rather than a water solution such as 5% dextrose in water. "Piggybacking" allows regulation of the oxytocin drip without interrupting the main intravenous line. Infusion pumps deliver more accurate doses and minimize the possibility of overdosage.
b. Administer oxytocin intramuscularly, immediately after delivery of the placenta.	To prevent excessive postpartal bleeding
c. With intravenous infusion of ritodrine, have the client lie in the left lateral position.	To decrease risks of hypotension
2. Observe for therapeutic effects	Therapeutic effects depend on the reason for use.
a. When oxytocin is given to induce or augment labor, observe for firm uterine contractions at a rate of 3 to 4 per 10 minutes. Each contraction should be followed by a palpable relaxation period. Examine periodically for cervical dilatation and effacement.	Oxytocin is given to stimulate the normal labor process. Contractions should become regular and increase in duration and intensity.
b. When oxytocin, ergonovine, or methylergonovine is given to prevent or control postpartal bleeding, observe for a small, firm uterus and minimal vaginal bleeding.	These agents control bleeding by causing strong uterine contractions. The uterus can be palpated in the lower abdomen.
c. When prostaglandins are given to induce abortion, observe for the onset of labor and the expulsion of the fetus and placenta.	Abortion usually occurs within 8 to 24 hours with dinoprost and within 24 to 48 hours with dinoprostone. Uterine contractions may be perceived by the client as abdominal cramping or low back pain.
d. When ritodrine is given in threatened abortion or premature labor, observe for absent or decreased uterine contractions.	The goal of drug therapy is to stop the labor process.
3. Observe for adverse effects	
a. With oxytocin, observe for	
(1) Excessive stimulation of uterine contractility (hypertonicity, tetany, rupture, cervical and perineal lacerations, fetal hypoxia, arrhythmias, death or damage from rapid, forceful propulsion through the birth canal)	Most likely to occur when excessive doses are given to initiate or augment labor

Nursing Actions	***Rationale/Explanation***
(2) Hypotension or hypertension	Usual obstetric doses do not cause significant changes in blood pressure. Large doses may cause an initial drop in blood pressure, followed by a sustained elevation.
(3) Water intoxication (convulsions, coma)	Unlikely with usual doses but may occur with prolonged administration of large doses (more than 20 mU/minute)
(4) Allergic reactions, including anaphylactic shock	
(5) Nausea and vomiting	
b. With ergot preparations, observe for	
(1) Nausea, vomiting, diarrhea	These drugs have a direct effect on the vomiting center of the brain and stimulate contraction of gastrointestinal smooth muscle.
(2) Symptoms of ergot poisoning (ergotism)—coolness, numbness and tingling of the extremities, headache, vomiting, dizziness, thirst, convulsions, weak pulse, confusion, anginalike chest pain, transient tachycardia or bradycardia, muscle weakness and pain, cyanosis, gangrene of the extremities	The ergot alkaloids are highly toxic; poisoning may be acute or chronic. Acute poisoning is rare; chronic poisoning is usually a result of overdosage. Circulatory impairments may result from vasoconstriction and vascular insufficiency. Large doses also damage capillary endothelium and may cause thrombosis and occlusion. Gangrene of extremities rarely occurs with usual doses unless peripheral vascular disease or other contraindications are also present.
(3) Hypertension	Blood pressure may rise as a result of generalized vasoconstriction induced by the ergot preparation. Hypertension is most likely to occur when ergonovine or methylergonovine is administered to postpartal women with previous hypertension or toxemia of pregnancy, or to those who have had regional anesthesia with vasoconstrictive agents (*e.g.,* epinephrine).
(4) Hypersensitivity reactions—local edema and pruritus, anaphylactic shock	Allergic reactions are relatively uncommon.
c. With prostaglandins, observe for	
(1) Nausea, vomiting, and diarrhea	These are the most common adverse effects. They occur with all routes of prostaglandin administration and result from drug-induced stimulation of gastrointestinal smooth muscle.
(2) Fever, cardiac arrhythmias, bronchospasm, convulsive seizures, chest pain, muscle aches	These effects occur less frequently and are not clearly related to prostaglandin administration. Bronchospasm is more likely to occur in clients with asthma. Seizures are more likely to occur in clients with known epilepsy.
d. With ritodrine, observe for	
(1) Change in fetal heart rate	This is a common adverse effect and may be significant if changes are extreme or prolonged.
(2) Maternal effects such as changes in heart rate, arrhythmias, palpitations, nausea and vomiting, tremors, hypokalemia, transient hyperglycemia and glucosuria, dyspnea, chest pain, and anaphylactic shock	
4. Observe for drug interactions	
a. Drugs that alter effects of oxytocin	
Vasoconstrictors (*e.g.,* ephedrine, epinephrine, phenylephrine)	Additive vasoconstriction with risks of severe, persistent hypertension and intracranial hemorrhage
b. Drugs that alter effects of ergot preparations	
(1) Propranolol (Inderal)	Additive vasoconstriction
(2) Troleandomycin (TAO)	Increased risk of ergotism due to inhibition of metabolism of ergot alkaloids and derivatives
(3) Vasoconstrictors	See oxytocin, above.

Nursing Actions	Rationale/Explanation
c. Drugs that alter effects of prostaglandins Aspirin and other nonsteroidal anti-inflammatory agents (*e.g.,* ibuprofen [Motrin]; indomethacin [Indocin])	These drugs inhibit effects of prostaglandins. When given concurrently with prostaglandins for abortion, the abortive process is prolonged.
d. Drugs that alter effects of ritodrine	
(1) Beta-adrenergic blocking agents (*e.g.,* propranolol)	Decreased effectiveness of ritodrine, which is a beta-adrenergic stimulating (agonist) agent
(2) Corticosteroids	Increased risk of pulmonary edema
5. Teach clients Purpose and expected effects of the drugs	The drugs discussed in this chapter are indicated for short-term use, with close supervision by a physician or nurse.

Selected References

Brengman SL, Burns M: Ritodrine hydrochloride and preterm labor. Am J Nurs 83:537–539, April 1983

Facts and Comparisons. St. Louis, J B Lippincott (Updated monthly)

Guyton AC: Textbook of Medical Physiology, 7th ed. Philadelphia, W B Saunders, 1986

Malseed RT: Pharmacology: Drug Therapy and Nursing Considerations, 2d ed. Philadelphia, J B Lippincott, 1985

Rall TW, Schleifer LS: Oxytocin, prostaglandins, ergot alkaloids, and other drugs; tocolytic agents. In Gilman AG, Goodman LS, Rall TW, Murad F (eds): The Pharmacological Basis of Therapeutics, 7th ed, pp 926–945. New York, Macmillan, 1985

Szigeti E, Sagraves R: Women's health care. In Wiener MB, Pepper GA (eds): Clinical Pharmacology and Therapeutics in Nursing, 2d ed, pp 891–933. New York, McGraw-Hill, 1985

INDEX

Page numbers followed by *f* indicate figures; *t* following a page number indicates tabular material.